# WOUND, OSTOMY, AND CONTINENCE NURSING SECRETS

# WOUND, OSTOMY, AND CONTINENCE NURSING SECRETS

**Catherine T. Milne, APRN, MSN, CWOCN, CS, ANP**
**Lisa Q. Corbett, APRN, MSN, CWOCN, CS**
*General Editors*
Partners, Connecticut Clinical Nursing Associates, LLC
Clinical Nurse Specialists, Bristol Hospital
Bristol, Connecticut

**Debra L. Dubuc, MSN, APRN, CS, CWCN, COCN**
*Ostomy Section Editor*
Comprehensive Wound Care
Westbrook, Connecticut

Nursing Secrets Series Editor

**Linda J. Scheetz, EdD, RN, CS, CEN**
Assistant Professor, College of Nursing
Rutgers, The State University of New Jersey
Newark, New Jersey

**HANLEY & BELFUS, INC.**/Philadelphia

Publisher:     HANLEY & BELFUS, INC.
               Medical Publishers
               210 South 13th Street
               Philadelphia, PA 19107
               (215) 546-7293; 800-962-1892
               FAX (215) 790-9330
               Web site: http://www.hanleyandbelfus.com

*Note to the reader:* Although the techniques, ideas, and information in this book have been carefully reviewed for correctness, the authors, editors, and publisher cannot accept any legal responsibility for any errors or omissions that may be made. Neither the publisher nor the editors make any guarantee, expressed or implied, with respect to the material contained herein.

This book is designed to provide information on the background and modalities used frequently in wound, ostomy, and continence nursing and how they are applied by practitioners in the field. It is not intended to be exhaustive, nor should patients use it as a substitute for the advice of their physician. It is strongly recommended that you talk with your own physician about any treatments you use personally, and research the area further for safety as it applies to the person you are treating. Before trying/recommending any treatment, the reader should review dosages, accepted indications, and other information pertinent to the safe and effective use of the therapies described.

Library of Congress Control Number: 2002110416

**WOUND, OSTOMY, AND CONTINENCE NURSING SECRETS**      ISBN 1-56053-523-7

Last digit is the print number:   9   8   7   6   5   4   3   2   1

# CONTENTS

# CONTRIBUTORS

**Sharon A. Aronovitch, PhD, RN, CETN**
Assistant Professor, School of Nursing, Florida State University, Tallahassee, Florida

**Theresa M. Bachhuber, BSN, RNC**
Director, Bristol Hospital Home Care Agency, Bristol, Connecticut

**Mona M. Baharestani, PhD, NP, CETN, CWS**
Director of Wound Healing, Division of Plastic and Reconstructive Surgery, Long Island Jewish Medical Center, New Hyde Park, New York

**Jane Ellen Barr, RN, MSN, CWOCN, ANP**
Wound, Ostomy, Continence Nurse Practitioner, Mercy Medical Center, Rockville Centre, New York

**Lynn Wentland Batchelder, ARNP, MSN**
Family Nurse Practitioner, Monadnock Community Hospital, Peterborough, New Hampshire; Adjunct Professor, Mount Wattchusett College, Gardner, Massachusetts

**Carole Bauer, BSN, RN, OCN, CWOCN**
Enterostomal Therapy Nurse, Barbara Ann Karmanos Cancer Institute, Detroit, Michigan

**Patricia Krawiec Bozeman, RN, MSN, CVN**
Clinical Nurse Specialist, Windham Community Memorial Hospital, Willimantic, Connecticut

**Marie Brown-Etris, RN, CWOCN**
President, Etris Associates, Inc., Philadelphia, Pennsylvania

**Diane E. Bryant, RN, MS, CWOCN**
Enterostomal Therapy Clinical Nurse Specialist, Department of Nursing, Brigham and Women's Hospital, Boston, Massachusetts

**Patricia E. Burns, MSN, RN, CWOCN**
Medical Education Manager, Smith & Nephew, Inc., Largo, Florida

**Mary Beth Canham, RNC**
Director, Clinical Division, Regenesis Biomedical, Inc., Scottsdale, Arizona

**Wai Yuen John Chen, BSc, PhD**
Principal Scientist, ConvaTec Global Development Centre, Flintshire, United Kingdom

**Armann O. Ciccarelli, MD, FACS**
Clinical Instructor, Department of Surgery, University of Connecticut School of Medicine, Farmington, Connecticut; Attending Senior Surgeon, Bristol Hospital, Bristol, Connecticut; Federal Hill Surgical Group, Bristol, Connecticut

**Ovleto William Ciccarelli, MD, FACS**
Clinical Professor of Surgery, University of Connecticut School of Medicine, Farmington, Connecticut; Attending Senior Surgeon, Bristol Hospital, Bristol, Connecticut; Federal Hill Surgical Group, Bristol, Connecticut

**Janice C. Colwell, RN, MS, CWOCN**
Wound, Ostomy, and Skin Care Clinical Nurse Specialist, Department of Patient Services, University of Chicago Hospitals, Chicago, Illinois

**Teresa A. Conner-Kerr, PhD, PT, CWS(D)**
Associate Professor, Department of Physical Therapy, School of Allied Health Sciences, East Carolina University, Greenville, North Carolina

**Patricia J. Conwell RN, BSN, CWCN**
Administrative Director of Outpatient Services, Department of Patient Care Services, William W. Backus Hospital, Norwich, Connecticut

**Lisa Q. Corbett, APRN, MSN, CWOCN, CS**
Clinical Nurse Specialist, Bristol Hospital, Bristol, Connecticut; Partner, Connecticut Clinical Nursing Associates, LLC, Bristol, Connecticut

**Debra L. Dubuc, APRN, MSN, CS, CWCN, COCN**
Wound and Ostomy Specialist, Comprehensive Wound Care, LLC, Westbrook, Connecticut

**Paula Erwin-Toth, MSN, RN, ET, CWOCN, CNS**
Director of Enterostomal Therapy, Department of Colon and Rectal Surgery, Cleveland Clinic Foundation, Cleveland, Ohio

**Deborah E. Ferretti, MS, RN, APRN, CS, CWOCN**
Clinical Nurse Specialist, Surgery and Enterostomal Therapy Nursing, New Britain General Hospital, New Britain, Connecticut

**Gail and Jim Fitzpatrick**
Bristol, Connecticut

**Ilene R. Fleischer, RN, MS, CWOCN**
Enterostomal Therapy Clinical Nurse Specialist, Department of Nursing, Brigham and Women's Hospital, Boston, Massachusetts

**Mary Ellen Franklin, PT, EdD**
Associate Professor, Department of Physical Therapy, Medical College of Georgia, Augusta, Georgia

**Robert Charles Franklin, MD**
Tuomey Regional Hospital, Sumter, South Carolina

**Gerald J. French**
Vice President, Global Sales and Marketing, Cook Urological, Inc., Spencer, Indiana

**Ruth Gallegos, RN, WOCN**
Regenesis Biomedical, Inc., Scottsdale, Arizona

**Joyce G. Genna, RNC, BSN, CDE**
Medical Education Manager, Smith & Nephew, Inc., Largo, Florida

**Joan Halpin-Landry, RN, MS, CWCN**
Clinical Support Specialist, Wound Care Division, Augustine Medical, Eden Prairie, Minnesota

**Heather R. Hamilton, MPT**
Physical Therapist, Department of Anatomy and Neurobiology, Medical College of Virginia at Virginia Commonwealth University, Richmond, Virginia

**Sean L. Hansen, BS, CRA**
Burn Research Coordinator, Senior Burn Trauma Technician, Saint Elizabeth Regional Burn and Wound Care Center, Lincoln, Nebraska

**Shirley M. Harkins, RN, BS, CWOCN**
Enterostomal Therapy Nurse Clinician, Department of Surgery, Waterbury Hospital Health Center, Waterbury, Connecticut

**Dawn M. Himes, MS, RD**
Director, Division of Training and Education, Morrison Management Specialties, Marietta, Georgia

**Judy Hoelscher, RN, MSN, EdD**
Team Manager, Calhoun County Health Department, Battle Creek, Michigan

**Tracy L. Houle, APRN, MSN, CCCN, COCN**
Staff Nurse, Wound Care Service, Interim Health Care, Farmington, Connecticut

**Lynette Jamison, MOT, OTR/L, CDP**
Lymphedema Specialist and Director of Aquatics and Rehabilitation, Desert Pain Institute, Mesa, Arizona

**Jeffrey C. Karr, DPM, ACCPPS, CWS**
Chief, Podiatry Section, Bartow Memorial Hospital; Private Practice, Lakeland, Florida

**Karen Lou Kennedy, RN, CS, FNP**
Family Nurse Practitioner, Bynon Health Center, Fort Wayne, Indiana

**Donald H. Lalonde, BSc, MD, MSc, FRCSC**
Associate Professor of Surgery, Division of Plastic Surgery, Dalhousie University, Saint John Regional Hospital, Saint John, New Brunswick, Canada

**Janice Lalonde, RN, CPSN, CPN(C)**
Saint John, New Brunswick, Canada

**Liz Lemiska, CWOCN, BSN, RN**
Wound, Ostomy, Continence Nurse Specialist, Middlesex Hospital, Middletown, Connecticut

**Janice A. Lexton, RN, BC, BSN**
Director of Nursing Services, Waterbury Extended Care, Watertown, Connecticut

**Michelle B. Mayer, PT, OCS, ATC**
Director, Rehab Dynamics, Bristol, Connecticut

**Rebecca E. McBride, RN, BSN, CWOCN**
Wound Care Specialist, Kendall Healthcare, Mansfield, Massachusetts

**Eileen M. McCann, RN, BSN, CWOCN**
Wound, Ostomy, Continence Nursing Specialist, The Stamford Hospital, Stamford, Connecticut

**Diane Merkle, RN, BSN, MSHSA, CWOCN**
Program Coordinator, Griffin Hospital Comprehensive Wound Center, Derby, Connecticut

**Lisa Mikulski, RN, BSN**
Clinical Coordinator, Wound Care Center of Eastern Connecticut, William W. Backus Hospital, Norwich, Connecticut

**Catherine T. Milne, APRN, MSN, CWOCN, CS, ANP**
Partner, Connecticut Clinical Nursing Associates, LLC, Bristol, Connecticut; Clinical Nurse Specialist, Bristol Hospital, Bristol, Connecticut

**Diane M. Morgan, BSN, RNC, CWOCN**
Director of Clinical Services, Lifespan Home Health and Hospice, Battle Creek, Michigan

**Ann D. Navage, APRN, MSN, CETN, CS**
Clinical Nurse Specialist, Center for Clinical Excellence and Professional Development, St. Francis Hospital and Medical Center, Hartford, Connecticut

**Denise Henry Nix, RN, BAN, MS, CWOCN**
Associate Director, WebWOC Nursing Education Program, Department of Nursing, Metropolitan State University, St. Paul, Minnesota

**Lisa M. Oliveira, APRN, MSN**
Nurse Practitioner, Department of Urology, Urology Specialists, Waterbury, Connecticut

**Liza G. Ovington, PhD, CWS**
President, Ovington & Associates, Inc., Pittsburgh, Pennsylvania; Adjunct Instructor, Department of Dermatology and Cutaneous Surgery, University of Miami School of Medicine, Miami, Florida

**Julie M. Peinhardt, MS, PT**
Physical Therapist, Bristol Hospital Wellness Center, Bristol, Connecticut

**Mary C. Ritz, PhD**
President and Chief Executive Officer, Regenesis Biomedical, Inc., Scottsdale, Arizona

**Joseph J. Robles, MD**
Clinical Instructor, Section of General Surgery, University of Connecticut School of Medicine, Farmington Connecticut; Chief of General Surgery, Bristol Hospital, Bristol, Connecticut

**Tamara L Roehling, MPT**
Physical Therapist, Tempe, Arizona

**Jody L. Schmidt, RN, BSN, CWOCN**
Product Specialist, Cook Biotech, Inc., Spencer, Indiana; Home Hospital Home Health Consultant, Lafayette, Indiana

**Daniel J. Scoppetta, MD**
Clinical Associate, Department of Surgery, University of Connecticut School of Medicine, Farmington, Connecticut; Chief of Staff, Bristol Hospital, Bristol, Connecticut; Bristol Surgical Associates, Bristol, Connecticut

**Patricia A. Slachta, PhD, RN, CS, CWOCN**
Chair, Division of Health Sciences, Technical College of the Low Country, Nursing Department, Beaufort, South Carolina

**Bonnie J. Sparks-DeFriese, PT, RN, CWS**
Wound Management Institute, Peoria, Arizona

**P. Karen Sullivan, PhD, MT(ASCP), SM(ASCP)**
Associate Professor, Department of Clinical Laboratory Sciences, School of Allied Health Sciences, East Carolina University, Greenville, North Carolina

**Nancy Tomaselli, RN, MSN, CS, CRNP, CWOCN, CLNC**
President and Chief Executive Officer, Premier Health Solutions, Cherry Hill, New Jersey

**James E. Tracy MS, PT, CDP, MLD**
Clinical Associate Professor, Department of Physical Therapy, School of Allied Health, East Carolina University, Greenville, North Carolina

**Ashley E. Webb, MPT**
Physical Therapist, Department of Biochemistry and Molecular Biophysics, Medical College of Virginia at Virginia Commonwealth University, Richmond, Virginia

**Pamela A. Wiebelhaus, RN, BSN**
Director of Burn Services, Saint Elizabeth Regional Burn and Wound Care Center, Lincoln, Nebraska

# PREFACE

As editors and authors, we were honored to have the opportunity to add wound, ostomy, and continence knowledge to the Nursing Secrets Series®. But don't let the term *nursing* fool you. Caring for patients with wound, ostomy, or continence issues is a multidisciplinary effort. Chapter contents are useful not only for nurses but also for their colleagues in medicine, surgery, podiatry, physical therapy, and nutrition.

The contributors to this book come from a variety of disciplines. This text would not have been possible unless the authors believed, as we do, that a comprehensive multidisciplinary approach to wound, ostomy, and continence care achieves the best patient outcomes. To the contributors, some of the finest practitioners in their specialties, we offer our gratitude.

Support from our friends and families is greatly appreciated. Of course, without the executive administrative talents of Carrie Gonzalez, who kept us organized, fixed computer glitches, made phone calls, and tackled every other problem that arose, this project would not have been possible.

Catherine T. Milne, APRN, MSN, CWOCN, CS, ANP
Lisa Q. Corbett, APRN, MSN, CWOCN, CS
Debra L. Dubuc, MSN, APRN, CS, CWCN, COCN

# I. Wounds

## 1. ANATOMY AND PHYSIOLOGY OF THE SKIN

*Joan Halpin-Landry*, RN, MS, CWCN

**1. What is the largest organ of the body?**
The skin, which serves many complex functions.

**2. List the three layers of the skin.**
1. The **epidermis** is the dry, outermost layer.
2. The **dermis** is the innermost, moist layer.
3. The **hypodermis** is the layer composed of subcutaneous fat and tissue.

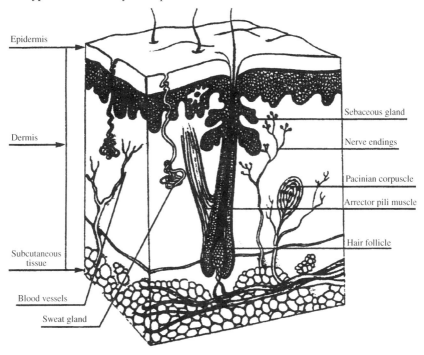

Anatomy of the skin. (From Macklebust J, Sieggren M (eds): Anatomy and Physiology of the Skin, 2nd ed. Philadelphia, Lippincott Williams & Wilkins, 1996, with permission.)

**3. Why is the skin unique? What purposes does it serve?**
The epidermis is a water-repellent layer of skin that contains no blood vessels and is composed of five distinct layers. The epidermis varies in thickness, depending on location. For example, the skin on the soles of the feet is thicker than the skin covering the eyelids. Dead cells on the surface are constantly being removed and replaced by new skin cells—approximately every 3–6 weeks. The purposes of the skin include the following:

1

- Protection from outside elements
- Sensation
- Vitamin D production

- Thermoregulation
- Maintenance of a homeostatic environment
- Mechanism for social interaction

### 4. How does the skin provide protection?

If the skin is unbroken, it offers barrier protection from both mechanical and chemical trauma as well as pathogenic organisms. It also maintains the hydration of the underlying tissue. Constant shedding of the epidermis keeps pathogens from remaining on the skin for an extended period.

### 5. Describe the process of thermoregulation.

Thermoregulation is provided by the skin, which acts as a barrier between the outside and inside environment to maintain body temperature. The two primary thermoregulatory mechanisms are circulation and sweating. Blood vessels can either dilate to dissipate heat or constrict to shunt heat to underlying body organs. Vasodilation increases blood flow and release of heat when internal or external heat is excessive. Sweat glands regulate temperature by secreting fluids, which evaporate from the skin surface, leading to skin cooling. When the outside temperature is cold, vasoconstriction and shivering assist the body in maintaining temperature. Under normal circumstances, the skin temperature is always lower than the core body temperature, and the temperature of wound surfaces may be even lower by 5–6°F.

### 6. How does the skin eliminate waste products?

Fluids containing sodium chloride, urea, sulfates, and phosphates are excreted by sweat glands.

### 7. How does skin sensation occur?

Nerve receptors in the skin are sensitive to pain, touch, temperature, and pressure. Combinations of these four types of sensation result in burning, tingling, and itching.

### 8. What does the skin need to synthesize vitamin D? Why is vitamin D important?

Sunlight. Vitamin D participates in calcium and phosphate metabolism. It is important in the formation and maintenance of bone structure and strength.

### 9. What role does the skin play in social interaction?

The skin is the organ of nonverbal communication (smiling, frowning, and pouting) and identification (facial characteristics, internal and external assessments of beauty and acceptance). The sensation of touching can also communicate feelings of comfort, concern, friendship and love. Injury to the skin can affect body image. Scarring can lead to changes in clothing choices, avoidance of public exposure, and a decrease in self-esteem.

### 10. What is the epidermis made of?

The epidermis consists of five layers of different cells. The top layer is the stratum corneum, a thin layer of keratinocytes without a nucleus. The bottom layer consists of basal cells, which are cube-shaped keratinocytes with a nucleus. A single cell begins as a basal cell and moves upward to the outer surface during its lifespan. During this time, both function and structure change. The basal cell layer contains the infant cells, and the stratum corneum contains the geriatric keratinocytes. In the middle, the keratinocytes change shape and become packed down as they move outward. These stages are akin to infancy, adolescence, and middle age.

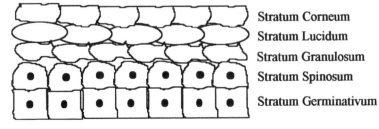

Stratum Corneum

Stratum Lucidum

Stratum Granulosum

Stratum Spinosum

Stratum Germinativum

Cell layers of the epidermis.

### 11. Describe the functions of the layers of the epidermis.

The basal cell layer makes melanin. The stratum corneum keeps out bacteria and excessive moisture while retaining moisture and electrolytes. The middle layers support these activities and houses chemicals made elsewhere.

### 12. Describe the blood supply to the epidermis.

The avascular epidermis gets its blood supply from capillary loops in the dermis. Dermal papillae (fingerlike projections of the dermis) house an abundance of capillary loops. Playing a major role in maintaining skin moisture, this vast blood supply is responsible for fluid, electrolytes, and oxygenation of the epidermis.

### 13. What separates the epidermal and dermal skin layers?

The basement membrane.

### 14. By what other name is the basement membrane known?

The epidermal-dermal junction (the site where the epidermis connects to the dermis).

### 15. How is the epidermis anchored to the dermis?

Rete pegs, or convolutions in the epidermal-dermal junction, interdigate with the dermal papillae much like a post-and-beam construction style. They provide a tight fit of two separate structures without glue, nails, or duct tape!

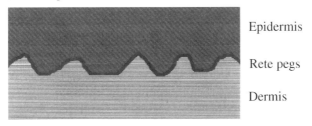

Rete pegs anchor the epidermis to the dermis.

### 16. What else is the basement membrane made of?

A number of proteins are located in the area: fibronectin, type II collagen, laminin, and heparin sulfate proteoglycans.

### 17. What is sebum?

Sebum is a substance secreted by the sebaceous glands via the hair follicles and shafts onto the skin surface. It provides an acidic coating to the skin. The acid coating is a natural antibacterial substance that retards the growth of microorganisms. Resistance to pathogenic microorganisms is also provided by normal skin flora via bacterial interference.

### 18. Describe the function of the dermis.

The dermis provides support and nourishment to the epidermis by housing a vascular system, nervous innervation, and sweat and sebaceous glands. Its tensile strength is provided by connective tissue consisting of collagen, elastin, glycosaminoglycans, and water. Fibroblasts are the cell types located in the dermis.

### 19. What is collagen?

Collagen is the protein that gives skin its tensile strength. The role of collagen in wound healing is discussed in Chapter 6.

### 20. What is elastin?

Elastin is a protein that provides the skin with elastic recoil. It prevents the skin from being permanently reshaped.

**21. What are fibroblasts?**

Fibroblasts are the cells that secrete the proteins elastin and collagen.

**22. Besides housing a blood supply for the epidermis, what else is important about the dermal layer?**

The dermis is composed of proteins, primarily elastin, collagen, and ground substance. Nerves, sebaceous glands, hair follicles, small muscles called arrector pili, and sweat glands are located in the dermis. Each of these structures serves a purpose.

**23. What is an acid mantle?**

The acid mantle, with a pH of 4.5–6.5, is the sebaceous substance secreted onto the skin via the emptying of sebum gland contents into the hair follicle. The sebum travels upward and onto the outer layer of the epidermis. Besides providing a natural bacteriostatic effect, sebum helps to lubricate the skin and provides a protective coating to reduce fluid loss.

**24. Define ground substance.**

Ground substance is another multiprotein material. Large proteins, primarily proteoglycan (PG) and glycosaminoglycan (GAG), compose the majority of ground substance.

**25. What is the role of PG and GAG?**

Although their function is not entirely appreciated, both PG and GAG have a role in wound healing and dermal ability to regulate moisture content. Both PG and GAG can bind fluid up to 1,000 times their weight. This ability has an impact on the volume and recoil of skin.

**26. What other components make up the dermis?**

Cellular elements, including macrophages (white blood cells), fibroblasts, mast cells (cells that cause vasoconstriction in response to an injury), and Langerhans cells.

**27. Does the skin have an immune system?**

Yes. The skin provides protection against invading microorganisms and antigens. The cells of the skin that provide the immune protection are the Langerhan cells, tissue macrophages that digest bacteria, and mast cells that cause vasoconstriction.

**28. What is the effect of temperature on the skin immune system?**

A lower temperature has an adverse effect on immune system function. Lowered temperature leads to a decrease in subcutaneous oxygen tension, which impairs the oxidative killing of neutrophils (white blood cells) as well as decreases collagen deposition and wound strength. These effects can affect wound healing. Mild perioperative hypothermia may promote surgical wound infections by triggering thermoregulatory vasoconstriction that decreases subcutaneous oxygen tension.

**29. What layer of tissue is found under the dermis?**

Beneath the dermis is a layer of loose connective tissue, called the hypodermis or superficial fascia, that forms the subcutaneous skin layer. It is composed of connective tissue and adipose. Deeper tissue layers consist of the fascia, a thin membrane covering muscle.

**30. What is the function of the hypodermis?**

The hypodermis attaches the dermis to the underlying structures. The larger arteries within this layer branch out with capillaries that supply the dermis with oxygen and nutrients.

**31. List the major normal skin flora.**

Staphylococci, diphtheroids, and yeast.

**32. What constitutes abnormal skin flora?**

Any gram-negative bacteria.

### 33. Discuss the role of skin pigmentation and melanin.

Pigmentation protects the skin from ultraviolet radiation. Skin pigmentation results from the synthesis of the pigment melanin. Melanin is found in all the layers of the epidermis in dark skin, but it is not found in large quantities in all layers of light skin.

### 34. How does aging affect skin?

| PHYSIOLOGICAL CHANGE | EFFECT |
|---|---|
| Flattening of the epidermal-dermal junction | Skin becomes more prone to tears and less pliable; the potential for trauma is increased. |
| Reduced dermal proteins | Increased fluid loss |
| Increased epidermal turnover time | Decrease in skin moisture content |
| Degeneration of elastin | Wrinkles |
| Decrease in sebum | Decreased bacteriostatic ability |
| Changes in sebum chemical make-up | Decreased bacteriostatic ability |
| Thinning of epidermis | Skin tears |
| Changes in capillary loop structure | Bruising |
| Reduction in mast and Langerhans cells | Decreased inflammatory response, impaired wound healing |

### BIBLIOGRAPHY

1. Bryant RA, Rostad B: Examining threats to skin integrity. Ostomy Wound Manage 47(6):18–27, 2001.
2. Fitzpatrick JE, Aeling JL (eds): Dermatology Secrets. Philadelphia, Hanley & Belfus, 1996.
3. Nix DH: Factors to consider when selecting skin cleansing products. J Wound Ostomy Contin Nurs 27:260-268, 2000.
4. Wysocki A: Anatomy and physiology of skin and soft tissue. In Bryant RA (ed): Acute and Chronic Wounds: Nursing Management, 2nd ed. St. Louis, Mosby, 2000, pp 1–15.

# 2. MAINTAINING SKIN INTEGRITY: GENERAL PRINCIPLES OF CARE

*Janice C. Colwell, RN, MS, CWOCN*

**1. Why is it important to maintain skin integrity?**

A break in skin integrity predisposes the patient to infection, increases caloric requirements, contributes to pain and suffering, and increases the cost of care. Vigilant care may not prevent skin breakdown in high-risk patients. Care must be aimed at reducing risk factors and at preventative measures. The estimated prevalence rate of skin breakdown in acute care settings ranges between approximately 8% and 12%.

**2. What are the major external causative factors of skin breakdown?**

Skin breakdown can be caused by external factors such as unrelieved pressure, shear, friction, or excessive moisture. Other causes may include stripping from adhesive removal or effluent from draining wounds. Pressure is the major cause of pressure ulcer formation. Shear (the pulling of the skin in one direction while the skeleton pulls the body downward) causes damage in deep tissues. Friction (the rubbing of two forces together) causes the top layer of skin, the epidermis, to become denuded. Friction is always present with shear. Moisture due to urinary or fecal incontinence, wound drainage, and perspiration softens the skin, making it susceptible to damage.

**3. What are the major internal causative factors of skin breakdown?**

Impaired nutritional status, immobility, altered level of consciousness, and fecal and/or urinary incontinence are patient-specific factors contributing to skin breakdown. Poor nutritional status, a factor in edema formation, causes protein deficiency, which makes tissues more susceptible to injury. An immobile person is unable to reposition on a frequent basis or to reduce or redistribute the amount of pressure exerted over bony prominences. Altered level of consciousness interferes with the person's ability to recognize discomfort and change position. Urinary/fecal incontinence can damage skin, causing possible loss of the epidermis.

**4. How can patients at high risk for skin breakdown be identified?**

Patients at risk must be identified so that risk factors can be reduced through appropriate interventions. The use of a systematic risk assessment tool is the backbone of any breakdown prevention program. Numerous risk assessment tools are available. One of the more frequently used tools is the Braden Scale for Predicting Pressure Sore Risk. The Braden Scale has been tested in diverse settings, and interrater reliability is good. This tool, as well as several others, allows identification of individual risk factors. Your practice setting should use a tool with well-established reliability and validity. "Home-grown" forms can be problematic in a legal setting, not to mention their possible inability to assess reliably the very data that they are designed to collect.

**5. How is the Braden Scale used?**

The Braden Scale has five subscales that reflect degrees of sensory perception, moisture, activity, mobility, nutrition, and friction and shear. Each subscale has a brief description. The user rates the patient, assigning a numerical score on each subscale. Potential scores range from 4 to 23. High-risk scores vary among clinical settings. For example, a hospitalized adult with a score of 16 or below is considered to be at risk for skin breakdown. It is recommended that the Braden Scale be used on admission and at frequent intervals thereafter. Once the patient has been assessed to be at risk, interventions should be tailored to the specific risk factors. For example, in a patient with a subset risk of moisture due to incontinence, care is aimed at reducing the contact of moisture with the skin. This goal can be accomplished by applying a barrier cream or ointment. Determining the cause of incontinence and initiating appropriate treatment also are indicated.

The Braden Scale is protected by copyright, but it can be viewed in its entirety in the Agency for Healthcare Research and Quality (AHRQ) Clinical Practice Guidelines for the prevention of pressure ulcers (available at www.ahrq.gov). Permission for use can be obtained from the author.

**6. What interventions can reduce the risk of moisture, specifically urinary and fecal incontinence?**

Before attention is given to skin protection or collection of the effluent, the cause of the incontinence should be investigated. Frequent causes of incontinence include infection, impaction, antibiotic administration, infrequent toileting, and intolerance of tube feedings. Once the cause is addressed, one of two approaches can be attempted: protection or containment.

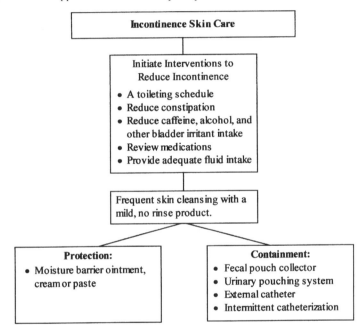

**7. How can the skin be protected?**

The affected skin should be protected with moisture barrier cream, ointment or paste, which should be reapplied after each cleansing. A thick layer of the moisture barrier is applied, providing a barrier between the skin and the moisture source. Skin cleansing should occur at the time of soiling, using a mild, no-rinse product. The moisture barrier is replaced after each cleansing.

**8. How can containment of incontinence be achieved?**

The effluent can be contained by use of fecal incontinence collectors (also known as fecal containment devices), which are pouches that fit around the rectum. They are usually most effective with loose stools. Urinary pouching systems, indwelling urinary catheters, or external catheters can be used to protect the skin from urine.

Indwelling catheters should not be used as a containment device unless all other options have been exhausted. The high rate of morbidity and mortality due to urosepsis in patients with catheters makes the risk-to-benefit ratio hard to justify. Intermittent straight catheterization should be attempted before placement of an indwelling device.

Although few urinary pouching systems for women are on the market, there are many options for male patients. Condom catheters, also known as Texas catheters, are available in adhesive latex or latex-free forms as well as in a nonadhesive apparatus. Penile clamps provide external pressure to the penile shaft to prevent incontinence. A retracted penile pouch looks much like an ostomy pouching system. Applied in a similar manner, this type of product can contain urine in patients whose anatomy is not well suited for a condom catheter. To facilitate pouching, it is best to clip the surrounding pubic hair first. By pressing gently, just above the symphysis pubis, the penis is moved outward, allowing more of the penile shaft to be contained in the pouch and thus ensuring an effective seal.

Underpads and briefs are not considered true containment devices. If used, they should be made of materials that absorb moisture and present a quick drying surface to the skin.

**9. What protective interventions are appropriate if the source of moisture is wound drainage?**

If the skin at risk for breakdown is located around a draining wound, several interventions may be warranted. A liquid skin barrier may be applied to the intact periwound skin. The liquid skin barrier provides a protective covering to the skin. If the periwound skin is denuded, a liquid skin barrier with no alcohol is recommended. Alcohol-containing products irritate denuded skin, causing a burning sensation. A solid pectin-based skin barrier can be fitted to the wound edges to provide a strong barrier between the wound drainage and the skin. The barrier acts as a "second skin," protecting the skin from the drainage. An absorptive dressing such as a calcium alginate or hydrofiber can be packed into the wound to collect the excessive drainage. If appropriate, a pouching system can be applied over the wound to contain the drainage. These devices are known as wound drainage collectors. They are applied like their ostomy pouch cousins. Most have "port-holes," a window-like feature that allows clinicians access to the wound through opening and closing motions. The pouch can be hooked to a drainage bag or capped tight for intermittent emptying. A nonadhesive pouching system also can be used to contain wound drainage.

**10. What interventions can decrease the risk associated with reductions in mobility, sensory perception, and activity?**

Because these risk factors relate to unrelieved pressure, the interventions are aimed at decreasing the amount and duration of pressure. The following interventions should be considered:

- Reposition the patient at least every 2 hours.
- Post a written turning schedule.
- Place the patient in a 30° lateral position, which avoids direct pressure on the trochanter.
- Limit the elevation of the head to 30° to decrease the amount of pressure and reduce shear on the sacrum.
- Positioning devices should be used to avoid direct contact with bony prominences.
- Use pillows under the length of the lower leg, suspending the heels, to protect them from pressure.
- Use a pressure reduction device such as foam, static air, alternating air, gel, or water.
- Chair-bound patients should use an air, foam, gel, or combination of these products to reduce pressure.
- Keep the number of layers between the patient and the pressure reduction device to a minimum. These devices decrease tissue surface interface pressure by allowing patients to sink into the surface and redistributing their weight. Too many layers between the support surface and the patient make the surface ineffective.
- Provide adequate nutrition and hydration.

**11. How can the risk factors of shear and friction be addressed?**

Shear and friction injuries generally occur when the skin remains stationary and the underlying tissues are moved or when the skin moves over a rough surface. Shear forces are reduced by using bed linen to move, rather than drag, the patient who cannot assist with transfers. A trapeze can be used if the patient can assist in the transfer using his or her upper body. Limit the amount of time that the head of the bed is elevated, and use the knee gatch to reduce pull and sliding down in bed. For protection from friction injuries, consider using lubricants, liquid skin barriers, and extra-thin hydrocolloids. These products provide a barrier between the skin and the corresponding surface.

**12. What interventions can be instituted to prevent skin breakdown due to adhesives?**

All adhesives should be removed by releasing the skin from the tape, using a finger to press the skin away from the tape as the adhesive is gently released. Porous tapes should be used when possible because they allow the skin to breathe, decreasing moisture build-up and preventing maceration. Paper tape is the most porous of all. To reduce adhesive injury, a liquid skin barrier can be placed on the skin before adhesive application. An extra-thin hydrocolloid also may be used under the tape. The extra-thin hydrocolloid can remain in place for an extended period and act as a skin barrier. Thicker, pectin-based barriers can act in a similar manner.

Perhaps the best way to avoid skin damage from adhesives is to avoid adhesives entirely. Orthopedic stockinettes, cloth binders, gauze wraps, tubular elastic netting, and even sports bras can be used to secure dressings and devices without adhesive application.

**13. When a patient is identified as at risk for skin breakdown because of a nutritional deficit, what interventions should be planned?**

A nutritional assessment should be done to assist in identifying the presence of malnutrition and to serve as a baseline to help assess the effectiveness of nutritional interventions. If the dietary intake is found to be inadequate, a plan of nutritional support and/or supplementation should be implemented. Evaluate the patient for factors that compromise intake and offer support with eating (see Chapter 8). As with all actions aimed at prevention, the role of early identification of specific risk factors, coupled with aggressive intervention, is crucial in maintaining skin integrity.

**14. Besides using a risk assessment tool and planning interventions based on specific risk factors, what else can be done to maintain skin integrity?**

All patients at risk should have a systematic skin inspection at least once a day. This inspection should include examination of all bony prominences as well as skin surfaces. Document the findings of the inspection to identify areas of potential skin breakdown and to allow daily comparison of results.

**15. What is an effective approach to educating health care providers about the importance of maintaining skin integrity?**

The development of a skin care team has proved effective in various health care settings. A skin care team is charged with implementing standards of care that are well documented in the literature. Some of the functions of skin care teams include product selection, development of a risk assessment program, planning standard interventions, and conducting prevalence and incidence studies. Education for the staff as well as the patient and family about the various aspects of skin care maintenance and skin alteration prevention is key to the success of a wound care team. The model of the skin care team varies from setting to setting, depending on patient and facility needs. Most skin care teams are multidisciplinary.

BIBLIOGRAPHY

1. Bates-Jensen BM: Pressure ulcers: Pathophysiology and prevention. In Wound Care: A Collaborative Practice Manual for Physical Therapists and Nurses. Gaithersburg, MD, Aspen, 1998, pp 235–270.
2. Bergstrom N, Braden BJ, Laguzza A, Holman A: The Braden Scale for predicting pressure sore risk. Nurs Res 36:205–210, 1987.
3. Braden BJ: Risk assessment in pressure ulcer prevention. In Krasner D, Kane D (eds): Chronic Wound Care, 2nd ed. Wayne, PA, Health Management Publications, 1997, pp 29–36.
4. Bryant RA: Skin pathology and types of damage. In Bryant RA (ed): Acute and Chronic Wounds, 2nd ed. St. Louis, Mosby, 2001, pp 125–156.
5. Panel for Prediction and Prevention of Pressure Ulcers in Adults: Pressure Ulcers in Adults: Prediction and Prevention. Clinical Practice Guideline No. 3. AHCPR Publication No. 92-0047. Rockville MD, Agency for Health Care Policy and Research, Public Health Service, U.S. Department of Health and Human Services, 1992.
6. Pieper B: Mechanical forces: Pressure, shear and friction. In Bryant RA (ed): Acute and Chronic Wounds, 2nd ed. St. Louis, Mosby, 2001, pp 125–156.
7. Rappl LM: Management of pressure by therapeutic positioning. In Wound Care: A Collaborative Practice Manual for Physical Therapists and Nurses. Gaithersburg, MD, Aspen, 1998, pp 271–299.

# 3. MAINTAINING SKIN INTEGRITY: CLEANSERS, CREAMS, AND LOTIONS

*Denise Henry Nix, RN, BAN, MS, CWOCN*

**1. What is the difference between cleansers, creams, and lotions?**

**Cleansers** are used to remove dirt and contaminants from the skin surface. They should not be confused with wound cleansers because the ingredients differ. Creams and lotions are intended to moisturize the skin. **Creams** are traditionally thicker than lotions, but have similar ingredients. **Lotions** are more aesthetically palatable to apply. They are manufactured by thinning a cream preparation through the addition of an alcohol component. Mentioned frequently in nursing literature, but seldom emphasized, is the importance of appropriate selection and use of cleansers, creams, and lotions in the maintenance of a healthy skin barrier.

**2. What are the best cleanser, cream, and lotion on the market today?**

It depends on the need of the person intended to use the product. The goal of an ideal skin cleanser is the removal of unwanted microorganisms while maintaining, as best as possible, the skin's barrier function. Required characteristics vary according to the needs of the population expected to use the product. For example, the resident in a nursing home requires a different product for general body bathing than the nurse with frequent exposure to contaminants requires for hand-washing. Product selection decisions should be made while keeping in mind the intended users, clinical goals, and concepts associated with ingredients and formulation.

**3. What are the determinants of a healthy, normal skin barrier?**

Normal skin flora, pH, and transepidermal water loss (TEWL) measurements. The healthy epidermis provides an effective barrier against noxious agents and infectious organisms. A familiar analogy for a normal skin barrier is the "brick-and-mortar" concept. The epithelial cells act as bricks, and the skin lipids act as mortar. Any substance that comes into contact with the skin and strips away its lipids produces a defect within this barrier. Such defects can allow invasion by pathogens or environmental irritants. Species of bacteria normally found on human skin (normal flora) provide bacterial interference to control pathogenic microorganisms. Examples of species normally found on human skin include *Staphylococcus, Brevibacterium, Proprionibacterium, Streptococcus, Micrococcus, Neisseria, Peptoococcus, Corynebacterium*, and *Acinetocacter* spp. Not all species are found on one person, but most people carry at least five of these species as normal flora.

Healthy skin is acidic with a pH of 5.5 The acid mantle discourages bacterial colonization and promotes moisture retention. The integrity of the skin's barrier function is typically measured by TEWL. TEWL is the evaluation of changes in the rate of passive evaporation (moisture loss) through the skin. TEWL values rise as the barrier function declines and the skin becomes dry. A decrease in TEWL values can be related to an improvement in the ability of the skin to act as a barrier against moisture loss. Normal TEWL varies according to the area of the body.

**4. How do I know if a particular product is safe to use on skin?**

Before marketing, the product may be tested for safety and function. If safety testing is not done, a warning statement must be applied to the package. Provided that testing has been completed, the manufacturer can supply a summary of the safety tests that have been performed on a specific product. These tests should evaluate stability, potential for allergy, dermal irritation, and preservative efficacy.

Preservative effectiveness can be demonstrated by using an in vitro minimal inhibitory concentration technique or an in vivo time-kill study technique in human subjects. It should be clarified that although a preservative is an antimicrobial, its function is *not* to kill bacteria on the skin but to prevent bacterial growth within the product's package or container.

*Examples of Product Tests*

| TEST | FEATURE TESTED | BASIC DESCRIPTION |
|---|---|---|
| Stability test | Odor, pH, viscosity | In vitro test that measures the degree of resistance to chemical changes of formula |
| Potential for allergy | Potential for allergy | Human repeat-insult patch test (HRIPT) in vivo on healthy humans or animals |
| Dermal irritation potential | Dermal irritation potential | In vivo test on healthy humans; 14-day cumulative irritation with challenge test |
| Preservative challenge | Prevention of microbial contamination | Microorganisms are introduced in vitro to the product and evaluated over 28 days. Preservatives efficacy is $\geq$ 99.9% reduction of viable bacteria at 14 days and maintenance of these levels for remainder of test period. |
| Time-kill study | Rapid microbial kill rate | Measures the time that antimicrobial product takes to reduce microbial contamination of skin to acceptable level. |

From Nix DP: Factors to consider when selecting skin cleansing products. J Wound Ostomy Contin Nurs 27:260–268, 2000, with permission.

**5. In addition to safety testing, what are key aspects of a high-quality product?**

**Therapeutic activity.** Health care workers have been examined for factors leading to compliance with handwashing policies. Persons complaining of dermatitis related to a skin cleanser were less likely to comply with handwashing policies. User acceptability, in this case, outweighs therapeutic activity.

**Convenience.** The Centers for Disease Control and Prevention (CDC) recommends placement of bar soap on drainable racks. Because bar soap users can include patients, staff, and visitors, all require education or notification of this policy. This policy can present a variety of teaching challenges, such as language barriers, age and developmental differences, varied educational and literacy levels, and differing motivation. In contrast, education about the proper installation and filling of liquid cleansers can be limited to specific departments trained in the performance of this task. Appropriate use of a pump dispenser is self-explanatory and more convenient.

**6. What specific ingredients should I look for in a skin care product?**

There are at least two good reasons for identifying specific ingredients in a product. First, a specific ingredient needs to be identified in selecting a product for a person allergic to the ingredient. Second, understanding the function of a specific ingredient can help achieve the intended outcome. For example, if a desired outcome is to repel enzymes and moisture off the perineal skin of a patient with incontinence, the clinician should select a product with a skin protectant such as petrolatum, dimethicone, or zinc oxide.

It is also essential to consider the total formulation and combined effect of individual ingredients. For example, a highly effective cleanser (surfactant) may achieve the goals of removing soil and reducing bacteria counts, but it also may strip away lipids and compromise cutaneous barrier function. Instead of selecting a less effective cleanser, the clinician may be able to combine the cleanser with a compatible moisturizer/conditioning product that restores the lipid content of the skin.

**7. Should alcohol be avoided?**

Not always. Alcohols are a diverse group of products and have a variety of effects, depending on their specific formulation. For example, isopropyl alcohol acts as an antimicrobial agent, whereas benzyl alcohol acts as a preservative. Cetyl or stearyl alcohols serve as emollients and thickening agents when added to moisturizers or lubricants. Used in this context, they safely enhance the total formula of the product and are not drying to the skin.

### 8. What are surfactants? How are they used in skin products?

Surfactants, also known as surface-acting agents, are chemical substances that adhere to skin surfaces to decrease the amount of friction required to remove unwanted material from the skin. They are incorporated into cleansing agents because the dirt that collects within the lipid barrier is not effectively removed by water alone, even with reasonably vigorous mechanical washing. The area of the surfactant molecule that provides the greatest detergent effect is its hydrophilic or polar region. Surfactants are generally categorized into four major groups based on their net charge. Anionic surfactants have a net negative charge, and cationic surfactants have a net positive charge. In addition, amphoteric surfactants have both positive and negative charges, and nonionic surfactants have no electrical charge.

*Categories of Surfactants*

| CATEGORY | CHARGE | EXAMPLES | COMMENTS |
|---|---|---|---|
| Anionic | Negative | Sodium lauryl sulfate, triethanolamine lauryl sulfate, ammonium lauryl sulfate, sodium lauryl sulfoacetate, triethanolamine lauryl sarcosinate | Excellent cleansing, foaming |
| Cationic | Positive | Benzalkonium chloride, benzathonium chloride | Used as preservative |
| Nonionic | None | Polysorbate 80, sorbitan oleate, sucrose oleate, polyethylene glycol (4) sorbitan laurate, poloxamer 407, dihydroxyethyl cocamine oxide | Excellent solubilizers, emulsifiers |
| Zwitterionic | Both | Lecithin | Mild |

From Zatz JL: The quality of skin care products and their ingredients. Ostomy/Wound Manage 47:25, 2001, with permission.

*Typical Uses of Surfactants in Skin Care Products*

| USE | MECHANISM | TYPE OF PRODUCT | EXAMPLES |
|---|---|---|---|
| Cleanser | Wet, disperse, emulsify lauryl solubilize oils | Cleanser bar, liquid, shampoo | Sodium lauryl sulfate, triethanolamine sulfate, sodium lauroamphoacetate |
| Emulsifier | Lower oil/water, interfacial tension; hinder coalescence of dispersed droplets | Lotion, cream | Polysorbate 80, sodium lauryl sulfate, lecithin, cholesterol |
| Wetting agent | Lower surface tension of water | Aqueous suspension | Polysorbate 80 |
| Foam stabilizer | Lower surface tension of water; hinder coalescence of dispersed air cells | Shampoo | Sodium lauryl sulfate, sodium laureth sulfate, sodium lauroamphoacetate |
| Solubilizer | Forms micelles, which can dissolve hydrophobic substances | Certain clear gels, aqueous solutions | Polysorbate 80, sucrose oleate, polyethylene glycol (4) sorbitan laurate |

From Zatz JL: The quality of skin care products and their ingredients. Ostomy/Wound Manage 47:25, 2001, with permission.

### 9. Can I delete additional lotion use if the cleanser contains moisturizer?

Humectants are substances used to obtain a moisturizing effect. Nevertheless, these ingredients only partially compensate for lipid stripping during hand washing, and an additional compatible moisturizing agent (lotion or cream) should be applied immediately after cleansing.

### 10. What is a humectant?

Examples of humectants include glycerin, methyl glucose esters, lactates, lanolin derivatives, and mineral oil. Humectants play an important role in maintaining and restoring skin barrier function by sealing in the skin's natural moisture. Frequent cleansing with any soap or detergent can reduce the lipid content of the stratum corneum. As a result, the barrier function of the skin is compromised and its TEWL rises. This depletion leads to dry, chapped hands. In some instances, eczema occurs as the skin develops a sensitivity to the chemicals used in skin products. To avoid this adverse outcome, a humectant or moisturizer may be added to the skin cleansers to minimize the loss of lipids.

**11. Why is the pH in a skin care product important?**

As stated previously, healthy skin has an acidic pH of 5.5 to discourage bacterial colonization. The pH of a skin care product influences the skin's pH. For example, repeated washings with an alkaline soap increase the pH of the skin. A product with a pH of 4–7 is recommended for skin cleansing, particularly for elderly patients because their skin is dryer, more prone to cracking, and slower to recover from the effects of alkaline substances compared with the skin of younger adults.

Most bar cleansers have a pH of 7–11. Ingredients can be added to products to adjust or compensate for a high pH. Common pH adjusters are citric acid, phosphoric acid, sodium hydroxide, and triethanolamine. Ingredients added to lower pH may cause the bar to form a gelatinous material on and below its surface. This material serves as an excellent media for bacterial growth. There is an attempt to compensate by adding a filler such as dextrin or starch. Drawbacks to fillers are a rough surface texture and loss of slip. Unfortunately, the pH is not usually listed on the product package. It is often necessary to ask for the pH of a particular product. This information is often available on the Material Data Safety sheets required by OSHA in employment settings. The manufacturer can also supply this information.

**12. Should skin care products include preservatives?**

Yes. Preservatives help prevent the product from breaking down and becoming contaminated with bacteria. Chloroxylenol (PCMX), triclosan, methyl acid, benzoic acid, and sorbic acid are just a few examples of preservatives. It is worth repeating that these products are effective against bacteria in the package but *not* on the skin.

**13. What about antimicrobial additives in skin products?**

The use of antimicrobial agents for skin care products is controversial. Some researchers suggest that the use of antimicrobial-based skin products may be beneficial in the management of patients colonized with methicillin-resistant *Staphylococcus aureus* (MRSA). Others contend that little convincing evidence supports routine use of an antimicrobial product. These researchers raise concerns that regular use of an antimicrobial may increase the risk of selecting organisms that are resistant to the agents used. The area of greatest agreement is in the use of antimicrobial agents for handwashing by health care personnel. Several studies have compared the benefits of antimicrobial cleansers in handwashing among health care personnel. Based on these results, an antimicrobial cleanser is recommended for healthcare providers with a high frequency of handwashing (8 or more times/day). The advantage, however, seems to disappear when handwashing frequency is low (≤ 6 times/day).

**14. What controversies are related to bar and liquid skin cleansers?**

Much has been debated about the use of bar vs. liquid skin cleansers. Some experts on infection control state that bar soaps are frequently misused because they are stored carelessly in contact with moisture. In some cases, this may be responsible for the transfer of bacteria from one user to another. In one study, researchers isolated strains of *Pseudomonas* spp. from environmental samples in a hospital. The study affirmed that hands are a method for the transfer of pseudomonal bacteria, and bar soap was implicated in its spread. Another study found that bacteria survived on soap bars used in public lavatories, even when cultured 48 hours after the last use. Soap dishes also have been cultured in hospitals units and labs. Cultures revealed gram-negative bacteria even when medicated iodophor bar soap was used. In contrast, liquid cleansers have been found to be negative for bacteria as long as they remain in a closed unit until it is replaced or cleaned and filled with fresh product. Researchers from the Dial Corporation dispute claims that bar soap is likely to transfer bacteria. They studied 16 adults who washed with *Escherichia coli*-inoculated bars using normal handwashing procedure. Even after noncoached washing, none of the 16 panelists had detectable levels of the bacterium on their hands.

**15. Are there any distinct advantages to using liquid soaps instead of bar soaps?**

Control over the volume of cleanser dispensed has been cited as a possible advantage of liquid over bar soap. Skin cleanser quantity has been examined as a variable in reducing bacterial colonization. Larson and associates compared bacterial colony counts on the hands of 40 subjects randomly assigned to one of four products in aliquots of 1 vs. 3 ml. Compared with those using 1 ml, subjects using 3 ml of cleanser had a significant reduction in bacterial colonization. Liquid cleansers have the potential to dispense a predetermined amount of product. Bar soap volume cannot be measured with any degree of accuracy.

**16. So no one product is the best?**

The primary factors that the clinician should consider when offering advice for the selection of skin care products must begin with the purpose, the clinical goals, and the people expected to use the product. Clearly one product will not meet all needs. Products purchased for general bathing, for example, may not be the correct perineal cleanser. Factors such as ingredients, acceptability, safety, and therapeutic activity can have a significant impact on how skin care products perform.

BIBLIOGRAPHY

1. Centers for Disease Control: Guideline for Handwashing and Hospital Environmental Control. Washington DC, U.S. Government Print Office, 1985.
2. Cosmetic Ingredient Handbook, Chemical Classes, 2nd ed. Washington DC, CTFA, 1994, pp 476–508.
3. Fiers S, Thayer D: Management of intractable incontinence. In Doughty DB (ed): Urinary and Fecal Incontinence: Nursing Management, 2nd ed. St. Louis, Mosby, 2000, pp 183–207.
4. Fitzpatrickk JE, Aeling JL (eds): Dermatology Secrets. Philadelphia, Hanley & Belfus, 1996.
5. Friedman M, Wolf R: Chemistry of soaps and detergents: Various types of commercial products and their ingredients. Clin Dermatol 14:/–14, 1996.
6. Kabara JJ, Brady MB: Contamination of bar soaps under 'in use' conditions. J Environ Pathol Toxicol Oncol 5:1–14, 1984.
7. Kirsner R, Froelich, C: Soaps and detergents: Understanding their composition and effect. Ostomy/ Wound Manage 44(3A):62S–70S, 1999.
8. Larson EL, Eke PI, Wilder MP, Laughon BE: Quantity of soap as a variable in hand washing. Infect Control 8:371–375, 1987.
9. Nix DP: Factors to consider when selecting skin cleansing products. J Wound Ostomy Contin Nurs 27:260–268, 2000.
10. Yosipovitch G, Maibach H: Skin surface pH: A protective acid mantle. Cosmetics & Toiletries Mag 111:101–102, 1996.
11. Zatz JL: The quality of skin care products and their ingredients. Ostomy/Wound Manage 47:22–33, 2001.

# 4. MECHANISMS OF WOUNDING

*Catherine T. Milne, APRN, MSN, CWOCN, CS, ANP, and*
*Lisa Q. Corbett, APRN, MSN, CWOCN, CS*

**1. Why is it important to know why and how a wound occurs?**

Wound healing occurs in an orderly fashion. Unfortunately, wounding does not. There are a number of reasons why a wound develops. Determining and eliminating these factors aid in healing. Knowing causative factors allows the clinician to teach the patient how to avoid new open areas and prevent a healed lesion from reopening.

**2. Name the most common factors contributing to the development of a wound.**
- Pressure and shear
- Friction
- Moisture
- Heat
- Cold
- Radiation
- Trauma
- Ischemia
- Malignancy
- Chemical contact
- Surgical intervention
- Vasculitic injury
- Factitious injury

**3. How is pressure defined?**

Pressure = Force/area

Clinically, pressure is defined as the perpendicular force applied to soft tissues, compressing them between bone and an external object. This form of mechanical injury contributes to a variety of wounds. Decubitus ulcers are caused by pressure. Pressure also forces a delay in wound healing.

**4. How does pressure cause tissue damage?**

The exertion of pressure sets into motion a number of damaging physiologic events leading to ischemia and possible necrosis. Normal capillary flow exerts an outward pressure of 32 mmHg in the arterioles. In patients with hypovolemia, shock, or other critical illness, this pressure is significantly less—possibly as low as 17 mmHg. Any external pressure exceeding the internal pressure causes vessel collapse. This phenomenon is called capillary closing pressure. When capillary closing pressure is reached, the vessel closes and ischemia results. If circulation is not restored in a timely fashion, necrosis results.

**5. Are certain tissues more susceptible to pressure than others?**

Yes. Muscle is a metabolically active tissue with tremendous blood flow. Fat, on the other hand, has less blood flow. Because of inherent anatomic and physiologic differences, both of these tissues are more susceptible to ischemia and necrosis than the dermis. This process explains how an ulcer with a small surface level involvement increases in size and severity as it progresses into deep tissues.

**6. What occurs physiologically when capillary closing pressures are exceeded?**

Fluid leaks from the capillaries into the interstitial tissue. Fluid build-up around the vessels further impedes circulation. Waste products produced by ischemia add to acidosis and the downward cycle of additional cell permeability with edema that leads to vessel thrombosis and cell death. If perfusion is restored before necrosis, reperfusion injury can occur. The release of oxygen free radicals produces damage to vascular endothelial cells, impairing normal function.

**7. What is the relationship between time and pressure intensity?**

High pressures over a short time are as damaging as low pressures over a long time. Intermittent pressures also affect tissue by reperfusion injury. Ischemia can occur in microvascular areas in as little as 2 hours of continuous pressure; necrosis may be noted in as little as 6 hours. The amount of time to injury is markedly reduced in patients who are acutely ill or hypovolemic.

**8. Define hyperemia.**

Hyperemia is a form of reactive vasodilation in response to pressure. It can occur in as little as 30 minutes and is seen clinically as a bright red, blanchable area over a bony prominence. The bright red area disappears within 1 hour after all pressure is relieved.

**9. What is the clinical significance of hyperemia?**

Hyperemia should be treated like a blinking red light. Stop and look around. It is a warning of troubled waters ahead. Take the opportunity to assess the patient fully, noting risk factors that predispose the patient to a pressure ulcer. Now is the time to implement a stepped-up plan of care to prevent further deterioration.

**10. Since pressure equals force divided by area, what effect does positioning have?**

A supine position allows the maximal amount of body area in contact with the bed. Unfortunately, not all body parts touch the surface of the bed. As a result, pressure is redistributed to certain body surfaces, including the heel, buttock, scapular, and occipital areas. Pressures can exceed 70 mmHg and even 100 mmHg in the heel—well above capillary closing pressures. The increased intensity is an example of high pressure. Remembering the relationship between time and pressure, the clinician can make the connection that in this situation, little time is needed to cause damage.

Sitting positions increase force and reduce body area in contact with a surface. The entire weight of the body is situated on the coccyx, posterior thighs, and the ischial tuberosities. Pressure on the ischial tuberosities have been recorded at 300 mmHg. Another example of the high pressure–short time relationship necessitates a more frequent repositioning schedule. Published clinical practice guidelines suggest that shifts in position should occur every 15 minutes in at-risk chair-bound patients.

Soft tissue compression at contracture sites is abnormally greater because of the increased internal forces and misalignment of bone as a result of the deformity.

**11. What is a pressure ulcer?**

The traditional definition of a pressure ulcer is a lesion caused by local tissue necrosis when soft tissues are compressed between a bony prominence and an external surface. Ulcers can develop, however, anywhere soft tissues are compressed at a force great enough to cause cell death. An example is the catheter tube compressed between the thighs.

**12. What is the staging system for pressure ulcers?**

In the attempt to improve communication about the severity of the wound, clinicians devised a system to classify pressure ulcers. The staging system is used only for pressure ulcers. Recommended by clinical practice guidelines and the National Pressure Ulcer Advisory Panel (NPUAP), the system describes pressure ulcers by anatomic depth of tissue damage. It is used as the basis for developing treatment protocols, selecting reduction support surface for individual patients, and obtaining reimbursement for a variety of wound-related products.

**Stage I:** a definitive area of color changes, skin temperature variations, induration (hardness), edema, or intact skin that may or may not be blanchable compared with surrounding tissue.

**Stage II:** a blister or open, shallow, abraded, ulcerated area involving the epidermis and dermis.

**Stage III:** an ulcerated area involving damage of epidermis, dermis, and subcutaneous tissue. The depth may extend to the fascia but does not include loss of integrity of the fascia.

**Stage IV:** an ulcerated open lesion involving epidermis, dermis, and subcutaneous tissue as well as damage to fascia, muscle, tendon or bone.

**13. What other wound classification systems have been devised?**

| CLASSIFICATION | DESCRIPTION |
| --- | --- |
| Partial-thickness wound | Non–pressure-related wound involving the epidermis and dermis |
| Full-thickness wound | Non–pressure-related wound involving the epidermis and dermis and extending into the subcutaneous tissue or deeper |

*Table continued on following page*

| CLASSIFICATION | DESCRIPTION |
|---|---|
| First, second, or third degree | Relates to severity of a burn wound |
| Wagner grades 0–5 | Neuropathic and arterial/ischemic classification of foot wounds |
| Red, yellow, black | Simplistic approach aimed at directing treatment based on the color of the wound bed |

**14. Why is anatomy rather than depth the framework for NPUAP staging of ulcers?**

Knowing anatomy allows us to properly stage pressure ulcerations. For example, if oxygen tubing causes an ulcer at the junction of the ear and skull, a depth of 0.5 cm or less makes this wound a stage IV ulcer because penetration to muscle is involved. On the other hand, a 2.0-cm wound on the trochanter of a morbidly obese patient may involve only subcutaneous tissue and thus is classified as a stage III wound.

**15. What are the disadvantages to using the NPUAP staging system?**

In a stage I ulcer, one cannot determine the severity and anatomic depth involved in the nonvisible tissue underneath the skin. Identifying a stage I ulcer is more difficult in non-Caucasian patients because of the variety of skin tones. Ulcerations that are covered with nonviable tissue, such as slough or eschar, cannot be staged until the tissue has been completely removed.

Most importantly is the misuse of the staging system for documentation. Clinicians inadvertently use the staging system to quantify healing. For example, documentation in the medical record may describe the wound as "once a stage IV, but now markedly improved to a stage III." The clinician is mistakenly looking at depth and trying to communicate that the wound is near or at the surface of surrounding skin. The NPUAP system, however, is based on anatomy. Because of the principles of wound healing (see Chapter 5), it is physiologically impossible to regrow muscle, fascia, or subcutaneous tissue. Wounds with full-thickness involvement heal by the deposition of granulation tissue. "Once a stage III, always a stage III, and once a stage IV, always a stage IV" is the motto among savvy wound care clinicians.

Unfortunately, some systems currently in place do not support this concept. In long-term care, the minimum data sheet (MDS), a form required by the federal government that affects reimbursement to the facility, forces a clinician to "back-stage" a pressure ulcer. This approach certainly places undue pressure on a clinician who truly understands wound healing.

**16. What does "back-staging" or reverse staging mean?**

Back-staging or reverse staging refers to the inappropriate staging of pressure ulcers based on wound healing rather than anatomic depth and the physiology of healing, as originally intended by the staging system.

**17. How can pressure be reduced?**

A number of devices are available (see Chapter 53). One caveat, however, should be remembered: no device can reduce heel pressures below capillary closing pressures unless the heel is suspended in air. For this reason, placing a pillow under the calf can be one of the most effective (and inexpensive) ways to decrease the incidence of heel pressure ulcers (see Chapter 44).

**18. What predisposes patients to the development of heel pressure ulcers?**

The anatomic ratio of soft tissue to bone is almost equal in the heel area, whereas the tissue-to-bone ratio in the buttocks can be considerably higher than 1:1. In addition, risk factors such as nutrition, hydration, mobility, vascular status, and macro- or microvascular disease contribute to the development of pressure ulcers in the heel. As one ages, fat pads in the feet become thinner. Less cushioning means less protection against mechanical forces.

**19. What other mechanical forces influence the wounding process?**

Shear and friction.

### 20. What is shear? When does it occur?

Shearing forces are more detrimental in the wounding process than pressure because shear, like pressure, has the intensity to exceed capillary closing pressures but also adds force. A stretching movement in the deep tissue layers in one direction is counteracted by pushing the superficial tissues in an opposite, but parallel, direction. This process is far more detrimental to tissue because the powerful grinding, twisting, and stretching movements produce far more damage than pressure alone.

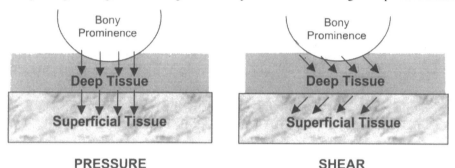

Mechanical forces of pressure and shear.

The nursing intervention that most often places the patient at greatest risk for shearing is raising the head of the bed to a semi-Fowler position. As the head of the bed is raised, the patient is typically drawn toward the foot of the bed by gravity, ultimately resulting in shear forces. The best intervention is to have the patient get out of bed and into a chair with 90° of flexion at the hips and knees.

### 21. Clinically, how can I tell the difference between shear force and pressure?

Shear wounds are irregularly shaped and positioned over a bony area. The coccyx is the most frequent area exposed to shear. Pressure wounds, on the other hand, are round and take the shape of the bone directly beneath. Shear forces contribute to the extensive undermining seen in the wound—something not usually seen in ulcers with exposure to pressure alone.

### 22. How does friction contribute to the wounding process?

Unlike shear, friction affects only the outermost skin layers by movement of the epidermis against an external surface. Clinically, friction presents as a superficial abrasion.

### 23. How can friction injuries be prevented or reduced?

Frequent use of lubricating oils, creams, or lotions lowers the surface tension on the skin to reduce friction injuries. A well-hydrated patient is less likely to succumb to friction because cells can better weather the external force. During physical care, avoid rubbing motions without lubricants. Teach caregivers and unlicensed personnel to lift rather than drag the patient during repositioning. This technique also has the added benefit of reducing shear forces.

Numerous items can be placed over the skin. Most are available as arm or leg sleeves. Elbow and heel devices also can be used. A frequent mistake that clinicians make is to assume that these products have pressure-reduction abilities. Most do not. If the goal is to reduce pressure and friction, seek out clinical proof that the product can reduce tissue interface pressures to an acceptable level while simultaneously decreasing friction.

### 24. How does moisture cause wounding?

Although not associated with the physical opening of a wound, excessive moisture weakens dermal integrity and destroys the outer lipid layer. Less intense mechanical force is needed to cause physical opening. Incontinence is by far the most frequent source of moisture. Wound drainage is the other phenomenon causing deterioration of intact skin. General skin care and prevention strategies were covered in Chapters 2 and 3.

**25. Why is heat a mechanism of injury?**

Intense heat causes burns. It is probably one of the first dangers that parents taught us to avoid: "Hot! Don't touch!" Heat can take many forms: solar, gas, liquid, and solid. Thermal injury shares the same characteristics as the pressure–time relationship. High heat over a short period can be as devastating as lower levels over a long period. Heat first desiccates tissue. If exposure continues, it causes extensive devitalization of all tissue layers by coagulation, thrombosis, and cell destruction. Altered capillary permeability leads to interstitial edema and initiation of the downward cycle of tissue destruction previously described. Burn injury and treatment are discussed in Chapter 55.

**26. How does cold cause injury?**

Cold produces a low-flow state via vasoconstriction. If exposure continues or extreme cold is encountered, cells and tissues freeze and never recover from the ensuing necrosis.

**27. Is radiation a form of heat?**

Ultimately, yes. Initial damage in patients receiving radiation therapy includes erythema and warmth, much like a first-degree burn. Deep tissues are also affected, causing cellular destruction that affects all types of tissue. Permanent cellular changes and scarring result. Normal cellular responses to injury, coupled with impaired nutrient and oxygen delivery to tissues, result in wound healing that is markedly delayed and sometimes absent.

Damaged tissues can range from hyperemic to ischemic to necrotic. Necrosis is often insidious and may occur decades after radiation exposure. A current injury may have been caused by a traumatic event, but the nonhealing quality of the wound can be attributed to the patient's distant history of radiation exposure. Fortunately, radiation therapy is much safer than it was 20 years ago because the ability to target specific cancerous cells has improved markedly.

**28. Are some types of trauma worse than others?**

Yes. Blunt trauma is often worse than penetrating trauma. In penetrating trauma, moist wound edges can be approximated and sutured, assuming no major organ damage lies beneath. Blunt trauma is more devastating, with crush injuries the most destructive and underappreciated. Crushing force adds shear and pressure to initiate the downward spiral of inflammation, capillary leak, edema, and tissue necrosis seen immediately in obvious injuries. Peak effect is noted in about 3 days.

Most crush wounds are best repaired after edema has subsided and tissue damage has been fully evaluated. In this case, time is an ally. Wounds that are not obvious crush injuries usually present as a laceration. Always consider crush forces as an assessment factor before approximating wound edges. The application of sutures, staples, or tissue adhesives to approximate wound edges on initial presentation is detrimental and inhibits healing.

**29. How is ischemia different from external forces?**

Ischemia eventually results from external forces but can arise from internal pathophysiologic events. The negative effects on tissue of the inability to supply oxygen and nutrients as well as remove cellular wastes are well documented.

**30. What four pathophysiologic events lead to ischemia?**

1. **Microvascular disease.** Involvement of arterioles and capillaries, narrowing of vessels due to calcification, endothelial dysfunction, and atherosclerosis are significant factors leading to ischemia.

2. **Diabetes mellitus.** Thickening of the basement membrane inhibits diffusion of vital nourishment to surrounding tissue.

3. **Macrovascular disease.** Calcification and atherosclerosis narrow large-vessel lumens. Claudication and physical changes such as the absence of hair and cool temperatures indicate macrovascular disease. Detailed information can be obtained in Chapters 41–48.

4. **Low-flow states.** Hypovolemia, shock, and multisystem organ failure lead to the shunting of blood from skeletal muscle and dermal tissues to major organs. Lowering blood flow reduces delivery of oxygen and nutrients. Waste removal is diminished, and if low flow continues, lactic acidosis ensues. Reperfusion injury in tissue is high after low-flow states are reversed. It is commonly thought that low flow contributes to occipital pressure ulcers after open-heart procedures.

### 31. How is a malignancy a mechanism of wounding?

Malignant tumors are highly vascular and occasionally invasive enough to "eat through" skin. Lesions that appear to look like the garden-variety ulcer in fact may be a malignancy. Even the most experienced clinician has been fooled at one time or another. Obtaining a wound biopsy is a valuable adjunct to wound care. Cancerous changes also occur, although rarely, in chronic nonhealing wounds.

### 32. How does chemical exposure promote wounding?

Characteristics of the offending agent, including pH, toxicity, chemical structure, exposure time, and method of application, influence how tissues and cells are damaged. Cell wall destruction, enzymatic inhibition, impairment of receptor cells, mitrochodria disruption, and protein denaturation are just a few of the insults that chemical injury can initiate. Although we appreciate the toxicity of the items kept in our household, almost anything can cause wounds in the wrong concentration or with prolonged exposure. Our own waste, in the form of stool or urine, is an example of a normal chemical capable of great damage.

### 33. What is important about surgical wounds?

The purposeful creation of a wound in controlled circumstances has its advantages. Such wounds often heal faster because healthy tissue is cut. Surgical wounds in unhealthy tissue usually result in prolonged, difficult healing.

### 34. How are surgical wounds closed?

**Primary closure.** Wound edges are approximated and closed using sutures, staples, tissue adhesives, or tape strips. Depth and location of the wound help determine what is used to close it.

**Secondary closure.** This technique allows the wound to be left open so that granulation tissue and subsequent development of scar tissue fill the wound to the level of the surrounding skin.

**Tertiary closure.** Combining the aspects of both primary and secondary methods, tertiary wound closure leaves the wound open for a certain period. Then the edges are approximated and closed. The decision to leave the wound open depends on various factors. With significant edema, questionable vascular integrity, need for aggressive cleansing because of contamination, or patient comorbidity that places the wound at high risk for dehiscence, the surgeon may choose tertiary closure.

### 35. What is a factitious wound?

A factitious wound is caused deliberately by the patient or caregiver. In its mildest and most socially acceptable form, ear and body piercing can be considered factitious. Münchausen's disease and Münchausen's by proxy are perhaps the most severe examples. Various methods are used to create a wound (heat, cold, chemical exposure, surgical scalpels, razors, other blunt and sharp instruments). Suspicion should be high in the following circumstances: (1) multiple wounds in unusual locations; (2) repeated wounding, always with a different story; (3) a different story each time for the same wound; (4) "doctor-hopping" because "no one can help" and a reported history of "nobody can find the cause"; (5) reports of abuse by others; (6) admission of self-abuse; or (7) attempts to split the team approach (evidenced as "he said...she said." statements)

### 36. What can be done about factitious wounds?

Applying the principles of wound healing is paramount. In addition, a collaborative unified team approach, consultation with a psychiatric nurse specialist. and limit-setting are helpful. Frank discussion about the nature of the wounds, done appropriately and professionally, is advocated.

### BIBLIOGRAPHY

1. Bryant RA: Acute and Chronic Wounds: Nursing Management, 2nd ed. St. Louis, Mosby, 2000.
2. Krasner D, Rodeheaver G, Sibbald G (eds): Chronic Wound Care: A Clinical Source Book for the Healthcare Professional, 3rd ed. Wayne, PA, HMP Communications, 2000.
3. Rolstad BD, Harris P, Fahey CB, Evans J, Alvarez O: Contemporary Wound Care: A Desk Reference. Arlington, TX, Johnson & Johnson Medical, Division of Ethicon, 1996.
4. Maklebust J, Sieggreen M: Pressure Ulcers: Guidelines for Prevention and Nursing Management, 2nd ed. Springhouse, PA, Springhouse Corp., 1996.
5. Sussman C, Bates-Jenson BM (eds): Wound Care: A Collaborative Practice Manual for Physical Therapists and Nurses. Gaithersburg, MD, Aspen, 1998.

# 5. PHYSIOLOGY OF WOUND HEALING

Marie Brown-Etris, RN, CWOCN, *and*
Catherine T. Milne, APRN, MSN, CS, CWOCN, ANP

### 1. Define wound healing.

The pure definition of wound healing is the orderly, complex process of tissue closure. Other ways of looking at this phenomenon include closure methods, stages of wound healing, and healing by regeneration or repair.

### 2. How does the closure method define wound healing?

**Primary intention.** The wound, full thickness in depth, is closed using sutures, staples, skin closure adhesive strips, or tissue adhesives.

**Secondary intention.** The wound, either partial or full thickness in depth, is left open for healing via the deposition of granulation tissue.

**Tertiary intention.** A full-thickness wound is left open to allow debridement or edema reduction or until optimal conditions are met for active closure. Wound edges are then approximated, and sutures, staples, tissue adhesives, or skin closure adhesive strips are used to close the wound.

### 3. How many stages of wound healing are generally recognized?

Four: coagulation, inflammatory, proliferative, and remodeling stages. These are physiologic descriptions, and the four stages overlap in a time continuum.

### 4. Describe what happens during the coagulation stage of wound healing.

Platelet activation results in fibrin formation. If blood vessels are transected, the body attempts to control bleeding by contracting the circular smooth muscle in the vessel. Unfortunately, if vessels are not completely transected, as in crush injuries, pressure ulcers, or ischemic wounds, this protective mechanism does not occur.

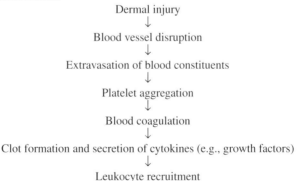

Dermal injury
↓
Blood vessel disruption
↓
Extravasation of blood constituents
↓
Platelet aggregation
↓
Blood coagulation
↓
Clot formation and secretion of cytokines (e.g., growth factors)
↓
Leukocyte recruitment

Coagulation stage of wound healing. (From Etris-Brown M: Measuring healing in wounds. Adv Wound Care 8(Suppl):53–58, 1995, with permission.)

### 5. What happens when platelet activation occurs?

Platelet activation is both a mechanical and a physiologic event. The platelets arrive at the area immediately after injury. As first responders, it is their job to achieve hemostasis and set up a "communications tent" with the other cells that arrive shortly thereafter. On contact with collagen in the wound, the platelets become sticky and clump together, producing a fibrin clot. This is the mechanical event of platelet aggregation.

Platelet activation also signals the release of adenosine diphosphate to enhance aggregation. Platelets secrete platelet-derived growth factors (PDGFs) and other chemical signals that initiate the wound-healing process, including transforming growth factor beta (TGF-$\beta$), transforming growth factor alpha (TGF-$\alpha$), fibroblast growth factor (FGF), epidermal growth factor (EGF), and insulin-like growth factor 1 (IGF-1).

### 6. When does the inflammatory phase start?

The inflammatory stage starts when leukocytes first enter the wound.—normally, at the time of injury. Simultaneously, histamine is released from mast cells in the dermis. Within 10 minutes, histamine-induced vasodilation occurs in the area of injury to facilitate the arrival of leukocytes.

### 7. Does histamine cause other physiologic responses?

Yes. The vasodilation is responsible for the redness and warmth typically seen in the wound area during the inflammatory stage. Increased vascular permeability, needed to deliver leukocytes into tissue, also results in localized edema.

### 8. How can edema be harmful?

Edema can place excessive force on injured tissue and compress blood flow, negating the physiologic purpose of inflammation. Excessive edema can result in nerve compression, adding to pain. Compartment syndrome is an example of the deadly forces of edema.

### 9. In what type of wounds should edema be managed?

In acute traumatic injuries, crush wounds are known to produce insidious edema, which peaks as long as 3–5 days after the event. Early management with ice and elevation and a high clinical suspicion for an impending compartment syndrome are essential. Chronic lower extremity wounds caused by venous insufficiency also are associated with edema. Compression of the tissue from the base of the toes to the tibial tuberosity is the mainstay of treatment.

### 10. What functions do white blood cells perform in the inflammatory stage of wound healing?

White blood cells, namely neutrophils and macrophages, function in a mechanical as well as chemical manner. Macrophages arise from monocytes. Both cell types depend on a healthy bone marrow. Normal wound healing is impaired without an adequate circulating number of these cells.

### 11. Describe the mechanical role of the white blood cells in the inflammatory stage.

Both neutrophils and macrophages have distinct functions. **Neutrophils**, the first of the white blood cells to arrive at the wound, have the immediate task of killing bacteria in the injured tissue by phagocytosis. They then "stand ground" to kill additional bacteria and assist in the removal of dead tissue. **Macrophages** arrive later. Besides having a phagocytic action on bacteria, they secrete collagenase, which autolytically debrides the wound of devitalized tissue.

### 12. Describe the chemical role of neutrophils in the inflammatory stage.

Neutrophils produce a sticky substance on their cell walls so that platelets can adhere to it. As the neutrophils infiltrate the injured site, platelets and platelet growth factors are brought along. Neutrophils also secrete PDGFs and IGF-1. These cells stay in the wound for 3–4 days and perform apoptosis. Remaining cell fragments are removed by the macrophages as they arrive into the wound.

### 13. What is apoptosis?

It is the cell equivalent of what secret agents do with classified information (preprogrammed self-destruction of all material when it is no longer useful).

### 14. Can neutrophils be harmful?

Neutrophils, for some unknown reason, remain active in chronic wounds. Turning from Dr. Jekyll into Mr. Hyde, they produce enzymes called metalloproteinase 8 (MMP8) and elastase in an excessive amount. These enzymes are responsible for the destruction of the extracellular matrix that acts as a scaffold for granulation tissue. Growth factors present in the wound are rendered ineffective.

**15. Can anything stop these wound-healing "sandbox bullies"?**

Yes. Tissue inhibitors of metalloproteinase (TIMPs) can offset the drainage caused by MMPs. TIMPs and MMPs should not fight in the sandbox but instead play on the see-saw. In normal wound healing when one goes up, the other pushes off (upregulates) to lower the higher one and achieve a natural balance of homeostasis.

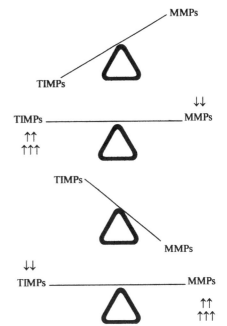

The TIMP–MMP seesaw, which achieves a natural balance of homeostasis.

**16. Describe the chemical actions of the macrophage.**

The macrophage is seen as the most essential cell in wound healing because of its ability to synchronize events and orchestrate numerous chemical processes; its absence is devastating to wound healing. Macrophages produce and secrete the following growth factors: TGF-β, PDGF, TGF-α, interleukin (IL)-1, and heparin-binding epidermis growth factor (HB-EGF). These chemicals are responsible for collagen deposition and encourage fibroblasts to proliferate. Lactate, needed for the production of tumor necrosis factor alpha (TNF-α), IL-1, and basic fibroblast growth factor (bFGF), is also produced by the macrophage. Collagen synthesis, the vital step in the next phase of wound healing, depends on the production of lactate.

**17. Can macrophages be harmful?**

Like its neutrophil cousin, the macrophage releases inflammatory mediators. When released in the wrong time sequence or in excessive amounts, the inflammatory process becomes chronic and impedes wound healing.

**18. How long does the inflammatory phase last?**

5–7 days.

**19. Clinically, how can a normal inflammatory stage be identified?**

It is easiest to begin by describing what is abnormal. The cardinal signs of inflammation gone awry are pain, redness, swelling, and heat. A normal inflammatory phase is characterized by mild diffuse pinkish-red hues at the wound edges, not extending beyond 1 cm. In melanin-rich skin, these edges have a slightly different color tone and may be bluish or purple. The absence of edema, heat, and induration (hardness) can be assessed by feeling the wound edges.

**20. What is the goal of the proliferative stage?**

In normal wound healing, the clinical outcomes expected are revascularization, deposition of new tissue, and wound closure. These goals are accomplished by angiogenesis formation of the extracellular matrix with granulation tissue and epithelialization.

**21. How is angiogenesis accomplished?**

Angiogenesis is the formation of a new vascular network in the wounded area. Endothelial cells from nearby intact vessels are recruited to the injury by enzymes secreted from macrophages. These cells are worker-cells that follow the strict instructions of the growth factors FGF, TNF-β, EGF, and wound angiogenesis factor (WAF). Vessel tubes are formed, capillaries sprout, and the building blocks of the extracellular matrix are laid down.

**22. Do endothelial cells produce growth factors?**

Yes. IGF, PDGF, and bFGF are secreted. These growth factors are essential for the extracellular matrix formation and manufacture of fibronectin and collagen.

**23. How is the extracellular matrix formed?**

The macrophages continue to play an important role by removing debris, destroying bacteria, and recruiting fibroblasts (a critical step) and supporting their proliferation.

**24. What role does the fibroblast play in the proliferative stage?**

Fibroblasts make collagen, elastin, glycosaminoglycans (GAGs), and proteoglycans, the components of a healthy extracellular matrix. Some differentiate into myofibroblasts, which are responsible for wound contraction. Fibroblasts also secrete essential growth factors to continue the wound healing process.

**25. What is granulation tissue?**

Named for its granular appearance, it is a combination of blood vessels and connective tissue. It should look beefy red and slightly moist.

**26. How does wound contraction occur?**

As the wound fills with granulation tissue to the surface of skin surrounding the wound, the myofibroblasts begin to secrete elastin. Much like the tension created by a stretched rubber band, whose natural tendency is to contract, the elastin imbedded throughout the wound pulls the wound edges closer together. This process facilitates epithelialization, the last step in the proliferation stage.

**27. Describe the events occurring during the epithelialization phase.**

The goal of the epithelialization phase is to resurface the wound and give it a protective covering. This process requires migration of keratinocytes located in adjacent intact epidermis. The first step is detachment of a leading edge of keratinocytes from the basal layer. These cells flatten out and become phagocytic as they move toward the wound center (much like a pack of wolves surrounding and closing in on their prey). A new basement membrane is created behind the leading edge of cells. The keratinocytes then produce and differentiate into the sublayers of the epidermis previously discussed in Chapter 1. This process is known as the sliding model of wound closure.

**28. What is the leapfrog model of epithelialization?**

The keratinocytes jump over the cell in front of them. After "leapfrogging" (also known as epiboly), they stick to the fluids and tissue in the wound bed. A wound may use both models to resurface itself.

**29. In addition to the mechanical process of keratinocyte movement, what chemical interactions occur?**

Keratinocytes produce IL-1, keratinocyte-derived autocrine factor (KAF), vascular endothelial factor (VEGF), TGF-α, TGF-β, MMPs, and enzymes. These growth factors are needed under the surface of the new epithelium to complete remodeling, the final stage of wound healing.

**30. What can go wrong in the proliferative stage?**

Because of its naturally complex nature, this stage of wound healing can be affected by a number of mechanical and chemical factors that impede wound healing. Absence or blunting of an immune response, excessive inflammation, overcolonization of the wound bed (bioburden), frank infection, inadequate numbers of macrophages, host factors, location and nature of the wound, and out-of-sequence physiologic steps at the cellular level can delay or stop the proliferative stage from progressing normally.

**31. How can a normal proliferative stage be identified clinically?**

In the early phase, the wound base should move from a clean, red or pink smooth surface to a surface that has puffy mounds of beefy red tissue. Next, the granulation tissue should fill in the defect toward the surface of the surrounding skin. Simultaneously, the wound dimension should diminish as contraction occurs. Epithelialization onset is observed by a small mound (0.1–0.2 cm) of pink tissue surrounding the open wound on its margins. This mound is known as the epithelial ridge. As migration occurs, the ridge flattens out and disappears as the wound is paved over with a new epidermis.

**32. Once the wound is closed, is healing complete?**

A frequent faux pas by inexperienced clinicians is underappreciation of the remodeling process. Failure to respect the physiology of this phase of wound healing can result in a reopening of the wound.

**33. How long does the proliferative stage last?**

The proliferative stage may last between 7 and 70 days, depending on the size of the wound.

**34. In terms of time, how does one clinically observe an impaired proliferative stage?**

No improvement in wound dimensions over a 2-week period is characteristic of a stalled wound.

**35. What is the goal during the remodeling stage?**

The creation of tensile strength of collagen scar tissue.

**36. Sounds simple. Is it?**

No. Like other wound-healing stages, this is a complex mechanical and chemical process.

**37. What mechanical processes occur in the remodeling stage?**

Collagen deposited in the wound in the proliferative stage is randomly scattered. In this stage, old collagen is destroyed and replaced with collagen bundles that are thicker and organized in a physical fashion to provide tissue strength. This process is known as cross-linking.

**38. What chemical processes occur?**

The degradation of the old collagen occurs through enzymatic activity. Collagenase, aided by MMPs, splits the randomly placed collagen fibers into fragments. Then the rebuilding process begins. During this time, TGF-β, PDGF, FGF, and TIMPs via residual fibroblasts and macrophages synthesize new collagen to replace the old.

**39. How long does the remodeling process last?**

As long as 2 years.

**40. Does the tensile strength of the skin return to prewound intensity?**

Unfortunately, no. The maturing scar has only 60–80% of the strength of the original skin.

**41. What are the clinical implications of reduced tensile strength?**

Scar tissue can reopen with less mechanical force. External factors such as friction, shear, pressure, or moisture and intrinsic factors such as edema in minimal amounts can cause rewounding. Nursing interventions should be aimed at reducing these factors.

**42. Describe the clinical appearance of the remodeling stage.**

Scar tissue first appears as a slightly raised pink mound of intact skin. As it flattens, it changes from pink to white and continues to contract.

**43. What is a keloid scar?**

A keloid scar is a dense overgrowth of scar tissue extending well beyond the margins of the original wound. Keloid scars are often pruritic. The excessive production of TGF-β may contribute to keloidal scarring. Prophylactic application of silicone to the area may reduce keloid formation.

**44. How is a hypertrophic scar different from a keloid scar?**

As with their keloid counterpart, a complication of the overexpression of growth factors contributes to development of hypertrophic scars. Hypertrophic scars are less pruritic, stay within the confines of the original wound margin, and resolve somewhat over a period of 1 year.

**45. Do all wounds heal in the exact same manner?**

No. Wounds heal by regeneration, repair, or as a hybrid of regeneration and repair.

**46. What makes tissue regeneration different from tissue repair?**

Only epithelial tissue can regenerate itself. Once the wound is resurfaced, there is no scar or loss of function or change in the physical structure of the wounded area. Tissue repair involves "filling" of the wound with connective tissue. This method always results in a scar. Sebaceous glands, hair follicles, and subcutaneous tissue are not reformed during the healing process, resulting in loss of normal function of these and other structures present before the injury occur.

**47. What dictates whether tissue is regenerated or repaired?**

Depth of the wound. Partial-thickness wounds extending from the epidermis into the upper levels of the dermis heal strictly by regeneration. Full-thickness wounds extending to a minimum of the subcutaneous tissues heal by repair.

**48. What characteristics of a wound lead to a combination of regeneration and repair?**

Only deep dermal wounds combine the two methods. Because the deep dermis is highly vascular, it goes through the traditional wound-healing stages of coagulation, inflammation, and proliferation. These stages occur at an exceptionally fast rate. Because wound depth is minimal, epithelial regeneration and migration occur simultaneously from the wound margins and from the epithelial cells lining the hair follicles. Scarring is minimal or absent. There may be some functional loss if complete structures such as the arrector pili muscle or sweat glands were destroyed in the upper dermis.

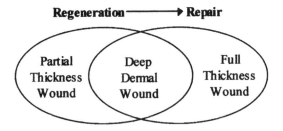

Combination of regeneration and repair. (Adapted from Etris-Brown M: Measuring healing in wounds. Adv Wound Care 8(Suppl):53–58, 1995, with permission.)

**49. What are the ideal conditions for wound healing?**

To facilitate the varied and highly complex physiologic process of wound healing, optimal internal and external conditions for tissue repair must be present.

| **Internal** | **External** |
|---|---|
| Adequate oxygenation | Minimal bacterial contamination |
| Optimal nutrition/hydration | Avoidance of mechanical forces |
| Bacterial control | Refrain from smoking |
| Intact immune systems | No medications known to affect wound healing |
| Wound bed moisture control | Wound not exposed to cytotoxic chemicals |
| Control of necrotic tissue | |
| Concomitant disease absent | |
| Edema absent | |

## 50. Why is moist wound healing beneficial?

Moist wound healing is defined as the right amount of wetness so that the wound glistens. Excessive moisture harms intact tissue around the wound. A dry wound bed does not allow the metabolic functions of cells to occur. Moist wound healing provides several advantages:

- Improved healing rate
- Increased epithelialization
- Reduced infection
- Enhanced collagen synthesis
- Macrophages appear earlier in wound and in greater numbers

### BIBLIOGRAPHY

1. Cohen IK, Diegelmann RF, Lindblad WJ: Wound Healing: Biochemical and Clinical Aspects. Philadelphia, WB Saunders, 1992.
2. Durham C: Laceration assessment and management. Patient Care Nurse Pract 4(6):17–23, 2001.
3. Etris-Brown M: Measuring healing in wounds. Adv Wound Care 8(Suppl):53–58, 1995.
4. Greenhalgh DG: The role of growth factors in wound healing. J Trauma 41:159–167, 1996.
5. Rolstad B, Harris A, Fahey CB, et al: Contemporary Wound Care: A Desk Reference. Arlington, TX, Johnson & Johnson Medical, Division of Ethicon, 1996.

# 6. THE ROLE OF COLLAGEN IN WOUND HEALING

*Liza G. Ovington, PhD, CWS*

### 1. What is collagen?

Collagen is a specific type of fibrous protein characterized by its unique structure and its ability to aggregate into complex arrangements of individual molecules. A single collagen molecule consists of three strands of protein. Each strand is twisted individually, and all three are twisted around each other. This unique twisted-triple-twist structure is known as the triple helix. Through chemical reactions, collagen molecules can line up end to end and side by side to create larger structures known as fibrils, which can then associate to form larger fibers. The twisted structure and multimolecular aggregates give collagen its characteristic strength. Collagen is the most abundant protein in the human body.

### 2. Is there more than one type of collagen?

Nineteen different types of collagen have been identified in the human body (designated type 1, type 2, type 3, and so on). However, 90% of all collagen in the body is type 1. Type 1 collagen is the predominant type found in soft tissues, bones, tendons, and ligaments. Certain types of collagen are localized to specific tissues. For example, cartilage contains predominantly type 2 collagen.

### 3. Where does collagen come from?

Collagen is made by different cells, depending on the type of tissue in which it is found. The fibroblast makes collagen in soft tissue, the osteoblast in bone, and the chondroblast in cartilage.

### 4. What role does endogenous collagen play in the wound-healing process?

Endogenous collagen plays a role in all three phases of the normal wound-healing process: inflammation, proliferation, and maturation. In the inflammatory phase of healing, collagen acts as the chemical signal that causes platelets to degranulate and release growth factors and other chemicals that initiate the healing process. Collagen also plays an important role in hemostasis. During the proliferative phase of healing, new collagen is produced by the fibroblasts and forms a three-dimensional matrix that serves as a scaffolding for the ingrowth of cells and new blood vessels that make up granulation tissue. Collagen synthesis by fibroblasts creates protein fragments that are chemotactic for more fibroblasts and for macrophages. In the maturation or remodeling phase of healing, the collagen fibers created in the proliferative phase grow thicker and become more directionally oriented, resulting in increased tissue tensile strength.

### 5. What clinical data address the use of collagen in wound management?

Collagen dressings have been evaluated in a number of randomized, controlled trials in both acute and chronic wounds. In trials of pressure ulcers, diabetic foot ulcers, and surgical wounds, collagen dressings appeared to result in enhanced granulation, increased incidence of wound closure, or decreased time to closure. In trials of venous leg ulcers, collagen dressings did not appear to enhance the healing rate (with compression bandages being the same in both treatment groups), but one study suggested that the collagen dressing resulted in reduced ulcer recurrence at 12-month follow-up.

## BIBLIOGRAPHY

1. Rao KP: Recent developments of collagen based materials for medical applications and drug delivery systems. J Biomater Sci Polym Educ 7:623645, 1995.
2. Baxter C: Collagen in the treatment of chronic wounds of the lower extremity. Biomechanics 4(6):24–28, 1997.
3. Van Gils CC, Roeder B, Chesler SM, Mason S: Improved healing with a collagen-alginate dressing in the chemical matricectomy. J Am Podiatr Med Assoc 88(9):452–456, 1988.
4. Donaghue V, Chrzan J, Rosenblum B, et al: Evaluation of a collagen-alginate wound dressing in the management of diabetic foot ulcers. Adv Wound Care 11:114–119, 1998.

# 7. THE ROLE OF HYALURONAN IN WOUND HEALING

Wai Yuen John Chen, BSc, PhD

### 1. Define hyaluronan.

Hyaluronan (hyaluronic acid [HA]) is a carbohydrate macromolecule. It is a linear copolymer of glucuronic acid and N-acetylglucosamine. Hyaluronan is found in most parts of the body and is almost ubiquitous; it is found in all vertebrates and in some lower marine organisms and bacteria. The structure of hyaluronan is identical across species except for molecular-weight variations. Its molecular weight can be as high as $5 \times 10^6$. Hyaluronan has been used in medicine for many years, primarily in ocular and joint surgery. More recently hyaluronan-based biomaterials have been developed for tissue repair processes.

### 2. In which tissue of the body is hyaluronan found?

Hyaluronan is a major component of the extracellular matrix. Most cells in the body have the capability to synthesize hyaluronan during some points in their cell cycles, implicating its functions in fundamental biologic processes. Hyaluronan is found in particularly high levels in the vitreous humor of the eye, cartilage, synovial fluid and skin (predominantly in the basal layer of the epidermis). Enrichment of hyaluronan in early granulation tissue matrix during wound healing probably is due to increased hyaluronan synthesis.

### 3. What are the biologic functions of hyaluronan?

The biologic functions of hyaluronan are many and depend on the interplay between its physicochemical and biologic properties. The main physicochemical property of hyaluronan is its ability to absorb up to 3000 times its own weight in water. As a result, it has unique osmotic, viscoelastic, permeability, and ionic properties that are central to its many biologic functions. These physicochemical properties are further tailored to the body's needs by specific binding to body cells and other body components. Hyaluronan binds to body cells via three main classes of cell surface receptors: CD44 (the major cell surface receptor for hyaluronan), RHAMM, and ICAM-1. Hyaluronan can also bind to extracellular matrix components such as collagen, fibronectin, and fibrin. The many biologic functions of hyaluronan include the following:
- Control of tissue hydration in the skin and other organs as well as an osmotic buffer in the kidney.
- Control of hydration in the cellular microenvironment to facilitate cell proliferation and migration.
- Cushioning and lubricating functions, especially in the eye and synovial joints.
- Possible effect on cellular signaling through membrane ion channels.
- Free radical scavenging and antioxidant properties, which may be particularly important in skin physiology as a protectant against solar radiation and in the control of inflammation.
- As an integral part of the extracellular matrix, it forms the backbone for the organization of proteoglycans in cartilage. It also binds with collagen, fibrin, and other matrix molecules.
- Mediation of the assembly of extracellular matrices, cell-matrix, and cell-cell interactions.
- Breakdown products affecting cells through direct receptor-mediated cell signaling involving the CD44 and ICAM-1 receptors.
- Promotion of angiogenesis has been demonstrated in a variety of models.

### 4. How and where is hyaluronan made?

Hyaluronan is made by body cells via a class of enzymes known as hyaluronan synthase. Most body cells studied so far have these enzymes. Hyaluronan synthase, located on the cell membrane, catalyzes the synthesis of hyaluronan. Newly synthesized hyaluronan is secreted directly into the extracellular matrix, thus providing a highly hydrated microenvironment at the sites of synthesis and facilitating cell detachment during mitosis and migration.

**5. In the repair and regeneration of skin after traumatic wounding, what functions does hyaluronan fulfill? In which stages of healing is it most evident?**

Wound healing follows a series of tightly regulated, sequential events: inflammation, granulation, reepithelialization, and remodeling. Hyaluronan is thought to be involved in every stage of the wound repair process.

*Summary of Tissue Repair Processes Involving Hyaluronan*

| STAGE | PROCESS | MECHANISM |
|---|---|---|
| Inflammatory phase | Inflammation activation | Enhancement of cell infiltration |
| | | Increase of proinflammatory cytokines, including tumor necrosis factor (TNF), interleukin (IL)-1, and IL-8, via a CD44-mediated mechanism |
| | | Facilitates primary adhesion of cytokine-activated lymphocytes to endothelium |
| | Inflammation moderation | Free radical scavenging and antioxidant properties |
| | | TSG-6– and IαI–mediated inhibition of inflammatory proteinases |
| Granulation phase | Cell proliferation | Hyaluronan synthesis facilitates cell detachment and mitosis |
| | Cell migration | Increased hyaluronan synthesis |
| | | Hyaluronan-rich granulation tissue provides open, hydrated matrix that facilitates cell migration |
| | Angiogenesis | Receptor-mediated cell migration (e.g., CD44, RHAMM) |
| | | Angiogenic properties of low-molecular-weight hyaluronan oligosaccharides |
| Reepithelialization | Keratinocyte functions | Hyaluronan-rich matrix is associated with proliferating basal keratinocytes |
| | | Facilitates keratinocyte migration via CD44-mediated mechanism |
| Remodeling | Scarring | Hyaluronan-rich matrix may reduce collagen deposition, leading to reduced scarring as seen in fetal wound healing |

Adapted from Chen WYJ, Abatangelo G: Functions of hyaluronan in wound repair. Wound Rep Reg 7:79–89, 1999, with permission.

Endogenous hyaluronan is synthesized by many types of cells on stimulation by a variety of factors and on cell division and cell migration. It appears early in the healing process and is associated with fibrin in the early provisional matrix. Levels then decline concurrently with blood vessel growth. Endogenous hyaluronan is also associated with the scarless embryonic healing quality.

**6. Can healing be enhanced by supplementation of endogenous hyaluronan with an extrinsic source?**

Many reports have attested to the beneficial effects of exogenous hyaluronan on wound-healing outcome. In animal experiments, topically applied hyaluronan has been shown to accelerate skin wound healing in rats and hamsters. Similar results have been observed in the healing of perforated tympanic membranes in rats. Corneal epithelial wound healing is also reported to be stimulated by applied hyaluronan.

Hyaluronan also has been reported to affect beneficially the quality of tissue repair. The lack of fibrous scarring in fetal wound healing has been attributed, at least in part, to hyaluronan, the levels of which remain high for longer periods than in adult wounds. This leads to the suggestion that hyaluronan, at least in part, may reduce collagen deposition and therefore results in reduced scarring.

Hyaluronan also may have a protective effect on chronic wounds, many of which have been shown to be highly inflammatory. Hyaluronan prevents free radical damage to granulation tissue in rats. Additional clinical data demonstrate the inflammation-moderating effect of hyaluronan.

**7. What future development potential is there for hyaluronan in wound repair and other medical applications?**

Much work still needs to be done to elucidate the biologic mechanisms of hyaluronan in tissue processes. Because of its ubiquitous nature and unique physicochemical properties, hyaluronan has already seen biomedical applications. In tissue repair, its physicochemical properties, the promising results shown in in vivo experimental studies, and its currently known biologic properties, strongly indicate applications in mediation of the wound-healing process as well as a biomaterial for bioengineering purposes.

Products already have been developed for antiadhesion, wound healing, tissue implants, and moisturizing purposes. These products are based on either pure hyaluronan or derivatives of hyaluronan, using cross-linking, esterification, or other chemical modification techniques to improve physical handling and stability characteristics. Derivatives of hyaluronan can be manufactured into many physical forms, including powders, fleece, fibers, semisolid gels, and microspheres; biocompatibility, for the most part, is preserved. Currently, hyaluronan-based medical products are designed to function as medical devices; without doubt, however, when the biology of hyaluronan becomes better known, applications will be developed to utilize its biological functions.

## BIBLIOGRAPHY

1. Aruffo A, Stamenkovic I, Melnick M, et al: CD44 is the principal cell surface receptor for hyaluronate. Cell 61:1303–1313, 1990.
2. Balazs EA, Laurent TC: New applications for hyaluronan. In Laurent TC (ed): The Chemistry, Biology and Medical Applications of Hyaluronan and its Derivatives. London, Portland Press, Wenner-Gren International Series 72, 1998, pp 325–336.
3. Chen WYJ, Abatangelo G: Functions of hyaluronan in wound repair. Wound Rep Reg 7:79–89, 1999.
4. Cortivo R, Brun P, Cardarelli L, et al: Antioxidant effects of hyaluronan and its alpha-methyl-prednisolone derivative in chrondrocyte and cartilage cultures. Semin Arthritis Rheum 26:492–501, 1996.
5. Ellis I, Banyard J, Schor SL: Differential response of fetal and adult fibroblasts to cytokines: Cell migration and hyaluronan synthesis. Development 124:1593–1600, 1997.
6. Ialenti A, Di Rosa M: Hyaluronic acid modulates acute and chronic inflammation. Agent Act 43:44–47, 1994.
7. Toole BP: Proteoglycans and hyaluronan in morphogenesis and differentiation. In Hay ED (ed): Cell Biology of Extracellular Matrix, 2nd ed. New York, Plenum Press, 1991, pp 305–341.
8. Wang C, Tammi M, Tammi R: Distribution of hyaluronan and its CD44 receptor in the epithelia of human skin appendages. Histochemistry 98:105–112, 1992.

# 8. NUTRITION AND WOUND HEALING

*Dawn M. Himes, MS, RD*

### 1. Why is nutrition important?

Many studies have reported a link between the importance of nutrition and the wound-healing process as well as between deteriorating nutritional status and development of pressure ulcers. Nutrition assessment and monitoring are critical to ensure adequate intake to support wound healing.

### 2. When should the dietitian become involved?

In the acute- or long-term care setting, federal and state regulations require screening of every patient or resident for potential nutrition intervention. Ideally, the dietitian should be consulted at the first sign of problems, hopefully before the development of pressure ulcers or more blatant signs of malnutrition. Generally, the request for a consultation is made by the physician. The involvement of the interdisciplinary team is key in identifying and addressing nutritional issues. Early intervention prevents additional losses, decreases costs associated with hospitalization, and improves quality of life by contributing to a positive treatment outcome.

### 3. What assessment parameters should be obtained in patients with a wound?

In conducting any type of physical assessment, it is important to explore thoroughly all parameters that contribute to nutritional status and to assess the patient as a whole. The table below summarizes the four primary areas that should be reviewed during a nutrition assessment.

| PARAMETER | COMPONENTS |
| --- | --- |
| Physical | Condition of hair, skin, nails, oral cavity, dentition |
| Anthropometric | Height/weight |
| Biochemical | Albumin, prealbumin, blood urea nitrogen, electrolytes, hemoglobin/hematocrit |
| Intake/diet history | Comparison with calculated needs |

### 4. What is the most reliable way to obtain a patient's height?

Obtaining the patient's accurate height helps to determine calculations related to energy needs as well as ideal body weight. Both of these measures are key to a dietitian's assessment and ultimately determine needs for nutritional intervention. The most accurate means of obtaining height is the traditional ruler provided on most physician's scales. However, if the patient is unable to stand, knee height index is suggested as an accurate alternative. After obtaining a measurement of the distance between the flexed knee and the flexed foot, the measurement can be put into the appropriate formula for calculation of total height. Another alternative for obtaining an approximate height is the wingspan technique. Although less accurate than the techniques described above, measurement of the distance from index finger to index finger between horizontally outstretched hands can provide an estimation of height.

### 5. What medications commonly affect nutritional status or appetite?

Many medications cause detrimental nutritional effects by affecting intake or absorption of nutrients. General categories known to have adverse effects on nutrition include psychotropics, chemotherapy medications, some antibiotics, and cathartics. Specific information about these effects can be obtained from the *Physicians' Desk Reference* or a nutrient and drug interaction reference.

### 6. What laboratory measures should be assessed?

Always review specific laboratory measures in reference to other values. For example, albumin is affected by hydration status, infection or other disease processes, and medication interactions. When possible, current laboratory values also should be compared with historical baselines. It is possible that what may be considered deficient for one patient may be normal for another, considering his or her medical condition. The following areas, at a minimum, should be reviewed during nutritional assessment.

| MEASURE | RISK INDICATOR* |
|---|---|
| Albumin | < 3.5 mg/dl |
| Total lymphocyte count | < 1,800/mm$^3$ |
| Transferrin | < 200 mg/dl |
| Cholesterol | < 150 mg/dl |
| Prealbumin | < 15 mg/dl |

* Refer to specific ranges as listed by local laboratory standards.

**7. On what criteria should frequency of assessment be based?**
- Acuity of the patient's condition
- Standards for general medical management
- Nutritional intervention approaches
- Lab value being measured

In general, laboratory measures used for traditional nutritional assessment should be obtained once per month. However, it is appropriate to assess measures (e.g., prealbumin) with a significantly short half-life on a more frequent basis. In addition, lab values should be obtained if a patient's nutritional status deteriorates for comparison with baseline assessment.

**8. What is albumin? What does it tell you about a patient?**
Albumin is a serum protein that measures visceral protein stores (those available to respond to metabolic stress, such as wound healing). Low albumin results in impaired exchange of cellular nutrients, interstitial edema, and decreased skin elasticity and resiliency, all of which impair wound healing. A direct relationship exists between the severity of albumin depletion and the severity of pressure ulcers. Albumin is considered a long-term measure of protein status, with a half life of 18–21 days. In evaluating albumin, it is important to note that it is strongly affected by hydration status, renal function, and infection.

**9. What is prealbumin? What does it tell you about a patient?**
Prealbumin is used to provide a more current picture of protein status because its half-life is 1–2 days. Although generally a more expensive test, it provides a better means of tracking protein repletion, especially in patients requiring nutritional support.

**10. What is transferrin? What does it tell you about a patient?**
Transferrin is an iron transport protein that may be used to measure visceral protein status. Use of transferrin is not recommended in patients with an iron deficiency. As iron deficiency worsens, transferrin levels decrease and provide a false indicator of nutritional status.

**11. Why is total lymphocyte count (TLC) important?**
TLC provides a measure of immunity proteins (required to elicit the immune response necessary for wound healing). The formula to calculate TLC is WBC × 10 × % of lymphocytes in the complete blood count. A score < 1800 mm$^3$ indicates nutritional risk, depressed immune response, and poor wound-healing outcomes.

**12. What role does blood sugar play in wound healing?**
Elevated blood sugar levels, as seen with poor management of diabetes mellitus or metabolic stress, impair wound healing by impairing lymphocyte function and, ultimately, the immune response.

**13. What other observations during physical assessment may indicate a nutritional problem?**
General indicators of nutritional deficiencies include overt emaciation, fluid retention, poor skin turgor, and overall condition of the hair, nails, and skin.

**14. What is the difference between starvation and cachexia wasting syndrome?**
**Starvation** results from the selective loss of fat due to inadequate caloric intake and can be reversed simply with refeeding. **Cachexia** is generally associated with either a disease state (e.g.,

cancer, AIDS) or metabolic stress and is not effectively managed by refeeding. Cachexia also tends to result in a significant loss of protein rather than fat, leading to reduction of lean body mass (LBM).

**15. What causes a catabolic state?**

A catabolic state results when the body's protein stores are broken down via an acute metabolic response resulting in LBM deterioration. Extreme physiologic stress such as sepsis, certain disease processes, and medical conditions like burns or surgery, and trauma can lead to a net catabolic response.

**16. Is a catabolic state the same as a negative nitrogen balance?**

A negative nitrogen balance indicates that protein intake is less than protein breakdown. A catabolic state results in a negative nitrogen balance due to the rapid breakdown of LBM, despite what may appear to be adequate protein intake. Increasing protein intake may not completely reverse a negative nitrogen balance if the metabolic cause of catabolism is not also addressed.

**17. Why is monitoring a patient's weight important?**

Unplanned weight loss is a key indicator of altered nutritional status. Weight loss, particularly loss of LBM, predisposes patients to decreases in functional status, mobility, and muscle strength (all of which contribute to the development of pressure ulcers and impaired wound healing).

**18. When should one become alarmed at weight loss?**

According to most guidelines, a 5% loss of weight from the previous month indicates a significant decline in nutritional status. In addition, a 10% loss in 6 months is an equivalent indicator. It is important to investigate thoroughly the accuracy of the weight change to determine quickly the most appropriate and effective approach for intervention.

**19. Define ideal body weight.**

Ideal body weight (IBW) is an average of an acceptable weight range based on height. IBW is calculated as follows:

Male: 106 lb for the first 5 feet plus 6 lb for each additional inch

Female: 100 lb for the first 5 feet plus 5 lb for each additional inch

It is also important to obtain a weight history to determine if the IBW calculation is an accurate measure of usual body weight (UBW) for individual patients. If UBW is inconsistent with IBW ranges, the primary goal should be to reach consistency with UBW standards; then assess the appropriateness of using IBW ranges for establishing weight goals.

**20. How many calories does it take to heal a wound?**

The guidelines of the Agency for Healthcare Policy and Research recommend a minimum of 30–35 kcal/kg and 1.25–1.5 gm protein/kg to heal a wound. In general, the deeper the wound, the greater the nutritional need. Nutritional intervention for full-thickness wounds should be aimed at target values of 35 kcal/kg and the 1.5 gm protein /kg. Calorie and protein calculations may need to be higher for patients who are already malnourished or who have higher needs, such as surgical and burn patients. Some patients may require in excess of 4,000 kcal/ day and 200 gm of protein.

**21. What is the role of vitamins and minerals in wound healing?**

All vitamins, minerals, and trace elements are necessary for cellular metabolism; thus, all are important to wound healing. Generally, a deficiency in only one of these nutrients is rare. Studies recommend overall supplementation with a multivitamin/mineral supplement if nutritional deficiency is suspected. Some studies have supported the additional supplementation of vitamin C (500 mg 2 times/day) and zinc sulfate (220 mg/2 times/day) but only if calorie and protein intake has been adequately addressed. The over-the-counter equivalent of zinc sulfate is elemental zinc (50 mg/day). Heavy metals, such as zinc, interfere with the absorption of some antibiotics and antilipemic agents. Discuss with a pharmacist the best way to administer medications with heavy metals to avoid drug–drug interactions. Recent research supports the necessity of supplementation of vitamin A in patients who receive glucocorticoid medications, but more studies are needed to support this intervention as a standard protocol.

### 22. Should protein supplements be given routinely to patients with wounds?

In developing nutritional intervention strategies for patients with wounds, foods should be the first approach to supplementing the traditional diet. However, the use of supplements may be warranted because of very high caloric or protein needs or observed poor intake. It is important to educate and involve the patient in the process of selecting a supplement.

### 23. In what forms are protein supplements available?

Fortunately, the variety of supplements has tremendously increased over the past few years. Soups, beverages, ice creams, puddings, bars, and powders help to prevent boredom and provide options to patients who require long-term supplements or are particular about what they eat.

### 24. How does one decide which protein supplement to use and in what form?

The choice of supplement should be based first on nutritional need, then on the patient's food preferences. Ideally, the patient should be given a choice of form and/or flavors as well as supplements to increase consumption.

### 25. When should total parenteral nutrition (TPN) be used for wound healing?

TPN should used for wound healing or, more specifically, as a nutritional intervention only when the oral route is unavailable and the gut is not functioning because of surgery, malformation, or malabsorption. Specific guidelines are available for the route of TPN administration. The decision to start TPN should be discussed with the patient by an interdisciplinary team.

### 26. When should a feeding tube be placed to facilitate wound healing?

A feeding tube should be placed only after all other types of oral supplementation have been exhausted or oral intake is not possible because of surgery or dysphagia. In addition, appropriate permission from the patient or healthcare power of attorney must be documented to allow tube placement. Generally, if long-term tube feeding is anticipated, a more permanent G-tube may be placed instead of a nasogastric tube. Increase tube feedings gradually to provide adequate nutritional support. Dramatic increases in feeding may result in refeeding syndrome, as evidenced by hypokalemia and reflux.

### 27. What are arginine and glutamine?

Arginine and glutamine are obligatory amino acids involved in protein anabolism. Inadequacies of one or both can delay the wound-healing response Studies of glutamine supplementation demonstrate their potential role in treating patients with pressure ulcers. Studies of arginine supplementation, although supportive, are few. Further research is needed in these areas.

### 28. What should the patient with a wound be taught about nutrition?

The patient should be instructed about the role of adequate nutrition in wound healing and specifically about the minimal intake requirements necessary to meet calculated caloric and protein needs. In some cases, discussion about the role of additional food items or supplements is helpful to encourage consumption.

### 29. What can be done for patients who are not hungry?

For patients whose appetites are not ideal, the dietitian and interdisciplinary team should first investigate the causative factors, which may include limited food preferences, environmental factors, anorexic effects of medications, or physiological reasons, such as gastric reflux or slow gastric motility. It is important to identify these factors before proceeding with an intervention. In some cases, it is appropriate to recommend an appetite stimulant. Two currently available drugs are megestrol acetatae (Megace) and dronabinol (Marinol).

### 30. How is the nutrition plan altered for diabetic patients with a wound?

The nutrition plan, which must take into consideration the control of blood glucose levels, is based on the severity of the diabetes. Increases in caloric need should be addressed by adding protein to the diet on a moderate basis and monitoring renal function, which may be reduced in diabetic patients. Carbohydrate calories may result in hyperglycemia, which decreases immune response and delays wound healing.

**31. How is the nutrition plan altered for renal patients with a wound?**

The challenge with developing nutritional plans that address pressure ulcers and other wounds in renal patients is balancing the appropriate amount of protein so that the renal load is not increased. When protein intake is increased, it is important to monitor blood urea nitrogen and creatinine levels. Protein intake should be increased gradually in renal patients.

**32. How is the nutrition plan altered for cardiac patients with a wound?**

Cardiac patients with wounds should receive appropriate calories and protein but not at the expense of excessive sodium or fat.

**33. Is there a difference in treating patients in a hospital or nursing home or at their own home in regard to nutrition and wound healing?**

Each environment presents its own challenge. It is important to conduct a clinical evaluation of each patient, using previously discussed parameters, despite clinical location.

The **hospital environment** may present challenges based on the patient's clinical condition. Consideration of disease processes and acute responses are key to addressing nutritional needs. Conditions such as sepsis, surgery, burns, and trauma have significant impact on energy and protein needs in addition to requirements for wound healing. Long-term disease processes (e.g, diabetes, cardiac disease, renal dysfunction) require additional consideration as nutrition therapies are developed and administered.

In the **nursing home environment**, different challenges exist. Initially, one must consider the effects of aging and their manifestation as nutrition analysis is conducted. Historical information about weight and laboratory levels becomes more important for accurate evaluation of nutritional status. Nutrition intervention may present its own challenges in relationship to barriers to adequate intake (e.g,. polypharmacy, dysphagia or other oral problems, self-feeding deficits, chronic disease processes).

In the **home care environment**, extra emphasis should be placed on educating the patient about the importance of nutrition and the expectations of adequate intake. It also may be necessary to have the patient keep a food intake record for subsequent evaluation. Measures must be taken to ensure that the patient has access to the proper foods and is able to prepare the food.

**34. What is oxandrolone?**

Oxandrolone is an oral anabolic agent that has been documented to be useful in the repletion of lean body mass losses secondary to cachexia and wasting secondary to extensive surgery, chronic infections, or severe trauma. Studies correlating the closure of nonhealing wounds with repletion of LBM have demonstrated success, and additional studies of the appropriate use of oral oxandrolone for patients with pressure ulcers or other wounds and significant loss of LBM are under way.

## BIBLIOGRAPHY

1. American Healthcare Association: Resident Assessment Instrument for Long Term Care Facilities, Version 2.0. Washington, DC, American Healthcare Association, 1994.
2. Chang DW, Demling RH, DeSanti L: Anticatabolic and anabolic strategies in critical illness. Shock 10(3):155–160, 1998.
3. DeHoog S: In Mahan LK et al (eds): Krause's Food, Nutrition, and Diet Therapy, 9th ed. Philadelphia, W.B.Saunders., 1996, pp 361–386.
4. Demling RH, DeSanti L: Closure of the non-healing wound corresponds with correction of weight loss using the anabolic agent oxandrolone. J Ostomy/Wound Manage 44(10):58–68, 1998.
5. Demling RH, DeSanti L: The stress response to injury and infection: Role of nutritional support. Wounds 12:3–14, 2000.
6. Himes, DM: Protein calorie malnutrition and involuntary weight loss: The role of aggressive nutrition intervention in wound healing. J Ostomy/Wound Manage 45(3):46–54, 1999.
7. Himes DM: Nutrition supplements in the treatment of pressure ulcers: Practical perspectives. Adv Wound Care 10:30–31, 1997.
8. Kotler D: Dilemmas in the Treatment of Weight Loss. Iselin, NJ, BTG Pharmaceuticals, 1996.
9. U.S. Department of Health and Human Services: Agency for Health Care Policy and Research. Clinical Practice Guideline 15:27–30, 1994.
10. Whitney EN et al: Understanding Normal and Clinical Nutrition, 5th ed. Belmont, CA, Wadsworth Publishing, 1998.

# 9. ASSESSMENT OF PATIENT AND WOUND

*Tracy L. Houle,* APRN, MSN, CCCN, COCN

### 1. What are the components of wound assessment?

A complete wound assessment entails a full nursing assessment of the patient to evaluate the effect of the patient's clinical condition on the wound and its ability to heal. Additional components of wound assessment include:

- Determination of physical characteristics, including size and depth
- Presence of undermining, tunneling, sinus tracts, foreign bodies, and exposed or palpable bone
- Identification of anatomic landmarks, such as dermis, subcutaneous tissue, fascia, tendon, muscle or bone
- Tissue type noted in wound bed, such as granulation tissue, eschar, or slough
- Amount of drainage and characteristics of the exudate
- Skin around the wound

### 2. When looking at the patient, what assessment components should be performed?

Perform a thorough patient history. The nurse must evaluate each patient and his or her wound(s) by identifying:

- Cause of the wound, such as trauma, pressure, venous insufficiency, or diabetes
- Treatment history of wound to date
- Wound duration: acute (< 12 weeks old) or chronic (> 12 weeks old)
- Adequacy of oxygen saturation (use noninvasive testing, if available)
- Identification of systemic factors affecting wound healing: medications that affect healing (e.g., prednisone, tamoxifen, nonsteroidal anti-inflammatory drugs) and laboratory data (consider obtaining albumin, prealbumin, and complete blood count with differential. Calculate the total lymphocyte count.)
- Age
- Acute and chronic illnesses, multisystem failure: cardiac disease, peripheral vascular disease, respiratory compromise, severe anemia, diabetes, renal failure, sepsis, dehydration, nutritional compromise (see Chapter 8), pain (see Chapter 56)
- Environmental factors: The goal of tissue load management (distribution of pressure, friction, and shear on the tissue) is to create an environment that enhances soft tissue viability and promotes healing of the wound. Observe where the patient spends the day: in bed? in a chair? (see Chapter 53.) Does shearing occur during transfer from one surface to the next? Are the patient's shoes tight? Is the oxygen tubing loosely draped around the ears or anchored snugly like a child's cap? Play detective, and an environmental factor contributing to the wound may be readily found.
- History of travel or known epidemic exposure (helps to focus on fungal or parasitic causes)

Investigating and obtaining a good history help to identify the correct cause and facilitate management. Periodic assessment of patient factors keep you on the right track for wound healing.

### 3. What are the components of a psychosocial assessment of the patient with a wound?

All patients treated for a wound, as well as their caregivers, should undergo a psychosocial assessment to determine their ability and motivation to comprehend and adhere to the treatment regimen. The assessment should include, but need not be limited to, the following elements:

- Mental status
- Ability to learn, barriers to learning, learning styles
- Depression
- Social support
- Polypharmacy

- Alcohol/drug abuse
- Goals, values, and lifestyle
- Sexuality
- Culture and ethnicity
- Stressors

#### 4. When should wound assessment be performed?

Most regulatory agencies and facilities have set standards based on the setting. In general, all patients are assessed on admission.

In **acute care** settings, the patient should be assessed every shift for the presence of new wounds. A thorough assessment should be performed daily to every 3 days based on the cause of the wound and the patient's condition. For example, complete assessment would be done less often in a patient admitted with pneumonia and a stage 4 pressure ulcer that has been present on the trochanter for 2 years than in a patient admitted with necrotizing fasciitis.

In **long-term care** settings, in addition to weekly assessments, any change in the patient's condition warrants a complete reevaluation.

In the **home**, the patient is traditionally evaluated on a weekly basis. In other outpatient settings, such as physician offices, clinics, and wound care centers, in-depth assessments are performed at each visit.

In each of these settings, it is important to note that, although the documentation of the wound assessment is formally done at these times, it is prudent to evaluate the current clinical picture with chart documentation to see whether they are still the same! Remember that small changes in the wound should prompt early intervention to avoid or minimize wound deterioration.

#### 5. What is the first step in performing wound assessment?

Wound cleansing is an overlooked and underappreciated part of the assessment. The benefits of wound cleansing are well described in Chapter 11. In short, reduction of bioburden, assistance in removing nonviable tissue, and promotion of optimal chemical composition of wound fluid by reduction of metabolic waste are keys to success in wound healing.

#### 6. Name the "three rights" essential to optimal wound irrigation.

The right solution, the right pressure,and the right volume.

#### 7. What is the right solution for wound cleansing?

For acute wounds due to traumatic injury, an antiseptic solution with or without surfactant generally should be used. Such wounds may or may not contain visible oil, dirt, or grease. In nontraumatic wounds, chronic wounds, pressure ulcers, leg ulcers, and wounds in the proliferative stage of healing, avoid cytotoxic solutions. Normal saline is the agent of choice.

#### 8. What about the commercially available wound cleansers?

Carefully examine the ingredients of these solutions. Most are cytotoxic and must be diluted a minimum of 10 times to avoid injury to granulation tissue. If in doubt, ask the manufacturer for cytotoxicity data.

#### 9. What is the optimal pressure?

The literature demonstrates that optimal pressures range from 4 to 15 pounds per square inch (psi). Pressure < 4 psi does not remove material from the wound bed, whereas pressure > 15 psi may move surface bacteria into the wound tissue and possibly cause trauma.

#### 10. Which devices used for irrigation are in fact inadequate?

Bulb syringes deliver a pressure of only 2 psi. If you have decided to use a commercially available wound cleanser, check with the manufacturer to determine the psi delivered through the spray device on the bottle or can.

#### 11. What is the right volume to use for wound cleansing?

Some clinical judgement should be used. In general, the bigger the wound, the more volume is needed. For a surface wound smaller than 1.5 cm × 1.5 cm without depth, 60 ml of normal saline is usually sufficient. All other wounds, including those with depth, require a minimum of 100 ml of normal saline. In large wounds, 500 ml or more of normal saline may be used.

**12. After wound cleansing, what is the next step in wound assessment?**
     Determine location. The anatomic location of existing skin breakdown should be documented. Location of a wound is a key assessment finding, because it is often diagnostic of the cause. Consider a whole-body assessment, as lesions on the scalp or in the mouth are important findings that aid in diagnosis. Do not forget to look between toe web spaces; fissures resulting from athlete's foot (tinea pedis) are often the cause of lower extremity cellulitis.

**13. How is the wound measured?**
     The literature discusses many ways to measure wounds. In clinical research, planimetry, Jeltrate molds, and complex computer models using digital photography are used. At bedside, most clinicians simply measure wound dimensions with or without the use of simple tracings onto acetate film.

**14. What are the components of bedside measurement in clinical practice?**
     Size is determined by measuring length, width, and depth in centimeters (cm), followed by determining the presence of undermining or tunneling in the wound. Length and width should be measured as linear distances from wound edge to wound edge. Look at the wound as if it were the face of a clock. The top of the wound (12 o'clock) points toward the patient's head, whereas the bottom of the wound  6 o'clock) points toward the patient's feet. Therefore, length can be measured from "12 to 6," using the patient's head and feet as guides. Width can be measured from side to side, or from "3 to 9." Document the longest "12 to 6" and "3 to 9" measurements in the patient's record.
     This method is somewhat controversial, because irregularly shaped wounds located on the extremity are difficult to measure consistently due to clinician disparity in determining the 12 o'clock location. Using a wound sheet with an outline of the body and drawing the wound shape, in conjunction with acetate tracings or digital photography, can improve documentation and uniformity.

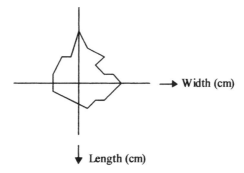

**15. How is wound depth best measured?**
     The depth of a wound can be described as the distance from the visible surface to the deepest area in the wound. If the depth varies, measure different areas of the wound bed to confirm the deepest. Insert a cotton tip applicator into the deepest portion of the wound that you can see. Grasp the applicator with the thumb and forefinger at the point corresponding to the wound's margin. Carefully withdraw the applicator while maintaining the position of the thumb and forefinger. Measure from the tip of the applicator to that position against a centimeter ruler. Record the depth in centimeters.

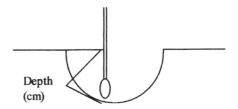

**16. What are tunneling and undermining?**

Tunneling is a course or pathway that can extend in any direction from the wound and results in dead space with potential for abscess formation. It is also called a sinus tract. Undermining is tissue destruction underlying intact skin along the wound margins.

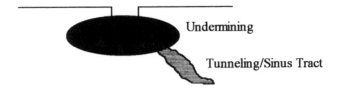

**17. How are undermining and tunneling best determined?**

Both the direction and the depth of tunneling and undermining should be documented using the face of the clock. With a cotton tip applicator, probe around the wound margins. Progressing in a clockwise direction, document the deepest sites where the wound undermines, using the clock-face method. Wound measuring sticks, specifically designed for this purpose. are commercially available. To measure the depth of tunneling, insert the applicator into the tunneling area. Grasp the applicator where it meets the wound edge. Pull the applicator out, place it next to a measuring guide, and document the measurement in centimeters. For example, the undermined sites in the wound below should be documented as "x" centimeters from 2–4 o'clock.

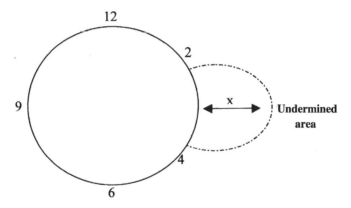

Tunneling in the figure below should be described as "x" centimeters at 9 o'clock.

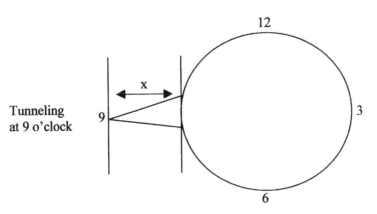

**18. After wound measurements are described, what is the next step in wound assessment?**

Describe the appearance of the wound. Examination of a wound includes determining wound bed color, tissue type and amount, characterization of the skin around the wound, and observation for the presence of objects in the wound. Assessment of surrounding skin is covered in Chapter 10.

**19. What colors can be seen in the wound bed?**

All colors of the rainbow have been described, but only certain colors are associated with good outcomes. Color is often lumped together with tissue type to best describe the wound. The color and tissue type of the wound should always be documented.

| COLOR | SIGNIFICANCE |
| --- | --- |
| Red | Healthy; good blood flow |
| Pale pink | Poor blood flow; ischemia; anemia |
| Purple | Engorged; edema; excessive bioburden; trauma |
| Black or brown | Nonviable tissue |
| Yellow | Nonviable tissue; also may indicate dermatitis |
| Gray | Nonviable tissue |
| Green | Infection; nonviable tissue |
| White | Ischemia; maceration; may be confused with bone or fascia |

**20. How is tissue type described?**

The four most common tissue types and their appearances are as follows:
• Granulation tissue: beefy red with a puffy or mounded appearance
• Clean wound base: pink or red with a smooth, flat appearance
• Slough: yellow, green, or gray nonviable tissue; may be wet and stringy
• Eschar: black, dry, nonviable tissue; usually with leather-like appearance

**21. Should the amount of tissue be quantified?**

Yes. Amount of each tissue type attached to the wound bed is assessed and documented. Using percentages, the amount of each tissue type and its location in the wound bed are described. The determination of success or failure of debridement can be facilitated with this method.

**22. What else should be assessed in the wound bed?**

The presence of foreign objects as well as the presence or absence of exposed or palpable bone should be determined. Assess the wound for foreign material such as sutures, staples, or environmental debris. If these are found or, even worse, left in the wound, delayed healing, abscess formation, and nonhealing sinus tracts can result. If foreign material is present, document the findings and make arrangements with the physician to determine the best method to remove it. Bone, when palpated in the wound bed just under tissue or when exposed and visible to the naked eye, correlates with a high probability of osteomyelitis (see Chapter 16).

**23. What about drainage?**

Determine amount, color, consistency, and odor of drainage.

**24. Is drainage amount a subjective measurement?**

Yes, unfortunately. Amount should be documented as light, moderate, or heavy. Some clinicians note the percentage of drainage on the removed dressing to quantify the amount. This technique can be used only if the same dressing in the same amount is applied with the same procedure. When using some wound-healing modalities, such as negative pressure therapy, wound drainage can be measured in a canister. Dressings can be weighed, but infection control issues, availability of equipment, and clinician technique confound results or make it impractical for the everyday clinician.

**25. What is an acceptable way to assess drainage?**

Do not assess drainage on the dressing that has been on the wound bed. One way to assess drainage is as follows:

1. Irrigate the wound.

2. Using fingers, palpate the wound periphery circumferentially, pushing fingers toward the wound edge. The drainage expressed into the wound bed is the amount to be assessed and documented.

Another way is to place a preweighed gauze pad in the wound and return in 1 hour to reweigh it. Although this technique gives a quantified amount, it is impractical for the bedside clinician. You know that drainage is heavy if the patient has a secondary dressing that is saturated in several hours or walks around with towels strapped to the wounds.

**26. How can drainage color and consistency best be described?**
- Serous: clear, watery plasma
- Sanguinous: bloody (fresh bleeding)
- Serosanguinous: plasma and red blood cells
- Purulent: thick, possibly with a yellow, green, or brown color

**27. Summarize the clinical significance of drainage color.**

| CHARACTERISTIC | SIGNIFICANCE |
| --- | --- |
| Serous | Seen in partial-thickness wounds and venous ulcerations. Moderate-to-heavy amounts may indicate heavy bioburden or chronicity due to subclinical inflammation. Serous drainage is normal in the acute inflammatory stage of wound healing but also can indicate seroma collection. |
| Sanguinous | Seen in deep partial-thickness wounds and full-thickness wounds during angio-genesis. Moderate-to-large amounts may represent heavy bioburden, chronic inflammation, or hematologic disorder (endogenous or drug-related). Small amounts of sanguinous drainage are normal in the acute inflammatory stage of wound healing. |
| Purulent | Never normal/ indicates acute or chronic infection. |

**28. Some wounds really smell. Is a "sniff test" helpful?**

The presence of necrotic material and external contaminants such as feces makes the wound odoriferous. Determine the presence of odor in wound after irrigation. A wound that still smells after irrigation is suspicious for the continued presence of necrotic material, infection, or a sinus tract to another body cavity (frequently the bowel). As in identifying *Clostridium difficile* colitis by smell, some clinicians can "smell" certain types of infection, such as methicillin-resistant *Staphylococcus aureus* (MRSA) or *Pseudomonas* spp. No literature evaluates the accuracy of clinician olfactory sense in the specific diagnosis of the offending organism. What a great research study for a graduate student!

Many occlusive dressings give off an odor when first removed, and many clinicians mistake the interaction between wound fluid and dressing as infection. If proper wound cleansing is performed before the "sniff test" is done, this problem is less likely.

**29. Is there a standardized framework for all of this information?**

Many agencies use a wound documentation flow sheet. This practice makes clinical sense because one can see whether the wound is deteriorating at a glance. Numerous flow sheets are available commercially, and some are offered by wound care companies without charge. The Agency for Health Research and Quality (AHRQ) has an example of the wound care flow sheet at its website (www.ahrq/clinic/cpgonline.htm) in the guideline section on pressure ulcer treatment.

The Wound, Ostomy, Continence Nurses Society also has published guidelines for the definition of a nonhealing, early partially granulating and fully granulating wound (available at www.wocn.org). This tool is extremely helpful for the OASIS data sheet required by federal agencies in the home health arena.

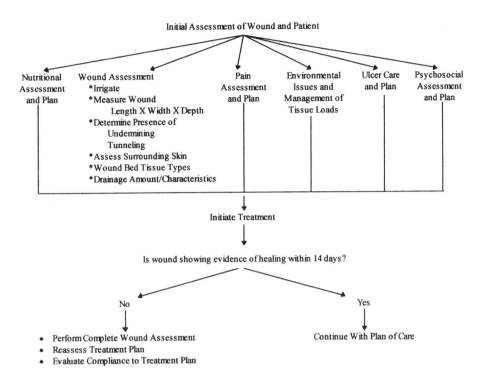

Algorithm for wound assessment. (© Connecticut Clinical Nursing Associates, LLC, 2001; used with permission.)

### 30. What about wound photos?

Photos are an adjunct for documentation in wound assessment. Following guidelines for health-care documentation and confidentiality, photographs of the wound, done in a serial fashion, can aid the clinician in looking at improvement or deterioration of the wound. Some cameras are available with a grid on the film to aid in measurements, but their accuracy is highly user-dependent. Clinicians should use a wound measurement guide or centimeter measuring tape next to the wound for size reference. A uniform procedure for placing the patient in the same position with the clinician at a uniform distance from the wound assists in getting the same angle and, hopefully, a similar picture for ongoing documentation. Digital photography has improved enough so that the average clinician with access to a personal computer can "shoot, store, and download" with ease.

A picture is worth a thousand words when coupled with a full assessment of the patient. Wound photographs can be used for case reviews, education, obtaining and maintaining services and reimbursement for patients, and legal purposes. Just be sure that a consent for photography is signed by the patient or significant other. In this document, which can be added to any general consent for treatment form, the intended use for the pictures should be clear and conform to the Health Insurance Portability and Accountability Act (HIPAA). Most agencies have access to a lawyer familiar with healthcare law, who can review a proposed photo consent form.

### 31. What about outcome measurements?

Wound outcomes are important to measure and flow naturally from individual wound and patient assessment factors into data management that, when used in a quality improvement program, can enhance patient outcomes. Various outcomes and tools are reported in the current literature. No one tool or outcome measurement is universal. Several of the tools in use are designed for specific types of wounds, such as pressure ulcers. Unfortunately, no predictive wound-healing scale is available with validated statistical significance that can be generalized to all types of wounds.

Traditional outcomes in wound management are measured in wound size, with success determined by complete wound closure. There is an increasing trend to quantify pain and functional outcomes along with standard tools. Visual analog scales for pain management and the SPF-36, a quality-of-life measurement, have been use with increasing frequency in conjunction with physical dimensions to monitor and report wound healing.

### 32. What are the more common wound-healing scales used?

Five wound-healing scales have been used: the Pressure Sore Status Tool (PSST), the Sessing Scale, the Pressure Ulcer Scale for Healing (PUSH), the Wound Healing Scale (WHS), and the Sussman Wound Healing Tool (SWHT). More are currently under development.

*Comparison of Wound-healing Tools*

| | |
|---|---|
| Physical characteristics | Included in all tools; but type of data collected varies. |
| Surrounding skin | Evaluated in PUSH, Sessing Scale, SWHT, but type of data documented varies; not evaluated in PUSH or WHS scale. |
| Host factors | Not consistently evaluated in any tool. |
| Identification of wound-healing | SWHT only. |
| Evaluation | Varies from Likert scale 0–5 in PSST; numerical value (0–6) in Sessing Scale, weighted scores in PUSH; letter modifiers to clarify subsections in WHS. SWHT delineates presence or absence of physical attributes of wound and measures healing by noting characteristics that are labeled "good" or "not good" for healing. |

### 33. Which tool is recommended?

No one tool is favored over the other. Much depends on the agency in which you work. Some institutions have developed their own tool. Some measure percent of healing, and in others third-party payors dictate what outcomes measures are collected. The important point is to determine what you want to accomplish and measure it. Analysis of data can be an important learning tool to improve your practice and the patient's overall status.

### BIBLIOGRAPHY

1. Agency for Health and Care Policy and Research: Treatment of Pressure Ulcers (AHCPR Publication No. 95-0652). Washington, DC, Agency for Health and Care Policy and Research, U.S. Dept. of Health and Human Services, 1994.
2. Bates-Jensen B: The pressure sore status tool: A few thousand assessments later. Adv Wound Care 10:78–80, 1997.
3. Ferrel B: The Sessing Scale for measurement of pressure ulcer healing. Adv Wound Care 10(5):78–80, 1997.
4. Sibbald R: An approach to leg and foot ulcers: A brief overview. Ostomy Wound Manage 44:28–35, 1998.
5. Sussman C, Bates-Jensen BM: Wound Care: A Collaborative Practice Manual for Physical Therapists and Nurses. Gaithersburg, MD, Aspen, 1998.
6. Valencia I, Falabella A, Kirsner R, Eaglstein W: Chronic venous insufficiency and venous leg ulceration. J Am Acad Dermatol 44:401–421, 2001.
7. Wills S: Ankle brachial index: Calculating your patient's vascular risk. Nursing 29(10):58–59, 1999.
8. Woodbury M, Houghton P, Campbell K, Keast D: Pressure ulcer assessment instruments: A critical appraisal. Ostomy Wound Manage 45(4):42–55, 1999.

# 10. ASSESSMENT OF PERIWOUND SKIN

*Deborah E. Ferretti, MS, RN, APRN, CS, CWOCN, and Shirley M. Harkins, RN, BS, CWOCN*

**1. What elements of the surrounding tissue can give information about the cause of the wound?**

The surrounding skin can reveal a great deal about the patient, including general health status, age, nutrition, and medications. In addition, it can validate or assist in the determination of cause of the wound and effects of treatment. The following pathologies have distinct periwound features.

**Venous stasis.** The surrounding skin has a ruddy-to-brawny discoloration because of hemosiderin deposits, which result from capillary leakage over time. The skin also demonstrates edema, unless concurrent arterial disease is present. The skin may be thickened and wrinkled from chronic edema. Severe cases have lipodermatosclerosis, which is due to hardening of the dermis and underlying subcutaneous fat and presents as a woody, hard texture. It is also common to see stasis dermatitis characterized by erythema, edema, scaling, and weeping of the lower leg. Another possible finding may be *atrophe blanche* areas of avascular, sclerotic white tissue from previous trauma.

**Arterial disease.** The surrounding skin is pale and cool because of reduced perfusion. Dependent rubor may be appreciable. Hair distribution is sparse or absent. Skin may be atrophic, taut, thin, dry, and shiny. Nails often have a thickened appearance.

**Infection.** Signs of infection include erythema, tenderness, heat, and swelling. Edges of erythema or skin discoloration may be diffuse and indistinct. One may see intense erythema or discoloration with well-demarcated and distinct borders. Streaking from the wound is also indicative of infection. The infected area is hotter to palpation than the unaffected skin nearby.

**Pressure.** External forces generate a variety of skin changes that are clinically important, including reactive hyperemia, blanch or nonblanch response, local edema, heat, induration, crepitus, and discoloration(blue, purple, or black). Redness of the surrounding skin may indicate unrelieved pressure. Irritation can result from exposure to feces or urine. In addition, a dermatitis-like reaction to traumatic removal of the dressing or tape may cause erythema.

**Peripheral neuropathy.** Neuropathy makes the skin insensate. The patient does not perceive touch. This condition can lead to edema, cellulitis, erythema, and possibly induration. When cellulitis is present, it may be accompanied by osteomyelitis. Peripheral neuropathy tends to induce callous formation, cracks, and fissures. Foot deformities, such as Charcot foot, may be present.

**Dermatologic disorders.** Changes in the skin may be observed: dryness, oiliness, pruritus, lesions, rashes, lumps, change in color or texture, and increased or decreased hair distribution. Lesion distribution, a clue to some disease processes, may be asymmetric or symmetric.

**2. What are the components of periwound assessment?**

Examination of the periwound skin is performed by inspection and palpation. Assess tissues within 4 cm of wound edges. The most important tools are your own eyes and powers of observation. As you inspect, palpate the skin for moisture, temperature, texture, turgor, and mobility. Assess color, induration, warmth, and edema of the skin around the wound. Note any areas of tense brawny edema, hyper- or hypopigmentation, and presence or absence of hair. Palpate pulses bilaterally on limbs. Pain also must be evaluated, including the wound and the surrounding tissue. The following are possible findings on exam.

**Erythema.** Redness can be noted from infection, irritation from drainage, exposure to urine or feces, or a dermatitis-like reaction to traumatic removal of the dressing or tape. Inflamed wounds usually present with well-defined borders. In dark-skinned persons, this may be seen as skin discoloration (e.g., purple or gray hue to the skin or a deepening of normal ethnic color). In infected wounds, edges of erythema or skin discoloration may be diffuse and indistinct. Infection also may present as intense erythema or discoloration with well-demarcated borders. Red stripes streaking superiorly or inferiorly from the wound area also may indicate infection. A halo of erythema around an arterial ulcer over the malleolus and pressure ulcers is frequently seen; however, the restriction of blood flow inhibits wound progression.

**Edema and induration.** Seen as slight swelling and firmness at the wound edge, these clinical findings may indicate infection if they are localized and accompanied by warmth. Induration is also an indication of deeper tissue damage. It is often present before deep tissue opens and can be fully assessed. Deep tissue damage sometimes takes many days to evolve fully because of tissue ischema and cell death. Such wounds look a lot worse before they improve. It is more useful to know that the problem is present than to think that the wound "got worse" despite good treatment. Aggressive interventions to reduce ischema and tissue edema are necessary, including maximal pressure reduction, optimal nutrition, pain management, and adequate hydration.

**Other skin color changes.** Inflammation produces a reddish skin tone, whereas pallor or bluish tones indicate poor vascularity. Brown staining around the gaiter area on the leg is indicative of venous disease. Darkly pigmented skin does not blanch, and, when inflamed, the area becomes darker and bluish or purple. Changes are often subtle, with shading slightly lighter or darker than the surrounding skin. Palpation is crucial to identifying changes in skin temperature and texture.

**Texture.** Is the skin dry or moist? Hyperkeratosis, seen as excessive dryness and scaling, is a chronic condition associated with venous disease. Weeping skin is often associated with an acute condition. A woody, hard feel indicates the presence of lipodermatosclerosis.

**Maceration.** Moisture from wound drainage, dressings, and urinary and fecal incontinence can cause maceration and overhydration of the epidermis. The skin tissue becomes less tolerant to pressure and shear forces. The involved areas may look white and wrinkled.

**Temperature.** Normal skin temperature may range from cool to warm. Skin temperature depends on the amount of vasoconstriction or vasodilation. Localized inflammation causes dilation of blood vessels and warmth. Vasoconstriction, with cool or cold skin, occurs as the body tries to conserve heat.

**Lesions or rashes.** Skin lesions are divided into two major categories: primary and secondary. Primary lesions are present at the initial onset of the problem. Secondary lesions result from changes over time due to disease progression, treatment, or manipulation via scratching, rubbing, or picking. Primary lesions such as bullae and pustules can develop into secondary lesions such as erosions and, ultimately, ulcers. Skin lesions should be described in terms of type, size, color, distribution, and configuration.

**Scar.** Scarring is formation of connective tissue that implies dermal damage. After injury or surgery, scars are initially thick and pink. Over time, they become white and atrophic. Scars are more susceptible to repeated injury.

**Wound edges.** Wound edges should be palpated for firmness and texture. This area may be attached to the wound bed or rolled downward into the wound. The wound edges may be diffuse, indistinct, or fibrotic.

**Ecchymosis.** Surrounding skin may be red to purple. Nonblanchable discoloration of variable size may be caused by vascular wall destruction, trauma, or vasculitis.

### 3. Describe findings that indicate the presence of cellulitis in the surrounding tissue.

Many methods to remember signs of infections are in use, but the clinician is cautioned that careful consideration of the patient's health status and illness is necessary. Many patients do not display typical indicators of infection, including those with diabetes, neutropenia, and arterial insufficiency. Many other processes and medications can interfere with the normal inflammatory response responsible for the signs and symptoms that we assess. The classic symptoms evaluated in surrounding tissue include:
- Induration on palpation of surrounding tissue
- Fever (tissue is hot compared with unaffected skin)
- Erythema extending beyond wound margins
- Edema of the surrounding tissue

4. **When is a dermatologic consultation indicated for a patient with a wound?**

Whenever rashes of an undetermined etiology are present, a dermatologist may help to diagnose and treat the area. In addition, if lesions are present, if the wound has an atypical appearance or location, or if the wound has not responded to treatment over time, a dermatologic consultation may be indicated. Various infectious or autoimmune processes may mimic or complicate the wound and surrounding skin. Cancers in the wound are one reason for chronic nonhealing and should be investigated. Descriptions of commonly encountered dermatologic conditions include:

**Pyoderma gangrenosum.** Ulcer borders are ragged, elevated, and dusky red or purple. A halo of edema spreads circumferentially at the advancing edge of the ulcer. The borders often are raised with undermining and boggy to palpation. Perforations may surround the primary lesion and drain pus.

**Fungating lesions for cancer.** Surrounding tissue is often red, edematous, and nodular to palpation. Areas of bogginess may also be palpable from trapped wound drainage.

**Squamous cell cancer in chronic wounds.** Erosions or growths may be indistinguishable from surrounding wound tissue.

**Vasculitis.** Palpable purpura in the skin may be associated with petechiae. Nodules and vesicles may be present. Vasculitis often follows a regional distribution. Purpura lesions do not blanch.

**Bullae** from conditions such as pemphigus. Surrounding skin may be erythematous or normal. Erosions and crusts from other lesions may be present.

**Calciphylaxis.** This finding often is associated with renal disease. Dusky, purple, and palpable nodules progress to necrosis and ulceration. Characteristics also include violaceous, mottled, reticulated patches and plaques with focal central necrosis.

**Herpetic ulcerations.** Discrete lesions on an erythematous base are the hallmark findings. Varicella is often described as "dewdrops on a rose pedal" to depict the erythematous appearance with a raised, central lesion.

**Psoriasis.** Hallmark findings are plaques with silvery, scaly appearance.

**Eczema.** Lichenified plaques, erosions, or excoriations may appear brown, black, or red, depending on natural skin pigmentation.

**Candidiasis.** Confluent and discrete, erythematous, and sometimes eroded areas with pustular and erythematous satellite lesions on the periphery of the rash.

5. **What impact can periwound assessment have on the wound treatment plan?**

Ongoing evaluation of the chosen treatment for the care of the surrounding skin should always be considered, because modifications may be needed if conditions change. If, despite appropriate treatment, the response is less than adequate, consider altering your treatment plan. Identification of dermatologic issues can save many lost days of treatment.

6. **What can be done to improve periwound skin alterations?**

**Macerated skin.** Change wound dressing to a more absorptive one, such as calcium alginates, foams, or absorptives. Topical skin protectants can be applied before dressings. Protecting the surrounding skin of a venous ulcer with a skin-barrier cream before application of a compression dressing can be quite beneficial.

**Skin stripping from tape injury.** Use of a skin protectant wipe helps to reduce epidermal injury. A thin hydrocolloid can be used to frame the wound, thus allowing dressings to be anchored to the surface of the barrier. Alternative securing devices can also be used, including wraps, Montgomery straps, mesh tubing, and cotton garments. Stretch cotton undergarments for holding dressings in place work well on the trunk, buttock, and leg areas. They are also comfortable for patients. This practice is particularly beneficial for patients who cannot tolerate the use of adhesives on their skin (e.g., tape allergy, epidermolysis bullosa).

**Erythema.** Identification of infection and initiation of treatment can greatly affect the success of wound intervention and shorten healing time. Persistent erythema of skin also may indicate the need to alter the plan of care for pressure relief and to provide a better pressure-relieving surface or increase the frequency of repositioning to prevent further damage.

**Callus.** Removal of the callus assists the ulcer in re-epithelializing the wound. Because callus build-up recurs rather quickly unless mechanical forces such as pressure and shear are completely eliminated, frequent paring of the callus is essential. Callus is frequently seen on plantar foot surfaces surrounding the wound.

**Evidence of vascular changes.** Venous changes may indicate the need for compression therapy to assist in edema management and wound closure. Arterial disease may need referral to a vascular surgeon for work-up and possible intervention for revascularization.

**Dryness.** The addition of a moisturizer to the skin helps to maintain skin health and prevent cracking and introduction of bacteria, which may lead to cellulitis.

## BIBLIOGRAPHY

1. Fitzpatrick TB, Johnson, RA, et al: Color Atlas and Synopsis of Clinical Dermatology: Common and Serious Diseases, 2nd ed. New York, McGraw-Hill, 1992.
2. Bryant R: Acute and Chronic Wounds: Nursing Management, 2nd ed. St. Louis, Mosby, 2000.
3. Sussman C, Jensen B: Wound Care: A Collaborative Practice Manual for Physical Therapists and Nurses. Gaithersburg, MD, Aspen, 1998.
4. Krasner D, et al: Chronic Wound Care: A Clinical Source Book for Healthcare Professionals, 3rd ed. Wayne, PA, HMP Communications, 2001.
5. Dealy C: The Care of Wounds. Cambridge, MA, Blackwell Scientific Publications, 1994.
6. Oh DH, et al: Five cases of calciphylaxis and a review of the literature. J Am Acad Dermatol 40:979–987, 1999.

# 11. WOUND CLEANSING

*Jane Ellen Barr, RN, MSN, CWOCN, ANP*

**1. What is wound cleansing?**
Wound cleansing, in its broadest definition is the process of mechanically breaking the bond between the tissue and bacteria, debris, contaminants, and inflammatory and necrotic tissue on the surface of the wound and then removing or flushing these materials from the wound surface. Defined in these terms, wound cleansing is interchangeable with mechanical debridement. In clean granular wounds, wound cleansing is the process of using fluids to gently flush or remove organic and inorganic debris and inflammatory material from the wound surface before the application of a dressing.

**2. What are the components of wound cleansing?**
Wound cleansing is achieved by using an appropriate cleansing solution in the proper amount and an adequate mechanical means of delivering the solution to the wound. The cleansing solution must be safe and effective. The volume of the solution must be adequate to properly cleanse the wound. Generally speaking, the larger the wound, the larger the volume of solution needed to remove debris, bacteria, or nonviable tissue. The mechanical force must be able to break the bond between the tissue and the bacteria, debris, and necrotic tissue on the surface of the wound and then flush it from the wound environment. Clinical research has shown that a mechanical force of 8–15 psi (pounds per square inch) is needed to cleanse wounds properly. Wounds in the proliferative phase of healing with a clean and granulating base should be cleansed more gently with a lower pressure stream so that fragile cells are not damaged.

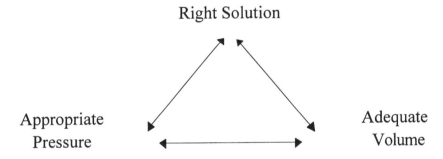

Components of wound cleansing. (From Milne C, Corbett L. Connecticut Clinical Nursing Associates, LLC, 1997; with permission.)

**3. What are the objectives of wound cleansing?**
The primary objectives of wound cleansing are as follows:
- Facilitate the process of phagocytosis by loosening, softening, and removing devitalized tissue, debris, contaminants, and toxic residue from the wound surface
- Separate eschar from fibrotic tissue and fibrotic tissue from granulation tissue
- Remove organic and inorganic debris and inflammatory material from the wound surface
- Reduce bacterial load of the wound surface and reduce incidence of wound infection and over-colonization
- Rehydrate the surface of a wound providing a moist environment
- Minimize wound trauma when removing adherent dressing materials
- Facilitate wound assessment by optimizing visualization of the wound surface

## 4. Can wound cleansing cause any negative effects on the wound healing process?

The benefits of obtaining a clean wound must be weighed against the potential trauma to viable tissue. Wound cleansing has the potential of causing either mechanical or chemical trauma to the wound bed. Mechanical trauma occurs when the mechanical forces used to cleanse the wound damage or injure viable tissue. Chemical trauma occurs when the fluids used to cleanse the wound damage or injure viable tissue or are toxic to the wound tissue.

## 5. What are the characteristics of an ideal wound cleansing solution?

- Nontoxic to viable tissues
- Effective in the presence of organic material such as blood, slough, or necrotic tissue
- Able to reduce the number of microorganisms from the surface of the wound
- Hypoallergenic and does not cause sensitivity reactions
- Readily available, cost-effective, and stable

## 6. What are the best cleansing solutions to use?

**Normal saline** or water is sufficient for cleansing the surface of most wounds. Normal saline, applied at room temperature, is the most common and cost-effective wound cleansing agent. It has no adverse effects on healing tissue. For home care, an acceptable saline solution can be made by adding two teaspoons of salt to 1 liter of boiling water or 8 teaspoons per gallon.

**Tap water** is an acceptable alternative in the home environment. Showering and bathing are becoming common practices for care of chronic wounds. During showering and bathing, wounds should not be allowed to soak for long periods. Open tissue has a tendency to absorb water. Water is hypotonic and causes cells within the tissues to swell and eventually rupture because of the effect of osmotic pressure. This process increases the amount of exudate produced over the next few days and often necessitates more frequent dressing changes.

**Commercial wound cleansers** can be used on wounds that require more aggressive cleansing. Commercial wound cleansers contain surface active agents (surfactants) that facilitate the removal of wound contaminants. The benefits of using surfactants for wound cleansing must be weighed against the cytotoxicity to viable tissue. Many surfactants have been shown to be toxic to cells. This toxicity delays wound healing by prolonging the inflammatory phase and inhibiting the wound's natural defenses against infection. Commercial skin cleansers should never be used on wounds. Skin cleansers are much more toxic than wound cleansers.

## 7. What mechanical forces can be used to cleanse a wound?

The most common mechanical forces used to cleanse a wound are scrubbing devices, irrigation methods, whirlpool therapy, and soaking. Several of these methods are discussed in the debridement chapters. Irrigation is the most common method used to deliver the solution to the wound surface. The clinician must choose how much mechanical force is to be used as well as the type and amount of solution based on the wound bed tissue type (clean and granulating or covered with necrotic tissue) and the presence or absence of infection. Necrotic and infected wounds should be cleansed with high-pressure irrigation (8–15 psi), whereas a low-pressure irrigation stream (< 8 psi; often as low as 1 psi) should be used to clean granulating wounds (see table below).

*Wound Cleansing Protocol*

| PHASE OF HEALING | WOUND ASSESSMENT FINDINGS | MECHANICAL FORCE | DELIVERY SYSTEM* |
|---|---|---|---|
| Inflammatory phase | Necrotic tissue, debris, contaminants, significant bacterial contamination or infection | High-pressure irrigation (8–15 psi) | 35-cc syringe and 19-gauge angio-catheter (8 psi) Irrijet DS Syringe with tip (Akrad Laboratories; 8 psi) Pulsatile irrigation (8–15 psi) Saline squeeze bottle (250 cc) with Baxter Tip (6 psi) |

*Table continued on following page*

### Wound Cleansing Protocol (Continued)

| PHASE OF HEALING | WOUND ASSESSMENT FINDINGS | MECHANICAL FORCE | DELIVERY SYSTEM* |
|---|---|---|---|
| Proliferative phase | Granulation tissue, epithelial tissue, wound care product residual on clean wound | Low-pressure irrigation | Pouring saline from bottle Piston syringe (4.2 psi) Bulb syringe (2.0 psi) |

• This is not an all-inclusive list of available delivery systems. Inclusion does not imply endorsement. Amount and type of fluid required depend on wound assessment findings.

**8. How often is wound cleansing done?**

At each dressing change.

**9. Is there any difference in the effect of wound cleansing on acute vs. chronic wounds?**

The efficacy of high-pressure irrigation in removing bacteria decreases with the age of the wound. For acute wounds, the majority of bacteria are surface contaminants. The number of bacteria on the surface of the wound is known as bioburden. If bacterial bioburden is not controlled, as is often the case in chronic wounds, the surface bacteria invade the tissue and cannot be removed without antibiotics or surgical debridement. The goal of cleansing is to keep the bioburden at an acceptable level and prevent tissue involvement.

**10. How does the temperature of the wound cleansing solution affect healing?**

The phagocytic and mitotic cellular activity within a wound is significantly decreased at temperatures below 28°C. The application of cool cleansing solutions can theoretically have similar local effects. It can take as long as 40 minutes for a wound to regain its original temperature after cleansing and up to 3 hours for mitotic division and leukocytic activity to return to normal. Cleansing solutions should be stored at room temperature. If cold, the solution should be warmed before application by immersion in warm water.

**11. What is the conflict in the use of antiseptics in wound cleansing?**

One of the objectives of wound cleansing is to remove bacterial contamination from the wound surface. The practice for many years in topical wound management has been to use antiseptics to prevent and treat infection. Over the past decade, especially since the publication of the *Clinical Practice Guidelines for Pressure Ulcers*, there has been a great debate about the clinical effectiveness and safety of topical antiseptics. The guidelines emphasize that no controlled studies have shown the effectiveness of antiseptics in decreasing the bacterial levels within chronic wound tissue. Numerous studies have documented the cytotoxicity of antiseptics to viable tissue. The management of bioburden and infection is discussed in other chapters. Wound cleansing should not be confused with treatment of infection. Wound cleansing is just what the name implies—cleansing!

**12. How does bacterial bioburden affect wound healing?**

Although it is known that all chronic wounds are contaminated with bacteria, the patient's natural defenses along with the standard wound management procedures of cleansing and debridement should be able to handle bioburden. Wounds that are covered with necrotic tissue and debris, especially moist necrotic tissue, are more likely to harbor high levels of bacteria. Debridement is the method of choice to decrease the bioburden of these wounds.

In immunocompromised patients, high levels of bacterial contamination may inhibit the healing process even in a granulating wound. The high level of bacteria in the wound competes with the healing cells for nutrients and oxygen. Bacteria prolong the inflammatory phase by producing inflammatory agents such as metabolic wastes, reactive enzymes, and toxins.

In addition to the level of bacterial contamination, the type of bacteria has an effect on wound healing. Nonhealing wounds, when cultured, often present with gram negative organisms such as *Proteus mirabilis, Pseudomonas aeruginosa, Escherichia coli,* and *Bacteroides* species. Studies showed that *Proteus* is probably the bacterial species that most inhibits wound healing. Nonhealing granulating wounds with a high bioburden can be identified by assessing the quality of their granulation tissue and healing outcomes. These wounds may present as:

- Granulating wounds that show no healing within 2–4 weeks, even though appropriate care has been implemented
- Granulating wounds that bleed easily, even though patient is not on anticoagulation therapy
- Granulation tissue that appears as exuberant or hypergranulated

**13. Discuss the optimal management of wound bioburden.**

When high levels of bacteria are suspected as the cause of nonhealing, culture and sensitivity testing should be done. If the wound is free of necrotic tissue and further debridement is not indicated, a regimen of topical antimicrobial agent should be considered. The agents of choice are topical antibiotics, not antiseptics. Antiseptics do not have selective antibacterial mechanism and on contact can damage viable cells. Antibiotics selectively kill bacteria. Systemically administered antibiotics should not be used topically to prevent the risk of developing increasing resistant strains of bacteria. The common topical antimicrobials used include mafenide acetate, metronidazole, mupirocin, nitrofurazone, Polysporin, silver sulfadiazine, nanocrystalline silver, cadexomer iodine, and ionic silver.

If considering the use of antiseptics, the clinician must take into account the cytotoxicity of the bacteria in relation to the cytotoxicity of the antiseptics. Because of the cytotoxicity of antiseptics, their use should be limited to specific clinical indications. There are several clinical situations in which the clinicians may consider using antiseptics. Dakin's solution is an antiseptic that, at the discretion of the clinician, can be used as a chemical method of debridement to dissolve the necrotic tissue in large contaminated wounds. The removal of necrotic tissue, not its antiseptic effects, is correlated with the reduction in wound bioburden.

Literature about hydrogen peroxide ($H_2O_2$) has been reviewed by the American Medical Association (AMA). The AMA concluded that $H_2O_2$ has little bactericidal effect, but its effervescence may provide some mechanical benefit in loosening necrotic tissue and debris. Its clinical use as an irrigant in close cavities is limited because it can cause air emboli and surgical emphysema.

Acetic acid (diluted vingear soak) is frequently used for topical treatment of pseudomonal infection, which is extremely sensitive to an acidic environment. Because *Pseudomonas* spp. often do not penetrate tissue deeply, topical management can be effective. In addition, because *Pseudomonas* spp. can develop antimicrobial resistance, acetic acid compresses for 15 minutes per day may be preferable to antibiotic therapy if the infection has not become systemic. Diluted vinegar soaks are also effective in odor control because of their antianaerobic activity. Acetic acid is also an effective management regimen for the palliation of distal gangrene in patients with marked vascular insufficiency who are not surgical candidates. Newer technologies to address safer ways of using antiseptics in chronic wound management to control bioburden are discussed in other chapters.

**14. What newer technologies allow safe and effective topical delivery of antimicrobials and antiseptics?**

One newer product used to decrease bacterial levels in a wound is **cadexomer iodine**. The iodine is trapped in a three-dimensional starch lattice within spherical microbeads. The cadexomer iodine is available at the concentration of 0.9% as a paste or ointment. One of the key properties of cadexomer iodine is its high absorption capacity. One gram of cadexomer iodine can absorb up to 7 ml of water or body fluid. As cadexomer iodine absorbs fluid, it slowly releases iodine. In clinical studies, cadexomer iodine was shown to be beneficial in controlling exudate, cleansing the wound, reducing bacterial levels, and improving healing. In this delivery method and at this concentration, iodine is not cytotoxic to granulation tissue, unlike its cousin povidone-iodine.

Another new technology has allowed for the **slow release of silver** from a wound care dressing. This silver functions as an antimicrobial barrier by preventing exogenous organisms from contaminating wounds. Silver is an excellent antimicrobial because it is nontoxic to viable tissue and does not develop bacterial resistance. Previously, delivery systems for silver were of limited usefulness in the clinical setting. For example, sulfur was proinflammatory, decreased bone marrow function, and damaged fibroblasts. Newer technology allows delivery of silver's antimicrobial properties to the wound without cytotoxicity to viable tissue.

## BIBLIOGRAPHY

1. Agency for Health Care Policy and Research: AHCPR Pressure Treatment Guideline Clinical Practice Guideline, No. 15. Rockville MD, U.S. Department of Health and Human Services, Public Health Service, AHCPR Publ. No. 95-0652, 1994.
2. Barr JF: Principles of wound cleansing. Ostomy Wound Manage 41(7A Suppl):15–21, 1995.
3. Barr JF, Van Rijswijk: Principles of Wound Cleansing: The Role of Therapy. Charleston, SC, Hill Rom, 1994.
4. Edlich RF, Rogers W, Kasper G, et al: Studies in the management of contaminated open wounds. I: Optimal time for closure of contaminated open wounds. II: Comparison of resistance to infection of open and closed wounds during healing. Am J Surg 117(3):323–329, 1969.
5. Flannagan M: Wound cleansing. In Morrison M, Moffatt C, Bridel-Nixon J, Bale S (eds): Nursing Management of Chronic Wounds. Philadelphia, Mosby, 1997, pp 87–101.
6. Hellewell TB, Majors DA, Foresman PA, Rodeheaver GT: A cytotoxicity evaluation of antimicrobial and non-antimicrobial wound cleansers. Wounds 9:15–19, 1997.
7. Lawrence JC: Wound irrigation, an update on irrigating fluids and their effect on wounds. J Wound Care 6:23, 1997.
8. Robson M, Edstrom LE, Krizek T, et al: The efficacy of systemic antibiotics in the treatment of granulating wounds. J Surg Res 16–229, 1997.
9. Robson M: Wound infection a failure of wound healing caused by an imbalance of bacteria. Surg Clin Noth Am 77:637, 1997.
10. Rodeheaver GT: Wound cleansing, wound irrigation, wound disinfection. In Krasner DL, Rodeheaver GT, Sibbold RG (eds): Chronic Wound Care: A Clinical Sources Book for Healthcare Professionals, 3rd ed. Wayne, PA, HMP Communications, 2001, pp 369–381.
11. Schultz G: Molecular regulation of the wound healing. In Bryant RA (ED): Acute and Chronic Wounds: Nursing Management, 2nd ed. St. Louis, Mosby, 2000, p 413.
12. Stotts A, Whitney J: Identifying and evaluating wound infection. Home Healthcare Nurse 17(3):159–164, 1999.

# 12. AUTOLYTIC, MECHANICAL, CHEMICAL, AND SHARP DEBRIDEMENT

*Jane Ellen Barr, RN, MSN, CWOCN, ANP*

## 1. What is debridement?

Debridement is a naturally occurring event in the wound-healing process. During the inflammatory phase of healing, neutrophils and macrophages digest and remove devitalized tissue, cellular debris, blood coagulum, cross-contaminants, and toxic residue from the wound. In chronic wounds, there is often an accumulation of a significant amount of damaged tissue. This natural debridement process becomes overwhelmed and insufficient. The build-up of necrotic tissue places considerable phagocytic demand on the wound. For the wound to progress in a timely fashion through the normal phases of healing, the natural debridement process needs to be augmented by topical management techniques. In wound management, debridement is the process by which the clinician facilitates the natural debridement process by implementing measures to remove the nonviable tissue and foreign matter from the wound surface.

## 2. Why is debridement beneficial?

Debridement of necrotic material is beneficial from both a physiologic and mechanical standpoint. Necrotic tissue or foreign matter in the wound provides a medium for bacterial growth. Colonization of $10^5$ organisms per gram of tissue by pathogenic bacteria results in delayed wound healing. Bacterial contamination results in protease production, which impairs the host response and makes the patient more susceptible to infection. Bacterial contamination and infection can actually increase tissue destruction, which increases the severity of the wound. Removing necrotic tissue and foreign matter by debridement reduces bioburden and wound infection, especially in the deteriorating wound. At the cellular level, debridement interrupts the cycle of the chronic wound so that protease and cytokine levels more closely approximate those of the acute wound to promote wound healing in a timely and organized fashion.

Necrotic tissue and debris serve as a mechanical barrier that prevents granulation tissue formation, wound contraction, and re-epithelialization. Debridement is necessary to remove this mechanical barrier so that the wound can progress through the natural phases of healing.

Debridement facilitates visualization of the wound base, promoting a more accurate and thorough assessment of viable tissue. Once the base of the wound is free of necrotic tissue, moist interactive wound healing can begin with a variety of topical treatments.

## 3. How does necrotic tissue present in the wound bed?

When tissue has been injured, an ischemic process occurs. In a sense, at this time the tissue can be considered to be in the "dying phase." During the ischemic process the tissue begins to change in color and consistency. Depending on the depth of injury, tissue can present in various forms: non-blanchable erythema, pallor, or ecchymosis. In patients with melanin-rich pigmentation, it begins as a darkened area or a change in pigmentation or hue. The consistency of the tissue during this ischemic phase also changes; the tissue feels "woody" to touch, hardened, and indurated. At this time the injured area needs to be monitored for further changes in tissue type as a result of avascularization.

As tissue dies, it changes in color, consistency, and adherence to the wound bed. The clinician may not initially be able to assess the extent of tissue damage but, by using assessment skills of visualization and palpation, often can determine whether the injury is superficial or extends to subcutaneous tissue, muscles, tendons, ligaments, or bone. The death of tissue often suggests the presence of a full-thickness injury. The necrotic tissue that forms is called either eschar or slough.

**4. What is eschar?**

Eschar is dry, desiccated, necrotic tissue. It has a firm, dry, leathery, black or gray appearance. It may be firmly attached to the wound base and edges. During the debridement process, eschar begins to soften as it becomes hydrated. It separates first from the wound edges and eventually from the base of the wound. Once the eschar is removed, slough is often visible covering the wound bed.

**5. What is slough?**

Slough is hydrated necrotic tissue. As the eschar is moistened or hydrated, the devitalized tissue becomes soft and may be brown, gray, yellow, or tan. Often a percentage of avascularized tissue may remain hydrated beneath the upper layers of eschar. If the black eschar is surgically removed, the base of the wound often presents as moistened necrotic tissue. The consistency of slough is often described as thin, fibrinous, stringy, or mucinous. Slough may be adherent or loosely adherent to the wound edges and base. Components of this material include fibrin, bacteria, intact leukocytes, cell debris, serous exudate, and significant quantities of deoxyribonucleic acid (DNA). If slough is continuously exposed to air, it may dehydrate and return to the hard, leathery state of eschar.

**6. List other names for slough and eschar.**

Nonviable tissue, devitalized tissue, and necrotic material. What is dead is dead, no matter the name.

**7. When is debridement indicated or contraindicated?**

Debridement is indicated for any acute or chronic wound when necrotic tissue, foreign bodies, or infection is present and the goal for treatment is to heal the injured tissue and/or to control infection. Once the wound bed is clean and viable tissue present, debridement is no longer indicated.

Wound debridement in a clinical setting may be delayed based on the judgment of the clinician. For example, with a noninfected, necrotic wound in a critically ill, unstable, or severely immunocompromised patient, it may be prudent to delay the debridement process until the patient's condition improves. Dry, desiccated eschar is not a medium for bacterial growth. As the eschar is hydrated, softens, and becomes moist slough, bacteria can proliferate and overwhelm the patient's immune system. Postponement of debridement in such situations can help reduce the likelihood of infection.

When eschar covers a stable, noninfected wound on an ischemic extremity or a pressure ulcer located on the heel, debridement is contraindicated until an overall plan of management in terms of revascularization has been decided. Any ischemic wounds of the lower extremities should not be debrided unless the clinician is certain of collateral circulation by vascular studies or the presence of an adequate ankle brachial index (see Chapters 37–39 for more detail). Ischemic wounds of the lower extremity or pressure ulcers on heels that are covered with black, hard eschar and left intact should be inspected daily for signs and symptoms of infection. Infection presents locally with periwound erythema, tenderness or pain, and elevated temperature. An infected wound often has an increased amount of exudate or purulent exudate. The ischemic or necrotic area may have a boggy or mushy consistency. Infection requires reevaluation of the plan of care, and debridement is indicated.

When blood supply to a wounded area covered with eschar is compromised, the most appropriate management often consists of painting the eschar with povidone-iodine to reduce bacterial bioburden on its surface and applying a dry, sterile dressing.

**8. How are methods of debridement classified?**

Debridement is described by physiologic and methodologic mechanisms. **Physiologic methods** are classified as selective or nonselective. Selective debridement removes only nonviable tissue from the wound, whereas nonselective debridement indiscriminately removes both viable and nonviable tissue.

**Methodologic debridement** is based on the actual mechanism of action (autolysis, chemical, mechanical, or sharp). Sharp debridement can be subdivided into surgical or conservative categories. The sharp, autolytic, and chemical methods are considered selective forms of debridement. Necrotic tissue is removed selectively by the clinician using surgical instruments, or the necrotic tissue is digested by exogenous or endogenous proteases in the wound. Chemical debridement with hypochlorite (Dakin's) solution and mechanical debridement methods are nonselective.

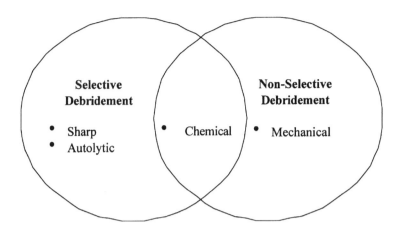

Methods of debridement.

**9. Can you combine debridement methods or must you only use one type at a time?**

Although one method of debridement may be the primary approach, debridement typically combines a variety of methods. For example, the surgeon may surgically debride the wound and remove black eschar. After surgical debridement it is not unusual for the wound base to be covered with slough. Further debridement may be accomplished mechanically via high-pressure irrigation or pulsatile lavage, chemically through the application of enzymes, or autolytically by moisture retentive dressings.

**10. How does one decide which method of debridement is best suited for an individual patient?**

An individual approach is required in selecting the proper debridement method. Clinicians must assess treatment goals, patient status or comorbidities, wound characteristics, and their own clinical experience and competence. Factors to consider include the following:
- Presence of infection or advancing cellulitis often dictates the need for surgical debridement.
- Cause of the wound. Diabetic foot ulcers often require early surgical excision of nonviable tissue because of the increased risk of infection in diabetic patients.
- Size of the wound and amount of necrotic tissue. Surgical debridement remains the quickest method of removing large amounts of devitalized tissue. Autolytic, enzymatic, and mechanical debridement are most effective for wounds with small-to-moderate amounts of necrotic tissue.
- Type of tissue exposure. When tendons and ligaments are exposed, autolysis with moisture retentive dressings prevent desiccation of vital tissue and provide a nontraumatic form of debridement.
- Availability of resources. Access to different methods of debridement, time availability, cost-effectiveness, patient comorbidities, and potential for and ability to treat complications in the healthcare setting in which the debridement will take place influence the choice of method.
- Care setting: hospital, long-term care, home care, or office/clinic.

**11. How does the clinician monitor and evaluate the effects of debridement?**

Several clinical outcomes can be used to assess the effectiveness of the debridement process:
- Transition in the type of necrotic tissue in the wound base. The wound should progress from black (dry eschar becomes hydrated, moist, softened, and soggy eschar) to yellow (slough changes from fibrinous or stringy to mucinous) to red (granulation and re-epithelialization).
- Decrease in the adherence of necrotic tissue to the wound base and edge. Progress from the adherence of the necrotic tissue of the wound should proceed as follows: firmly attached to the edge and base of the wound → lifts or loosens from the edge of the wound → separates from the granulation tissue at the base of the wound.

- Decrease in the amount of erythema, induration, heat, pain, or tenderness in the periwound area of an infected wound.
- Decrease in the amount of drainage as necrotic tissue is removed.

## AUTOLYTIC DEBRIDEMENT

**12. Define autolytic debridement.**

The process of autolysis is a natural physiologic process. Autolytic debridement uses the body's own white blood cells and proteolytic, fibrinolytic, and collagenolytic enzymes to soften and break down necrotic tissue. It is a selective form of debridement that results in natural degradation of devitalized tissue. The body's white blood cells and enzymes enter the wound site during the inflammatory phase of healing and liquefy the necrotic tissue. With autolytic debridement, adequate cleansing is essential to flush the wound of degraded tissue and toxic materials.

**13. When is autolytic debridement indicated?**

Autolysis as the primary method of debridement is recommended for the noninfected wound with a minimal-to-moderate amount of necrotic tissue. It is generally considered a slow process of debridement. The time frame for effective autolytic debridement varies with the size of the wound as well as the amount and type of necrotic tissue. Autolysis should demonstrate effective clinical outcomes within 72–96 hours after treatment is initiated, although complete debridement may take considerably longer.

**14. What are the primary requirements for effective autolytic debridement?**

The primary requirements are the presence of a moist wound environment, adequate neutrophil count, and intact leukocyte function. Autolysis is enhanced and supported by the proper use of moisture-retentive dressings that must be allowed to remain intact and undisturbed for a reasonable length of time. By maintaining a moist environment, the neutrophils and macrophages essential for phagocytosis remain intact and are not prematurely destroyed by improper wound care practices or desiccation of the wound.

**15. What are the advantages of autolytic debridement?**

Autolysis is a painless method of debridement that is easy to perform and requires minimal technical skills. It is a selective, noninvasive form of debridement that does not disrupt healthy tissue. Autolysis maintains a moist wound environment that facilitates granulation tissue formation and re-epithelialization while preventing ambient air exposure that would desiccate the wound surface. It is an excellent adjunctive form of debridement when other primary methods are used. Autolysis is often used in combination with high-pressure irrigation, sharp surgical, or sharp conservative debridement.

**16. Discuss the necessary precautions when autolysis is used to debride a wound.**

1. The amount of wound fluid and odor often increases under moisture-retentive dressings during the autolytic process. As a result, dressings may have to be changed more frequently. There is a potential risk for periwound skin maceration. Liquid skin barriers, solid skin barriers, barrier ointments, or pastes should be applied to the periwound skin prophylactically in moderately-to-highly exudative wounds when autolysis is used.

2. Autolysis can be an extremely slow method of debridement and is not the method of choice in the presence of infection or advancing cellulitis. In the presence of infection the goal is always to debride the wound as quickly as possible. Most infections in chronic wounds are due to polymicroorganisms, including some anaerobic bacteria. Dressings that maintain a moist environment create a layer of fluid between the base of the wound and the dressing and provide varying degrees of occlusiveness that may promote further growth of the anaerobic bacteria. At the discretion of the clinician, autolysis may be used if there is no sign of systemic or local clinical infection and the patient has been treated with appropriate antibiotics.

3. Immunocompromised patients do not meet the requirement for autolytic debridement because they lack adequate neutrophil count and leukocyte function. A patient who is neutropenic is at

risk for infection and sepsis. When occlusive dressings for debridement are used, there is an increased risk of bacterial overgrowth under the dressings. In neutropenic patients, in whom the number of viable neutrophils available in the wound fluid may be diminished, even the slightest increase in the number of bacteria at the wound site can overwhelm the immune system.

### 17. What dressings are most often used to promote the process of autolytic debridement?

Autolytic debridement is often facilitated by the use of semiocclusive dressings. Dressings support autolysis if they add or maintain moisture at the wound surface. The specific type of dressing selected for wound management is based on tissue type in the wound bed, depth of the wound, amount of exudate, and the patient's general condition. When the wound base is dry, dressings that add moisture, such as hydrogels, or that may trap enzyme-rich wound exudate at the wound site, such as thin films, are used. When moisture-retentive dressings are used for the management of hard, dry, black eschar, cross-hatching of the eschar is recommended to expedite the autolytic process. If the wound has mild-to-moderate amounts of exudate, a hydrocolloid is often an appropriate dressing of choice. Wounds with moderate-to-heavy drainage require dressings that provide maximal absorption, such as hydrofibers, hydropolymers, alginates, and foams.

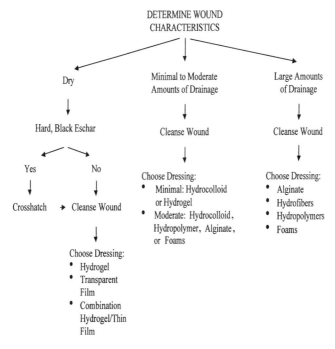

Autolytic debridment using moisture-retentive dressings.

### 18. What is cross-hatching?

Cross-hatching is the procedure of increasing the surface area of necrotic tissue to allow more moisture contact. This technique speeds the autolytic process. It is accomplished with a scalpel. The area of hard black eschar is incised slightly in a criss-cross pattern.

### 19. Is a wound at greater risk for infection when moisture-retentive dressings are used to facilitate autolysis?

Autolytic debridement, when used properly and for the appropriate patient, does not promote an environment that places the patient at greater risk for wound infection. Wounds treated with semi-occlusive or occlusive dressings are less likely to become infected than wounds treated with conventional gauze dressings. Semiocclusive and occlusive dressings are impermeable to exogenous bacteria, create an environment in which the neutrophils in the wound fluid remain viable, inhibit bacterial growth, and decrease the amount of necrotic tissue, which is the medium for bacterial proliferation.

## MECHANICAL DEBRIDEMENT

**20. Define mechanical debridement.**

Mechanical debridement is achieved by applying an external force that is great enough to separate or break the adhesive forces between the necrotic tissue and the base of the wound. Mechanical methods of debridement include wound scrubbing, wet-to-dry dressings, and varied forms of hydrotherapy, such as high-pressure irrigation, whirlpool therapy, and pulsatile lavage. Mechanical forms of debridement are nonselective. Therefore, they are best used on wounds with moderate-to-large amounts of necrotic tissue or debris. As granulation tissue becomes more prevalent, a more selective method of debridement is required to prevent injury to viable tissue.

**21. How does wound scrubbing mechanically debride a wound?**

Wound scrubbing mechanically dislodges loosely adherent slough and surface debris from a wound. The wound should be scrubbed using circular motions from the center of the wound outward to the wound margins for minimum of 2–3 minutes. Wound scrubbing is a nonselective form of debridement and thus should be used on wounds with moderate-to-large amounts of necrotic tissue. Try to avoid healthy granulation areas as much as possible, because scrubbing is harmful to viable tissue.

**22. What principles should be followed for mechanical debridement of the wound bed by scrubbing?**

1. The wound must be properly irrigated after scrubbing to remove the dislodged devitalized tissue, particles, and bacteria from the wound surface.

2. Scrubbing increases the risk for mechanical trauma to the wound surface. To minimize this risk, the scrubbing should be done gently with devices that are soft and nonabrasive.

3. Scrubbing should be used only on wounds with a large percent of loose necrotic tissue.

4. The most common scrubbing devices are gauzes and sponges designed specifically for wound cleansing.

5. Use only nonwoven gauze, which is less likely to leave fine, fibrous particles on the wound surface that may result in a prolonged inflammatory phase of healing.

6. Surfactants are the solution of choice when a wound is mechanically cleansed by scrubbing. Properties of surfactants reduce the coefficient of friction between the scrubbing device and the wound tissue.

**23. When are wet-to-dry dressings an appropriate form of mechanical debridement?**

Wet-to-dry dressings are a nonselective mechanical method of debridement. They are most appropriate for wounds covered with a large amount of moistened necrotic tissue, such as fibrin slough. It is not effective on dry, black eschar. Once more than 50% of the wound bed is covered with granulation tissue, wet-to-dry dressings are no longer appropriate because they can destroy viable tissue.

**24. How does the clinician appropriately apply a wet-to-dry dressing?**

A wet-to-dry dressing consists of applying saline-moistened gauze to the wound bed and allowing it to dry, trapping the necrotic tissue and debris. The process is continued until viable tissue is apparent; it may take several days to weeks. For wet-to-dry dressings to work effectively, the clinician must follow the following guidelines:

1. Premedicate the patient with analgesia before the dressing change, which can be a painful experience.

2. Irrigate the wound with high-pressure irrigation and an adequate amount of solution. This technique hydrates the necrotic tissue and allows it to be easily trapped in the gauze dressing.

3. Use an appropriate type of dressing material. The gauze for wet-to-dry dressings needs to be an open-weave cotton fabric that provides a combination of mildly abrasive qualities with adherent properties. Nonwoven gauze is not as effective because the fiber composition does not allow tissue adherence.

4. The gauze needs to be moistened—not wet—and allowed to dry thoroughly between dressing changes. Once dry, usually 4–6 hours after application, the dressing is pulled off the wound along with the necrotic tissue and debris that have become trapped in the open holes of the gauze.

5. The gauze used as the primary dressing, which touches the wound surfaces, must be opened so that the small holes in the gauze come into direct contact with the necrotic tissue at the base of the wound. This approach allows the hydrated necrotic tissue and debris to be trapped in the gauze dressing as it dries. After the initial contact layer is applied to the base of the wound, the remaining depth of the wound can be filled with moist, fluffed gauze.

6. An appropriate secondary dressing should be applied.

7. Dressings should be changed every 4–6 hours.

### 25. What methods of irrigation are considered mechanical forms of debridement?

Irrigation with pressurized fluids is another method of mechanically removing debris, necrotic tissue, and bacteria from the wound surface. For wound irrigation to be effective, the hydraulic force generated by the stream of fluid has to be greater than the adhesive forces holding the debris or necrotic tissue to the wound surface. Two common types of wound irrigation are used for debridement: high-pressure irrigation and pulsatile high-pressure lavage (see Chapters 13 and 14).

### 26. What are the benefits of using high-pressure irrigation or pulsatile lavage as a mechanical action to deliver the cleansing solution to the wound?

- Assists the process of phagocytosis by loosening, softening, and removing devitalized tissue and debris, blood coagulum, gross contaminants, and toxic reside from the surface of the wound.
- Promotes the separation of eschar from fibrotic tissue and fibrotic tissue from granulation tissue.
- Reduces the bacterial load of the wound surface and the incidence of infection.

### 27. What is considered high-pressure irrigation?

Irrigation of a wound with fluid delivered at a pressure of 8–15 psi is considered high-pressure irrigation. This amount of pressure provides adequate force to remove debris without damaging healthy tissue or inoculating the underlying tissue with bacteria. Pressures below 8 psi are considered low-pressure irrigation, such as that provided with bulb syringe or piston syringe. Low-pressure irrigation is not effective in removing necrotic tissue from the wound base.

### 28. How can a force of 8–15 psi be attained for irrigating a wound?

Research has shown that a force of 8 psi can be attained by delivering the fluid from a 35-ml syringe and an 18- or 19-gauge needle or angiocatheter. Angiocatheters are safer than needles because of the hazard of accidental needlesticks. If catheters and syringes of other sizes are used, it is important to remember that as the size of the syringe increases, the pressure decreases because the force applied to the plunger is distributed over a larger cross-sectional area. Other devices developed to irrigate wound with varying degrees of high pressure include products that attach to saline bags so that a continuous flow of irrigation solution can be delivered to the wound at a consistent high-pressure stream. Prepackaged canisters of pressurized saline and tips attached to 250-cc bottles of irrigant also are available commercially. Normal saline is the recommended irrigant.

### 29. What precautions related to high-pressure irrigation need to be addressed?

Although the mechanical action of wound irrigation must be sufficient to remove debris and necrotic tissue, it should not traumatize the healing tissue. Pressures above 25 psi are unnecessarily high. Ideal pressures are between 8 and 15 psi.

Health care professionals should adhere to universal precautions while irrigating wounds with high pressure, including the use of protective eye wear, face shields, gloves, and water-resistant gowns. Commonly used high-pressure irrigation methods result in the splatter of blood and body fluids. The use of splash shields on irrigation equipment has been shown to reduce splatter significantly. If mist is expected (e.g., with pulsatile lavage), treatment should be delivered in an enclosed area separated from other patients to avoid cross-contamination.

## CHEMICAL DEBRIDEMENT

**30. Define chemical debridement.**
Chemical methods of debridement remove necrotic tissue or debris from the wound base through a chemical process. They may be a selective or nonselective form of debridement, depending on the chemical used. Wounds can be debrided chemically with the use of enzymes, sodium hypochlorite (Dakin's solution), maggots, or hypertonic saline.

*Chemical Debriders*

| DEBRIDER | MANUFACTURER | ACTIVE AGENT | FREQUENCY |
| --- | --- | --- | --- |
| Accuzyme | Healthpoint | Papain/urea | Once daily |
| Panafil | Healthpoint | Papain/urea–chlorophyllin Copper–sodium complex | Once daily |
| Ethezyme Ethezyme 830 | Ethex | Papain/urea | Once daily |
| Mesalt | Molnlycke Health care | Hypertonic saline | Once or twice daily |
| Curasalt | Kendall | | |
| Hypergel | Molnlycke Health Care | | |
| Santyl | Smith and Nephew | Collagenase | Once daily |

From Corbett L, Milne C, Houle T. 2001; with permission.

**31. How are enzymes used to debride the wound?**
Enzymatic debridement, a selective form, is achieved by applying exogenous enzymes to devitalized tissue on the wound surface. Enzymes are selective for eschar, protein, and nucleic acids. They cause minimal damage to healthy tissue when applied properly. The enzymes work in one of two ways:
1. Papain/urea agents directly digest the components of slough, fibrin, bacteria, leukocytes, cell debris, serous exudate, and DNA.
2. Collagenase agents dissolve the collagen that attaches the avascular tissue to the wound surface.

 Enzymes debride slowly, depending on the size of the wound and amount of necrotic tissue. They may take 14–30 days or longer to clean the wound. Enzymatic debridement may be combined with other methods, such as sharp debridement and high-pressure irrigation. Enzymatic debridement should be stopped when the wound is clean. Although enzymes do not damage viable tissue, more appropriate and cost-effective dressings are available for the clean granulating wound.

**32. When are enzymatic debridement agents indicated?**
Enzymatic debriding agents are indicated for wounds with small-to-moderate amounts of necrotic tissue and debris and wounds prone to eschar formation, such as burns and friction-type injuries. Because of its ease of use, enzymatic debridement is well suited to settings in which sharp debridement is not readily available.

**33. How often do enzymes need to be applied to the wound?**
Enzymatic debridement agents usually require application once or twice daily depending on the type of enzyme used. The product insert is a valuable guide for safe use.

### 34. What secondary dressings should be used with enzymes?

Most dressings can be used safely with enzymes, including gauze, hydrogels, absorptive dressings, and transparent films. Manufacturer guidelines should be followed carefully because enzymes require specific conditions to be effective. For example, papain/urea products work best in a moist environment, whereas a dry, sterile dressing should be used with collagenase. Because enzymes are typically applied once or twice daily, dressings that are intended to remain in place for several days are not cost-effective in combination with enzymes.

### 35. What specific conditions are required for enzymes to be most effective?

The heavy metals that are found in many wound cleansers and other topical wound products inactivate the enzymes. The most common heavy metals used in wound care products include silver and zinc. Enzymes also require a specific pH range to be effective. Collagenase works best at a physiologic pH range of 6–8 to dissolve and liquefy necrotic wound debris, whereas papain/urea agents work well in a broader pH range of 4–12.

Acidic solutions that alter the pH inactivate some enzymes. Enzymatic ointments are not active in a dry environment. Papain/urea-based products function best in a moist environment and require a slightly moist saline gauze or a hydrogel dressing. Enzymes are more effective when used on eschar if the dry, black eschar is cross-hatched with a scalpel before the enzyme is applied.

### 36. What important factors should be considered when enzymatic debridement is used?

- Enzymatic agents are available by prescription only.
- Enzymatic debridement agents can be used alone or in combination with other debridement methods.
- Clinicians should always refer to the package insert or *Physicians' Desk Reference* for specific recommendations related to the different types of enzymes available for debridement.
- In the presence of hard, dry eschar, cross-hatching allows the enzyme to penetrate to the softer tissues of the wound and to act more effectively.
- Enzymatic agents do not cause injury to healthy granulation tissue.
- Enzymatic agents may cause a local dermatitis as the result of inflammation due to pH differences with surrounding skin. The dermatitis is evidenced by pain, erythema, or rash. If it occurs, the enzymes should be discontinued.

### 37. How does Dakin's solution work as a chemical debriding agent?

Dakin's solution (diluted sodium hypochlorite solution) is a nonselective form of chemical debridement that denatures the protein of the necrotic tissue, promoting its removal from the wound surface. Dakin's solution also exerts an antimicrobial effect and controls wound odor.

### 38. When is Dakin's solution indicated as a chemical debriding agent?

Dakin's solution is used most appropriately when there is a large amount of necrotic tissue on the wound surface, the wound is infected or malodorous, and surgical debridement is contraindicated. Because of its cytotoxic properties, it can damage healthy granulation tissue. Therefore, Dakin's solution should be used as a debridement agent only on wounds covered with more than 50% necrotic tissue. It should be considered a short-term treatment (5–7 days). Once infection and odor are under control, another method should be selected to complete the debridement process.

### 39. How is Dakin's applied to the wound when it is used as a chemical debriding agent?

Dakin's solution is applied by saturating gauze with the solution, lightly packing it into the wound, and applying a gauze or pad secondary dressing. It is changed 2 or 3 times daily, depending on the size of the wound and the amount and type of exudate. Periwound skin protection should be provided with a barrier ointment, liquid skin barrier, or solid skin barrier wafers.

### 40. How is therapeutic maggot therapy used as a form of chemical debridement?

Therapeutic maggot therapy involves the use of sterilized fly eggs. Once the eggs hatch, the sterile larva are introduced into the necrotic wound bed. It is theorized that the larvae secrete proteolytic enzymes, including collagenase. that break down the necrotic tissue. The larva also functions as an antimicrobial in the wound by ingesting microorganisms and decreasing the wound's bioburden and odor. Maggot therapy also has been called biologic debridement or biosurgery (see Chapter 15).

## SHARP DEBRIDEMENT

**41. Define sharp debridement.**

Sharp debridement is a selective method of debridement using sterile instruments, such as a forcep, scissor, scalpel with a no. 10 or no. 15 blade, or laser, to remove macroscopically identified nonviable necrotic tissue from a wound. Sharp debridement is classified as  sharp surgical debridement or conservative sharp debridement. Sharp surgical debridement is performed usually as a one-time process in which all or a significant amount of necrotic tissue is removed from the surface of the wound. Sharp surgical debridement is often done by a surgeon in the operating room. Conservative sharp debridement is a sequential debridement of necrotic tissue. Sharp conservative debridement is usually done at the bedside by a trained clinical practitioner or physician and is usually less invasive.

**42. What are the indications for sharp surgical debridement?**

Sharp surgical debridement is considered the quickest and most effective form of debridement. It is indicated for wounds requiring the removal of large amounts of necrotic tissue. It is always the method of choice when an infectious process is present because effective treatment requires immediate removal of the necrotic tissue. It is also the method of choice when the wound bed is being prepared for surgical flaps or skin grafts.

**43. What are the risks of sharp surgical debridement?**

The potential risks include bleeding, sepsis, and risks associated with anesthesia. It is possible for a transient bacteremia to develop after the wound is debrided. Many patients are not candidates for surgical debridement because of comorbidities, associated risk factors, and complications of anesthesia.

**44. How is sharp conservative debridement used?**

The procedure is usually not done aggressively enough for immediate exposure of all viable tissue. Rather, the removal of necrotic tissue is done sequentially and in combination with other debridement methods, including high-pressure irrigation, enzymes, or moisture-retentive dressings. Risks to the patient are minimal. Conservative sharp debridement is done at the bedside and is less invasive than sharp surgical debridement. It is less likely to cause excessive bleeding than surgical debridement, although some bleeding may occur.

**45. When is sharp conservative debridement indicated?**

Sharp conservative debridement is indicated as a selective debridement method for the removal of loosely adherent, nonviable tissue.

**46. Describe a potential complication of sharp conservative debridement.**

Although less likely than with sharp surgical debridement, bleeding is a potential complication. Before performing sharp conservative debridement, the clinician should evaluate the patient for any bleeding disorders or conditions that may result in an inability to clot properly. Examples include patients taking medication such as heparin, warfarin, or high doses of aspirin or nonsteroidal anti-inflammatory drugs and patients with pathologic conditions such as thrombocytopenia, impaired liver function, vitamin K deficiency, and malnutrition.

**47. Who is qualified to perform sharp conservative debridement?**

Sharp conservative debridement is the most aggressive type of debridement performed by non-physician health care practitioners. Its performance requires basic technical training. Practitioners should take a course or workshop on sharp conservative debridement method and demonstrate clinical competency. The nonphysician health care practitioner who is certified to do sharp conservative debridement should have his or her job description privileges extended to cover this method of wound debridement in the employment setting. In addition, the licensing board of his or her state must consider the procedure within the scope of practice of the person's professional license.

### 48. When is sharp conservative debridement contraindicated?

Sharp conservative debridement should not be performed on an ischemic limb because it may lead to invasive sepsis due to poor blood supply. In such a situation, revascularization measures are necessary. If the patient is not a candidate for revascularization, amputation may be indicated. It should be used cautiously in patients who present with bleeding disorders or in the presence of infection or advancing cellulitis.

### 49. How can the clinician control bleeding if it occurs during sharp conservative debridement?

If bleeding is encountered, the debridement process should be stopped. Application of a dry, sterile gauze and gentle pressure should stop the bleeding. Bleeding can also be stopped by the use of topical agents such as thrombin or surgical gelfoam. The use of a calcium alginate dressing may stop the bleeding since the calcium is thrombogenic. Silver nitrate sticks have also proved to be helpful in cauterizing superficial capillary bleeding.

### 50. What basic principles should be followed in performing sharp conservative debridement?

1. Prepare the site of debridement with an antimicrobial, such as povidone iodine.
2. Use sterile instruments and sterile technique to decrease the likelihood of infection.
3. Establish a plane of dissection by holding the necrotic tissue taut to visualize clearly the planc of dissection.
4. Avoid all vascular tissues and tissues that are not clearly identified. Know your anatomy!
5. Irrigate the wound after the procedure.

### BIBLIOGRAPHY

1. Bates-Jensen B: Management of necrotic tissue. In Sussman C, Bates-Jensen B (eds): Wound Care: A Collaborative Practice Manual for Physical Therapists and Nurses. Gaithersburg MD, Aspen, 1998, pp 139–158.
2. Barr JF: Physiology of healing: The basis for the principles of wound management. MedSurg Nurs 4(5):387–392, 1995.
3. Baxter C, Mertz P: Local factors that affect wound healing. In Eaglstein, Baxter C, Mertz P, et al (eds): New Directions in Wound Healing. Princeton, NJ, F.R. Squibb, 1990.
4. Fatabella A: Debridement of wounds. Wounds 10(Suppl C):1C–9C, 1998.
5. Gordon B: Conservative sharp wound debridement. J Wound Ostomy Continence Nurses 23(3):137, 1996.
6. Harding K: Wound care: Putting theory into clinical practice. Wounds 2:21–32, 1990.
7. Loehne HB: Pulsatile lavage with concurrent suction. In Sussman C, Bates-Jensen B (eds): Wound Care: A Collaborative Practice Manual for Physical Therapists and Nurses. Gaithersburg MD, Aspen, 1998, pp 389–393.
8. Mosher BA, et al: Outcomes of 4 methods of debridement using a decision analysis methodology. Adv Wound Care 12(2), 1999.
9. Sieggreen M, Maklebust J: Debridement choices and challenges. Adv Wound Care 10(2):32–37, 1997.
10. Sherman R: A new dressing for use with maggot therapy. Plast Reconstr Surg100:451, 1997.
11. Wheeler C, et al: Side effects of high pressure irrigation. Surg Gynecol Obstet 143:775, 1976.

# 13. PULSED LAVAGE

*Diane M. Morgan,* BSN, RNC, CWOCN, *and Judy Hoelscher,* RN, MSN, EdD

**1. Define pulsed lavage.**

Pulsed lavage, also known as pulsatile lavage, is a form of hydrotherapy that is delivered by a hand-held device. The device provides a pressurized, pulsed solution to a wound bed for the purpose of irrigating and debriding.

**2. What is the purpose of pulsed lavage?**

Pulsed lavage treatment is an efficient, cost-effective, user-friendly way to provide wound debridement that prepares the wound bed for healing. Hydrodebridement is an effective treatment for cleaning and debriding when the wound contains thick exudate, slough, or necrotic tissue. The high-pressure delivery softens and mechanically debrides devitalized tissue. By softening necrotic tissue, it also facilitates sharp debridement .

**3. What is the difference between pulsed lavage and pulsed lavage with suction?**

Pulsed lavage delivers irrigating solution for cleaning purposes, whereas pulsed lavage with suction is a form of mechanical debridement. The negative pressure exerted by the suction device removes irrigating solution and debris as well as promotes granulation tissue. Negative pressure (suction) dilates arterioles, which may increase flow to tissues.

**4. Who can use pulsed lavage?**

Physical therapists have been using pulsed lavage since the late 1980s for irrigation and mechanical debridement. Nurses are becoming more accustomed to pulsed lavage and are integrating it into their practice.

**5. In which clinical setting is pulsed lavage beneficial?**

Pulsed lavage is beneficial in numerous settings, including acute care, long-term care, and home health. A pulsed lavage unit is small and can be easily transported to a patient's home. For home-bound patients receiving skilled home care services, this treatment option is significantly less expensive than outpatient whirlpool.

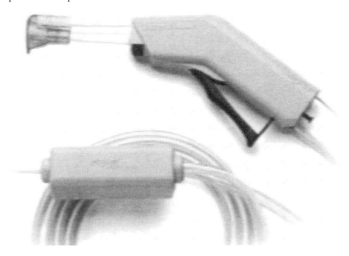

Stryker InterPulse.

**6. In what situations can pulsed lavage be used?**
- When there is significant necrotic or foreign material
- As an adjunct to other debridement methods
- To minimize cost and avoid unnecessary surgical intervention
- In the home when the patient is homebound
- To remove debris from the wound bed in preparation for wound healing
- To prepare the wound bed for placement of negative-pressure dressing or grafting

**7. What are the advantages and benefits of using pulsed lavage?**
- It decreases the bioburden of the wound.
- It is a noninvasive, safe, conservative treatment.
- There is no trauma to the tissues because the pressure (pounds per square inch) is < 15.
- Cytotoxic agents are avoided.
- Positive patient outcomes are achieved.
- It prepares the wound bed for healing.
- One study suggests a 20% reduction in debridement time.

**8. What are the precautions for pulsed lavage with suction?**
- Do not perform over exposed blood vessels, nerves, tendons, or bone.
- Intensity should be between 4 and 15 pounds per square inch (psi).
- Patients on anticoagulation medication may exhibit excessive bleeding.
- Improper technique may harm wound bed
- Patients with sensory impairment are unable to provide accurate feedback needed to guide the clinician if improper technique is used.
- Cover IV sites and other open areas to protect from splashing.

**9. What are the steps in the decision making process for choosing pulsed lavage?**
1. **Assess the patient.**
   - General health history
   - Cause of the wound and wound history
   - Healing potential
   - Use of medications (e.g., anticoagulant therapy, steroid therapy, agents for pain management)
   - Nutritional status (obtain 24-hour food recall or 3-day food diary)
   - Pressure reducing surfaces
2. **Assess the wound(s).**
   - Location
   - Size (length, width, depth, undermining, tunneling)
   - Wound bed
   - Surrounding derma
   - Amount, color and odor of drainage
   - Presence and description of necrotic tissue
3. **Assess the patient's environment and clinician availability and training.**

**10. What equipment is needed?**
- Hand-held pulsed lavage equipment (see question 13)
- Tubing and tips (check with manufacturer regarding recommendations for use)
- Suction equipment or absorbent product to collect irrigant
- Sterile saline (1000 cc) in bag format
- Gloves, mask, goggles, gown
- Dressings

**11. Summarize the steps in the procedure.**
1. Adhere to the manufacturer's guidelines.
2. Obtain the physician's order, which should include the following:

- Manufacturer's instrument with sterile saline suggested
- Discontinue pulsed lavage when wound bed is free of necrotic debris
- Post-lavage wound care dressing

3. Document assessment findings.
4. Observe standard precautions.
5. Spike the solution and flush the tubing with irrigation solution.
6. Attach the tubing to the suction machine if negative therapy is to be used.
7. Remove the soiled dressing.
8. Assess the wound bed.
9. Reposition the patient comfortably.
10. Place pulsed lavage unit against wound and begin treatment.
11. Apply wound dressing.
12. Carry out standard precautions for dressing disposal.

## 12. What are some "tricks of the trade"?

1. If suction is not used, pad bedding with absorptive pads.

2. With extremities, use a clean plastic biohazard bag to line a clean container designated for procedure and to collect irrigation solution.

## 13. What vendors offer products for pulsed lavage?

- Davol Simpulse Solo (1-800-556-6275)
  Adjustable flow rates available
- Stryker Instruments Interpulse (1-800-253-3210)
  Flow rate: psi established at < 15
- Zimmer Pulsavac Plus (1-800-348-2759)
  Adjustable flow rates available

## 14. What research has been done to identify outcomes of pulsed lavage?

Luedtke-Hoffman and Schafer summarize the research in *Pulsed Lavage in Wound Cleansing*. The authors indicate that the research is scant and has produced less than clear results. However, research indicates that pulsed lavage appears to be a safe method for wound cleansing. Research has demonstrated no evidence of bacteremia after treatments, regardless of the pressure used. More research is needed to validate outcomes.

### BIBLIOGRAPHY

1. Loehne H: Pulsatile lavage with concurrent suction. In Sussman C, Bates-Jenson BM (eds): Wound Care: A Collaborative Practice Manual for Physical Therapists and Nurses. Gaithersburg MD, Aspen, 1998, pp 389–403.
2. Luedtke-Hoffman KA, Schafer DS: Pulsed lavage in wound cleansing. Phys Ther 80:292–300, 2000.
3. Morgan D, Hoelscher J: Pulsed lavage: Promoting comfort and healing in home care. Ostomy Wound Manage 46(4):44-49, 2000.
4. Scott RG, Loehne H: Treatment options: Five questions and answers about pulsed lavage. Advances in Skin and Wound Care 13(3):133–134, 2000.
5. Wound/skin care: Pulsed lavage procedure. Lifespan Home Health and Hospice Care, Battle Creek, MI, Section 7-10, 1999.

# 14. HYDROTHERAPY FOR CLEANSING AND DEBRIDEMENT

*Tamara L. Roehling, MPT, and Bonnie J. Sparks-DeFriese, PT, RN, CWS*

**1. After a dressing change does a noninfected, granulating wound need to be cleaned?**

The purpose of wound cleansing is to remove inflammatory contaminants from the wound surface. While cleansing, the practitioner should minimize trauma to a granulating wound bed. Gentle flushing with water or saline is appropriate.

**2. Should wounds be cleaned with normal saline or a wound cleanser?**

Isotonic saline solution is the preferred wound cleanser. Commercial wound cleansers contain surfactants that help lift debris from wound surfaces. Many of these surfactants have been shown to be toxic to cells and may delay wound healing. Wound cleansers may be appropriate for wound covered with necrotic tissue or nongranulating wounds with heavy debris. For the majority of wounds, normal saline is the appropriate choice.

**3. What is the reason for selecting whirlpool treatments?**

Whirlpool with agitation is a form of mechanical debridement that softens and removes necrotic tissue and foreign contaminant. Wound cleansing is enhanced in the whirlpool because of the extended soaking time along with the pressurized streams of water. Softening hard eschar and blood coagulum during whirlpool can facilitate sharp wound debridement. If the extremity is in the dependent position in the whirlpool and the water is warm, whirlpool treatment may vasodilate vessels, thus increasing blood flow to the wound and enhancing oxygen perfusion and nutrition.

**4. Are physical therapists the only health care providers who can give whirlpool treatments?**

No. Historically, physical therapists were the primary providers who conducted whirlpool treatments. However, with reimbursement changes resulting from the Balanced Budget Act of 1997, nurses are performing more whirlpool treatments. Medicare continues to reimburse physical therapists conducting whirlpool treatments, if the goal is to soften necrotic tissue for subsequent sharp debridement.

**5. How long should a patient remain in the whirlpool tank?**

Research has established that 10–20 minutes is the optimal time to soften necrotic tissue and reduce bacteria. Whirlpool treatments lasting longer than 20 minutes may increase the risk of maceration (softening of the skin due to liquid soaking), which can cause further tissue compromise.

**6. After a whirlpool treatment, should the wound be rinsed with water?**

Definitely. When the extremity is removed from the whirlpool tank, a visible ring of residue remains on the extremity, similar to the bathtub ring following a bath. Rinsing of the wound and surrounding skin with clean water is recommended to remove residual bacteria.

**7. Are whirlpool treatments indicated for patients with venous insufficiency?**

Venous insufficiency is a relative contraindication for whirlpool treatments. Venous insufficiency ulcers are most commonly found in the gaiter area of the leg, distal to the knee, and at or above the malleolus. Extremity whirlpool tanks are used with the patient in the 90-90 position (90° of hip flexion and 90° of knee flexion). Thus, the leg is in a dependent position, which facilitates edema in the lower extremity. Patients with venous insufficiency generally have edema, which delays wound healing. The combination of vasodilation and dependent sitting further increases the edema. If a patient must have hydrotherapy, consider pulsatile lavage with suction. If this option is not available, perform the whirlpool with caution. Limit the patient's treatment time in a dependent position to 10 minutes, and decrease the temperature of the water to a nonthermal temperature of 92°F.

8. **What are the systemic effects of whirlpool treatment?**

The "thermal response" of whirlpool treatments includes the following:
- Increased heart rate
- Increased respiratory rate
- Increased muscle relaxation
- Increased sedation and analgesia
- Impaired temperature regulatory system

9. **What temperature should the water be?**

Necrotic tissue is softened in water, regardless of its temperature. Select water temperature according to the patient's medical condition. If in doubt, nonthermal water temperature is the safest temperature for wound healing.

*Whirlpool Temperature Selection*

| TEMPERATURE CLASSIFICATION | TEMPERATURE | INDICATIONS | PRECAUTIONS |
| --- | --- | --- | --- |
| Nonthermal | 80–92°F 27–33.5°C | Venous insufficiency Peripheral vascular disease Single limb | Hypothermia: limit treatment time to 10 min and increase room temperature |
| Neutral | 92–96°F 33.5–35.5°C | Larger body areas Cardiopulmonary disease Most commonly used temperature range for chronic wounds | Patients may become chilled; increase room temperature |
| Thermal | 96–104°F 35.5–40°C | Muscle relaxation Vasodilation | Significant stress on circulatory, nervous, and cardiopulmonary systems |

Because patients with autonomic neuropathy and pulmonary compromise have difficulty in cooling body temperature, observe the following guidelines:
- Use cooler water temperatures.
- Limit the amount of body surface area submersed in the whirlpool.
- Decrease treatment time to lessen physiologic demands induced by thermal effects of whirlpool.

10. **Should whirlpools be used to soak off dried dressings?**

Wet-to-dry dressings, a form of mechanical debridement, are applied wet and removed when dried to lift off necrotic tissue between gauze interstices. Therefore, if mechanical debridement is the goal, do not soak off dried dressings. If wet-to-moist dressings are intended, dried dressings can be soaked off with caution. First, be sure that whirlpool agitators are turned off to avoid entanglement of gauze dressing in the agitator. Secondly, be sure to remove all dressing components. If a small part of dressing gets caught and lost in the whirlpool components, it may become a source of infection.

11. **Is cross-contamination a serious threat with whirlpool treatment?**

Yes. Studies have shown that whirlpool treatments are often a cause of nosocomial infection. *Pseudomonas aeruginosa* (52.9%), *Staphylococcus aureus* (25.5%), and *Candida albicans* (5.2%) are the most prevalent agents. In general, warm water and mechanical agitation facilitate festering of bacteria in whirlpool tanks, motors, water pipes, drains, and around the thermometer. Tub-cleaning routines and disinfection protocols should be followed carefully to avoid contamination.

12. **What are the disadvantages of whirlpool treatment?**
- Increased risk of infection due to cross-contamination
- Maceration

- Increased edema
- Nonselective debridement (debrides viable and nonviable tissue)
- Not cost-effective because of time needed to fill whirlpool tank with water, transport patient to and from hydrotherapy room, treatment time, emptying of whirlpool tank, and tank cleaning

### 13. Should stable heel ulcers covered with black eschar be put in a whirlpool?

A stable heel ulcer should not be placed in the whirlpool. Placing a stable heel ulcer in the whirlpool may open the wound and increase the likelihood of infection. The *Treatment of Pressure Ulcers* guideline from the Agency for Health Care Policy and Research (AHCPR) states, "Heel ulcers with dry eschar need not be debrided if they do not have edema, erythema, fluctuance, or drainage." However, if the wound is infected or already open with necrotic tissue that requires debridement, whirlpool treatment is not contraindicated and may assist with the debridement process.

### 14. Summarize the contraindications and precautions for whirlpool treatment.

- Clean, granulating tissue. Whirlpool treatment damages viable cells needed for wound healing. Rule of thumb: Do not place wounds that have more than 50% viable tissue into a whirlpool.
- New skin grafts, which may float away.
- New tissue flaps, which do not tolerate shearing forces caused by the agitator.
- Callus on diabetic foot. A macerated callus increases wound size. In addition, moisture under the callus is a source of infection
- Moderate-to-severe edema, which increases in the whirlpool.
- Severe neuropathy
- Unresponsiveness
- Fever> 101.9°F
- Acute phlebitis
- Renal failure
- Bladder or bowl incontinence (if there is a chance that urine or feces may enter the whirlpool and contaminate the wound).
- Dry gangrene, which may be converted to wet gangrene when soaked. Wet gangrene facilitates bacterial proliferation, which can enter the circulation and cause sepsis.
- History of cardiopulmonary disease, cardiac disease, cerebrovascular accident, or hypertension: vital signs should be monitored closely before, during, and after whirlpool treatment.

### 15. Are twice-daily whirlpools needed?

Twice-daily whirlpool treatments are not recommended for the following reasons:
- Increased exposure to possible infection
- Disruption of optimal wound environment and temperature
- Not cost-effective

### 16. Which personal protective equipment (PPE) should be worn during a whirlpool or pulsatile lavage treatment?

Because of splashing and aerosolization, the following PPE is recommended:
- Gloves
- Hair coverings
- Face shields or goggles with mask
- Water-resistant gowns
- Shoe coverings

### 17. Is pulsatile lavage with suction preferable to whirlpool treatments?

The advantages of pulsatile lavage over whirlpool are as follows:
- Debridement is more selective, because the pulsatile lavage is site-specific.
- Cross-contamination is eliminated because the units are disposable.
- Less expensive due to lower labor costs (minimal set-up and clean-up with less treatment time).

- Periwound maceration (overhydration of surrounding skin) is avoided.
- Often can be used when whirlpool is contraindicated (e.g,. venous insufficiency, unresponsiveness, cardiopulmonary disease, febrile, and incontinence).
- Can be used on patients when whirlpool tank is inaccessible, including patients in intensive care unit or isolation room.

## CONTROVERSY

**18. What is the role of cytotoxic agents in the whirlpool?**

Physicians often order cytotoxic agents for use in the whirlpool. Common examples include povidone-iodine (Betadine), sodium hypochlorite (Dakin's solution), chlorhexidine (Hibiclens), and chloramine T (Chlorazene). An order that reads, "Whirlpool with Betadine," is common but controversial in the literature. Cytotoxic agents are not recommended, because toxicity, even in diluted concentrations, destroys cells that are needed for wound healing. Some clinicians argue that cytotoxic agents should never be used, because they impair the body's immune system and facilitate cytotoxic resistance. Other clinicians believe that the use of cytotoxic agents is justified only when the wound is infected.

## BIBLIOGRAPHY

1. Bryant RA (ed): Acute and Chronic Wounds: Nursing Management. St. Louis, Mosby Yearbook, 1992.
2. Haynes LJ, Brown MH, Handley BC, et al: Comparison of Pulsavac and sterile whirlpool regarding the promotion of tissue granulation. Phys Ther 74:54, 1994.
3. Luedtke-Hoffman K, Schafer DS: Pulsed lavage in wound cleansing. Phys Ther 80:292–300, 2000.
4. Morgan D, Hoelscher J: Pulsed lavage: Promoting comfort and healing in home care. Ostomy Wound Manage 46:44–49, 2000.
5. Rodeheaver GT: Pressure ulcer debridement and cleansing: A review of current literature. Ostomy Wound Manage 45:80s–85s, 1999.
6. Sparks BJ: Physical therapy and wound care: What's the connection? Ostomy Wound Manage 40:76–81, 1994.
7. Sussman C, Bates-Jensen B: Wound Care: A Collaborative Practice Manual for Physical Therapist and Nurses. Gaithersburg, MD, Aspen, 1998.

# 15. BIOTHERAPY DEBRIDEMENT: MAGGOT THERAPY

*Catherine T.Milne, APRN, MSN, CWOCN, CS, ANP,
and Lisa Q. Corbett, APRN, MSN, CWOCN, CS*

**1. Define biotherapy.**

Biotherapy describes the use of live organisms to assist in the medical regimen. Maggots and leeches are commonly accepted forms of biotherapy in wound care settings.

**2. What is maggot debridement therapy (MDT)?**

MDT is a form of biotherapy that uses maggots to remove necrotic and devitalized tissue from wounds. MDT is also known as larval therapy and biosurgery.

**3. Why maggots?**

Maggots have been used in the practice of medicine for centuries. In the Civil War, maggots in war wounds actually improved the patient's outcome. This finding led physicians to use maggots for the treatment of necrotic wounds until the 1940s, when antibiotics became the standard of care.

**4. Is MDT a gross concept?**

Only because society associates maggots with filth and unsanitary conditions. Only sterile, medicinal-grade maggots are used for MDT. There is no spread of disease or bacteria. Many health care practitioners can think of patients who have obtained MDT from unconventional sources. Many such patients were surprised to learn that their wounds were inhabited by maggots, as they could not feel or see them.

**5. How does MDT work?**

Live *Phaenicia sericata*, *Phormia regina*, or *Lucilia illustris* larvae are placed into the wound. These organisms digest necrotic tissue. Bacteria are destroyed, and wound healing is facilitated by this method. Only certain kinds of maggots can be used, as other species can digest healthy tissue.

**6. How are maggots used in forensic medicine?**

Forensic medicine uses the natural life cycle of the fly to determine the time of death. In some cases, maggots can add missing details about the nature or a location of a crime.

**7. On what kind of wounds should MDT be used?**

Wounds with devitalized tissue such as eschar or slough may undergo MDT therapy. Studies have shown that MDT has been successful in burns, severe skin infections, pressure ulcers, and venous stasis ulcers.

**8. When should MDT not be used?**

Patients who do not consent or who are uncomfortable with the prospect of biotherapy should be counseled about other debridement options. Persons with allergies to chicken eggs or soybeans should not receive MDT.

**9. How does one prepare the patient for MDT?**

The importance of having an open, frank discussion with the patient and significant others about debridement options is the best way to prepare the patient for MDT.

**10. What procedure is used to apply the maggots?**

**Step 1.** Medicinal maggots should be obtained from reputable sources. Information can be found at www.ucihs.uci.ed/path/sherman/home_pg.htm. The maggots are ready for use on arrival. Kept at room temperature, several thousand eggs are imbedded on a gauze in a sterile vial. Of these,

72

a quarter or so of the eggs will have hatched. It is important to keep the gauze slightly moist. A few drops of sterile saline or water should be added daily to the vial.

**Step 2.** It is important to ensure the patient, family, staff and others involved in the patient's care (either directly or peripherally) that measures will be taken to prevent the maggots from getting into the environment. Sometimes simply using the phrase *biotherapy organisms* can greatly relieve everyone's anxiety. To prevent inadvertent escape, the wound must be dressed properly. The literature defines several techniques, all involving layering of dressings to keep the maggots where they belong. Generally, a hole slightly larger than the wound opening is cut in the center of an adhesive dressing, such as a hydrocolloid; transparent film or thin foam product is the bottom layer closest to the skin.

**Step 3.** Prepare the containment dressings. A breathable layer of cloth, such as chiffon or Owen's gauze (parachute silk), should be cut to the size of the adhesive dressing but without the hole that is placed over the first dressing. The last, or top layer, is a semi-permeable dressing, such as a transparent film, foam, or hydropolymer, with a hole the same size as the bottom dressing. These dressings, prepared ahead of time, should be available and ready to be placed at the time of application of MDT. The purpose of the top and bottom layer is to hold the middle dressing in place. The middle dressing keeps the biotherapy organisms where they belong. It is important to use a breathable dressing so that the maggots do not suffocate. Gauze should be available to be placed over the layered dressing to collect any drainage coming through the hole. This gauze can be changed every 4 or 6 hours, depending on the amount of drainage.

**Step 4.** The maggots should be removed from the vial using forceps and placed on an area of approximately 5–8 square centimeters of slightly dampened normal saline gauze. Some people use the gauze from the vial in which the maggots were delivered. Although this method is more palatable for squeamish clinicians, sometimes more maggots are delivered to the wound bed than one would like. This method is suitable for wounds that may need only one or two treatments.

**Step 5.** Place the biotherapy gauze into the wound. Cover the wound with the bottom layer of the designed environmental control dressing. Follow the layering technique previously discussed. Place gauze on top to collect any drainage. The maggots are left in the wound for 48 hours. At this time, all dressings are removed, and the wound is irrigated in the standard fashion. All wound irrigant is considered infectious material and disposed of in a sealed bag or container. Many clinicians place a plastic bag under the wound; as the wound is irrigated, the material naturally flows into it.

## 11. How long does MDT take to debride the wound?

Most wounds need only one treatment to achieve total debridement. Wounds with thick eschar may need several weeks; thus, other methods such as a surgical debridement or a mechanical process (e.g., pulsatile lavage) may be more suitable.

## 12. Can the patient feel the maggots?

Some, but not all, patients report a tingling or other sensation. At times, this sensation can lead to premature discontinuation of therapy. Because other debridement options are available, the patient's psychological well-being takes first priority. An open discussion with patients about their willingness to continue with therapy is in order.

## 13. Has the literature compared this method of debridement with chemical, surgical, or mechanical techniques?

No randomized, controlled clinical trials have compared MDT with the more commonly used debridement methods. Anecdotal reports describe complete debridement in 1–3 days without adverse sequelae.

### BIBLIOGRAPHY

1. Rund C: Alternative topical therapies for wound care. In Krasner DL, Rodeheaver GT, Sibbald RG (eds): Chronic Wound Care: A Clinical Source Book for Healthcare Professionals, 3rd ed. Wayne, PA, HMR Communications, 2001, pp 329–340.
2. Sherman RA: A new dressing design for use with maggot therapy. Plast Reconstruct Surg 100:451–456, 1997.
3. Stoddard SR, Sherman RA, Mason BE, Pelsang DJ: Maggot debridement therapy: An alternative treatment for nonhealing ulcers. J Am Podiatr Med Assoc 85(4):218–221, 1995.
4. Thomas S, Jones M, Shutler S, Jones S: Using larvae in modern wound management. J Wound Care 5:60–69, 1996.

# 16. DIAGNOSING WOUND INFECTIONS

*Teresa A. Conner-Kerr, PhD, PT, CWS(D), and*
*P. Karen Sullivan, PhD, MT(ASCP), SM(ASCP)*

### 1. Define wound infection.
A wound infection is the invasion of pathologic organisms into healthy tissue surrounding the wound. Fever, erythema, edema, and induration that clinically present as hard, firm tissue are classic signs of infection. Increased pain and a change in wound drainage to a purulent nature are also characteristics of a wound infection.

### 2. Is fever always a reliable sign?
Unfortunately, in elderly or severely immunocompromised patients, fever in wound infection is suppressed or minimal.

### 3. Is there a reliable way to diagnose wound infection?
Cultures can be helpful in confirming clinical suspicion, which should be raised if no improvement in wound healing is noted after 2 weeks of good wound care. Some clinicians empirically treat the patient without obtaining cultures, because it can be difficult to distinguish infection from colonization.

### 4. How should cultures be obtained?
The gold standard is a tissue culture. Using a punch biopsy device, tissue is extracted from the wound. It should be sent to the laboratory as soon as possible. The lab weighs the specimen, flames the surface to kill surface contaminants, and grinds the tissue before placing in culture medium. If the number of organisms per gram of tissue is $10^5$ or greater, infection is confirmed.

### 5. The Nurse Practice Act in my state allows only advanced practice nurses to perform tissue cultures. Physical therapists are not allowed to do so either. Are there any alternatives?
Yes. A quantitative swab culture can be obtained. The swab culture uses a different technique than the traditional swab method, which obtains information about surface colonization. Data show that the quantitative swab method is comparable to tissue cultures.

### 6. How is the quantitative swab method performed?
After wound cleansing is performed, swab 1 $cm^2$ of clean wound bed with sufficient pressure to obtain wound fluid and place into culture tube medium. Aseptic technique should be used.

### 7. What determines infection risk?
In addition to the ability of the vascular system to deliver oxygen, nutrients, and white blood cells to the area at risk, the following triad illustrates three significant factors that determine the risk of developing infection.

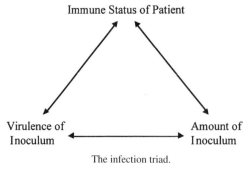

The infection triad.

**8. What is the difference between colonization and infection?**

Colonization occurs in any open wound, usually within 3 days. The pathogens attach themselves to the surface of the open wound. They do not invade healthy tissue surrounding the wound.

**9. So there is a fine line between colonization and infection?**

Absolutely. The goal of the clinician is to provide interventions that have a positive effect on the infection triad.

| INFECTION TRIAD DIMENSION | GOAL | INTERVENTION |
| --- | --- | --- |
| Immune status of patient | Enhance | Use noncytotoxic wound cleansing solutions. Provide adequate nutrition. Consider glutamine and arginine supplementation. Monitor complete blood count differential. Consider modalities to improve oxygenation perfusion, such as E-stim, hyperbaric therapy, NNWT. Treat neutropenia. Local periwound injections with antineutropenic agents. |
| Amount of inoculum | Reduce | Wound cleansing at each dressing change with adequate pressures and volume of solution. Protective dressings over wounds that prevent contamination from external source. Clean technique at dressing changes. Adjunctive therapies such as ultraviolet C light, pulsed electromagnetic field (PEMF), ultrasound. Caregiver to wash hands before and after wound care. |
| Virulence of inoculum | Minimize | Avoid exposure to inoculum. Reduce colonization. Caregiver to wash hands before and after wound care. Use topical antimicrobials not associated with the development of resistant organisms. Adjunctive modalities such as ultraviolet C light, PEMF, ultrasound. |

## BIBLIOGRAPHY

1. Feedar JA: Clinical management of chronic wounds. In McCulloch JM, Kloth LC, Feedar JA (eds): Wound Healing: Alternatives in Management, 2nd ed. Philadelphia, F. A. Davis, 1995, pp 137–185.
2. Sibbald RG, Williamson D, Orstead H, et al: Preparing the wound bed: Debridement, bacterial balance, and moisture balance. Ostomy Wound Manage 46(11):14–35, 2000.
3. Sussman C, Bates-Jensen BM (eds): Management of Exudate and Infection in Wound Care: A Collaborative Practice Manual for Physical Therapists and Nurses. Gaithersburg MD, Aspen, 1998, pp 166–177.

# 17. TOPICAL AGENTS FOR MANAGEMENT OF WOUND INFECTIONS

*Teresa A. Conner-Kerr, PhD, PT, CWS(D), and*
*P. Karen Sullivan, PhD, MT(ASCP), SM(ASCP)*

**1. What options are available for the treatment of infection?**
- Topical agents
- Systemic antibiotics
- Surgical debridement
- Hyperbaric oxygenation
- Ultraviolet C energy
- Electrical stimulation

**2. What topical agents are used commonly for open wounds?**
- Antiseptics
- Antimicrobials
- Enzymes
- Growth factors

**3. Which of the above agents are currently recommended for use in an open wound?**

The use of topical agents on an open wound, particularly antiseptics and antimicrobials, continues to be an issue of ongoing debate. Of interest, chronic wound management providers view the use of antiseptics and topical antimicrobials somewhat differently from burn wound clinicians. The utility of antiseptics and topical antimicrobials appears to be a more accepted practice for both prevention of infection and management of infected burn wounds. Clinicians in the chronic wound arena are beginning to appreciate the role that bioburden plays in delaying wound healing. Thus, the agents are finding greater acceptance in practice.

**4. Are antiseptics safe to use in an open wound?**

Currently, the traditional antiseptics are not recommended because of their associated cytotoxicity for wound cells. However, a new generation of antiseptics/antimicrobials appears to be effective in decreasing wound bioburden while sparing human cells (see question 7).

**5. What are antiseptics? Which ones have been used in the management of open wound infections?**

Antiseptics are chemicals used as disinfectants on the skin. Examples of antiseptics that have been used in the management of open wound infections include:
- Povidone iodine
- Iodophor
- Sodium hypochlorite (Dakin's solution)
- Hydrogen peroxide
- Acetic acid
- Chlorhexidine
- Hexachlorophene
- Quaternary ammonium (Cetrimide)

**6. What organisms are they effective against?**

| AGENT | SENSITIVE ORGANISMS |
| --- | --- |
| Povidone iodine | Gram-positive, gram-negative, yeast, fungi |
| Iodophor | Gram-positive, gram-negative, yeast, fungi |
| Sodium hypochlorite (Dakin's solution) | Gram-positive |
| Hydrogen peroxide | Not effective |
| Acetic acid | Gram-positive, gram-negative |
| Chlorhexidine (Hibiclens) | Gram-positive, gram-negative |
| Hexachlorophene (Phisohex) | Gram-positive |
| Quaternary ammonium (Cetrimide) | Gram-positive, gram-negative, yeast, fungi |

**7. What new antimicrobials are now available?**

Several relatively new agents have come on the market. All use a slow- or controlled-release approach. These products have been designed to take advantage of the antimicrobial properties of their traditional antiseptic cousins while having a low cytotoxic potential for human cells. They work by releasing low levels of either iodine or silver into the wound. These levels appear to be cytotoxic to microbes while sparing human cells. New antiseptics include the following:

- Iodosorb (cadexomer iodine)
- Arglaes (controlled-release film dressing): silver
- Acticoat (antimicrobial barrier dressing): nanocrystalline silver
- Silverlon (antimicrobial dressing): ionic silver

**8. What topical antibacterials have been commonly used in open wound management?**

| | | | |
|---|---|---|---|
| • Bacitracin | • Metronidazole | • Neomycin | • Mafenide acetate |
| • Gentamicin | • Mupirocin | • Silver sulfadiazine | • Nitrofurazone |

**9. What are their mechanisms of action? Which organisms are they effective against?**

| AGENT | ACTION | SENSITIVE ORGANISMS |
|---|---|---|
| Bacitracin | Interferes with cell wall synthesis | Gram-positive and anaerobes |
| Gentamicin | Inhibits protein synthesis | Gram-positive and gram-negatives |
| Metronidazole | Unclear | Anaerobes |
| Mupirocin | Interferes with cell wall synthesis | Gram-positive |
| Neomycin | Inhibits protein synthesis | Gram-positive, gram-negative |
| Silver sulfadiazine | Damages cell wall | Gram-positive, gram-negative, and fungi |
| Mafenide acetate | Unclear | Gram-positive, gram-negative, anaerobes |
| Nitrofurazone | Unclear | Gram-positive, gram-negative |

**10. Is there a particular topical antimicrobial/antiseptic recommended for use with antibiotic-resistant pathogens such as methicillin-resistant *Staphylococcus aureus* (MRSA)?**

Yes. Mupirocin (Bactroban) is recommended for treating MRSA infections. In fact, it is recommended that mupirocin be reserved for MRSA infections to limit the development of resistant forms. Cadexomer iodine and nanocrystalline silver agents have also been shown to be effective.

**11. Which of these agents have been associated with a decreased likelihood of generating antibiotic resistance? Why?**

Mupirocin (Bactroban). The unique mechanism by which mupirocin interferes with bacterial cell wall synthesis appears to convey some protection in preventing the generation of antimicrobial resistance. However, recent cases of mupirocin-resistant microbes have been reported. There is no reported resistance to the silver and cadexomer iodine products, most likely because of their recent introduction to the market. Experts contend that resistance is unlikely because both iodine and silver have been used for decades without reported resistance.

**12. Have any topical antibiotics been associated with allergic reactions?**

Yes. Neomycin is a common skin allergen, especially in people with venous insufficiency. Allergic reactions to neomycin are due to two separate chemical moieties, the deoxystreptamine backbone and the neosamine sugars A, B, and C. Currently, neomycin or neomycin-containing medications are not recommended for topical use because they are such potent skin allergens. Incidents of allergic reactions to bacitracin also have been reported.

**13. List five rules that help determine which topical agents are appropriate for managing high levels of wound bioburden.**

1. Do not use agents that are common skin sensitizers.
2. Patch tests for sensitivity(allergy) can be helpful in susceptible patients.

3. Do not use topically any agent that is used systemically.
4. Frequently reevaluate therapy, approximately at 2-week intervals.
5. Do not combine agents that have not been tested together.

**14. When should a systemic antibiotic be added to the treatment regimen?**
Wound experts suggest starting systemic antibiotics when a local infection spreads past the wound margin or if bone can be palpated or is exposed in the wound bed.

**15. Are topical enzymes or growth factors helpful in wound infection?**
No. Enzymes and growth factors should not be applied to infected wounds. Many clinicians assess for high levels of wound bioburden and then treat to reduce the number of bacteria before applying these agents.

## BIBLIOGRAPHY

1. Burrell RE, Heggers JP, Davis GJ, Wright JB: Efficacy of silver-coated dressings as bacterial barriers in a rodent burn sepsis model. Wounds 11(4):64–71, 1999.
2. Feedar JA: Clinical management of chronic wounds. In McCulloch JM, Kloth LC, Feedar JA (eds): Wound Healing: Alternatives in Management, 2nd ed. Philadelphia, F. A. Davis , 1995, pp 137–185.
3. Ovington LG: Nanocrystalline silver: Where the old and familiar meets a new frontier. Wounds 13(Suppl B):5–10, 2001.
4. Sibbald RG, Cameron J: Dermatological aspects of wound care. In Krasner DL, Rodeheaver GT, Sibbald RG (eds): Chronic Wound Care: A Clinical Source Book for Healthcare Professionals, 3rd ed. Wayne PA, HMP Communications, 2001, pp 273–285.
5. Voigt DW, Paul CN: The use of Acticoat as silver impregnated telfa dressings in a regional burn and wound care center: The clinician's view. Wounds 13(2 Suppl B):11–20, 2001.
6. Wright JB, Hansen DL, Burrell RE: The comparative efficacy of two antimicrobial barrier dressings: In-vitro examination of two controlled release silver dressings. Wounds 10(6):179–188, 1998.

# 18. ULTRAVIOLET C IN THE MANAGEMENT OF WOUND INFECTIONS

*Teresa A. Conner-Kerr, PhD, PT, CWS(D)*

### 1. Define ultraviolet (UV) radiation.

UV radiation or energy is a form of radiant energy that falls between x-rays and visible light in the 100- to 400-nm region of the electromagnetic spectrum. UV is commonly divided into three distinct bands: the region between 320 and 400 nm is designated as UVA, the region between 280 and 320 as UVB, and the region between 100 and 280 nm as UVC.

### 2. Is this the same type of radiation that people should avoid by using sun-screen?

The bands of UV radiation that are targeted with sunscreens are UVA and UVB. In fact, UVB is known as sunburn radiation and is thought to mediate most of the harmful effects of sunlight on human skin, including photoaging and carcinogenesis. On the other hand, UVC is effectively screened out by the ozone layer and does not reach the earth's surface.

### 3. Are short exposure times to UVC related to carcinogenesis?

The answer is not definitively known. The information available about the carcinogenic potential of UV is related to long- term exposure predominantly to UVB. Because UVC treatment involves extremely short exposure times (seconds) compared with the life-long exposure that is linked with skin cancers and because it is also targeted at subepidermal tissues, the risk is thought to be minimal for the induction of skin cancers. Furthermore, the periwound skin can be effectively screened from UVC exposure by applying ointments such as petrolatum or zinc or by using precisely cut drapes. Additional safety evidence comes from the differential sensitivity of eucaryotes (fungus, mammalian cells) compared with procaryotes (bacteria) to the detrimental effects of UVC. Treatment times that are highly effective at killing procaryotes such as bacteria are much less than those required for killing eucaryotes.

### 4. How does UVC work?

The killing effects of UVC are mediated by the induction of detrimental changes in cellular DNA through the interruption of thymine dimers.

### 5. Is UVC equally effective in killing both gram-negative and gram-positive organisms?

Yes. Both gram-positive and gram-negative bacteria tested in vitro demonstrated a 99.99% kill rate with only 5 seconds of UVC exposure. In addition, UVC treatment eradicated the methicillin-resistant form of the gram-positive bacteria, *Staphylococcus aureus*, in an animal model as well as significantly decreased the numbers of bacterial species (methicillin-resistant *S. aureus* [MRSA]) in chronic wounds during a clinical study.

### 6. Can this treatment be used with yeast and fungus?

Yes. An in vitro study using optimal growing conditions for both the common yeast, *Candida albicans,* and the fungus, *Aspergillus fumigatus*, demonstrated that short treatment times with UVC was effective in eradicating both pathogens. A 99.9% kill rate of *C. albicans* and *A. fumigatus* was detected at 15 and 30 seconds, respectively. In addition, testing of mixed cultures (fungus, yeast, and bacteria grown together) demonstrated an increasing sensitivity of the fungus, *A. fumigatus*, to UVC. Therefore, since most wound beds contain mixed flora, UVC may be even more effective in mixed culture conditions compared with pure isolates in vitro.

In a recent case study, UVC was effective in lowering skin surface numbers of *C. albicans* when applied for short treatment times once daily for 4 days. The skin surface was treated for 60 seconds on days 1 and 2 and then again for 30 seconds on days 3 and 4. The surface numbers decreased from $2.6 \times 10^6$ to undetectable levels after 4 days of treatment. Other case studies have demonstrated similar results but documented changes only in clinical symptoms.

### 7. Does UVC kill MRSA and other antibiotic-resistant bacteria?

Yes. Short exposure times have been shown to be effective in both in vitro and in vivo testing. Under optimal conditions in the laboratory setting, 99.99% of MRSA is killed by 5 seconds of exposure to UVC. Likewise, MRSA was totally eradicated in an infected animal model after 1 week of daily UVC treatments for 30 seconds. In this study, intratissue levels of MRSA decreased from $> 10^5$ to undetectable levels after treatment with UVC. A recent clinical study of 12 chronic ulcers demonstrated that UVC (more than two clinical applications) significantly decreased the numbers of MRSA in the wound beds with a treatment time of 180 seconds/exposure.

### 8. How long should an infected wound be treated?

As with any modality, treatment should be discontinued if no improvement is documented within a reasonable time. Because of the seriousness of infection, treatment should be discontinued if there is an escalation in pathogen numbers or dissemination of infection to adjacent tissues. Changes in wound size due to enhanced autolytic debridement and sloughing of necrosis should not be mistaken for increased levels of infection. Wound cultures before treatment and at selected intervals (~3 days) during treatment are recommended.

### 9. What are the contraindications to application of UVC?

- Diabetes
- Pulmonary tuberculosis
- Hyperthyroidism
- Systemic lupus erythematosus
- Cardiac, renal, and hepatic disease
- Acute eczema or psoriasis
- Herpes simplex

### 10. Are there any adverse effects to the application of UVC?

UVC treatment should be discontinued if severe pain, itching, or burning is reported. If excessive drying or burning of the tissue has occurred, hydrogel wound dressings or other products that have been shown to decrease burn wound pain are recommended.

### 11. How is UVC applied?

UVC is applied via a small hand-held device. The standard application method includes protection of periwound skin with drape or UVC-resistant ointment, limitation of treatment area overlap, and 1-inch spacing of the lamp from the highest point of the wound bed. Several devices are on the market. One is outfitted with a spacer bar that ensures a 1-inch placement from the wound surface. The benefit of this design includes reproducibility for lamp placement and prevention of the lamp from touching the wound bed. However, a drawback of this system is the possibility of client cross-contamination if the spacer bars are not adequately cleaned. Other lamps on the market can be fitted with a 1- inch space bar by simply taping sterile 1-inch sections of cotton swabs or tongue depressors (smooth edge down, of course) on the lamp base. These spacers can then be disposed of after treatment.

### 12. What are the treatment times for application of UVC?

In vitro and in vivo work indicates that 30-second treatments once daily are adequate for bacterial infection. However, a recent clinical study demonstrated significant decreases in MRSA in chronic wound beds only after more than two UVC applications with an exposure time of 180 seconds.

Although dose-response studies need to be performed to determine the optimal dose for microorganism reduction with sparing of the wound bed tissue, the above studies provide a framework that suggests that short treatment times (30–180 seconds for several sessions) are effective at reducing bacterial numbers.

In addition, in vitro studies indicate that eucaryotic organisms such as yeast and fungi are more resistant to UVC. As a result, treatment times greater than the above range and number of exposures described for bacterial pathogens may be necessary for reduction of yeast or fungi (see question 6).

### 13. Does UVC penetrate thin film dressings?

No. Using an in vitro assay, two representative plain film dressings were tested for UVC penetrability via a bioassay. Blood agar plates were inoculated with bacteria and then covered with a thin film dressing. UVC exposure times as long as 180 seconds resulted in no bacterial killing.

### 14. Should the periwound skin be treated with UVC?

This question and can be argued both ways—yes and no. If the periwound is infection-free and the tissue is healthy, it should be protected from UVC overexposure. Early information in an animal model suggests that the periwound skin can benefit from UVC because the epithelial edges progress in a more organized manner and with less rolling when treated. However, this issue requires further study.

If the periwound skin is infected, UVC can be used to reduce the bioburden so that the wound is not continually inoculated with high numbers of organisms. Case studies have demonstrated the efficacy of UVC in reducing skin infections.

### 15. How is the periwound skin protected?

The periwound tissue or skin can be protected by using a sterile drape or by coating the skin with a UV-blocking agent such as petrolatum or zinc oxide. The clinician should be careful to prevent petrolatum or zinc oxide from getting into the wound bed. Any residual ointment that remains can be left in place on the periwound skin or removed. Because of their multiple ingredients and potential for irritation, sunscreens are not recommended for use on the periwound skin.

### BIBLIOGRAPHY

1. Conner-Kerr TA, Sullivan PK, Gaillard J, et al: The effects of ultraviolet radiation on antibiotic-resistant bacteria in vitro. Ostomy Wound Manage 44(10):50–56, 1998.
2. Conner-Kerr TA, Sullivan PK, Keegan A, et al: UVC reduces antibiotic resistant bacterial numbers in living tissue. Ostomy Wound Managet 45(4):84, 1999.
3. Harm W: UV carcinogenesis. In Harm W (ed): Biological Effects of Ultraviolet Radiation. New York, Cambridge University Press, 1980, p 191.
4. Licht S: History of ultraviolet light therapy. In Licht S (ed): Therapeutic Electricity and Ultraviolet Radiation, 2nd ed. New Haven, CT, Elizabeth Licht, 1967, pp 191–212.
5. Licht S: History of ultraviolet therapy. In Stillwell GK (ed): Therapeutic Electricity and Ultraviolet Radiation, 3rd ed. Baltimore, Williams & Wilkins, 1983, pp 228–261.
6. Moseley H: Photomedicine. In Moseley H (ed): Non-ionising Radiation: Microwaves, Ultraviolet and Laser Radiation. Philadelphia, IOP Publishing, 1988, pp 155–182.
7. Moseley H: Sources of ultraviolet radiation. In Moseley H (ed): Non-ionising Radiation: Microwaves, Ultraviolet and Laser Radiation. Philadelphia, IOP Publishing, 1988, p 110.
8. Scott BO: Clinical uses of ultraviolet radiation. In Stillwell GK (ed): Therapeutic Electricity and Ultraviolet Radiation, 3rd ed. Baltimore, Williams & Wilkins, 1983, pp 228–261.
9. Stenback F: Health hazards from ultraviolet radiation. Public Health Rev 10:229, 1982.
10. Sullivan PK, Conner-Kerr TA, Smith ST: The effects of UVC irradiation on group A Streptococcus in vitro. Ostomy Wound Manage45(10):50–58, 1999.
11. Sullivan PK, Conner-Kerr TA: Effects of UVC irradiation on prokaryotic and eucaryotic wound pathogens. Ostomy Wound Manage 46(10):28–34, 2000.
12. Taylor GJS, Bannister GC, Leeming JP: Wound disinfection with ultraviolet radiation. J Hosp Infect 30:85–93, 1995.
13. Thai TP, Houghton PE, Keast DH, et al: Effects of ultraviolet light C on the bacterial burden in chronic ulcers. Ostomy/Wound Manage 47(11):51, 2001.
14. Weisberg J: Ultraviolet irradiation. In Hecox B, Mehreteab TA, Weisberg J (eds): Physical Agents: A Comprehensive Text for Physical Therapists. Norwalk, CT, Appleton & Lange, 1994, pp 377–378.

# 19. SYSTEMIC MEDICATIONS FOR INFECTIOUS WOUNDS

*Robert Charles Franklin, MD, and Mary Ellen Franklin, PT, EdD*

**1. What kinds of acute wounds are likely to develop infection? When are prophylactic antibiotics helpful for the prevention of infection?**

Initial and subsequent evaluation of a wound always includes an analysis of the risk of infection. Certain wounds are more prone to infection than others, and such wounds require prophylactic antibiotics. Any type of crush injury with extensive tissue injury and necrosis has an increased tendency for infection and usually requires parenteral antibiotics. Bite injury wounds also fall into this category. If exogenous debris, such as dirt, oil, or animal hair, is observed in a wound, antibiotic therapy is usually indicated, even if the debris has been removed.

Other wounds at high risk for infection include wounds with erythema > 2 cm in diameter, wounds with purulent material, wounds larger than 5 cm, underwater injuries, extremity injuries, gunshot wounds, and injuries in immunocompromised patients. Immunocompromised patients include patients with HIV infection, diabetes mellitus, or neutropenia and patients undergoing chemotherapy or corticosteroid therapy. Wounds complicated by fractures, ligamentous injury, or cartilaginous injury are usually treated with parenteral antibiotics. With more severe injuries, such as those that penetrate the pleural space, peritoneum, cranium, or any other vital organ, hospitalization and intravenous antibiotics are required.

**2. What types of prophylactic antibiotics are used for acute wounds? What pathogens should they cover?**

Amoxicillin/clavulanic acid (Augmentin) every 12 hours by mouth with food is adequate coverage for most wounds. Cephalosporins and clindamycin should be considered for patients who are allergic to penicillin. The more common pathogens that tend to infect wounds are *Staphylococcus aureus* and group A streptococci. Because *Pseudomonas* spp. have a high predilection for puncture wounds of the foot, ciprofloxacin is indicated. Ciprofloxacin also covers *Aeromonas hydrophilia*, a common pathogen in fresh water injuries, and *Vibrio vulnificus*, a pathogen in saltwater injuries. Guidelines for antibiotic usage can change rapidly. Consultation with a well known reference, such as the *Sanford Guide to Antimicrobial Therapy* or an infectious disease specialist, is often helpful.

**3. When acute wounds become infected, which antibiotics are used?**

Antibiotic selections should be based on the clinical exam and wound culture. Wound culture results may take several days to complete, but empirical antibiotic therapy should be started immediately after the Gram stain has been reviewed. When wound culture results are available, an antibiotic change may be necessary. If the patient is septic, blood cultures should be done and intravenous antibiotics given.

**4. How do you determine what tetanus prophylaxis is needed for a wound?**

First determine whether the patient has received the primary immunization series. Most patients receive tetanus immunization before starting elementary school—diphtheria, pertussis, tetanus (DPT) series. Next, determine whether the wound is at high risk for tetanus. Examples include wounds older than 6 hours or > 1 cm deep, wounds contaminated with foreign material, and wounds already showing evidence of necrotic tissue or infection.

If the patient has never completed the primary immunization series, tetanus toxoid plus tetanus immune globulin (TIG) should be given. For patients who have completed the primary immunization series and have sustained a tetanus-prone wound, tetanus toxoid is required unless they have had a booster within 5 years. If, however, the wound is not tetanus-prone, patients do not need a tetanus toxoid unless they have not had a booster in the past 10 years.

### 5. Which animals present a risk for rabies and what prophylaxis is needed?

The raccoon, bat, skunk, and fox present the highest risk for rabies after a bite wound. In fact, however, any unprovoked animal attack should be considered at risk for rabies. For domestic animal bites in which the risk of infection is low, the animal may be closely watched for 10 days to see whether it develops any signs or symptoms before prophylaxis is considered. If the vaccination status of the animal is unknown and the animal cannot be observed or tested for rabies, treatment with the rabies vaccination and passive immunization with immune globulin is needed. Remember that most people who get rabies from bats do not get the infection from bites; they get it from scratches, abrasions, or inhalation of the aerosolized virus.

### 6. What pathophysiologic conditions increase the vulnerability of diabetic patients to foot infections?

The combination of neuropathy, peripheral artery disease, and altered immune response is responsible for the increased incidence of foot infection. The poor immune response is multifactorial and not well understood, but there appears to be impairment of the polymorphonuclear leukocyte in the form of deficient chemotaxis, adherence, and phagocytosis.

### 7. In diabetic foot ulceration, what are the involved pathogens?

Most ulcerations have aerobic gram-positive cocci such as *S. aureus* or streptococci. Less commonly, aerobic gram-negative bacillus such as *Escherichia coli* or *Klebsiella* spp. may occur. Anaerobic infection must also be considered. More severe infections may have a polymicrobial etiology. Enterococci typically are found in 30% of all wound cultures, but they rarely are found as an isolated pathogen.

### 8. What antibiotics are used for diabetic foot ulcers?

Antibiotic selection is based on whether the ulcer is limb-threatening or non–limb-threatening. Most ulcerations are non–limb-threatening when the erythema is confined to a diameter of 2 cm or less from the edge of the ulcer and fever and significant necrotic tissue are absent. For such infections, a first-generation cephalosporin such as cephalexin (Keflex) or amoxicillin/clavulanic acid (Augmentin) may be used.

If the ulceration is limb-threatening with extensive erythema, necrotic tissue, full-thickness ulceration, abscess formation, bone involvement. or fever, more aggressive antibiotic therapy is indicated. For such infections, intravenous medication such as ciprofloxin (Cipro) or ofloxacin (Floxin) may be used in combination of clindamycin. In this case, clindamycin adds coverage for anaerobic infection. Other antibiotics such as ampicillin/sulbactam (Unasyn), ticarcillin/clavulanic acid (Timentin), or cefoxitin (Mefoxin) also may be used.

### 9. What is the role of antibiotics in the treatment of pressure ulcers?

Parenteral antibiotics have only a limited role in the treatment of decubitus ulcers. Even though most wound cultures show polymicrobial growth, antibiotics should be used only in patients with clinical evidence of infection, such as cellulitis or sepsis.

### 10. What systemic agents have been found to improve healing in venous ulcers?

Generally, infection is not a problem with venous ulcers. Other systemic agents that have proved somewhat useful in healing for venous ulcers include pentoxifyllin (Trental). In some studies, pentoxifyllin was found to improve healing time by 30%. This agent increases red blood cell deformity and therefore may improve perfusion to the tissues.

## BIBLIOGRAPHY

1. Bello YM, Phillips TJ: Recent advances in wound healing. JAMA 283:716–718, 2000.
2. Bunzli WF, Wright DH, Hoang AD, et al: Reviews of therapeutics: Current management of human bites. Pharmacotherapy 18:227–234, 1998.
3. Caputo GM, Joshi N, Weitekamp MR: Foot infections in patients with diabetes. Am Fam Physician 56:195–202, 1997.
4. Demling RH, DeSanti L: Management of partial thickness facial burns (comparison of topical antibiotics and bio-engineered skin substitutes). Burns 25:256–261, 1999.
5. Eaglstein WH, Falanga V: Chronic wounds. Surg Clin North Am 77:689–700, 1997.
6. Eron LJ: Antimicrobial wound management in the emergency department: An educational supplement. J Emerg Med 17:189–195, 1999.
7. Gilbert DN, Moellering RC, Sande MA: The Sanford Guide to Antimicrobial Therapy, 3rd ed. Hyde Park, VT, Jeb Sanford Publishing, Antimicrobial Therapy Inc., 2001.
8. Goodman CM, Cohen V, Armenta A, et al: Evaluation of results and treatment variables for pressure ulcers in 48 veteran spinal cord-injured patients. Ann Plast Surg 42:665–672, 1999.
9. Hansraj KK, Weaver LD, Todd AO, et al: Efficacy of ceftriaxone versus cefazolin in the prophylactic management of extra-articular cortical violation of bone due to low-velocity gunshot wounds. Orthop Clin North Am 26:9–17, 1995.
10. Hiatt WR: Contemporary treatment of venous lower limb ulcers. Angiology 43:852–855, 1992.
11. Presutti RJ: Bite wounds: Early treatment and prophylaxis against infectious complications. Postgrad Med 101(4):245–254, 1997.
12. Steed DL: Foundations of good ulcer care. Am J Surg 176(Suppl 2A):20S–25S, 1998.

# 20. DIAGNOSIS AND MANAGEMENT OF OSTEOMYELITIS

Jeffrey C. Karr, DPM, ACCPPS, CWS

### 1. Define osteomyelitis.

Osteomyelitis is defined, in general, as an infective inflammatory process of bone involving the cortex and cancellous portions. Osteitis refers only to the cortical involvement. The source of osteomyelitis is classified as either (1) spread to the bone from a source through the blood stream (hematogenous) or (2) spread to the bone from a source in nearby tissue (contiguous focus).

### 2. How is osteomyelitis classified?

The Cierny-Mader classification system takes into consideration the anatomic extent of bone involvement, the quality of the host, and treatment factors. It has been used as a staging system to describe extent and severity of osteomyelitis and compare effectiveness of treatment protocols.

*Cierny-Mader Classification System*

| **Anatomic Type** | | |
|---|---|---|
| STAGE | NAME | DESCRIPTION |
| Stage 1 | Medullary osteomyelitis | Confined to medullary canal |
| | | No cortical involvement |
| | | Results from hematogenous infection |
| | | Treated with antibiotics alone (children) or cortical unroofing and medullary reaming (adults) |
| Stage 2 | Superficial osteomyelitis | Exposed, necrotic outer surface of the bone |
| | | Results from adjacent soft tissue infection |
| | | Requires superficial debridement and coverage with local flap |
| Stage 3 | Localized osteomyelitis | Full-thickness cortical sequestration |
| | | Requires surgical debridement, possibly bone graft |
| Stage 4 | Diffuse osteomyelitis | Involves cortical bone at multiple cortices |
| | | Loss of bony stability |
| | | Requires debridement, stabilization, flap |
| **Host Type** | | |
| CATEGORY | DESCRIPTION | |
| Host A | Normal host with normal immunologic defenses, metabolic function, vascularity | |
| Host B | Host with local compromise | |
| | Venous stasis, lymphedema, major vessel compromise | |
| | Arteritis, radiation fibrosis, small vessel disease | |
| Host C | Host with systemic compromise | |
| | Malnutrition, diabetes; renal, liver, or immune disease | |
| | Malignancy, chronic hypoxia | |
| | Treatment of bone infection poses a greater risk than the disease | |

### 3. Describe the clinical staging of osteomyelitis according to the Cierny-Mader classification system.

The A host demonstrates normal systemic defenses, metabolic capacities, and vascularity. The B host demonstrates local, system, or combined deficiencies. The C host demonstrates high treatment morbidity; the treatment poses a greater risk to the patient than the disease process.

**4. Describe the four anatomic types of osteomyelitis according to the Cierny-Mader classification system.**

Stage one osteomyelitis is confined to the medullary canal without cortical involvement. Stage two osteomyelitis (osteitis) is confined to the cortical bone with no medullary involvement. Stage three osteomyelitis involves the cortical bone at one cortex as well as medullary bone; it is the most commonly encountered type of osteomyelitis. Stage four osteomyelitis involves the cortical bone at multiple cortices and the medullary bone as well.

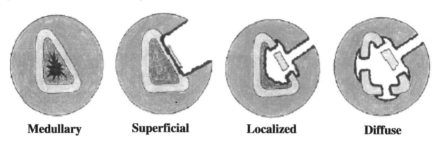

| **Medullary** | **Superficial** | **Localized** | **Diffuse** |

Anatomic classification of osteomyelitis.

**5. What wounds are suspicious for osteomyelitis?**

Suspicious wounds include those that probe to the bone, joint, or deep fascial compartments. In general, any wound in close proximity to bone and over 6 months duration should be suspect. When a history of a wound that heals and then opens again is preceded by an episode of extreme warmth and abscess formation, osteomyelitis should be suspected.

**6. What are the causative agents of osteomyelitis?**

**Bacteria.** The most common bacterial pathogen is *Staphylococcus aureus*. Other infective bacterial pathogens include *Staphylococcus epidermidis* and streptococci. These bacterial pathogens account for up to 73% of the cases of osteomyelitis diagnosed after musculoskeletal surgery. *S. epidermidis* has been more frequently the causative pathogen of osteomyelitis after implant arthroplasty. Diabetic patients, especially those with vascular disease, have a mixed polymicrobial infection of gram-positive and gram-negative bacteria. *Salmonella* species has a higher incidence in patients with sickle cell disease or other hemoglobinopathies. *Pseudomonas* species and other gram-negative bacteria have a higher incidence in drug addicts.

**Fungi.** Fungi involved in osteomyelitis include *Blastomyces, Cryptococcus*, and *Coccidioides* species. These pathogens usually occur in noncompromised hosts. Fungi pathogens that may be seen in compromised hosts include *Aspergillus* and *Candida* species. Fungal osteomyelitis may be rather recalcitrant to therapy and may require amputation of the affected body part.

**Mycobacteria.** Tuberculosis osteomyelitis is seen usually in the bacteremic phase of the mycobacterial infection and is generated by hematogenous spread. This type of osteomyelitis occurs in approximately 1% of patients with tuberculosis. Mycobacterial infection has a higher incidence in patients with renal transplant.Although it may occur at any age, it is seen most frequently in adults. Negative purified protein derivative (PPD) skin tests do not exclude the diagnosis. Patients generally respond well to oral therapy.

**7. What are the common bacterial pathogens in osteomyelitis due to a puncture wound?**

*Pseudomonas aeruginosa*, followed by *P. multocida* and other gram-negative rods. *P. aeruginosa* osteomyelitis secondary to puncture wounds is not uncommon. *P. aeruginosa* is inoculated in 2% of all puncture wounds and is the causative agent in 90% of cases. The phalanges, metatarsals, and calcaneus are the most commonly involved bones of the feet. Therapy for *P. aeruginosa* osteomyelitis includes surgical debridement and a minimum of 14 days of appropriate antibiotics.

8. **What are the two most common bacterial pathogens of neonatal osteomyelitis due to a puncture wound (e.g., repeated heel punctures for phlebotomy)?**

*S. aureus* and *P. aeruginosa.*

9. **Discuss the clinical findings of mycetoma in soft tissue wounds. How does this condition relate to outcome of osteomyelitis treatment?**

Mycetoma is a chronic infection of soft tissue structures and bone that is characterized by drainage from multiple sinus tracts of pus containing mycotic granules with an indurated swelling of the affected area. Treatment of mycetoma is difficult , and medical cure is rarely obtained. Men aged 20–40 years are more frequently involved than women. The lower extremities are involved in 56–70% of the patients. The most common site is the dorsum of the forefoot. Treatment with iatroconazole has been promising. Diagnosis is made by the clinical triad of mycotic granules, sinus tracts, and bacterial and fungal cultures. Surgical debridement alone is rarely curative. Treatment of mycetoma is difficult, and eventually amputation may be required.

10. **Discuss the cause and clinical findings of hematogenous osteomyelitis.**

Hematogenous osteomyelitis is the spread of bacteria from an internal source, such as an upper respiratory infection, through the circulation to an osseous location where bacteria reproduce and lead to an infective process. Hematogenous osteomyelitis is most commonly a disease of children. Other sources include colonized intravenous devices and dental and urinary tract infections. Foot involvement is rather uncommon compared with other sites. Foot bones are involved in 5–11% of children and 8% of adults. The most commonly affected foot bone is the calcaneus, followed by the metatarsal, tarsal bones, talus, and phalanges. *S. aureus* is the most common pathogen in children and adults, occurring in 60% of patients. Gram-negative rods are seen more commonly in adults. Polymicrobial infection is uncommon. Fungi and mycobacteria are also spread by dissemination with hematogenous osteomyelitis.

Classically, acute hematogenous osteomyelitis in a child presents with abrupt onset of high fever, sudden pain, systemic toxicity, and local signs of infection and suppuration along the affected bone. The presentation in adults is less definitive. Leukocytosis and elevated sedimentation rate are common.

11. **Discuss the cause and clinical findings of contiguous focus osteomyelitis.**

Contiguous focus osteomyelitis is the result of the spread of infection from an adjacent soft tissue focus. Commonly this focus is a wound, laceration, abscess, open reduction of a compound fracture, postoperative infection, or septic joint. Contiguous focus osteomyelitis is usually seen in adults over the age of 50. The phalanges and metatarsals are most commonly involved. The most common pathogen is *S. aureus*, but frequently a polymicrobial infection is encountered. Other pathogens encountered include *S. epidermidis*, gram-negative rods, and anaerobes.

Contiguous focus osteomyelitis in this age group usually coexists with significant comorbidities that must be considered in assessing possible outcomes. The more significant comorbidities include diabetes, vascular disease, hypertension, coronary vascular disease, hyperlipidemia, renal disease, venous insufficiency, and autoimmune disease. Osteomyelitis in conjunction with vascular insufficiency often occurs in diabetic patients. Patients with tobacco usage alone have higher rates of significant morbidity for wound/bone complications and limb loss.

12. **Describe the mechanism of development of osteomyelitis in the diabetic foot.**

Foot osteomyelitis typically develops by spread of infection in the patient with underlying polyneuropathies. The insensate foot receives increased repetitive microtrauma at high axial load areas, such as bony prominences. This process leads to localized tissue necrosis and ulcer formation. Diabetic patients usually have some degree of proximal arterial vascular disease. At times, proximal vascular disease can be segmental with high-grade stenosis or occlusions that severely impair the body's ability to heal this type of neuropathic ulceration. Uncontrolled hyperglycemia, especially in brittle diabetes, decreases the immune capacity to fight infection. Trauma, ulceration, and bacterial invasion, therefore, precede the development of osteomyelitis. This sequela leads to chronic ulcer formation with a bacterial load that colonizes and eventually infects the neighboring bone (contiguous focus). Underlying osteomyelitis is present in as many as two-thirds of patients hospitalized with a diabetic foot ulcer.

### 13. How can osteomyelitis develop in nonhealing wounds other than the foot?

In contiguous focus osteomyelitis, any deep soft tissue wound infection adjacent to bone can be the source of osteomyelitis. Bacteria from necrotic tissue, as seen with a stage IV pressure ulcer or non-stageable mal perforans ulcer, can invade the outer surface of bone. Wounds on the pretibial surface of the leg can quickly expose the bone to the environment and initiate the osteomyelitis process. The pretibial surface of the leg is rather dysvascular and has a thinner tissue depth than the other leg compartments.

### 14. Are blood cultures helpful in the diagnosis of osteomyelitis?

Blood cultures may be positive up to 60% of patients with acute hematogenous osteomyelitis. Blood cultures are rarely positive in other forms of osteomyelitis. A negative blood culture cannot prove that osteomyelitis is absent. To obtain an accurate sampling of the pathogen, a bone biopsy or deep aspirate is usually required. Blood cultures may be useful in reflecting the potential source of bone pathogens from origins such as urinary or upper respiratory tract infections.

### 15. Are radiographic findings helpful in the diagnosis of osteomyelitis?

Soft tissue swelling, subperiosteal elevation, and lytic/sclerotic changes of bone are the classic radiographic findings of osteomyelitis. Bone changes are usually not evident for 10–14 days or until 35–50% of the bone has been destroyed. Sequestrum, the segmentation of dead bone from living bone, is highly suggestive of chronic osteomyelitis. Sequestrum appears on x-rays as more dense than surrounding bone, which may be osteoporotic or hyperemic. It is usually not present for at least 3 weeks. Sequestrum findings on x-rays mimic the findings of osteoarthropathy (Charcot deformity) in diabetic patients. Involucrum or new bone formation at the periosteum is suggestive of osteomyelitis. Cloaca formation is found at the bone–periosteum interface from extrusion of sequestrum and dead bone products.

### 16. Discuss the differences between hematogenous and contiguous osteomyelitis on radiologic evaluation?

Initial findings of **hematogenous osteomyelitis** initially are limited to swelling of the soft tissue over the metaphysis. The first radiographic findings are one or more lytic areas surrounded by a wide area of radiolucency. This finding is followed by periosteal elevation with cortex that takes on a moth-eaten appearance. Radiographic evidence of subacute or chronic hematogenous osteomyelitis (i.e., Brodie's abscess) is a radiolucent area in the metaphysic surrounded by sclerotic or hypertrophic bone.

The radiographic features of **contiguous focus osteomyelitis** are bone destruction and reabsorption at the area of adjacent soft tissue focus. Bone involvement begins in the outer bone cortex and periosteum. Cortical and cancellous involvement follows the reverse of hematogenous osteomyelitis.

Radiographic findings of an infected arthroplasty are a progressively enlarging radiolucent zone at the bone–prosthesis interface, endosteal scalloping, and focal lytic areas. Sequential radiographic studies are always useful in the evaluation of either type of osteomyelitis.

### 17. What is the limitation of radiographic evaluation in osteomyelitis?

Findings consistent with osteomyelitis may not be evident for at least 10 days and may lag weeks behind the clinical presentation, because 50% of the bone matrix must be destroyed before lytic lesions are seen. Radiographic lytic lesions are seen 3–4 weeks after onset of symptoms in 90% of patients.

Initial radiographic findings of osteomyelitis, when present, are often vague and inconclusive. A periosteal elevation of a metatarsal may be the start of the infective process or an old stress fracture with exocallous bone. Wounds or nonstageable eschar at the posterior and plantar aspect of the heel with suspicious calcaneal cortical bone findings may be misleading. This type of calcaneal finding may represent an early infective process or the normal irregular cortical surface seen with the posterior calcaneus. A periosteal elevation of the tibia or fibula may represent an early infective process or normal findings associated with chronic venous insufficiency. The radiographic findings of osteoarthropathy (Charcot deformity) and atrophic or hypertrophic nonunions of the foot, ankle, and knee are usually the same as those seen with osteomyelitis. To confuse matters further, magnetic resonance imaging has similar pitfalls, and nuclear imaging is usually required. Reabsorptive or destructive changes to bone may be noted in such disorders as rheumatoid arthritis or gout.

**18. Describe the advantages and disadvantages of bone scan evaluation of osteomyelitis.**

A technetium bone scan is more sensitive than plain film imaging in detecting early infections and may be positive as early as 3 days after infection. Bone scans can clarify and distinguish osteomyelitis from a healed, old fracture with bone callus; irregular, chronic bone changes; periosteal reactions from venous insufficiency; and Charcot deformity. Indium-111 white blood cell scanning is useful in the early detection of osteomyelitis. In Charcot deformity, dual nuclear imaging scans are performed using technetium sulfur colloid and an indium-111–labeled white blood cell study.

Bone scans, in general, are sensitive for bone turnover but are generally not specific for osteomyelitis. There is a high incidence of false-positive nuclear medicine studies. These studies are less sensitive when contiguous foci or soft tissue infection is present. Gallium scans are less sensitive and also lack specificity in the presence of soft tissue infections.

**19. How is osteomyelitis treated?**

The treatment of osteomyelitis is controversial. Osteomyelitis is treated most effectively by surgical removal of infected bone. Debridement should remove infected bone back to solid bleeding bone. Dead space management is addressed with polymethylmethacrylate (PMMA) beads. Once the infected bone is removed, antibiotics are required only for control of infection in surrounding soft tissues.

If the patient is not a candidate for surgical bone debridement and/or resection, prolonged intravenous antibiotic therapy based on reliable culture methods and bone penetration ability of the antibiotic agent is started. Recent literature suggests that long-term oral therapy with high doses can be as effective as intravenous therapy for diabetic patients with osteomyelitis.

If a large dead space results from debridement with significant soft tissue deficit, a flap or graft placement may be indicated for closure. Patients that do not undergo a strict smoking cessation program have a high morbidity rate for treatment failure.

After treatment of infection, methods for healing a wound with osteomyelitis follow general wound-healing guidelines.

**20. Discuss the limitations of basing antibiotic therapy for osteomyelitis on sinus tract or wound culture.**

Less than 50% of the sinus tract or wound cultures contain the same pathogen as the infected bone. Culture of a sinus tract often provides a polymicrobial list that may not identify the true osteomyelitis pathogen or include other pathogens that are localized to the soft tissue but not the bone. If *S. aureus* is present, it usually can be assumed to be the causative pathogen of osteomyelitis. Bone biopsy or aspiration, when indicated, results in a reliable culture of the involved pathogen if properly done. Different pathogens may grow in isolated microenvironments within the bone. Therefore, there is a high probability that a needle biopsy will miss some of these microenvironments. The risk of potentially contaminating uninvolved bone must be considered before proceeding with a bone biopsy for pathogen identification.

**21. How do antibiotic-impregnated PMMA beads help?**

PMMA beads manage osseous dead space, reduce the incidence of secondary infections, and provide high local antibiotic concentration (10–100 times higher) without serious systemic effects. Gentamicin and tobramycin are commonly used. Other antibiotics that can be used are clindamycin and vancomycin. The antibiotic is released at bacteriocidal concentrations at the site of infection with only trace amounts detectable in the circulation. The antibiotic has been measured to diffuse up to 2 cm around the area of implantation. At levels 10–100 times greater, such antibiotics may be bacteriocidal against pathogens that were previously assessed as resistant in the routine antibiogram. The implantation of the beads allows primary closure when possible. In vitro studies demonstrated that fibroblast function is not inhibited with the high concentration of gentamicin from the PMMA beads.

**22. Explain why, even with appropriate wound care, a wound in an area of osteomyelitis may not heal or remain healed for a prolonged period if the osteomyelitis is not directly managed.**

The wound continues to be seeded by etiologic agents and will not close or stay closed if continually seeded from the neighboring bone. When a sinus tract is present, the pustular product of the deep bone infection maintains this structure. At times the lining of the sinus tract may become ep- ithelialized and remain open. A chronic sinus tract may result in a malignant neoplasm, which in turn maintains the sinus tract.

### 23. Bone osteitis (infection) refers to which stage of the Cierny-Mader anatomic classification system?

Bone osteitis in an infective process is localized to the cortex and thus is classified as stage 2. This infective process does not involve the cancellous or medullary bone. However, it can quickly progress and soon involve the cancellous bone, progressing to stage 3 osteomyelitis. Stage 3 os- teomyelitis is rather amenable to bone debridement and PMMA bead placement with good outcome and low rates of recurrence.

### 24. Which Cierny-Mader anatomic type is the most unstable and may require multiplane ex- ternal fixation, such as the Ilizerov system?

Stage 4 osteomyelitis that is the most unstable. It osteomyelitis may present as chronic os- teomyelitis with several draining sinus tract. Axial limb deviation may be present as a result of pre- vious trauma, such as an open compound fracture. This type of osteomyelitis, once debrided or partially excised, has a significant morbidity rate for fracture or dislocation because of the amount of bone substance removed. Once fractured, the bone is usually not amenable to open reduction and in- ternal fixation because of soft diseased bone and gross instability and requires below- or above-knee amputation. Closed treatment, such as casting and immobilization, generally yields poor results with a high incidence of nonunion, nonfunctional limb, significant pain, and recurrent osteomyelitis.

### 25. Discuss the advantages of tissue grafting for wound management in osteomyelitis.

The purpose of local muscle and free vascular transfers is to provide a soft tissue envelope, to cover large exposed osseous defects, and to improve the local biologic environment by bringing in a new source of blood supply for antibiotic delivery, improved host defense mechanisms, and promo- tion of soft tissue healing. Skin grafting is advantageous in patients with chronic soft tissue infection and a sinus tract that are responsible for recurrent infections. Viable periosteum that covers the bone or granulation tissue is mandatory to ensure graft survival.

### 26. When is hyperbaric oxygen therapy an appropriate adjunctive therapy?

Hyperbaric oxygen treatment is directed at the local hypovascularity and hypoxia associated with chronic bone and joint infections. In patients with decreased systemic blood flow, such as dia- betics, or decreased segmental blood flow, such as trauma patients, hyperbaric oxygen therapy may be beneficial (see Chapter 32).

### BIBLIOGRAPHY

1. Blaha JD: The use of antibiotic impregnated PMMA beads. Presented at the Annual Meeting of the American Academy of Orthopedic Surgery; Instructional Course Lecture, 1990, New Orleans.
2. Cierny G, Madner JT, Pennick JJ: A clinical staging for adult osteomyelitis. Contemp Orthop 10:17–37, 1985.
3. Gayle LB, Lineaweaver WC, Oliver A: Treatment of chronic osteomyelitis of the lower extremities with de- bridement and micro vascular muscle transfer. Clin Plast Surg 19:895–903, 1992.
4. Koval KJ, Meadows SE, Rosen H, et al: Posttraumatic tibial osteomyelitis: A comparison of three treatment approaches. Orthopedics 6(3):340–346, 1992.
5. Mader JT, Cripps MW, Calhoun JH: Adult posttraumtic osteomyelitis of the tibia. Clin Orthop 360:14–21, 1999.
6. Meadows SE, Zuckerman JD, Koval KJ: Posttraumatic tibial osteomyelitis: Diagnosis, classification, and treatment. Bull Hosp Joint Dis 52:11–16, 1993.
7. Patzakis MJ, Abdollahi K, Sherman PD, et al: Treatment of chronic osteomyelitis with muscle flaps. Orthop Clin North Am 24:505–509, 1993.
8. Patzakis MJ, Greene N, Holtom P, et al: Culture results in open wound treatment with muscle transfer for tibial osteomyelitis. Clin Orthop 360:66–70, 1999.
9. Patzakis MJ, Scilaris TA, Chon J, et al: Results of bone grafting for infected tibial non-union. Clin Orthop 315:192–198, 1995.
10. Seigel HJ, Patzakis MJ, Holtom PD, et al: Limb salvage for chronic tibial osteomyelitis: An outcome study. J Trauma 48:484–489, 2000.

# 21. TOPICAL DRESSINGS AND RATIONALE FOR SELECTION

*Joan Halpin-Landry*, RN, MS, CWCN

**1. What are the characteristics of the ideal wound dressing?**
The ideal dressing should maintain a moist wound environment, insulate the wound, protect the wound from external trauma and contamination, maintain an intact periwound skin, manage the wound exudate, and be free of particulate material.

**2. How many dressings are available on the market?**
Over 3,000—and increasing daily.

**3. How do you choose the right dressing for a wound?**
Dressing selection depends on several factors:
• Current characteristics of the wound.
• Goal of wound care (Is it to control drainage? promote epithelialization? debride?)
• Understanding that as wounds progress in the healing trajectory, their needs will change. Thus, a different dressing will be needed.
• Social and emotional state of the patient and caregivers. It is best to promote patient/caregiver self-care, even though it may sacrifice a week or two in healing time, by using a simple, one-step dressing rather than a complicated, four-step dressing.
• Appreciation of what the dressing is supposed to do. Although trade names of dressings are used frequently, one should group them into product categories. Understanding use, application, and contraindications by this organizational method facilitates correct selection.

**4. What is the difference between a primary dressing and a secondary dressing?**
The primary dressing is in contact with the wound. The secondary dressing covers the primary dressing.

**5. What are the most common primary dressing categories?**
• Gauze dressings
• Wet-to-dry or wet-moist saline gauze
• Alginates
• Foams
• Hydrofibers
• Hydropolymers
• Hydrocolloids
• Hydrogels
• Transparent films

## GAUZE DRESSINGS

**6. Are all gauze dressings composed of woven cotton fibers?**
No. Gauze dressings may be composed of cotton or cotton and synthetic blends. Gauze dressings may be woven or nonwoven in consistency.

**7. Are gauze dressings always sterile?**
No. They may be sterile or nonsterile and packaged as sponges, rolls, pads, ribbon or strips.

**8. For what kinds of wounds are gauze dressings appropriate?**
Gauze dressings can be used on either full-thickness or partial-thickness wounds.

**9. Why are gauze dressings used for wound care?**
Gauze dressings may be used to mechanically debride a necrotic wound, to pack a wound space, or to absorb wound exudate.

**10. What are the drawbacks to using gauze dressings?**

Gauze dressings require frequent changes, usually 2–3 times/day. They do not facilitate autolytic debridement, maintain a moist wound environment, or protect the periwound skin from maceration.

**11. Is it common for a gauze dressing to be impregnated with another substance?**

Yes. Gauze dressings may be impregnated with water, hypertonic sodium chloride, normal saline, hydrogel, or another substance.

**12. What kinds of wounds are appropriate for impregnated gauze dressings?**

Impregnated dressings are indicated for both partial- and full-thickness wounds. When gauze contains an additional ingredient, it is classified in that particular product category and no longer considered gauze.

## WET-TO-DRY SALINE DRESSINGS

**13. What is the purpose of a wet (moist)-to-dry saline dressing?**

The purpose of a wet (moist)-to-dry saline dressing is to mechanically debride necrotic tissue from a wound. This form of mechanical wound debridement may be painful and can be complicated by bleeding. In reality, saline dressings should be applied while moist and removed while still moist. This approach often necessitates dressing changes every 4–6 hours.

**14. Are there any situations in which a wet-to-dry dressing is not indicated?**

Wet (moist)-to-dry dressings should not be used if granulation tissue is present in the wound base. As the dressing is taken off the wound, granulation tissue is removed, slowing wound healing.

**15. If wet-to- dry dressings are indicated only for debridement, why do doctors order them?**

Because they were educated to do so and are unfamiliar with the myriad of currently available moist wound-healing techniques that are less painful and facilitate a wound healing environment. Carpe diem—teach them!

## ALGINATE DRESSINGS

**16. What are alginate wound dressings?**

Alginate dressings are primary wound coverings derived from brown seaweed. These spun fibers are available as nonwoven pads or ropes that are composed of calcium salts of alginate acid. The dressing forms a gel on contact with wound fluid. Alginates are nonadhesive, nonocclusive, conformable dressings that absorb moderate-to-large amounts of wound exudate. They promote a moist environment as well as autolytic debridement. Alginate dressings require a cover, also known as a secondary dressing.

**17. For what types of wounds are alginate dressings most appropriate?**

Alginate dressings are indicated for draining partial- and full-thickness wounds. Although they promote autolytic debridement, it is generally recommended that the wound have a clean wound bed for optimal effectiveness.

**18. How often should an alginate dressing be changed?**

Alginate dressings are usually changed every 1–3 days, depending on the amount of wound exudate.

**19. Can alginate dressings be used on clinically infected wounds?**

Yes—as long as the dressing is changed on a daily basis.

**20. Are there any wounds for which an alginate dressing should not be used?**

Alginate dressings are not indicated for third-degree burns. They are not recommended for minimally draining wounds because the bed may become desiccated with fibers embedded in the wound.

**21. What else is important to know about alginates?**

Inform the patient that many of the alginate products may turn a light green in contact with wound fluid. This color change is normal and not a sign of infection.

**22. When should an alginate dressing be changed to another product category?**

- After 3 days, if the product has not absorbed much or any wound fluid.
- The wound bed is dry and desiccated.
- The wound is re-epithelializing with no significant drainage.

## FOAM DRESSINGS

**23. What is a foam dressing?**

Foam dressings are composed of polymers that contain small open cells capable of holding fluids and pulling them away from the wound bed.

**24. For what kinds of wounds are foam dressings appropriate?**

Foam dressings can be used on either full-thickness or partial-thickness wounds. Most often used for draining wounds, foam dressings are also useful for moist wounds.

**25. How much wound exudate do foam dressings absorb?**

Foam dressings absorb varying amounts of wound exudate, depending on the thickness of the foam and the brand used. The manufacturer can usually provide specific information.

**26. Do foam dressings provide a moist wound environment?**

Yes. They also provide insulation.

**27. Do foam dressings promote autolytic wound debridement?**

Yes, but this type of debridement is slower than other available methods.

**28. What product considerations are relevant to foam dressings?**

Foam dressings are usually semipermeable, nonadherent, and easy to apply and may have an adhesive film border. Foam dressings are available in a variety of shapes, rolls, and cavity dressings as well as varying thickness. Some foam products need a secondary dressing; others do not.

**29. How frequently are foam dressings changed?**

Foam dressings are changed every 1–3 days, depending on the amount of wound exudate and the absorption characteristics of the specific dressing. When wound exudate is seen on the outer surface of the dressing, it is time to change it.

**30. Are there any situations in which a foam dressing is not indicated?**

Foam dressings are contraindicated for third-degree burns. They are not indicated for nondraining wounds because the dressing may adhere to the wound bed. They should not be used to fill in sinus tracts. Cavity foam dressings should not be cut, as small pieces of the foam can get trapped in the wound bed, precipitating abscess formation or foreign body inflammation.

**31. Anything else one needs to know about foams?**

There is a misconception that the foam also provides pressure reduction. Nothing can be further from the truth.

## HYDROPOLYMER DRESSINGS

**32. What are hydropolymer dressings?**

Multilayered synthetic products with a surface layer that expands into the contours of the wound as it absorbs wound exudate.

**33. For what kinds of wounds are hydropolymer dressings appropriate?**

They are indicated for partial- and full-thickness wounds that have a clean wound base. The wound can be moist or draining. In addition to flat wounds, the conformable characteristic of a hydropolymer also works well in shallow craters.

**34. Do hydropolymer dressings promote a moist wound environment?**

Yes. They also facilitate autolytic debridement and maintain optimal wound bed moisture. Some products are semipermeable, allowing escape of moisture vapor from the wound.

**35. How frequently are hydropolymer dressings changed?**

Usually changed every 1–3 days, according to amount of wound exudate absorbed.

**36. What are the major product considerations relevant to hydropolymer dressings?**

Hydropolymer dressings are available in multiple sizes and shapes conformable to the wound and absorb a moderate-to-large amount of wound exudate.

**37. What precautions are associated with hydropolymer dressings?**

Hydropolymer dressings are not indicated for third-degree burns and are not recommended for dry or minimally exudating wounds. If they are used on heavily exudating wounds or wounds with undermining or tunneling, an alginate may be required to help absorb drainage and pack dead space.

## HYDROFIBER DRESSINGS

**38. What are hydrofiber dressings?**

Nonwoven dressings composed of carboxymethyl cellulose, which forms a gel when exposed to wound fluid.

**39. For what kinds of wounds are hydrofiber dressings appropriate?**

Hydrofiber dressings are indicated for draining full- and partial-thickness wounds.

**40. Do hydrofiber dressings promote a moist wound environment?**

Yes. They also promote autolytic debridement.

**41. How are hydrofiber dressings packaged?**

Hydrofiber dressings are sterile and available as either pads or ribbons.

**42. Do hydrofiber dressings require a secondary dressing?**

Yes.

**43. What are the major product considerations relevant to hydrofiber dressings?**

Hydrofiber dressings are nonadhesive, nonocclusive, and conformable to the wound; they absorb a moderate-to-large amount of wound exudate.

**44. How frequently are hydrofiber dressings changed?**

Hydrofiber dressings are usually changed every 1–3 days, according to the amount of wound exudate absorbed. Some brands have been tested for up to 7 days without adverse events.

**45. What precautions are associated with hydrofiber dressings?**

Hydrofiber dressings are not indicated for third-degree burns. They are not recommended for dry or minimally exudating wounds.

**46. Do hydrofibers and alginates share similar characteristics?**

Yes. Like alginates, hydrofibers may turn a light green when they absorb wound fluid. A decision to discontinue the hydrofiber and use another product is based on the same clinical decision-making used with alginates.

## HYDROCOLLOID DRESSINGS

**47. Describe the composition of hydrocolloid dressings.**

Hydrocolloid dressings are formulated from elastomeric, adhesive, and gelling agents. They form a gel over the wound as the exudate is absorbed. Some formulations contain an alginate to increase absorption capabilities. Exudate absorption varies from product to product. Hydrocolloids are among the earliest categories of products introduced for modern moist wound healing.

**48. For what kinds of wounds are hydrocolloid dressings appropriate?**

Hydrocolloid dressings can be used for partial- and full-thickness wounds with a dry or moist wound bed. They are not indicated in wounds with a large amount of exudate.

**49. Do hydrocolloid dressings maintain a moist wound environment?**

Yes. They also promote autolytic debridement.

**50. Is there a risk of traumatizing the periwound skin on hydrocolloid dressing removal?**

As with any dressing using an adhesive, trauma to the periwound skin may occur. Each brand has a product insert in the package. Take the time to read it, because removal instructions vary.

**51. What are the major product considerations for hydrocolloid dressings?**

Hydrocolloid dressings are occlusive and available in multiple sizes and shapes as well as thin or thick depths. They are available in sheets, powders, pastes, and gel form. Hydrocollid dressings are easy to apply but can leave a residue on the wound and periwound skin at dressing removal. This residue is not harmful and can be removed by irrigation/wound cleansing in the usual fashion.

**52. Is there a risk of periwound maceration with hydrocolloid dressings?**

Yes. The periwound skin may become macerated, if the dressing is not changed as clinically indicated, because of the pooling of exudate under the dressing. If maceration is a problem, consider substituting a more absorptive product, such as alginate, hydrofiber, or foam.

**53. How frequently are hydrocolloid dressings changed?**

Usually every 3–7 days, depending on the amount of wound exudate.

**54. What precautions are associated with the use of hydrocolloid dressings?**

Hydrocolloid dressings are contraindicated for third-degree burns. They are usually not recommended for the management of wounds with dry eschar or for clinically infected wounds. Hypergranulation tissue may develop under hydrocolloid dressings.

**55. Describe hypergranulation tissue.**

Hypergranulation tissue, also known as "proud flesh," becomes mounded over and above the surface of the intact skin surrounding the wound. Often drainage is increased. Wounds with hypergranulation are unable to heal because the epithelial cells cannot resurface the wound bed.

**56. How is hypergranulation tissue treated?**

Usually the application of a silver nitrate stick to this aberrant tissue reduces its volume. Several daily applications may be needed.

**57. What can clinicians do to improve hydrocolloid wear time so that it does not "roll up into a ball" in the sacral area?**

To counter the roll-up effect, a minimum of a 6 cm × 6 cm piece should be used. Applying a liquid skin adhesive to the intact skin before application of the dressing also helps. Some manufacturers recommend taping the edges of the dressing to the skin.

**58. What common mistakes occur with hydrocolloid use?**

1. The active portion of the dressing must be in contact with the entire wound base. Therefore, if there is any depth to the wound, a hydrocolloid sheet should not be used. Instead, hydrocolloid in a gel, paste, or powder form should be considered.

2. The wound fluid, when mixed with the hydrocolloid meltdown, frequently looks like pus and has an odor. It is frequently interpreted as a wound infection and the dressing is inappropriately discontinued. Before pushing the panic button, irrigate/cleanse the wound and perform a systematic assessment. Hydrocolloid use is associated with a low infection rate—even lower than wet-to-dry dressings.

3. Inexperienced clinicians want to observe the wound daily and remove the hydrocolloid prematurely. Unless there is a clinical indication, such as suspected infection, hydrocolloids should be left in place and not be disturbed.

4. Using creams, ointments or other wound care products under the hydrocolloids is not indicated. Many of these products are absorbed into the hydrocolloid, negating the intended effects. The adhesive properties of the hydrocolloid may be adversely affected, allowing premature removal or ineffective wear time.

**59. Are secondary dressings needed?**

A sheet hydrocolloid does not require a secondary dressing. Other forms require a covering.

## HYDROGEL DRESSINGS

**60. What are hydrogel dressings?**

Hydrogel dressings are three-dimensional networks of cross-linked hydrophillic polymers that trap water. Some formulations may add an alginate to increase wound exudate absorption. Available as a sheet, these formulations may be nonadhesive or may have an adhesive border.

**61. What are amorphous hydrogel dressings?**

Hydrogels that are either water- or glycerin-based without the cross-linked hydrophilic polymers. The viscosity of the dressing varies from product to product. Most clinicians consider hydrogels and amorphous hydrogels as one product category.

**62. How are amorphous hydrogels packaged?**

Amorphous hydrogel dressings are available in either tubes as a gel or in a spray form. Some products have impregnated gauze sheets or rope packing strips with hydrogel.

**63. For what types of wounds are hydrogel dressings appropriate?**

They are indicated for partial- and full-thickness granulating wounds that are dry or slightly moist. They are generally used in clean wounds but can be used to facilitate autolytic debridement.

**64. What precautions are associated with hydrogel dressings?**

Hydrogel dressings are not indicated for third-degree burns and are not recommended for moderately or highly exudating wounds. Except for impregnated hydrogel gauze, these dressings are not intended to fill wound spaces.

**65. Do hydrogel wound dressings promote a moist wound environment?**

Yes. They also facilitate autolytic debridement. Hydrogel dressings hydrate a wound and are helpful for dry or minimally exudating wounds. They also keep healthy, moist wounds in this condition—healthy and moist!

**66. Do hydrogel-impregnated gauze dressings absorb exudate?**

Yes, but the absorption rate varies from product to product. If the goal of wound care is to control drainage, another more absorptive dressing should be used instead.

**67. Is there a risk of periwound maceration with hydrogel wound dressings?**

Yes. If the dressing is not changed as clinically indicated, maceration may result from pooling of exudate under the dressing.

**68. How frequently are hydrogel wound dressings changed?**

Usually every 1–4 days, according to the amount of wound exudate absorbed.

**69. When are hydrogel dressings no longer indicated?**
A hydrogel should be discontinued if there is enough exudate to require a twice-daily dressing change. As the wound re-epithelializes, the hydrogel can still be used, but in this instance, a different form may be needed. The sheet form can be substituted for the gel.

**70. Do hydrogels require a secondary dressing?**
Yes.

## TRANSPARENT FILM DRESSINGS

**71. What are transparent film dressings?**
Transparent film dressings consist of a thin, transparent, polyurethane sheet coated on one side with acrylic hypoallergenic adhesive that will not adhere to a moist surface, allowing self-adherence without the use of tape.

**72. For what kinds of wounds are transparent film dressings appropriate?**
Transparent film dressings are indicated for flat, partial-thickness, nondraining wounds as a primary dressing or as a means of autolytic debridement of dry, nonviable tissue. They are useful as a secondary dressing to secure a primary dressing because they are easy to use and conform well to body contours.

**73. What are the major product considerations for transparent film dressings?**
These dressings are impermeable to fluids and bacteria, and waterproof. Because they allow one-way passage of oxygen and moist vapor away from the wound, they are not able to absorb wound exudate.

**74. Do transparent film dressings promote a moist wound environment?**
Yes. They also facilitate autolytic debridement.

**75. How frequently are transparent film dressings changed?**
Every 1–7 days.

**76. What precautions are associated with transparent film dressings?**
Transparent film dressings are not indicated for use in third-degree burns. Patients with thin skin, especially elderly patients and patients receiving steroids, may experience epidermal stripping or skin tears if the product is not removed with care. Take the time to read the product insert for each brand; the manufacturer describes the best way to remove the product with minimal epidermal damage.

**77. When should a transparent film dressing be switched to another product category?**
Transparent films do not hold exudate well. If there is drainage or maceration at the wound, they should be switched to a more absorbent product, such as hydrocolloid, hydropolymer, or foam.

## BIOSYNTHETIC DRESSINGS

**78. What are biosynthetic dressings?**
Wound dressings composed of both manmade ingredients, such as synthetic polymers, and biologic substances, such as amino acids or collagen. Because indications for their use vary, it is best to read the manufacturer's product insert. See also Chapters 22, 23, and 24.

## WOUND FILLER DRESSINGS

**79. What are wound filler dressings?**
Pastes, powders, beads, and strands that are used as wound fillers and exudate absorbers. They are made of a variety of substances, including dextrose and starches. Some of the common product

categories, such as hydropolymers, can also be considered wound fillers. This product category is aptly named because the product "fills" the wound as it absorbs drainage.

**80. For what kinds of wounds are wound filler dressings appropriate?**

Wound filler dressings are indicated for partial- and full-thickness wounds that are granulating or have minimal-to-moderate nonviable tissue as a base.

**81. Do wound filler dressings promote a moist wound environment?**

Yes. They also facilitate autolytic debridement.

**82. Do wound filler dressings require a secondary cover dressing?**

Yes.

**83. How frequently are wound filler dressings changed?**

Usually every 1–3 days, according to the amount of wound exudate and the absorbency of the secondary dressing.

**84. What are the major product considerations for wound filler dressings?**

Wound filler dressings absorb a moderate-to-large amount of wound exudate. They may be used in combination with other wound dressings to increase the absorption of wound exudate or to fill shallow wound defects.

**85. What precautions are associated with wound filler dressings?**

Wound filler dressings are not indicated for third-degree burns and are not recommended for dry or minimally exudating wounds or wounds with sinus tracts.

## ABSORPTIVE DRESSINGS

**86. What are absorptive dressings?**

Dressings that use superabsorbent materials to trap fluids within the dressing. Usually they are hybrids created by combining major product categories. The combination of absorbent layers using cellulose, alginates, or hydropolymers with an outer semiadherent layer defines this dressing.

**87. For what kinds of wounds are absorptive dressings appropriate?**

Absorptive dressings are indicated for partial- and full-thickness wounds with large amounts of exudate. The wound base should be clean, although placement on minimal, thin, nonviable tissue is acceptable.

**88. Do absorptive wound dressings promote a moist wound environment?**

Yes. They also facilitate autolytic debridement.

**89. How frequently are absorptive wound dressings changed?**

Usually every 1–3 days, according to amount of wound exudate absorbed.

**90. What are the major product considerations for absorptive wound dressings?**

They absorb a moderate-to-large amount of wound exudate.

**91. What precautions are associated with these dressings?**

Because no one uniform material is used, it is best to read the product insert before use.

## COMPOSITE DRESSINGS

**92. What are composite dressings?**

Dressings with a distinct structure that include at least one of the following: a bacterial barrier; an absorbent layer other than a foam, alginate, hydrocolloid. or hydrogel; a semiadherent or nonadherent surface that makes contact with the wound; an adhesive border; and a semiocclusive or non-occlusive fabric cover.

**93. For what types of wounds are composite dressings indicated?**

Composite dressings are indicated as a secondary or cover dressing for granulating full-thickness wounds or as a primary dressing for partial-thickness wounds.

**94. How frequently are composite dressings changed?**

Usually every 1–4 days, according to the amount of exudate produced by the wound.

**95. In which situations are composite dressings contraindicated?**

Composite dressings are not indicated for third-degree burns and are not appropriate for heavily exudating wounds or as a primary dressing for a full-thickness wound. Because of the wide range of materials used in composite dressings, it is best to read the product insert.

## CONTACT LAYER DRESSINGS

**96. What are contact layer dressings?**

Dressings composed of a single layer of woven or perforated material that acts as a low adherence material and is placed directly over the wound. They are made from silicone, nylon, rayon, or polyethelene.

**97. For what types of wounds are contact layer dressings appropriate?**

Contact layer dressings are indicated for both partial- and full-thickness wounds with a granulating wound base.

**98. What is the primary purpose of using a contact layer dressing?**

Contact layer dressings protect a wound from trauma and often are used initially over skin grafts.

**99. How long can a contact layer dressing remain in place?**

Depending on the material, contact layer dressings can remain in place for up to 7 days.

**100. What precautions should be taken?**

As with most miscellaneous product categories, the variety of materials used requires the user to be familiar with the product insert before use.

**101. Is there a simple way to choose a dressing from these various product categories?**

Selection of the best dressing depends on patient assessment and the goal of therapy. The dressings described above work best on clean wounds. If debridement is the therapeutic goal, consider all types of techniques for removal of nonviable tissue—not just the dressing. Once assessment is completed and the expected clinical outcomes are identified, one can refine dressing options based on other patient-specific factors: healthcare setting, availability of caregivers, skill level of patient and caregiver, cost, insurance and formulary restrictions, and ability to obtain the dressing with relative ease.

*Examples of Appropriate Dressings*

| WOUND DEPTH | DRAINAGE | EXAMPLES |
|---|---|---|
| Shallow | Dry-to-moist | Transparent films, hydrogel sheets, hydrocolloids, collagen |
| | Wet | Composite dressing, hydropolymers, absorptives, foams, collagen-alginates |
| Deep | Dry-to-moist | Hydrogels, hydrocolloid gels, collagen, hydropolymers |
| | Wet | Calcium alginates, hydrofibers, foams, collagen-alginates |

**102. Offer an algorithm for topical wound treatment.**

See algorithm on following page.

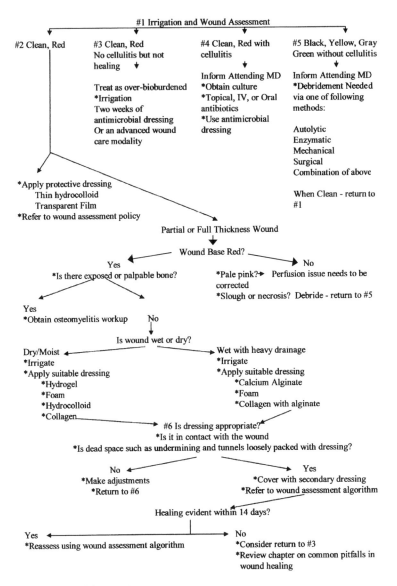

© 2001, Connecticut Clinical Nursing Associates, LLC. Used with permission.

## BIBLIOGRAPHY

1. Currence S: Product selection in the new millennium: Developing strategies for your practice setting. In Krasner DL, Rodeheaver GT, Sibbald RG (eds): Chronic Wound Care: A Clinical Source Book for Healthcare Professionals, 3rd ed. Wayne, PA, HMP Communications, 2001, pp 321–328.
2. Hess CT: Nurse's Clinical Guide to Wound Care. Springhouse, PA, Springhouse Corporation, 1995.
3. Krasner D: Resolving the dressing dilemma: Selecting wound dressings by category. Ostomy Wound Manage 40(4):35, 1991.
4. Ovington L: Wound care products: How to choose. Home Healthcare Nurse 19:224–231, 2001.
5. Ovington L, Peirce B: Wound dressings: Form, function, feasibility and facts. In Krasner DL, Rodeheaver GT, Sibbald RG (eds): Chronic Wound Care: A Clinical Source Book for Healthcare Professionals, 3rd ed. Wayne. PA, HMP Communications, 2001, pp 311–319.

# 22. COLLAGEN WOUND DRESSINGS

*Liza G. Ovington, PhD, CWS*

**1. What is the source of the collagen in collagen-based wound dressings?**

A common source of collagen for wound dressings is cowhide, but in some products the collagen is derived from chicken tendon or pig intestine.

**2. Are collagen dressings different from other wound dressings?**

Collagen dressings are different from other wound dressings in that they are composed of a material that is found naturally in tissues. This endogenous collagen plays a role in the normal wound-healing process. Exogenous collagen in wound dressings may play a similar role in promoting healing in chronic wounds.

**3. Is collagen from animal sources compatible with human wound tissue?**

Yes. Collagen is a highly conserved protein; it has changed very little over the course of evolution or between species. Collagen from a cow, pig, chicken, or human is essentially the same. As long as the collagen protein is purified and free of any cellular components from its original source, it is biocompatible with human tissues and will not cause an allergic reaction. A very small portion of the population, however, may have allergies to any products of bovine origin.

**4. Is the collagen-alginate dressing called Fibracol Plus similar to a calcium alginate dressing?**

No. Fibracol Plus (Ethicon, Inc., Somerville, NJ) is a specific dressing that contains 90% bovine collagen and 10% alginate to improve the absorbency and gelling behavior of the dressing. Calcium alginate dressings are 100% alginate and contain no collagen.

**5. How long can collagen-alginate dressings be left in the wound?**

The dressing can be left in a wound for up to 7 days.

**6. Should I worry about "mad cow disease" (bovine spongiform encephalitis) if the collagen dressing is derived from cowhide?**

No. Cowhide and tendons are low risk tissues for containing the bovine spongiform encephalitis (BSE) prion or transmission vector (usually found in brain tissues). In addition, the chemical processing of collagen from its tissue source is known to inactivate the BSE prion.

**7. What are the key benefits of collagen dressings for wound care?**

Because endogenous collagen plays such key roles in the healing process, it is thought that exogenous collagen may have similar effects in promoting hemostasis and granulation. It may even influence the orientation of new collagen created by wound fibroblasts, resulting in decreased time for tissue maturation.

**8. What types of wounds benefit most from collagen dressings?**

Collagen dressings are thought to work optimally on wounds that are free of necrotic tissues or recently debrided. Collagen is suitable for managing chronic wounds such as pressure ulcers, diabetic foot ulcers, and venous leg ulcers as well as acute wounds such as skin graft donor sites, dehisced surgical wounds and minor burns. Collagen is naturally absorbent and provides fluid management in draining wounds, but it may be used even on dry wounds if premoistened with saline.

**9. Can I use collagen-based dressings on infected wounds?**

Yes, as long as the infection is being managed locally or systemically.

**10. What happens if collagen dressings are degraded in the wound?**

Collagen may be broken down to some extent by enzymes present in chronic wounds; however, collagen dressings are usually changed before they are degraded completely. When collagen is degraded, it is broken first into gelatin and then slowly into individual amino acids. Studies have shown that when exogenous collagen is broken down in the body, about 80% of the resulting amino acids is used to create new proteins and 20% is excreted as urea.

**11. Does collagen go bad?**

Collagen dressings are labeled with an expiration date, as required by the Food and Drug Administration. Like most proteins, if collagen is in an aqueous state, such as a paste or gel, it is susceptible to heat denaturation. Dry forms of collagen—sheets, powders, and granules—are more heat stable.

### BIBLIOGRAPHY

1. Rao KP: Recent developments of collagen based materials for medical applications and drug delivery systems. J Biomater Sci Polym Ed 7:623–645, 1995.
2. Baxter C: Collagen in the treatment of chronic wounds of the lower extremity. Biomechanics 4(6):24–28, 1997.
3. Van Gils CC, Roeder B, Chesler SM, Mason S: Improved healing with a collagen-alginate dressing in the chemical matricectomy. J Am Podiatr Med Assoc 88(9):452–456, 1988.
4. Donaghue V, Chrzan J, Rosenblum B, et al: Evaluation of a collagen-alginate wound dressing in the management of diabetic foot ulcers. Adv Wound Care 11:114–119, 1998.

# 23. SMALL INTESTINE SUBMUCOSA DRESSINGS

*Jody L. Schmidt*, RN, BSN, CWOCN

**1. What is a small intestine submucosa (SIS) dressing?**

An SIS dressing is a collagen-based matrix material made from porcine small intestine submucosa. It is commercially available as Oasis in the form of a dry sheet.

**2. What is an extracellular matrix (ECM)?**

The ECM is the structural and space-filling part of tissue situated outside cellular boundaries.

**3. Does the SIS dressing use the ECM?**

Yes. The ECM is composed of proteins, carbohydrates, and lipids. The proteins consist predominantly of collagen. Fibroblast growth factor-2 has been identified as present and bioactive in this particular dressing.

**4. As an ECM, how can Oasis assist with wound management?**

It provides a natural scaffold for host tissues to migrate into during the wound management process.

**5. For what kind of wounds is SIS dressing appropriate?**

SIS can be used in the local management of partial- and full-thickness wounds, such as abrasions, burns, vascular ulcers, donor sites, and pressure ulcers.

**6. Is there any immune response to the SIS dressing?**

No harmful immunologic response indicating rejection or sensitization has been documented in any species, including humans. A mild-to-moderate localized inflammatory reaction may occur in the first few days and is a natural step in the body's healing process. If the inflammatory response does not resolve after 3 days, the dressing should be removed.

**7. Do any clinical data support the use of SIS dressings in wound care?**

At the time of publication, numerous clinical trials are under way. Early data from these trials suggest an improved healing rate in partial- and full-thickness wounds compared with traditional saline dressings.

**8. Can I use an SIS dressing on an infected wound?**

No. In addition, an SIS dressing should not be used in wounds with excessive exudate, bleeding, or acute swelling.

**9. Do I have to rehydrate the dry Oasis dressing before applying it to a wound?**

The wound dressing can be applied in a dry state to a fresh wound. The exudate from a fresh wound is usually sufficient to rehydrate the dressing. Cut the dressing slightly larger than the outline of the wound while it is dry. Typically the dressing is placed into the wound for rehydration to occur. If the wound does not have enough exudate to provide an optimal moist wound environment, the Oasis needs to be rehydrated by wetting it in sterile saline before application.

**10. Is a secondary dressing needed?**

Yes. An appropriate nonadherent secondary dressing is needed to maintain a most wound environment.

**11. How often does the SIS dressing need to be changed?**

SIS dressings become incorporated into the wound bed. If the SIS is visible on the wound bed at the dressing change, the wound is irrigated in the usual fashion and the secondary dressing is reapplied. Additional SIS is placed on the wound bed when the primary dressing is not visible. A caramel-colored gel is often seen when the secondary dressing is removed. This gel can be rinsed away with gentle irrigation.

BIBLIOGRAPHY

1. Cook Biotech: Oasis product insert. Cook Biotech, Spencer, IN, 2001.
2. Hodde J, Hiles M: Bioactive FGF-2 in sterilized extracellular matrix. Presented at the Symposium on Advanced Wound Care and Medical Research Forum on Wound Repair, Las Vegas, 2001.
3. Niezgoda J, Parmenter M: A clinical study to evaluate small instestine submucosa (SIS). Poster presentation at the Symposium on Advanced Wound Care and Medical Research Forum on Wound Repair, Las Vegas, 2001.
4. Brown-Etris M, Milne C, Corbett L, et al: A clinical study to evaluate small intestine submucosa (SIS) as a treatment for full-thickness pressure ulcers. Poster presentation at the Symposium on Advanced Wound Care and Medical Research Forum on Wound Repair. Las Vegas, 2001.

# 24. HYALURONAN WOUND DRESSINGS

*Wai Yuen John Chen, BSc, PhD*

### 1. What is the role of hyaluronan (HA) in the human body?

HA is a major carbohydrate component of the extracellular matrix of skin, most organs, and most tissues and of the fluid in joints and eyes (see Chapter 7). A derivative of HA for wound care applications is available as Hyalofill (ConvaTec, Princeton, NJ).

### 2. What clinical evidence supports the use of extrinsic hyaluronan in aiding wound repair?

Exogenous HA has been used successfully for many years in ophthalmologic applications, joint conditions, postsurgical wounds, and burn wounds. The following results have been reported:

- HA treatment reduced the incidence and degree of dehiscence macroscopically, increased the maturation of granulation tissue during the first postoperative days, and stimulated fibroblasts to synthesize procollagen shortly after surgery with topical treatments through the drains of the laparotomy suture.
- The efficacy and safety of HA in comparison with Dextranomer, the product of choice for this indication in France, was evaluated in a multicenter controlled clinical study of 50 patients with venous ulcerations. Both groups recorded significant wound improvements, but HA resulted in a faster and greater reduction in ulcer dimensions.
- A benzyl ester of HA was used as an adjunct to the standard treatment of diabetic foot ulcers (sharp debridement, pressure relief, and infection control). The control group received the standard treatment only.

Overall, the experimental and clinical data about the beneficial effects of HA are limited. However, the available data, although anecdotal, have already stimulated the exploration of HA and HA-derived materials as wound-healing products. Some of these are already available for clinical use.

### 3. Is topically applied HA active both physicochemically and biologically?

Because HA has many functions that depend on the interplay between its physicochemical and biologic properties, one may hypothesize that this, too, is the case for topically applied HA. At present, however, experimental or clinical evidence to support this hypothesis is insufficient.

### 4. Is HA absorbed intact or catabolized into its components before absorption?

In normal skin, endogenous HA is catabolized very rapidly. It is estimated that the total HA content in adults is about 15 gm, most of which is found in skin. "A few grams" can be degraded each day, representing a significant portion of total body HA. Using radiolabeled pulse-chase experiments, HA in the epidermis has a short half-life of about 1 day, indicating rapid metabolism of HA in epidermal tissue.

Since there is no difference between endogenous and exogenous HA, it is expected that topically applied HA is also catabolized rapidly and absorbed, utilizing the same metabolic pathways as endogenous HA. The principal pathways for HA degradation are via hyaluronidase. HA breakdown is also mediated by oxygen free radicals, generated by sunlight or local inflammatory conditions.

The partially degraded HA is taken into the lymph system and further broken down in the lymph nodes. Eventually it reaches the blood circulation and is taken up by the liver, where it is further metabolized into constituent sugars and eventually into carbon dioxide and water. In wounds, contaminating microorganisms also may contribute to the initial breakdown of HA through the action of microbial hyaluronidases.

### 5. How does Hyalofill function as a vehicle for HA?

When Hyalofill comes into contact with moisture and water from wound exudate, the action of water separates the benzyl alcohol moiety from the HA molecule by a chemical process known as hydrolysis. Hyalofill, therefore, can be seen as a vehicle for HA.

**6. For what type of wounds is the use of HA indicated?**

HA is indicated for use on chronic wounds such as venous ulcers, sinuses, and fistulas. It is also indicated for use in deep exuding wounds and donor skin graft sites.

**7. Can Hyalofill be used on a dry wound? Can it be premoistened?**

Hyalofill can be used on dry wounds. However, to create and/or contribute to an HA-rich wound interface, the Hyalofill needs to be moistened by application of water or saline. The aim is to achieve a moistening effect but not to result in excessive fluid. For ease of handling, it is recommended that the Hyalofill fleece be placed dry on the wound and then moistened. The wound can then be kept in its moist state by application of an appropriate occlusive secondary dressing.

**8. Does the wound have to be clean?**

Yes. Before application, the wound should be cleansed by any appropriate method. Debridement should be performed if necrotic tissue or eschar is present.

**9. Is it a problem when parts of Hyalofill remain in the wound during a dressing change?**

There is no problem if a small amount of Hyalofill remains in the wound after cleansing. If a large amount is left in the wound during dressing change, removal and replacement with fresh Hyalofill are recommended. Removal may be aided with forceps or gloved fingers.

**10. How do I know the product is ready for replacement?**

The dressing is ready for replacement when it has been completely dissolved in the wound. Other indicators for dressing replacement include heavy exudate, amount of slough, or any other clinical judgment that indicates the need for a dressing change.

**11. How is Hyalofill best covered?**

Hyalofill can be used together with a variety of secondary dressings and cover dressings, depending on the need to absorb wound exudate or to provide a moist healing environment. For a highly exudating wound, an absorptive secondary dressing placed on top of the Hyalofill is suggested. The use of a thin occlusive cover dressing to maintain the moist environment is recommended in wounds with less drainage.

**12. What is the longest amount of time that Hyalofill can be left in place to maximize uptake into the wound?**

Replacement of Hyalofill every 2–3 days in a moderately exuding wound is the recommended guideline. For heavily draining or minimally sloughing wounds daily application may be needed initially, but as healing progresses and the amount of exudate decreases, the interval between changes may be extended to 2 or 3 days.

**13. When do I stop using Hyalofill?**

Hyalofill may be used until full healing is achieved. However, when it is used as an adjunct to good wound care and management, one may consider discontinuing its use once a healthy bed of granulation tissue is established.

**14. What are the alternatives when Hyalofill does not give the desired results?**

Hyalofill needs to be in a moist state in the wound to provide an HA-rich environment supportive of moist wound healing. Other issues may be limiting wound improvement (see Chapter 49).

**15. Anecdotal case studies are favorable. How did compliance and follow-through with wound management play a part?**

Hyalofill is not a replacement for good basic wound management. Wound healing, particularly of chronic wounds, is a complex problem that requires a systematic approach to treat the causes and manage the symptoms. Hyalofill, like all other topical agents, is recommended for use as an adjunct to good clinical care and management. The cases were conducted by specialists focusing on a combination of continued good basic wound management supplemented with Hyalofill. These wounds previously had failed to respond to good clinical care and management alone. That these wounds responded favorably when Hyalofill was used as an adjunct is an indication of its benefits. This issue merits further clinical investigation and forms the main objectives of current clinical trials.

## BIBLIOGRAPHY

1. Chen WYJ, Abatangelo G: Functions of hyaluronan in wound repair. Wound Rep Reg 7:79–89, 1999.
2. Edmonds ME, Foster A: Hyalofill, a new product for chronic wound management. Diabetic Foot 3:29–30, 2000.
3. King SR, Hickerson WL, Proctor KG, Newsome AM: Beneficial actions of exogenous hyaluronic acid on wound healing. Surgery 109:76–84, 1991.
4. Ortonne JP: A controlled study of the activity of hyaluronic acid in the treatment of venous leg ulcers. J Dermatol Treat 7:75–81, 1996.
5. Trabucchi E, Forshi D, Marazzi M, et al: Prevention of wound dehiscence in severely obese patients with jejuno-ileal bypass: The role of hyaluronic acid. Pharmatherapeutica 5:233–239, 1988.

# 25. GROWTH FACTORS AND WOUND HEALING

*Teresa A. Conner-Kerr, PhD, PT, CWS(D)*

### 1. What are growth factors?

In a nutshell, they are small protein factors that are used by many different types of cells for communication. They provide a means for intercellular communication and also orchestrate numerous biologic phenomena, such as wound healing.

### 2. Are growth factors, interleukins, and cytokines the same thing?

Loosely, yes. This is a question asked by clinicians and scientists alike. The confusion started early in the discovery process of these grand chemical entities when cell culture fluid samples were found to induce a variety of biologic activities in different cell types. These chemicals or protein factors were named for the biologic response that they facilitated, induced, or inhibited. As a result, many factors received multiple names that included the descriptors of proteins, factors, or growth factors. As knowledge of these grand chemicals grew, it became apparent that many of them were the same entity with different names. In many cases, they had received different names because they responded differently under various culture conditions. Currently, the chemicals classified as cytokines are cellular messengers. Chemicals that play a role in communication between leukocytes are designated as interleukins. Some holdovers from the early days of the discovery process are still called growth factors.

### 3. How many cytokines are there?

More than 100 cytokines have been recognized, and the list continues to evolve.

### 4. How do cytokines work?

Cytokines, like neurotransmitters or hormones, interact with a specific receptor protein located on a target cell. Binding of a cytokine to its specific receptor results in the initiation of a cascade of cellular events that leads to altered gene expression. These cellular activities eventually culminate in a variety of physiologic responses that interest clinicians, such as induction of the inflammatory response or stimulation of hematopoiesis.

### 5. Do many cytokines have multiple actions and affect many different cell types?

The resounding answer is yes. Many cytokines interact with multiple different types of cells and also elicit multiple physiologic responses in varying degrees. For example, transforming growth factor beta (TGF-β—an example of a holdover) stimulates chemotaxis of monocytes and fibroblasts while inhibiting endothelial cell chemotaxis.

### 6. What are the roles of cytokines in wound healing?

Although their roles are too numerous and involved to outline fully, the basic actions of common growth factors involved in wound healing are shown below:

*Sources and Functional Activities of Growth Factors*

| GROWTH FACTOR | CELLULAR SOURCE | FUNCTIONAL ACTIVITY |
|---|---|---|
| TGF-α | Platelets, macrophages, keratinocytes | Activates neutrophils<br>Stimulates angiogenesis |
| TGF-β | Platelets, macrophages, lymphocytes | Stimulates fibroplasia and angiogenesis<br>Includes cell proliferation |
| PDGF | Platelets, macrophages, keratinocytes, endothelial cells | Elicits neutrophils and fibroblasts by chemoattraction<br>Stimulates mesodermal cell mitogenesis |

*Table continued on following page*

*Sources and Functional Activities of Growth Factors (Continued)*

| GROWTH FACTOR | CELLULAR SOURCE | FUNCTIONAL ACTIVITY |
|---|---|---|
| FGF | Macrophages, neural tissue | Stimulates mitogenesis of keratinocytes, endothelial cells, and fibroblasts |
| EGF | Platelets, keratinocytes | Stimulates mitogenesis of keratinocytes, endothelial cells, and fibroblasts |

TGFα = transforming growth factor alpha, TGF-β = transforming growth factor beta, PDGF = platelet-derived growth factor, FGF = fibroblast growth factor, EGF = epidermal growth factor.
From Mahl D: Growth factors in wound management. Fed Pract, July:14–19, 1998, with permission.

### 7. When are cytokines used for wound healing?

This question continues to be a topic of great debate. Since understanding of immunology and the processes involved in both acute and chronic wound healing are in their infancy, clinical recommendations for how to apply growth factors are still evolving. The current approach is to add growth factors to kick-start particular wound-healing processes that are thought to retard healing. However, this approach depends on the knowledge of the intricacies of wound healing. Wound healing has been likened to an orchestra in which each member (cytokine) knows when and what part to play. Since we do not know the exact musical score for wound healing, we can only estimate the correct times for growth factor application. As knowledge of wound healing grows, estimations will become more accurate. In addition, since it takes more than one player to make an orchestra, investigators of these processes are looking for the master plan or score that determines which cytokines play together and in what order.

### 8. What specific cytokines are available for therapeutic use in wound healing?

Several growth factors have been studied in clinical trials, including epidermal growth factor (EGF), granulocyte-macrophage colony stimulating factor (GM-CSF), interleukin 1 (IL-1), transforming growth factor 2 (TGF-2), and fibroblast growth factor (FGF). Keratinocyte growth factor (KGF-2) is currently in clinical trials. However, the first and only cytokine or growth factor approved by the Food and Drug Administration (FDA) for use in wound care is becaplermin (Regranex, Ortho-McNeil, Raritan, NJ) for diabetic neuropathic foot ulcers. The recommendation indicates that becaplermin is to be used "for diabetic neuropathic foot ulcers that extend into the subcutaneous tissue or beyond and have an adequate blood supply."

### 9. What type of growth factor is becaplermin?

Becaplermin is derived from the most active portion of the platelet-derived growth factor molecule, the B-chain. Its activity is similar to that of the parent protein; it facilitates chemotaxis and proliferation of wound cells and formation of granulation tissue.

### 10. How are growth factors produced? Are there any potential problems with allergies or carriage of harmful pathogens?

Regranex is produced by recombinant DNA technology. Since it is a recombinant human factor, allergies to animal proteins should not be a problem. However, the prescribing information indicates that Regranex should not be used in people with a known hypersensitivity to parabens, which are present in the product vehicle. In addition, since Regranex is a recombinant product generated in the yeast *Saccharomyces cerevisiae* and is not derived directly from a human donor, the potential for carriage or exposure to harmful pathogens is extremely minimal.

### 11. How are growth factors applied to wounds?

Recommendations for Regranex include application "to a clean wound bed once daily in a measured quantity." In addition, product representatives advocate using a quantity of dime-sized thickness. In the author's experience, Regranex can be applied to the wound with a sterile applicator such as a swab or tongue depressor or by placing the product on sterile saline-moistened gauze.

### 12. What kind of dressing should be used with Regranex?

According to the product guidelines, a saline-moistened dressing should be used. This type of dressing was used in the clinical trials; the interaction of Regranex with other moist wound dressings requires further study before other recommendations can be made.

### 13. Which types of wounds can be treated with growth factors?

Regranex has been approved for diabetic neuropathic wounds, and its use in pressure ulcers and venous stasis ulcers is currently under study.

### 14. Is Regranex cost-effective?

Models of cost have been constructed, but they need to be fully validated in different patient populations. In addition, patients must be appropriate candidates for growth factor therapy, and a 30% decrease in wound size by weeks 8–10 must be attained for growth factor application to be cost-effective.

### 15. Who can apply topical growth factors to wounds?

Always check the licensure laws in the state where you practice. Regranex must be prescribed by an appropriate health care provider. Appropriately licensed professionals providing wound management services may apply the product; caregivers and patients can be taught to do so.

### 16. Any other tips?

- Be familiar with the product insert. It is the guideline for proper use.
- Regranex is an expensive drug. Be sure to discuss cost with the patient and determine whether its use is covered by insurance. If not, the patient may spend over $350. As a result, some patients forego dressing supplies, other medications, and food to the detriment of the wound and themselves.
- Regranex must be refrigerated.
- Check the expiration date on the crimp of the tube because Regranex has a short shelf life.
- If the patient cannot afford the medication, call the local company representative, who can advise you and the patient about current policy for indigent patients.
- Always provide optimal wound care in conjunction with this medication, including offloading of pressure and shear forces, adequate cleansing, serial debridement of callus, control of blood sugar, and debridement of necrotic tissue.
- If there is no response or inadequate response, take a step back and determine why.

### BIBLIOGRAPHY

1. Mitchell RN, Cotran RS: Repair: Cell regeneration, fibrosis and wound healing. In Kumar V, Cotran RS, Robbins SL (eds): Basic Pathology, 6th ed. Philadelphia, W.B. Saunders, 1997, pp 47–59.
2. Kunimoto BT: Growth factors in wound healing. In Krasner DL, Rodeheaver GT, Sibbald RG (eds): Chronic Wound Care: A Clinical Source Book for Healthcare Professionals, 3rd ed. Wayne, PA, HMP Communications, 2001, pp 391–397.
3. Kunimoto BT: Growth factors in wound healing: The next great innovation? Ostomy Wound Manage 45(8): 56–64, 1999.
4. Mahl D: Growth factors in wound management. Fed Pract July:14–19, 1998.
5. Ortho-McNeil Pharmaceutical, Inc: New Regranex Gel (becaplermin) (0.01%). Raritan, NJ, Ortho-McNeil Pharmaceutical, Inc., 1998 [product insert].

# 26. PLASTIC SURGERY IN WOUND MANAGEMENT

*Armann O. Ciccarelli, MD, FACS*

**1. What is plastic surgery?**

From the Greek word *plastikos*, meaning "to mold," plastic surgery focuses on the restoration of form and function to the human body. Plastic surgery procedures have been described as far back as 800 B.C. with accounts of nose reconstruction via local skin flaps. Modern plastic surgery traces its roots to the early 20th century and the advent of modern warfare. The devastating injuries suffered by participants in World War I generated the need for surgeons specializing in complex reconstructive surgery. Contemporary plastic surgery includes wound care and management, reconstructive surgery for both congenital and acquired deformities and defects, soft tissue ablative surgery, esthetic surgery, and hand surgery.

**2. When is a plastic surgery consultation indicated?**

Consultation with a plastic surgeon is appropriate for any situation in which wound healing is expected to be difficult or delayed. Consultation should be considered strongly for any wound or wound closure that may create significant functional deficits or esthetic deformity.

**3. What is the reconstructive ladder? How does it relate to wound closure?**

The goal of wound management is to achieve wound healing, minimizing the required time and short- and long-term disability and morbidity. The reconstructive ladder is a concept for evaluating wound interventions in an ascending order of complexity.

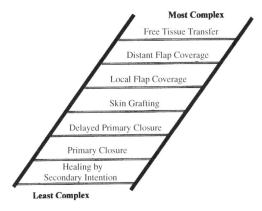

The reconstructive ladder.

**4. Define healing by secondary intention.**

Open wounds allowed to heal without surgical intervention may do so by a process of wound contracture, spontaneous re-epithelialization, and fibroplasia. This process is termed healing by secondary intention. Typically, smaller, more superficial wounds in areas of soft tissue laxity are the best candidates for healing by secondary intention. Larger wounds, particularly in areas of high mobility (e.g., over joints) or esthetically sensitive areas, are less favorable candidates for healing by secondary intention.

**5. What wounds are most appropriate for treatment via primary closure?**

Acute, clean wounds less than 12 hours old, whose edges can be approximated with minimal tension, are the best candidates for primary closure with sutures, staples, adhesive strips, or skin adhesives. Suturing or other direct closure of chronic open wounds is to be avoided. The combination of poor local vascular supply, tissue induration, high bacterial load, and debris found in chronic wounds is a recipe for disaster.

### 6. Define delayed primary closure.

When acute wounds cannot be immediately closed because of concerns about infection, tissue viability, or extensive contamination, delayed primary closure may be considered. The wound is treated in an appropriate open fashion until it is clean. The wound edges are then loosely reapproximated with sutures, clips, or adhesive tapes. This process of wound preparation and closure typically occurs over 3–5 days. Open wounds beyond 7–10 days typically develop tissue induration and bacterial colonization that make direct delayed closure less reliable. Alternatively, for smaller wounds, one can consider complete open wound excision and primary closure. This approach essentially converts the chronic open wound into a fresh wound that can be primarily closed.

### 7. What is a graft?

A graft is a portion of viable but avascular tissue that, when placed in an appropriate wound, is revascularized by new blood vessel growth from the wound bed. Grafts are essentially "parasitic" in relation to the wound. Grafts can be classified as either simple or composite. Simple grafts contain only one tissue type, such as skin or fat. Composite grafts contain more then one tissue type, such as dermal-fat or skin-cartilage grafts.

### 8. How do grafts survive?

Imbibition, inosculation, and vessel ingrowth are the steps of graft survival (also known as graft take). Initially, the viable but avascular tissue of the graft survives by diffusion of nutrients across the wound surface (imbibition). This stage typically lasts 1–2 days. Inosculation is the early blood flow across the existing capillary vessels in both the wound and the graft. During vessel ingrowth, the last phase of healing, vessel neogenesis occurs; new blood vessels cross from the wound bed into the graft to revascularize it completely. As a consequence, tissues closest to the active wound interface are first to be revascularized. Tissues the farthest from the wound surface are the last to be revascularized. Tissues too far away from the wound surface to be revascularized promptly undergo cell death and necrosis.

### 9. What causes graft failure and graft loss?

Any process that prevents rapid revascularization of the graft results in graft tissue death and loss. Common problems include the following:
- A poor wound bed. Poor wound vascularity, debris within the wound, and irregular wound contours prevent good contact between the graft and the wound bed, preventing prompt revascularization.
- Infection
- Subgraft seromas or hematomas, which prevent revascularization.
- Graft motion. Motion and shearing of the underlying wound in relation to the graft prevent adherence and revascularization.

### 10. What is the difference between split- and full-thickness skin grafts?

Skin grafts may be considered as either split-thickness or full-thickness grafts. Split-thickness skin grafts typically are 10–15 thousandths of an inch in thickness and include the epidermis and upper dermis. Skin appendages such as sweat glands and hair follicles are below the level of the graft and are not included in the graft. Full-thickness grafts encompass the complete thickness of skin from epidermis up to, but not including, subcutaneous fat. Skin appendages are included in a full-thickness graft.

Split-thickness grafts have a better survival ability. The contact area of the graft is high in proportion to the thickness of the graft, thereby allowing rapid revascularization and early survivability. In addition, the donor site for the skin graft can readily heal and re-epithelialize, typically in 7–10 days, because the remaining deep dermal elements and the dermal appendages contain epithelial cells. This allows rapid healing of the donor site, which can be reused for skin grafts after a short time.

The primary disadvantage of split-thickness skin grafts is the high degree of contracture after healing, which limits their use in certain areas (e.g., over joints and in the face). Esthetically they are also often a poor match to the surrounding skin. Split-thickness skin grafts can be applied either as a sheet or as a fenestrated (mesh) graft.

Full-thickness skin grafts tend to be limited in size because of the need to close the donor site. No dermal or epidermal elements remain in the donor site to allow spontaneous re-epithelialization or healing. Full-thickness skin grafts have less contraction during healing than split-thickness skin grafts and are more appropriate for joint and facial areas. In general, they are esthetically superior to split-thickness grafts. Initial healing is often less complete in full-thickness skin grafts than in split-thickness skin grafts because of the thickness of tissue that needs to be revascularized.

### 11. What technique can improve graft take?

Fenestrating or "meshing" the graft improves egress of blood and serum, thus preventing accumulation of fluid under the graft and subsequent "floating off" of the graft during healing. Mesh grafts are significantly esthetically inferior to sheet grafts when they heal. Fenestration can be achieved by using a device that punches uniform holes in the graft after harvest and before application to the wound bed.

### 12. Define xenograft, allograft, and cultured, and artificial skin grafts.

Skin **xenografts** (from other animal species, typically pigs) and **allografts** (from other people) may be applied to wounds as temporary coverage. They undergo biologic rejection and therefore are not suitable for permanent coverage. They are useful as a temporary wound covering to help a wound progress to the point that it can support an autologous graft. Xenografts also may be used in a temporary setting to maintain the wound in a healthy state when the patient is temporarily not a candidate for a surgical procedure. Typically they can be applied at bedside and may "take" in the wound for 5–14 days.

**Cultured autografts** consist of small pieces of autologous skin that are harvested, grown, and expanded in vitro and then applied to a wound. Their fragility and the time required for growth limit the use of these grafts. Cultured autografts are most useful in patients with extensive burn wounds. Nonallogenic cultured skin allografts are now available. This allogenic split-thickness skin graft appears to be incorporated into the recipient wound without rejection, although the current mechanism of healing is not completely clear. The use of these tissues is rapidly expanding.

**Artificial skin** in the form of a collagen dermal matrix with a silicone "epidermis" is currently available. It is used primarily for extensive burn wounds. It requires staged replacement of the silicone epidermis with a dermal split-thickness skin graft (see Chapter 28).

### 13. What are flaps?

Flaps differ from grafts in that they represent vascularized tissue transfers. By maintaining their own vascular supply, flaps are not directly dependent on the status of the wound for survival. A flap may augment the blood supply to a wound significantly with its own blood flow. A flap is distinct from the parasitic nature of a tissue graft. Flaps may be a single tissue type transfer, as in skin or muscle, or a composite transfer, such as a fasciocutaneous or musculocutaneous flap. Flaps may optimize wound closure by replacing a tissue defect with similar tissue.

### 14. Where are the flaps harvested?

Flaps may consist of tissues immediately adjacent to the wound (local flaps) or tissues from other areas (distant flaps). In all cases a vascular supply, called the vascular pedicle, must be maintained and protected to ensure the survival of transferred tissue. This vascular supply may consist of identifiable vessels or be based on random blood flow from the adjacent tissues (random pattern flap). In both types of flaps, the area of vascular perfusion maintained by the pedicle determines flap size, dimensions, and orientation.

### 15. How are local tissues formed into flaps?

Local adjacent tissues may be advanced, turned over, or rotated into the existing wound to provide wound closure. They are known as types of transposition flaps. An island flap is a local flap with an intervening intact tissue barrier between the flap donor site and the wound site.

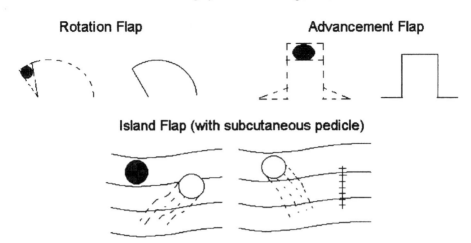

**Rotation Flap**          **Advancement Flap**

**Island Flap (with subcutaneous pedicle)**

Three basic types of flaps.

### 16. What is a Z-plasty? When is it used?

In closing wounds, it is preferable to have the line of closure fall parallel to or into a natural skin crease, particularly over joint surfaces. Creases are also known as relaxed skin tension lines. Incisions that perpendicularly cross relaxed tension lines tend to form thicker scars as they heal. Such wounds also cause formation of flexion contractures when the incisions are located on the flexor surfaces of joints. A Z-plasty is a method of using small local flaps to break up and reorient the scar line to prevent linear scar bands and scar contracture. Z-plasty should be used when possible for closing incisions across relaxed skin tension lines.

### 17. How are distant tissues used as flaps?

Distant flaps may be transferred as either pedicle or free tissue flaps. **Distant pedicle flaps** are infrequently used today because of the difficulty in transferring the flap to the wound site. Typically a multistage procedure is required. First the wound is brought into proximity to the donor flap site. The flap is then raised and transposed to cover the wound defect, and the flap donor site is closed directly or with a skin graft. The flap pedicle remains intact, and the flap remains attached to the donor site. As the flap heals into the wound, it establishes a blood supply through the wound, independent of the pedicle. Two to three weeks after transfer, the pedicle can be transected, leaving the flap free on the wound.

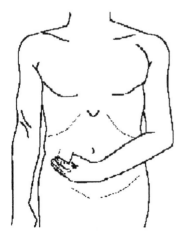

Distant abdominal wall-to-thumb flap–first stage. After 2–3 weeks, the base of the skin flap (pedicle) is cut, thereby freeing the hand from the abdomen and transferring the abdominal tissue to the thumb.

**Free flaps** are transfers in which the vascular pedicle is transected. The flap is then transferred to the wound site, and the vascular pedicle is anastomosed to a new vascular supply. In the above case, the tissues of the lower abdomen may be transferred directly to the thumb, using microsurgical techniques to "hook up" the cut pedicle blood vessels, thereby transferring the tissue directly to the thumb in one step. The disadvantage of free flaps is that they are technically demanding and lengthy procedures. In addition, depending on the site to be reconstructed, donor tissue options may be limited. Despite these limitations, however, free tissue transfers have become the gold standard for many types of reconstruction procedures.

### 18. What is the role of flaps in treatment of osteomyelitis?

Osteomyelitis, an invasive bone infection, and the more common local osteitis, an inflammatory destruction of local cortical bone with local bacteria colonization, complicate open wounds. The best treatment is often a combination of antibiotics, surgical debridement, and appropriate wound closure. Muscle or myocutaneous flaps have been shown to provide a definite advantage in wound closure in this setting. The bulk of muscle tissue can fill dead space left by the required extensive debridement, and the highly vascularized muscle tissue aids in bacterial clearance in the wound.

Cutaneous flaps with their subdermal element of adipose tissues are less reliable in this setting. The adipose component of cutaneous flaps is relatively poorly vascularized. Such flaps, therefore, are less effective in clearing bacterial loads and are at higher risk for secondary flap infection and local fat necrosis.

### 19. What are common causes of flap loss?

1. **Inadequate vascular inflow and ischemia.** Inappropriate flap design that fails to incorporate an appropriate vascular pedicle into a flap or elevates the flap with more tissue that can be adequately perfused results in ischemic flap loss. Careful planning and execution of flap surgery is of paramount importance.

2. Flap ischemia may also be secondary to **mechanical compromise of the vascular pedicle** secondary to twisting, kinking, or edema about the pedicle. In the case of free flaps that have undergone microvascular anastomosis, thrombosis of the pedicle can lead to ischemia. Postoperative recognition of decreased perfusion secondary to thrombosis or mechanical problems may allow timely surgical intervention and salvage of a flap.

3. **Poor venous outflow** also may compromise the flap by causing venous engorgement of the flap with secondary thrombosis and disruption of the microcirculation. Ensuring adequate venous outflow in the vascular pedicle, ensuring no mechanical obstruction of the vascular pedicle, and keeping the flap elevated assist in preventing this complication. As with arterial insufficiency, early recognition of a venous outflow problem allows timely secondary intervention and salvage of a compromised flap. When venous engorgement is seen in a vascular pedicle without compromise or thrombosis, use of medicinal leeches to reduce the venous engorgement may be considered.

4. **Infection.** Direct tissue destruction along with tissue edema and induration, followed by vascular embarrassment, may result from infection of the flap. As noted previously, muscle flaps are relatively resistant to infection and are the flaps of choice for dealing with infected or heavily colonized wounds.

5. **Hematoma** may potentiate flap loss both by direct pressure phenomenon on the vascular pedicles and microcirculation and by inducing vasospasm within the flap.

### 20. What are Vasconez's laws about flap survival?

1. Some do. Some don't.
2. All of the flap survives except the part needed to close the wound.
3. If plan A fails, don't make plan B the same as plan A.
4. It always happens to me.

### 21. What type of postoperative care is required after flap surgery?

Special patient care is needed during the postoperative period after flap reconstruction. Primary considerations are to ensure adequate arterial inflow and adequate venous drainage and to prevent secondary infection during the postoperative period. When possible, flaps should be kept warm to prevent temperature-induced vasoconstriction and slightly elevated to improve venous outflow drainage. All pressure is to be kept off the flap and its pedicles to avoid compromise of flap perfusion. Patients should be well hydrated, and blood pressure should be kept in a normotensive range. Use of vasoconstrictive medicines should be avoided. Antiplatelet or anticoagulant medications such as dexedrine, heparin, or aspirin occasionally may be used at the discretion of the physician, particularly in cases of vascular insufficiency of the flap or after microvascular anastomoses have been performed.

Flap motion and tension on the flap should be avoided to prevent suture line disruption and compromise of the vascular pedicle.

Positioning after closure of wounds with truncal flaps, particularly decubitus flaps, may be problematic. The use of an appropriate pressure reduction bed is mandatory. Air-fluidized beds remain the current gold standard, but alternating pressure beds are used with increasing frequency. Patients are typically kept at bed rest for 3–6 weeks until the flap is well healed. In general, when air-fluidized beds are used, patients are kept completely supine to maximize weight distribution and pressure reduction. Sitting in bed and wedging with pillows are kept to a minimum and used for short periods at meal time. Subsequently, patients are allowed to sit or apply pressure to the flaps in a limited fashion, with slow advancement as tolerated. Close monitoring of the flaps during this period is mandatory to prevent recurrent pressure injury.

A definitive program of long-term pressure reduction, using appropriate wheel chairs, mattresses, and cushions along with pressure reduction positioning and exercises, is essential.

**22. A 35-year-old, two-pack-per-day smoker presents with a 3 × 2 cm, full-thickness stage III posterior ankle ulcer with exposed Achilles tendon secondary to cast immobilization of an ankle fracture. Using the reconstructive ladder, discuss the most appropriate treatment options.**

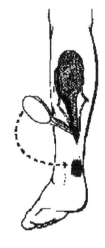

Inferiorly based sural fasciocutaneous flap.

1. **Secondary intention.** Tendons are relatively avascular structures and therefore tolerate open exposure poorly and tend to progress rapidly to dessication and necrosis. The nature and location of this wound make healing by secondary intention a poor choice with little likelihood of success.

2. **Primary closure.** The location of the wound makes this option impractical. There are insufficient tissue laxity and mobilization to allow primary closure.

3. **Skin grafts.** Exposed tendon in general provides a poor wound bed for grafts because it is relatively avascular. Skin grafts are expected to take poorly, if at all, over exposed tendon.

4. **Local flaps.** Flap coverage is the most appropriate choice for this type of wound. Local flaps are limited in number because of the limited availability of soft tissue in this area. Given the size of the wound, a local or regional flap with a fasciocutaneous nature—i.e., an inferiorly based sural fasciocutaneous flap—may be appropriate.

5. **Free flaps.** A free fasciocutaneous flap also may be used. A fasciocutaneous rather than a muscle flap is the most appropriate choice to avoid excessive bulk in the area. Alternatively, one also may consider a pure free fascial flap in combination with an overlying skin graft.

Regardless of flap selection, discontinuation of tobacco use is mandatory. Tobacco smoking has been well documented to impair microcirculation and increase the incidence of flap loss.

**23. A 67-year-old paraplegic with a 6-cm, stage IV right ischial decubitus ulcer with local osteomyelitis and undermining presents after 6 months. Using the reconstructive latter, discuss the most appropriate treatment options.**

1. **Secondary intention** is a feasible option but probably will require a prolonged period of labor-intensive care. The presence of exposed bone in the wound also presents difficulties. Without

appropriate treatment, the bone can readily desiccate, becoming nonviable and thus an impediment to healing. Secondary intention will result in significant scarring and accumulation of indurated tissue and cicatrix, placing the patient at higher risk for recurrence.

2. **Primary closure.** The chronicity of the wound and the presence of infection preclude primary closure. Direct, extensive debridement with or without excision of the wound would allow primary closure to be considered. The anatomic constraints and the size and location of the wound preclude simple direct closure. Delayed closure using a VAC device is a consideration. It is less labor-intensive than other open wound methods but does not recruit new tissue into the defect. Risk of recurrence of the decubitus ulcer after a VAC closure is high. It remains a viable option, however, for patients who are poor surgical candidates (see Chapter 29).

3. **Skin graft.** The presence of infection and the irregularity of the wound make skin grafting a poor choice. The placement of grafts directly on the bone, while technically feasible, is generally avoided because of the relative fragility of the graft. Recurrent wound breakdown is a significant issue. Skin grafts can be considered if one can reasonably expect no loading or additional trauma to the area. Overall, when bone is exposed, skin grafts are better considered as temporary wound closure.

4. **Local flaps.** Cutaneous, fasciocutaneous, and musculocutaneous flaps based on the gluteal skin and muscles, posterior thigh skin and muscles, or the tensor fasciae latae muscle and fascia are appropriate choices. The depth and volume of the wound as well as the presence of osteomyelitis make a musculocutaneous flap the best choice. The ability of the muscle component to provide soft tissue fill and to augment significantly the local wound bed vascularity is a major benefit. Given the typical high risk of decubitus recurrence rates for paraplegics, care must be taken in final flap selection to ensure that the surgery involved in raising and transposing the flap does not preclude other local flap use in the future.

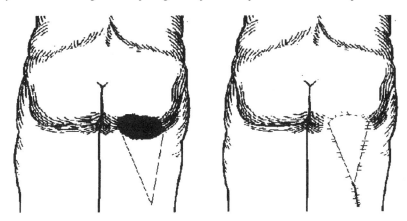

Posterior thigh biceps V-Y musculocutaneous advancement flap.

5. **Free musculocutaneous flaps**, like local pedicle flaps, can be adequately used to treat this wound. However, a free tissue transfer requires an increased operative time. It is technically more demanding and has a higher flap failure rate than local pedicle flaps. In addition, donor site selection is important. Given the patient's paraplegia, care must be taken that the loss of the donor muscle function does not impair upper extremity or trunk strength. Lower extremity donor sites can be used in paraplegic patients, but muscle bulk and vascularity may be diminished secondary to atrophy.

### BIBLIOGRAPHY

1. Georgade GS, Riefkoh LR, Levin LS (eds): Plastic, Maxillofacial and Reconstructive Surgery. Baltimore, Williams & Wilkins, 1997.
2. McCraw JB, Arnold PG: McCraw and Arnold's Atlas of Muscle and Musculocutaneous Flaps. Norfolk, VA, Hampton Press, 1986.

# 27. BIOTHERAPY: LEECHES

Donald H. Lalonde, BSc, MD, MSc, FRCSC, and Janice Lalonde, RN, CPSN, CPN(C)

### 1. In what types of cases should leeches be used?
Leeches have been useful primarily in assisting with replantation of small external body parts, such as fingers, ears, lips, and scalps. They also can be used in failing flaps, although this issue is controversial (see question 19).

### 2. How do leeches work?
Leeches have a sucker-like mouth and teeth. When a leech is attached to a designated body part, such as a replanted finger, its first action is to inject a substance that acts as a local anesthetic. Thus the patient does not feel the actual bite. The second substance injected by the leech is hirudin, which prevents the blood from clotting. This mechanism can last up to 24 hours, causing the bite wound to bleed long after the leech has detached. The leech feeds for 10–20 minutes and then falls off of the replanted digit, thus leaving the bite wound to bleed continuously.

### 3. How does a bleeding wound caused by a leech bite keep a finger alive after it has been replanted?
Leeches are used in replanted parts with good arterial inflow and poor venous outflow (usually because the veins are clotted). For a replanted body part to survive, blood must flow in and out. When the veins clot and cannot be repaired by a microsurgical procedure, leeches come into play. The leeches' bites drain blood out of the part for 3–7 days until the area regenerates its own veins, allowing outflow to occur.

### 4. Why not use surgery instead of leeches?
Leeches are generally used when surgeons have tried to repair the veins of a replanted part and have been unsuccessful. In some cases, the veins are simply too small to repair, whereas in other cases too much venous damage was caused by the initial injury.

### 5. How can you tell that a replanted area might need a leech?
A replanted body part that receives sufficient arterial inflow but no venous outflow is cool, bluish, swollen, and tense. When the end of the finger is stabbed (usually with an 18- or 20-gauge needle), dark blue blood drips out quickly. This means that the venous pressure is high, and in this circumstance a leech is required.

### 6. What does it mean when a leech will not bite a replanted finger or any other tissue?
Usually, when a leech will not bite a replanted area, it means there is no arterial inflow. If there is adequate arterial inflow, the leech will be quite responsive in its actions.

### 7. How do we attach leeches to the designated host part without getting bitten by them?
Leeches can be applied manually with gloves. They also can be placed in the barrel of a syringe with the tip cut off with a scalpel. They come out of the end of the barrel when placed on the host area. A specimen container also works well when placed close to the compromised area. The leech may wiggle and squirm for a few moments, but if arterial inflow is sufficient at the site, the leech will be quite accommodating. To prevent leeches from migrating to other tissues, simple cover those areas with a greasy petrolatum-based dressing. Leeches willingly stay clear of these slippery areas.

### 8. How do we get leeches off of a replanted body part?
Once a leech is sufficiently satisfied, usually in 10–20 minutes, it simply falls off by itself. Be sure that a medical staff person is nearby to retrieve it or everyone will be on a "leech hunt."

### 9. How do we dispose of leeches?

When the leeches' action is completed, they are bathed in a 70% alcohol solution, then are disposed of in the facility's biomedical waste department. Guidelines for disposal may vary from facility to facility.

### 10. Can leeches be reused?

Leeches are never used again on another patient because of the possibility of spreading blood-borne diseases. Medicinal leeches are raised in the laboratory under controlled conditions. They will not have the desire to feed for several months. The feeding schedule for leeches varies from 6 to 12 months.

### 11. Why do leeches have such long periods between feedings?

The ingested blood is stored in the intestinal tract of the leech. Leeches use the *Aeromonas hydrophila* bacteria to split the heme and the globin, which aids the leech in digestion. Leeches use only what they need to sustain life; therefore, time between feeding periods is very long.

### 12. How are leeches stored?

In medical facilities, leeches are kept in a specific leech tank purchased through specific leech suppliers. The medium is a solution consisting of 2 ml of Hirudo salt and 3 liters of sterile water; the solution is changed about once a month. Leeches can be kept alive in a controlled environment for up to 1 year. For facilities that do not house their own leeches on standby, they can be purchased 24 hours a day from leech suppliers within the United States. One such supplier is Leeches USA. More information is available at www.leechesusa.com.

### 13. How do you know when it is time to apply a new leech?

After the leech has finished feeding, the replanted part is usually pink in color. It will continue to ooze blood ,and the replanted part will stay pink. When the blood stops dripping because of clotting, the finger start to become bluish and purple again as well as cool to the touch. This is the time to apply another leech.

### 14. How many days does leech therapy last?

After the replanted part has generated its own veins between three and seven days on average, the finger will stay pink even after the leech bite clots. This is when you know the leech therapy has been successful and you can stop applying the leeches.

### 15. When should leech therapy not be used?

A leech should not be used in a setting associated with poor arterial inflow. With poor arterial inflow, bacteria contained in leech saliva are not flushed out through the bite wound, and infection can occur.

### 16. When an infection occurs from a leech bite, what organism is responsible?

The usual organism is *Aeromonas hydrophila*, a gram-negative organism. Another organism that has grown due to leech therapy is *Serratia marcescens*.

### 17. What antibiotics are effective in treating infectious organisms due to leech therapy?

Common first line antibiotics include cotrimoxazole, ciprofloxacin, gatifloxacin, levofloxacin, ofloxacin, cefotaxime, amikacin, gentamicin, netilmicin.

### 18. Are transfusions frequently required with leech therapy?

Although the authors are not aware of any studies of this issue, patients requiring leech therapy sometimes require transfusions because of the significant blood loss. However, if the leeches are used simply for a finger, ear, or other small body part, blood loss may not be significant enough to require transfusion.

## CONTROVERSY

### 19. Should leeches be used in failing flaps?

Leeches have been used successfully to treat failing flaps, and the flaps have survived. However, some people believe that leeches should not be used in failing flaps because often the flaps may be compromised by poor arterial inflow. If arterial inflow is poor, saliva is not flushed out through the leech bite wound, and a large section of avascular flap tissue is at the mercy of the bacteria in the leech saliva. The second reason is that, if the flap is large, a significant amount of venous outflow is required for leech therapy to be successful. Many leeches would have to be applied, and a large volume of blood would have to come out of the flap to keep it alive, which in turn may require large volumes of blood transfusion.

## BIBLIOGRAPHY

1. Graf J: Symbiosis of *Aeromonas* and the medicinal leech. ASM News 3:148–152, 2000.
2. Green C: The medicinal leech. Nature 323:494–496, 1986.
3. Hermansdorfer JW, et al: Antibiotic sensitivities of *Aeromonas hydrophila* cultured from medicinal leeches. Br J Plast Surg 41:649–651, 1988.
4. Lineaweaver WC, et al: *Aeromonas* infections following use of medicinal leeches in replantation and flap surgery. Ann Plast Surg 2238–2244, 1992.
5. Mackay DR, et al: *Aeromonas* species isolated from medicinal leeches. Ann Plast Surg 42:275–279, 1999.
6. Lalonde DH, et al: Salvage of three cases of class 2V ring avulsion injuries with medicinal leeches. Can J Plast Surg 4:169–171, 1996.
7. Weinfield AB, et al: Clinical and scientific considerations in leech therapy for management of acute venous congestion: An updated view. Ann Plast Surg 45:207–212, 2000.
8. Chao JJ, et al: Microsurgery, free tissue transfers and replantation. Sel Read Plast Surg 9:11, 2000.
9. Valauri FA: The use of medicinal leeches in microsurgery. Sel Read Plast Surg 8:10, 1999.

# 28. SKIN SUBSTITUTES

*Pamela A. Wiebelhaus, RN, BSN, and Sean L. Hansen, BS, CRA*

### 1. What is a skin substitute?

A skin substitute is a temporary or permanent covering to replace skin loss after a burn, trauma, or chronic wound. Unlike skin grafts taken from one area on the patient and placed elsewhere, the skin substitutes are manufactured using a variety of techniques and placed onto the wound. Some are designed for partial-thickness wounds, whereas others can be used in full-thickness wounds.

### 2. When should a skin substitute be used instead of the patient's own skin?

Much depends on individual patient characteristics and the underlying need for covering the wound with skin. In a burn patient, there may not be enough skin to harvest. In a patient with microvascular disease or severe immunocompromise, the harvest site may not heal, placing the patient at a greater risk for additional complications.

### 3. Define the term *take*.

*Take* describes the degree of viability of a skin graft at the wound site. It applies to autografts, allografts, and skin substitutes.

### 4. Describe the common skin replacement products used in the treatment of partial-thickness burns.

TransCyte, Biobrane, porcine, and bismuth-impregnated petroleum gauze are used in the treatment of partial-thickness burns. TransCyte, a temporary skin substitute derived from human fibroblasts, provides a transparent synthetic epidermis. Biobrane is a biosynthetic wound dressing constructed of a silicone film with a nylon fabric partially imbedded into the film. Porcine products are obtained from pigs. Bismuth-impregnated petrolatum cause is commonly called Xeroform. All of these products are most effective when applied to clean wounds.

### 5. How should Biobrane be applied to a partial-thickness burn?

Biobrane should be applied wet, using normal saline. The dull side of the dressing is placed toward the wound, and a moderate stretch is applied to the edges to prevent wrinkles. Steri-strips can be used to secure the dressing to the surrounding intact skin. A bulky dressing should be applied until the Biobrane is well adhered to the wound bed.

### 6. If partial-thickness burns eventually heal, why use a skin substitute?

Decreased pain, decreased wound healing time, and minimal dressing changes—in a nutshell, a happy patient. The skin substitute may protect the remaining dermis and minimize scarring caused by further manipulation of the wound.

### 7. What currently available skin substitutes provide a permanent dermal replacement?

Integra, AlloDerm, Apligraf (Graftskin), and Dermagraft. Integra and AlloDerm are approved for use in the treatment of full-thickness burns. Apligraf and Dermagraft are approved for use in the treatment of diabetic foot ulcers. Many clinicians use them in other scenarios, including trauma, venous stasis, and arterial wounds. Clinical trials are ongoing.

### 8. Describe Apligraf (Graftskin).

Apligraf is an allogenic, cultured skin equivalent that contains an epidermal and dermal layer. The dermal layer is formed by using bioengineered human fibroblasts. The epidermal layer is formed from bioengineered keratinocytes. Apligraf does not contain Langerhans cells, lymphocytes, macrophages, melanocytes, or blood vessels. It is nonallergenic and considered a permanent replacement. The human fibroblasts and keratinocytes are obtained from neonatal foreskins. The cells are removed from the tissue. Through a complicated bioengineering process, the cells are made into a bilayered skin product. One neonatal foreskin can make a skin substitute product about the size of a football field!

**9. Does the patient need any special preparation before the application of Apligraf?**

Yes and no. Careful attention to optimal wound care before the procedure is important. Control of bioburden of the wound bed improves graft take. However, antiseptics should not be applied for at least 48 hours before the procedure. Many clinicians use topical antibiotics such as mupirocin or silver sulfazadine, whereas others use antimicrobial agents such as nanocrystalline silver or cadexomer iodine to control bioburden.

Choosing the appropriate patient is also consideration. Patients with known noncompliance to the treatment plan are not the best candidates to receive an expensive skin substitute. In addition, some insurance carriers require notification before the procedure to approve payment. It is always best to check with third-party payors ahead of time.

**10. What happens during the application procedure?**

The product comes in a sterile container resembling a Petri dish. Using forceps, the Apligraf is teased off the container and placed onto the wound. Some clinicians staple or suture the edges; others do not. A silicone or petrolatum dressing is applied directly over the graft site, followed by a compression dressing. This dressing is left in place for 5–7 days. Graft take may be improved if a negative-pressure therapy dressing (see Chapter 29) is applied on top, but no studies have confirmed this practice. This procedure is remarkably simple and can be performed in just about any clinical setting.

**11. What issues are important after the procedure is done?**

Apligraf does not look like an autograft at the time of the first dressing change. A slimy, yellowish film appearance on the wound bed is normal, although the inexperienced clinician may be concerned. This appearance naturally fades over the next 2–3 weeks, and the wound looks more like an autograft take. Complications are rare and usually are related to infection or lack of graft take. Lack of graft take can be attributed to an excessive bioburden in the wound, acute infection, patient non-compliance, absence of a clean wound bed, or inadequate circulation to the wound bed. Optimal wound care and elimination of patient factors that retard wound healing before application cannot be overemphasized.

**12. How do AlloDerm and Integra differ?**

Both products provide a permanent dermal replacement, but they differ in application and biologic constitution. **AlloDerm** is a specially processed human cadaver allograft that is immunologically inert. It is used for surgically excised wounds, and an ultra-thin split–thickness autograft is applied during the same operation, thus providing complete wound closure. **Integra** is a bilayered dermal regeneration template. The dermal replacement layer is made of bovine collagen and serves as a matrix for the infiltration of fibroblasts, macrophages, lymphocytes, and capillaries. The outer silicone layer serves as a temporary epidermal covering. An autograft is still necessary.

**13. What are the indications for use of Integra?**

Integra is indicated for the postexcisional treatment of full-thickness or deep partial-thickness thermal injury when sufficient autograft is not available at the time of excision. Integra should not be used in patients with a known hypersensitivity to bovine collagen or chondroitin materials.

**14. How long should Integra remain in place before an autograft can be applied?**

Incorporation of the dermal components of the bilayered membrane with the patient's own cells with formation of a neodermis that will accept an epidermal autograft requires 14–21 days.

**15. What are the advantages of a product that promotes the formation of a neodermis?**

A neodermis allows harvest of a much thinner donor site, which results in shorter wound-healing time of the donor site. Healed wounds are often more pliable with improved range of motion.

**16. What if the patient does not have enough skin to perform an autograft after 21 days?**

After the neodermis has formed, the outer membrane can be left in place until sufficient autograft is available for definitive grafting. According to some reports, Integra has remained in place for 73 days before autografting.

**17. What potential postoperative problems are associated with Integra?**

Hematoma formation, fluid accumulation, premature silicone (outer layer) separation, invasive infection, areas of nonadherent graft, and wound colonization.

**18. Describe the postapplication care of Integra artificial skin.**

It is necessary to observe for signs and symptoms of infection on a daily basis. Any purulent drainage should be reported. Dressings should be changed daily, taking care not to remove the underlying elastic net dressing if at all possible. If Integra has been applied over a joint or in mobile areas, ambulation and physical therapy should be delayed for at least 10 days. Immersion hydrotherapy should be avoided as long as the outer silicone layer is still in place; however, spray table or shower cleansing can be used. Hematomas or fluid accumulations should be drained promptly.

**19. When should a cultured epidermal autograft be used?**

Traditionally, the use of cultured epidermal autografts has been reserved for patients with extensive full-thickness burns when adequate donor sites are not available and other treatment options have not proved successful. Cultured epidermal autografts are expensive to produce and are extremely fragile. In published studies, graft take has varied anywhere from 0% to 57%.

**20. What is the best product available for complete wound closure?**

The patient's own skin is still the best option for complete wound closure, as long as adequate donor sites are available and the patient is a suitable candidate for a surgical procedure.

**21. Is there a risk of disease transmission with the use of temporary skin substitutes?**

Not from synthetic substitutes, but the potential for disease transmission has been reported with the use of human cadaver allograft. After these reported events, the Food and Drug Administration (FDA) and the American Association of Tissue Banks issued extensive guidelines for the testing of donor skin.

**22. What permanent skin replacement products do not require additional autografting?**

Apligraf and Dermagraft do not require additional skin grafting. Apligraf (Graftskin) is used in conjunction with compression therapy in the management of venous insufficiency and standard care for diabetic foot ulcers that have persisted for longer than 3 weeks.

**23. Describe TransCyte.**

TransCyte is a bilayered temporary skin substitute derived from human fibroblasts. The outer layer serves as a synthetic epidermis, and the inner layer contains human structural proteins, glycosaminoglycans (versican, decorin), and growth factors (transforming growth factor-1, keratocyte growth factor, vascular endothelial growth factor, and insulin-like growth factor-1).

**24. What are the indications for use of TransCyte temporary skin substitute?**

Most often it is used as a temporary covering for burns of mid-dermal to indeterminate depth, which typically require debridement and may be expected to heal without surgery. TransCyte also may be used as a temporary covering of excised full-thickness burns.

**25. Describe the postapplication care of TransCyte.**

Twenty-four hours after application, the outer dressing is removed and the site inspected for air bubbles or fluid accumulation, which are aspirated or drained as necessary. If the TransCyte is adherent, it is left open to air. At this point, the patient may resume full range of motion. If the TransCyte is not adherent, the dry outer dressing is reapplied and reassessed in 24 hours. The use of moist dressings or ointments on or near TransCyte should be avoided.

Color changes are observed in the first days after application, from moist and clear to dry and crusty. Yellow, green, or brown coloration also may be observed. If dry and adherent, it is left in place. The patient should be observed closely for signs of infection. If exudate is present, TransCyte will slip and slide when touched.

After 24–48 hours, any nonadherent area where exudate is present is cut and removed. It is not necessary to remove the entire piece. As the wound epithelializes, TransCyte begins to lift. At this point, all loose edges are gently trimmed.

### 26. When TransCyte is used, how long does it take the wound to heal?

A partial-thickness burn treated with TransCyte should be healed in approximately 7–10 days.

### 27. Which skin substitutes can be used for which wounds?

Determine need for a temporary or permanent skin substitute. Then consider the following principles:

**Partial-thickness substitutes for temporary skin replacement**
Allograft: human cadaver skin
Biobrane: nylon mesh bonded to silicone
TransCyte: polymer membrane with bioengineered human fibroblasts
**Partial- and full-thickness substitutes for permanent replacement**
Integra: bilayered bovine collagen matrix on a silicone layer
Alloderm: cadaver allograft with an immunologically inert dermal matrix
Apligraf: bilayered with epidermal and dermal living bioengineered tissue
Epicel: epithelial autograft cultivated from patient
Dermagraft: cultured dermal fibroblasts on a biosynthetic scaffold

From Milne C, Corbett L: 2001, with permission.

### BIBLIOGRAPHY

1. Eaglstein WH, Iriondo M, Laszlo K: A composite skin substitute (graftskin) for surgical wounds. Dermatol Surg 21:839–843, 1995.
2. Hansbrough JF, Franco ES: Skin replacements. Clin Plast Surg 3:407–423, 1998.
3. Hansen SL, Voigt DW, Weibelhaus P, Paul CN: Using skin replacement products to treat burns and wounds. Adv Skin Wound Care 14:37–46, 2001.
4. Limova M, Mauro T: Treatment of leg ulcers with cultured epithelial autografts: Treatment protocol and five years experience. Wounds 7:170–189, 1995.
5. Livesey S, Herndon DN, Hollyoak MA, et al: Transplanted acellular allograft dermal matrix. Potential as a template for the reconstruction of viable dermis. Transplantation 60:1–9, 1995.
6. Naughton G, Mansbridge J, Gentzkow G: A metabolically active human dermal replacement for the treatment of diabetic foot ulcers. Artif Organs 21:1203–1210, 1997.
7. Noordenbos J, Dore C, Hansbrough JF: Safety and efficacy of TransCyte for the treatment of partial-thickness burns. J Burn Care Rehabil 20:245–281, 1999.
8. Sheridan RL, Hegarty M, Tompkins RG, et al: Artificial skin in massive burns-results to 10 years. Eur J Plast Surg 17:91–93, 1994.
9. Tompkins RG, Burke JF: Burn wound closure using permanent skin replacement materials. World J Surg 16:47–52, 1992.
10. Wainwright DJ: Use of an acellular allograft dermal matrix (AlloDerm) in the management of full thickness burns. Burns 21:243–248, 1995.

# 29. NEGATIVE-PRESSURE WOUND THERAPY

*Mona M. Baharestani, PhD, NP, CETN, CWS*

### 1. What is negative-pressure wound therapy?

Negative-pressure wound therapy (NPWT) is a noninvasive treatment by which controlled, localized subatmospheric pressure is delivered to a wide variety of acute, subacute, and chronic wounds.

The Vacuum-Assisted Closure (VAC) system (Kinetic Concepts, Inc., San Antonio, TX) is the only NPWT system available on the market. The VAC system entails placement of a sterile foam dressing into a wound defect. A noncollapsible, fenestrated evacuation tube exits the foam parallel to the skin surface and is connected to a microprocessor-controlled vacuum pump. The open wound is converted into a controlled, closed wound as the foam dressing/wound site is sealed with an adhesive transparent film dressing. For most wounds, a setting of 125 mmHg of negative pressure is applied continuously or cyclically (5 minutes on, 2 minutes off) with dressing changes at 48-hour intervals. The wound drainage evacuated during this time empties into a canister placed in the vacuum pump.

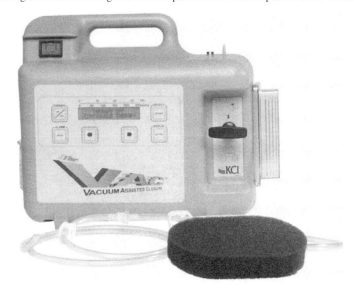

The Vacuum-Assisted Closure (VAC) system (Kinetic Concepts, Inc., San Antonio, TX).

### 2. Is the VAC approved by the Food and Drug Administration (FDA)?

Yes. The correct term for devices is *cleared*. The VAC was cleared by the FDA in 1995.

### 3. How does the VAC work?

The postulated mechanisms of action are as follows:
- Removal of excessive interstitial edema, thereby decompressing the small vessels and restoring local blood flow.
- Removal of chronic wound fluid rich in matrix metalloproteinases, which inhibit wound healing.
- Mechanical deformation of cells. As the VAC foam collapses, tractional forces are transmitted to the surrounding tissues, perturbing the cytoskeleton and stimulating proliferation of fibroblasts, endothelial cells, and vascular smooth muscle cells.

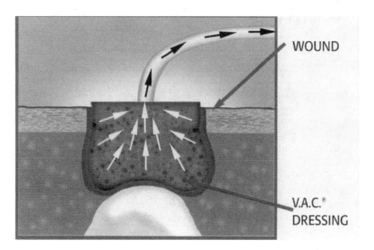

Theorized mechanisms of action of the VAC system.

### 4. What types of wounds are appropriate for VAC therapy?
• Dehisced surgical wounds
• Complex operative wounds left open to heal by secondary intention
• Meshed grafts & flaps
• Chronic open wounds
• Pressure ulcers (stages III and IV)
• Diabetic foot ulcers
• Stasis ulcers
• Degloving injuries
• Partial- and full-thickness burns within 12 hours of burn

### 5. What are the clinical benefits of VAC therapy?
• Removal of excessive interstitial fluid from the wound periphery
• Increased local vascularity
• Decreased bacterial colonization
• Quantification/qualification of wound drainage
• Increased rate of granulation tissue formation
• Maintenance of a moist wound environment
• Increased rate of contraction
• Increased rate of epithelialization

### 6. Under which circumstances is VAC contraindicated?
• Malignancy within the wound (because of the potential for increasing the mitosis of cancer cells)
• Insufficient vascularity to sustain wound healing
• Large amounts of necrotic tissue
• Untreated osteomyelitis (once osteomyelitis is treated with appropriate antibiotics, VAC can be initiated)
• Fistula(s) to organs or body cavities (although many clinicians, including the author, have successfully treated wounds with fistula[s])

### 7. Have randomized, controlled trials (RCTs) compared healing outcomes of VAC vs. moist dressings?
Yes. In a pilot study of postoperative diabetic foot wounds (n = 10), McCallon et al. reported healing at 23 days with VAC vs. 43 days with moist dressings. The small sample size precludes

statistical significance; therefore, no statistical analyses were performed. Similarly, in a study of 24 patients with 36 chronic, nonhealing wounds, Joseph et al. reported depth decreases of 66% in VAC-treated wounds vs. a 20% decrease in wounds treated with moist dressings (p < 0.00001). In the swine model (N = 10), Morykwas et al. reported a 63% increase in the rate of granulation tissue formation in wounds treated with continuous VAC therapy vs. wounds treated with moist normal saline dressings. Currently large, multicenter RCTs are in progress to compare VAC with moist wound dressings in the healing of pressure ulcers, venous stasis ulcers, and dehisced abdominal wounds.

### 8. Does VAC debride wounds?

Although VAC assists in the autolytic and mechanical debridement of surface slough, it should not be used as a primary means of debridement. Debridement of necrotic material should be performed before initiation of VAC.

### 9. Since VAC provides an occlusive wound environment, are anaerobic bacteria more likely to proliferate?

No. In studies by Morykwas and Argenta, bacterial colonization in VAC-treated wounds was decreased 1000-fold compared with wounds treated with normal saline dressings after 4 days of therapy.

### 10. How often are VAC dressings changed?

Typically 3 times a week. If the wound is actively infected, twice-daily or daily changes are recommended.

### 11. Does the wound become desiccated when VAC is used?

No. As long as there is an air-tight seal, a moist wound environment will be maintained

### 12. If more than one wound on a single patient is treated with VAC, are additional VAC units required?

No. Multiple wounds on a single patient can be treated with one VAC unit. The number of sponges and connections to the main vacuum pump is different.

### 13. Can patients ambulate while receiving VAC therapy?

VAC therapy alone does not limit the ability to ambulate; extension tubing or battery operation can be useful. Ambulation may be limited for medical reasons, such as the need for complete off-loading of a neuropathic ulcer or a newly grafted lower limb.

### 14. What is the difference between the two types of foam used with VAC therapy?

The black, polyurethane (PU) foam is reticulated and hydrophobic. It is clinically considered to be more effective at stimulating granulation tissue formation and wound contraction. It is the most frequently used foam.

White, polyvinyl-alcohol (PVA) Sof-Foam is a more dense, premoistened hydrophilic foam that is not reticulated. It is generally recommended when the rate of granulation tissue needs to be somewhat restricted or when the patient cannot tolerate the pain associated with the black foam. Because of its higher density, PVA foam requires higher pressure (125 mmHg) than PU foam to work effectively.

### 15. How do I know which setting—continuous or intermittent—to select?

Although faster rates of healing may be achieved by advancing patients from continuous to intermittent therapy after the first 48 hours, the conditions for switching to intermittent therapy may not be optimal. In the following situations, patients are best served by remaining on continuous therapy:

- Significant discomfort during intermittent therapy
- Technical difficulty in maintaining an air-tight seal with continuous therapy because of anatomic location. Frequently the perianal region, toe wounds, and wounds adjacent to drainage tubes, skin depressions, or ostomy sites are involved.
- Presence of sinus tracts or tunneled or undermined areas
- Use of VAC white foam

**16. Which skin problems are most commonly associated with VAC?**

1. **Candidiasis** (yeast overgrowth) within skin folds and when more than one layer of VAC drape is placed over the skin. Only a single layer of drape should be applied to the skin to avoid interference with moisture-vapor transmission. Candidiasis can be treated with an antifungal powder and sealed in with a liquid skin sealant. In some cases VAC therapy may be temporarily halted to treat the skin.

2. **Subepidermal granulation budding** can result from overlap of the VAC sponge dressing onto the periwound skin. This problem resolves with proper placement of the VAC sponge within the wound and/or placement of protective sheet skin barriers on the periwound skin.

3. **Skin stripping** from aggressive removal of VAC drape.

**17. What should the VAC dressing look like when it is properly functioning in the wound?**

When the VAC therapy is in progress, it should resemble a prune or raisin and should be hard and wrinkled on palpation. In addition, there should be no audible whistling sounds from the dressing.

**18. What options are available for patients who are ambulatory, work, or go to school?**

The Mini-VAC and the VAC Freedom are mobile, battery-powered units that fit in a carrying case. The Mini-VAC is used for minimally draining wounds (15 cc/day). The canister capacity is 50 cc. The VAC Freedom is used for moderately to heavily draining wounds and has a canister capacity of 300 cc.

**19. What should be done if the wound fluid has a really foul odor?**

1. Identify and treat the cause of the odor:
   - Is the wound infected? If so, appropriate antibiotic therapy needs to be initiated and VAC dressings should be changed once or twice daily.
   - Is necrotic tissue present? If so, debridement needs to performed.
   - Is a fistula present? If so, can it be surgically taken down? If not, can it be managed with bowel rest, total parenteral nutrition, and VAC therapy?
2. In addition, VAC canisters with Isolyser LTS can be used to address odor.

**20. Which Current Procedural Terminology (CPT) code can be used to bill for VAC applications?**

Although NPWT has no specific code, VAC application is categorized as a topical dressing under nonselective debridement (code 97602) in the 2001 *CPT Manual, Physical Medicine and Rehabilitation Section*. In 2001 the American Medical Association established CPT codes for active wound care management to provide nonphysician practitioners (nurses, physical therapists, physician assistants, occupational therapists) specific codes for wound care activities. The two codes and their definitions (CPT 2001, p. 299) are as follows:

97601: Removal of devitalized tissue from wound, selective debridement without anesthesia (e.g., high-pressure waterjet, sharp selective debridement with scissors, scalpel, and tweezers), including topical applications, wound assessment, and instructions for ongoing care per session.

97602: Nonselective debridement without anesthesia (e.g., wet-to-moist dressings, enzymatic treatment), including topical applications, wound assessment, and instructions for ongoing care per session.

**21. Who can apply the VAC?**

Health care professionals, home caregivers, and patients who can provide correct demonstrations of proper VAC application and removal techniques. Wound status should be monitored by a specialist in wound healing.

**22. How many hours per day must a patient remain on VAC therapy?**

For optimal results, VAC therapy is recommended 24 hours/day, but patients can be off therapy for a total of 2 hours per day to ambulate, be transported for tests, and perform other necessary activities of daily living. When VAC is placed over a split-thickness skin graft or a fistula, interruptions in therapy cannot occur.

**23. Should special precautions be taken with patients who have latex allergies?**

No. Neither VAC disposables nor the VAC unit has latex components.

**24. What special precautions are involved when VAC is used in neonates and children?**

VAC can be used in neonates, but given the rapid rate of ingrowth of granulation tissue into the foam dressing, white foam should be used and dressings should be changed daily. The amount of drainage must be closely calculated and intravenous replacements provided as medically indicated.

**25. Can the same wound-healing results be achieved by hooking the VAC dressing to wall suction?**

No. VAC dressings are to be used only with the VAC unit. VAC dressing attachment to wall suction is not an FDA-cleared modification. Because there are no alarms with wall suction, the caregiver would not be alerted to potential hazards. If VAC dressings are attached to wall suction, the following complications can occur:
- Exsanguination
- Air leaks that drive air across the wound bed and lead to desiccation and increased bacterial load
- Fluctuation in pressure

**26. What are the benefits of VAC therapy over split-thickness skin grafts?**

- Uniform stabilization
- Removal of wound transudate
- Prevention of bacterial contamination
- Increased neovascularization

**27. What should I do if blood vessels and tendons are exposed in a wound?**

Exposed blood vessels, vein grafts, and nerves should be protected by transposition of available fascia or muscle over them. Exposed tendon should be covered by a monolayer of a nonadherent dressing such as Xerform or Vaseline Gauze before application of black foam dressing.

**28. How are sinus tracts, tunnels, and undermining managed with VAC?**

When placing foam in sinus tracts, tunnels, and undermined areas, leave a "tail" of foam to allow visualization of the foam and facilitate retrieval. White foam should be used for sinus tracts and tunnels because it has a higher tensile strength and is easier to retrieve without breakage than the black foam. Record the number of foam pieces on the adhesive drape for removal during the next dressing change.

**29. How are stasis ulcers managed with VAC?**

Lower extremity ulcers secondary to venous hypertension generally do not require significant amounts of granulation tissue. PVA white foam can be used to reduce edema and bacterial load without producing large amounts of granulation tissue. If using black PU foam, pressures of 50–75 mmHg at a continuous setting are best tolerated initially. Gradual increases of 25 mmHg to a maximum of 100 –125 mm Hg are recommended. Pain, wound, and vascular responses must be monitored throughout the course of therapy; pressure settings and overall management plans should be adjusted accordingly.

**30. Can VAC be used in abdominal wounds over exposed mesh?**

Yes. VAC black foam can be placed directly over Vicryl, Prolene, Composix, or Marlex mesh; Gortex patch; and intact peritoneum.

**31. What should be done if areas of exposed bowel are present in the wound?**

If mesh does not cover the entire wound base and small areas of bowel are exposed, the greater omentum can be pulled down over the bowel and VAC therapy initiated. If the greater omentum is not available, VAC white foam or several layers of Xeroform or Vaseline Gauze can be placed over the exposed bowel, thus isolating it from the VAC dressing.

**32. Can VAC be used over skin substitutes or in conjunction with growth factors and topical proteolytic enzymes?**

Although many clinicians report excellent results with using VAC over skin substitutes and in combination with growth factors and topical enzymes, no controlled studies have examined the clinical efficacy of these combined therapies.

**33. How can a patient qualify for home NPWT?**

To meet Medicare B Criteria for NPWT in the home:
1. Patient must present with a qualifiable wound type.
   * Pressure ulcer (stage III or IV)
     *Subcriteria*
     * Patient has been appropriately turned and positioned
     * Patient has used group 2 or 3 support surfaces for ulcers on the posterior trunk or pelvis
     * Moisture and incontinence have been appropriately managed
   * Neuropathic (diabetic) ulcer:
     *Subcriteria*
     * Patient has been on a comprehensive diabetic management program
     * Off-loading of pressure over ulcer site has been accomplished with appropriate modalities
   * Venous hypertension ulcers
     *Subcriteria*
     * Compression bandages have been consistently applied
     * Leg elevation and ambulation have been encouraged
   * Chronic wound present for at least 30 days (of mixed etiology)
   * Complications of surgically created wounds/traumatic wounds:
2. Medical necessity for accelerated formation of granulation tissue that cannot be achieved by other available topical wound treatments must be documented.
3. Wound therapy program must include:
   * At least monthly documentation in the patient's medical record of evaluation, care, and wound management by a licensed medical professional
   * Application of a dressing to maintain a moist environment
   * Debridement of necrotic tissue, if present
   * Evaluation and provision of adequate nutritional status
4. Completion of the initial statement of the ordering physician (ISOP) form

**34. What are the fiscal responsibilities of acute care and skilled nursing facilities during the first 100 days?**

The facility is responsible for costs that are reimbursed under the diagnostic-related group (DRG) system in acute care and the prospective payment system (PPS) in long-term care.

**35. What about commercial payors?**

It is best to call the payor directly to determine coverage availability. Some insurance providers follow Medicare B criteria.

**36. Under which conditions should VAC be terminated?**
1. Goals of therapy have been attained.
   * Adequate granulation base achieved, allowing for change to conventional local care, split-thickness skin graft (VAC may be used over the graft, if needed), or flap closure (VAC may be used over compromised flaps).
   * Wound dimensions have decreased, making the wound more amenable to conventional dressing changes.

2. Wound exhibits no progress for 1–2 weeks despite all attempts at optimizing overall medical condition, nutritional status, perfusion status, and bacterial burden.

3. Wound requires assessment more often than every 24–48 hours.

4. Wound exhibits clinical deterioration.

5. Patient's overall physiologic status has deteriorated to a level that wound healing is no longer a treatment goal.

6. Continuous air-leak problems, when all potential solutions have failed secondary to anatomic location

## BIBLIOGRAPHY

1. American Medical Association: Current Procedural Terminology 2001, Standard Edition. Illinois, AMA Press, 2001.
2. Argenta LC, Morykwas MJ: Vacuum-assisted closure: A new method for wound control and treatment: Clinical experience. Ann Plast Surg 38:563–576, 1997.
3. Joseph E, Hamori CA, Bergman S, et al: A prospective randomized trial of vacuum-assisted closure versus standard therapy of chronic nonhealing wounds. Wounds Compend Clin Res Pract 12(3):60–67, 2000.
4. KCI Therapeutic Services: KCI's Vacuum-assisted Closure Manual. San Antonio, TX, KCI Therapeutic Services, Inc., 2000.
5. KCI Therapeutic Services: Vacuum-assisted Closure. Resources for Physicians. San Antonio, TX, KCI Therapeutic Services, Inc., 2000.
6. KCI Therapeutic Services: Vacuum-assisted closure: Recommended guidelines for use. In Physician and Caregiver Reference Manual. San Antonio, TX, KCI Therapeutic Services, Inc., 2001.
7. KCI Therapeutic Services: V.A.C.™ therapy information package. San Antonio, TX, KCI Therapeutic Services, Inc., 2001.
8. McCallon SK, Knight CA, Vallius JP, et al: Vacuum-assisted closure versus saline-moistened gauze in the healing of postoperative diabetic foot wounds. Ostomy Wound Manage 46(8):28-34, 2000.
9. Morykwas MJ, Argenta LC, Shelton-Brown EI, McGuire W: Vacuum assisted closure: A new method for wound control and treatment: Animal studies and basic foundation. Ann Plast Surg 38:553–562, 1997.
10. Schneider AM, Morykwas MJ, Argenta LC: A new and reliable method of securing skin grafts to the difficult bed. Plast Reconstr Surg 102:1195–1198, 1998.

# 30.  ANABOLIC AGENTS IN WOUND HEALING

*Catherine T. Milne, APRN, MSN, CWOCN, CS, ANP,
and Lisa Q. Corbett, APRN, MSN, CWOCN, CS*

### 1.  What are anabolic agents?

Anabolic steroids in oral form, given to patients to promote weight gain through the synthesis of protein.

### 2.  Why would patients with wounds need to gain weight?

Weight loss is an indicator of a hypermetabolic state. In patients with infection, major surgery, sepsis, burns, trauma, and severe chronic infections such as HIV, the stress response is activated. The increased energy demand for host survival requires use of muscle stores (lean body mass) as the supplier. It is more efficient for the body under stress to rapidly turn muscle into calories than to use fat stores.

### 3.  Does this mean that obese patients are at higher risk for loss of lean body mass?

Not really. All patients under stress revert to a catabolic state. Unfortunately, the detrimental effects are underrecognized in obese patients because of the preconceived and often ill-fated notion that they should "lose weight." Catabolism certainly causes weight loss in this population—but the wrong kind. Protein located in the viscera, connective tissue, and muscle is lost, while fat is spared. All stressed, catabolic patients, regardless of body habitus, will lose weight.

### 4.  What are the effects of a hypermetabolic state?

Catabolism is a lot like Audrey, the people-eating plant in *Little Shop of Horrors*. Audrey was never sated; she needed more frequent and larger feedings. Small effects of the stress response occur first—very early after injury. Hormonal balance is altered, with increased release of catecholamine, cortisol, glucagon, and insulin and decreased secretion of growth hormone.

Local and systemic mediators resulting from injury-induced inflammation add to the maladaptive response to rob needed energy from protein sources. The results are increases in body temperature, glucose production, and metabolic rate.

Weight loss, impaired wound healing, immunosuppression, and profound weakness are generally evident over a period of several weeks to months. Pneumonia is quite common. As weight loss progresses, more and more energy is required. Supply cannot keep up with demand, and, like Audrey, the whole system gets out of control. Once there is a 40% loss of lean body mass, there is no return. Death will occur even if a magic switch to turn off the catabolic state were to appear.

### 5.  What happens to a wound during this catabolic period?

The wound contributes greatly to catabolism. Increases in metabolic and cellular activity occur at the wound site. Not only does the wound need to rid its surfaces of unwanted debris, but the proliferative stage of rebuilding tissue requires a significant amount of calories. Large wounds, fistulas, and burns are added stressors because fluid losses add additional metabolic requirements. Impaired and markedly delayed wound healing results.

The immunocompromised patient is more likely to succumb to a wound infection. If more than 20% of lean body mass is lost, the body shifts its energy to maintain organ viability and all wound healing processes cease. Only when lean body mass is partially restored will wound healing resume.

### 6.  What is the role of anabolic agents in reversing the catabolic state?

Anabolism, defined as the synthesis of lean body mass, is the opposite of catabolism. It is the rebuilding mode. Exogenous use of an anabolic agent directly reverses catabolism by shunting available amino acids to rebuild tissue instead of being used as an energy supplier.

### 7. Do anabolic agents work alone?

No. A patient identified as a candidate for receiving an anabolic agent must also be able to receive and tolerate the nutritional requirements necessary to overcome the catabolic deficits. The ability to participate in resistance exercise is an additional prerequisite.

### 8. Why is exercise needed if the patient is extremely weak?

Exercise, in its own right, is a stimulus for anabolism. Resistance exercises, especially to large muscle groups, can promote weight gain. Consultation with a physical therapist to set up an exercise regimen early in the injury phase is paramount.

### 9. Discuss the three anabolic steroids on the market.

1. **Testosterone.** Metabolized in the liver and with a half-life of 10 minutes, this anabolic agent is not useful for wound healing.

2. **Human growth hormone** (HGH) is also metabolized in the liver. Exogenous supplementation in burn and trauma patients has shown its effectiveness in promoting anabolism and improving wound healing. The dosage, ironically, is based on weight: 0.1–0.2 mg/kg body weight. Unfortunately, HGH is associated with a number of complications, including hyperglycemia and hepatotoxicity.

3. **Oxandrolone** is the only anabolic steroid approved by the Food and Drug Administration for restoration of weight loss associated with HIV, trauma, sepsis, or surgery. It has a much more favorable side-effect profile than HGH. Available commercially as Oxandrin (Bio-Technology General Corp., Iselin, NJ), it is given in doses of 5–20 mg/day for 2–4 weeks. Although metabolized primarily in the kidney, oxandrolone can alter lipid profiles, suppress clotting factors, and increase edema. These effects are dose dependent. Absolute contraindications include prostate cancer, male breast cancer, female breast cancer associated with hypercalcemia, pregnancy, and the nephrotic phase of nephrosis. Clinical studies have shown that protein synthesis is evident in as few as 5 days.

### BIBLIOGRAPHY

1. Chang DW, DeSanti L, Demling RH: Anticatabolic and anabolic strategies in critical illness: A review of current treatment modalities. Shock 10:155–160, 1998.
2. Demling RH, DeSanti L: The stress response to injury and infection: Role of nutritional support. Wounds Compend Clin Res Pract 12(1):3–14, 2000.
3. Demling RH, DeSanti L: Closure of the "non-healing wound" corresponds with correction of weight loss using anabolic agent oxandrolone. Ostomy Wound Manage 44:58–65, 1998.
4. Himes D: Nutritional supplements in the treatment of pressure ulcers. Adv Wound Care 10:30–31, 1997.
5. Himes D: Strategies for managing involuntary weight loss. Adv Wound Skin Care 14(Suppl 1):7–12, 2001.

# 31. NONCONTACT NORMOTHERMIC WOUND THERAPY

*Joan Halpin-Landry, RN, MS, CWCN*

### 1. Define noncontact normothermic wound therapy (NNWT).

NNWT is a wound management system that provides controlled, radiant warmth to a wound within an optimal moist environment of 100% humidity. With NNWT, the skin and the subcutaneous tissues are returned to a temperature closer to normal. Warming encourages blood vessels to dilate, increasing blood flow and oxygen to the wound and periwound area. This process initiates a complex series of events that facilitates the migration of white blood cells into the wound. Fibroblasts increase in number and activity. These events bolster cellular function and the immune response to help fight infection and enhance wound healing. The only commercially available product to deliver NNWT is Warm-Up therapy (Augustine Medical, Eden Prairie, MN).

### 2. What is the most beneficial temperature to enhance healing?

Various temperatures have been tested, and 38°C (100.4°F) was found to be the most beneficial. Warming the wound bed affects a number of physiologic processes. There is a considerable increase in the measurement of transcutaneous partial pressure of oxygen and blood flow. The increase in capillary blood flow positively influences collagen formation in the wound bed.

### 3. What kinds of wounds are appropriate for NNWT?

NNWT is indicated for full- and partial-thickness wounds, including stage II–IV pressure ulcers; venous, arterial, and neuropathic/diabetic ulcers; and surgical wounds.

### 4. Does NNWT provide a moist wound environment?

Yes. It also facilitates autolytic debridement.

### 5. Can NNWT be used on clinically infected wounds?

Yes. NNWT may be used on clinically infected wounds with concurrent, appropriate antibiotic therapy to treat the infection.

### 6. What precautions are associated with NNWT therapy?

1. NNWT is not indicated for use in third-degree burns or stable arterial wounds with dry eschar.

2. The warming card or temperature control unit should never be used in the bath, shower, or other wet environments.

3. There is no risk of electrical shock from placing the warming card into a damp/wet wound cover. However, a damp/wet wound cover may damage the warming card.

### 7. Can a wound with nonviable tissue be managed effectively with NNWT?

Yes. It is not necessary to remove all nonviable tissue from a wound bed before beginning NNWT, although removal of such tissue favorably alters the healing environment. NNWT promotes autolytic wound debridement because the wound cover allows devitalized tissue to "self-digest" with the natural enzymes in the wound fluid.

### 8. Is clinical outcome improved if NNWT is used continuously throughout the day?

No. Intermittent warming was found to have the best outcomes with minimal risk. The subcutaneous tissue oxygen level was found to increase and remain elevated for 1 hour after the warming session was discontinued. Studies conclude that continuous warming is not beneficial to the wound.

**9. Can NNWT be applied to the wound if the periwound skin is macerated or traumatized?**

Yes. NNWT may be applied to a wound when the periwound skin is macerated or traumatized. The periwound skin should be protected with an appropriate skin protector or moisture barrier product. It is important that the wound cover be applied securely without causing additional skin trauma. The wound cover should be changed when the foam border becomes saturated with wound exudate.

**10. What are the components of an NNWT system?**

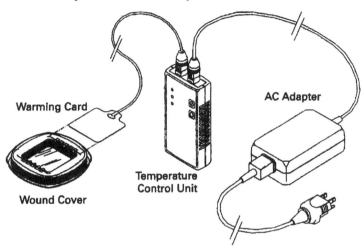

Warm-Up therapy is a stand-alone wound management system consisting of four components: a wound cover, warming card, temperature control unit, and AC adapter. (Courtesy of Augustine Medical, Eden Prairie, MN.)

**11. Can NNWT elevate tissue or skin temperature above normothermia?**

No. Warm-Up therapy will not elevate tissue temperature above normothermia. When inserted into the pocket of the wound cover, the warming card maintains a constant temperature of 38°C (100.4°F). The temperature control unit includes a microprocessor for safety and reliability and automatically shuts off after 2 hours of continuous use.

**12. Describe the wound cover.**

The wound cover is composed of a thin, transparent, semipermeable polyurethane film; a foam border to absorb wound exudate; and a water-based, hypoallergenic adhesive to secure the cover to the periwound skin. The wound covers are sterile and latex-free; they do not adhere to the wound surface. Some clinicians describe the dressing as looking and acting like a greenhouse. The wound covers allow trauma-free removal and are available in a multitude of shapes and sizes to accommodate different wounds.

**13. How frequently are wound covers changed?**

The wound covers are changed as clinically indicated, usually when the foam border of the wound cover becomes saturated with exudate. On average, they are changed every 3 days. More frequent changes are often necessary during the first 7–10 days of therapy because of the anticipated increase in wound exudate associated with enhanced tissue perfusion.

**14. What is the temperature of the warming card?**

The warming card will warm to 38°C (100.4°F).

**15. Where do you place the warming card?**

The warming card slips in a sleeve on the outside of the wound cover.

**16. Does the warming card come in contact with the periwound skin?**

No. When used according to proper protocol, the warming card never comes in contact with the wound or the periwound skin.

**17. Can the warming card be used for more than one patient?**

No. The warming card is for single patient use and is disposed of after therapy is discontinued.

**18. How do the warming card and temperature control unit work?**

The warming card connects to the temperature control unit port via a cable. The "on" button may be activated to initiate warming. The warming card is then inserted into the wound cover. When active warming therapy is completed, the temperature control unit is turned off and the warming card is removed from the wound cover. The warming card is then removed from the temperature control unit and placed into a patient-specific plastic pouch.

**19. What safeguards are associated with the temperature control unit?**

The operation of the warming card is controlled by a microprocessor in the temperature control unit. It will not exceed the recommended temperature of 38°C (100.4°F). An alarm will sound if the warming card becomes dislodged or if circuits in the warming card become damaged. There is also a low battery indicator on the temperature control unit. The temperature control unit can be run on either batter or AC power. The temperature control units and AC adapters may be used for more than one patient after the equipment has been cleansed according to the manufacturer's guidelines.

**20. How long can the temperature control unit run on battery power when the unit is fully charged?**

The battery charge life varies among different sizes of warming cards from 2.5 to 15 hours. The temperature control unit can power the warming card and simultaneously recharge the batteries when plugged into a wall outlet.

**21. How often is NNWT applied?**

Warming is initiated for a minimum of 1 hour 3 times/day. The interval between sessions should a minimum of 1 hour. The temperature control unit automatically shuts off after 2 hours of continuous use.

**22. Should the patient lie on the wound cover while the warming card delivers radiant warmth to the wound?**

No. While the warming card is in place, the patient should not be positioned on the affected area. NNWT is more effective and allows greater tissue perfusion when the treatment area is not exposed to pressure. The wound cover has been designed to withstand the normal activities of daily living. It will not be damaged if the patient lies on it after the warming card is removed.

**23. Why is it important to select a wound cover that will encompass an undermined or tunneled area as well as the open areas?**

NNWT needs to be applied to dermal and subcutaneous tissues that surround the wound. This approach increases capillary blood flow and oxygen perfusion to the whole wound.

**24. Can a liquid skin protector or skin barrier product be applied to the periwound skin to protect it from excessive wound exudate?**

Yes.

**25. Is it necessary to use any other wound products, such as hydrogels or wound fillers, with NNWT**

No. NNWT is a stand-alone therapy. Multiple treatment modalities are not necessary.

**26. What is the effect of showering with the wound cover in place?**

Showering or tub bathing with the wound cover in place may dislodge the wound cover or saturate its absorbent foam border.

**27. How is NNWT used with compression therapy?**

The patient removes the compression device (stocking, wrap, or pump sleeve) to expose the cover over the wound. The warming card is then inserted into the temperature control unit port. The warming card is placed into the outside pocket of the wound cover. The temperature control unit is turned on to begin the warming session. When the warming session is complete (approximately after 1 hour), the warming card is removed from the wound cover and the temperature control unit is turned off. The warming card is removed from the temperature control unit and stored in a plastic pouch. The compression stocking or wrap should then be reapplied. It is recommended that NNWT sessions be initiated 3 times/day.

**28. Does the patient need to off-load the neuropathic/diabetic wound if NNWT is used?**

Yes. Off-loading of the neuropathic/diabetic foot by eliminating pressure and shear is an essential component of wound management. NNWT has been shown to provide a beneficial wound healing environment for the neuropathic ulcer. It can be used with a removable walking cast, special half shoes, or individually designed orthotic footwear.

## BIBLIOGRAPHY

1. Ikeda T, Tayefeh F, Sessler DI, et al: Local radiant heating increases subcutaneous oxygen tension. Am J Surg 175:33–37, 1998.
2. Park HY, Shon K, Phillips T: The effect of heat on the inhibitory effects of chronic wound fluid on fibroblasts in vitro. Wounds 10(6):189–192, 1998.
3. Santilli SM, Valusek BA, Robinson C: Use of a noncontact radiant heat bandage for the treatment of chronic venous stasis ulcers. Adv Wound Care 12(2):89–92, 1999.
4. Whitney JD, Salvadalena G, Higa L, Mich M: Treatment: Pressure ulcers with noncontact normothermic wound therapy: Healing and warming effects. J Wound Ostomy Contin Nurs 28(5):244–252, 2001.
5. Xia A, Sato A, Hughes MA, Cherry GW: Stimulation of fibroblast growth in vitro by intermittent radiant warming. Wound Rep Reg 8:138–144, 2000.

# 32. HYPERBARIC OXYGEN AND TISSUE REPAIR

*Diane Merkle*, RN, BSN, MSHSA, CWOCN

### 1. What is hyperbaric oxygen?

Hyperbaric oxygen therapy ($HBO_2$) is inhalation of 100% oxygen delivered at pressures of more than 1 atmosphere (ATA). The term *atmosphere* describes an amount of prescribed pressure, with one atmosphere equal to pressure at sea level. Hyperbaric oxygen is provided in enclosed chambers in individual (monoplace) and group (multiplace) settings. A typical treatment consists of inhalation of 100% oxygen at pressures 2–3 times the pressure at sea level—the amount of pressure that a scuba diver encounters at approximately 33–66 feet below the ocean surface.

### 2. Describe the oxygen chamber.

The **multiplace chamber** is a large pressurized room in which multiple patients and staff are in attendance. Multiplace chambers are pressurized to the desired therapeutic level with compressed air, and the patient receives the oxygen via a mask or head tent. Multiplace chambers require special expertise to operate and maintain. They are large and expensive but have the flexibility of treating many patients at once. An additional advantage is the capability of direct hands-on care during therapy.

**Monoplace chambers** are the more common type. A monoplace chamber is a soundproof, cylindrical, acrylic tube in which a single, unaccompanied patient reclines on a stretcher. The entire monoplace chamber is pressurized with 100% oxygen. It can also be compressed with air, with the requirement of a mask to deliver the oxygen. Monoplace chambers are the least expensive type of hyperbaric chambers. They are portable and require only a small amount of floor space. Staff can be easily trained to operate the chambers safely. Monoplace chambers do not require "off-gassing" of nitrogen build-up because the patient is not breathing air. The drawbacks are patient fears of isolation and the lack of hands-on care while the patient is enclosed in the chamber.

### 3. When should $HBO_2$ be considered for wound patients?

The costs of a nonhealing wound are great. $HBO_2$ should be considered as an adjunctive modality to good wound care when traditional treatment plans fail. Irradiated tissue, the presence of certain infections, failure or exclusion of revascularization, and tissue hypoxia are conditions for which the practitioner may consider $HBO_2$ as an option.

### 4. Why is $HBO_2$ relatively uncommon?

Scientists have studied hyperbaric oxygen for over 100 years, but it is still misunderstood by many practitioners. Unfortunately, $HBO_2$ has a somewhat checkered past, with unscrupulous providers marring the reputation of those providing legitimate care. The Undersea and Hyperbaric Medical Society established practice guidelines in 1976 to standardize $HBO_2$ indications and protocols. These guidelines are updated every 2–3 years. Modern $HBO_2$ therapy has been used since the 1960s, when research focused on its effectiveness with gas gangrene and anemia. Randomized, double-blind studies exploring $HBO_2$ and wound healing are needed to support efficacy.

### 5. What specific conditions may benefit from $HBO_2$?

Clinical acceptance for $HBO_2$ is uncontested to treat decompression sickness ("the bends"), arterial gas embolism, clostridial myonecrosis, and carbon monoxide poisoning. Other less known indications for $HBO_2$ include chronic refractory osteomyelitis, acute traumatic ischemia (e.g., compartment syndrome), necrotizing soft tissue infection, soft tissue and osteoradionecrosis, intracranial abscess, exceptional blood loss anemia, thermal burns, and compromised flaps and grafts.

6. **How does HBO$_2$ affect tissue viability and wound healing?**

The mechanisms of HBO$_2$ are hyperoxygenation, increased pressure, vasoconstriction, and antimicrobial activity. Partial pressure of oxygen (PO$_2$) > 30 mmHg contributes to reduced ischemia in tissues with low oxygen delivery, formation of a collagen matrix, and increased angiogenesis. Breathing pure oxygen under pressure increases the tissue PO$_2$ from a normal value of 30–40 mmHg to values in excess of 200 mmHg. Two atmospheres of pressure at 100% oxygen lead to a proportional increase in angiogenesis. Increases of arterial oxygen up to 1500 mmHg or greater during hyperoxygenation result in greater distances of oxygen diffusion, reversing the hypoxia that leads to wound healing failure and tissue death. Mild-to-moderate ischemia responds best to HBO$_2$. Severe ischemia does not respond to HBO$_2$. Although cartilage can repair with a low oxygen tension, bone repair responds favorably in a high oxygen environment.

Vasoconstriction effects of HBO$_2$ intuitively seem counterproductive to tissue repair. However, the amount and diffusion distance of dissolved oxygen in the plasma are so greatly increased that oxygen-dependent wound healing mechanisms are unaffected. More importantly, vasoconstriction reduces interstitial edema. It also aids in management of compartment syndromes and acute ischemia of the limbs.

HBO$_2$ has a variety of microbiologic effects. Leukocyte function is oxygen-dependent, selected antibiotics (e.g., aminoglycosides) have a potentiated effect, and a variety of microbial metabolic reactions are inhibited. HBO$_2$ also has bacteriostatic and bactericidal effects on selected microorganisms due to an increase in the generation of oxygen radicals. Elevated tissue PO$_2$ increases the effectiveness of aminoglycosides, floroquinolones, trimethoprim, and vancomycin and potentiates the activity of some sulfonamides.

HBO$_2$ results in increased flexibility of red blood cells. It also prevents reperfusion injury in the endothelial linings of blood vessels by preventing adherence of polymorphonucleocytes to the endothelium. HBO$_2$ preserves adenosine triphosphate, contributing to edema reduction through cellular osmolarity control.

7. **How long does the effect last?**

The effect of therapy lasts approximately 2–4 hours after treatment and is cumulative over time.

8. **What are the contraindications to HBO$_2$?**

Absolute contraindications include the use of adriamycin, Antabuse, cisplatinum, and sulfamylon; terminal state of illness; and untreated pneumothorax. A history of bleomycin use is also an absolute contraindication. A history of leukemia, testicular cancer, or lymphoma may signal past bleomycin treatment. Relative contraindications include active malignancy, seizure disorder, congenital spherocytosis, pregnancy, emphysema, carbon monoxide retention, and as ear, nose, and throat complications. Such cases should be considered on an individual basis.

9. **Describe the typical HBO$_2$ treatment.**

Generally, the patient remains in the chamber for approximately 90–120 minutes at a pressure of 2–2.4 ATA, depending on the diagnosis and individual tolerance. An air break may be required. During this brief period the patient breathes room air through a mouthpiece to prevent oxygen toxicity complications, such as seizures. An example of an HBO$_2$ treatment plan is 40 treatments of approximately 120 minutes at 2.4 atmospheres for recalcitrant osteomyelitis. Emergent conditions such as an ischemic flap or clostridial infection may require twice-daily treatments.

10. **What other oxygen therapies are not hyperbaric?**

Breathing 100% oxygen that is not pressurized to more than 1 atmosphere is not hyperbaric. Oxygen applied topically or with an extremity in a chamber is not hyperbaric.

11. **What undesirable side effects may be seen with hyperbaric oxygen?**

Therapeutic oxygen and pressurized oxygen are drugs. Hyperoxia and the effects of increased pressure on the body can lead to potential undesirable side effects. Oxygen toxicity can result from oxygen tension > 40% over time, but normal hyperbaric protocols minimize this risk. A rare side effect is seizures. Barotrauma to ears can require temporary pressure equalization tube placement. Eyesight may temporarily be affected as a rare complication. Vision may become nearsighted but returns to normal 6–8 weeks after completion of treatment.

### 12. What diagnostic studies are done to prepare for hyperbaric oxygen treatment?

Transcutaneous oximetry (TCOM) is an excellent tool to measure the potential success of $HBO_2$. TCOM measures the level of hypoxemia in the periwound tissue as the patient breathes room air. A tissue $PO_2$ of 20 mmHg or less generally reflects a wound that will not heal; a tissue $PO_2$ of 30 mmHg or higher should result in healing. An oxygen challenge (breathing 100% oxygen via facemask) during TCOM reveals the potential of the periwound tissue for oxygen uptake. An increase of 10 mmHg or higher in TCOM during the oxygen challenge qualifies a patient for $HBO_2$.

Occasionally, a borderline TCOM result may lead to a diagnostic $HBO_2$ treatment. The tissue $PO_2$ is measured during $HBO_2$ pressurization. A tissue $PO_2$ augmentation in excess of 200 mmHg signifies potential therapeutic benefit.

Before treatment, a complete history and physical exam, review of medications, complete blood count, erythrocyte sedimentation rate (as needed in cases of infection), chest x-ray, and electrocardiogram are required. Vascular bypass should be ruled out as a viable option in ischemic wound cases. Smoking should be stopped, because it is counterproductive to the treatments and tissue healing. Smoking causes approximately a 30% reduction in perfusion.

### 13. Does hyperbaric oxygen affect soft tissue infections?

$HBO_2$ can affect a number of mixed aerobic and anaerobic gas-forming and necrotizing infections. Hypoxic conditions created by anaerobic organisms potentiate the infectious process. Necrotizing soft tissue infections can lead to devastating tissue loss and death if not identified quickly and aggressively treated. $HBO_2$ works in several ways as an adjunct to treatment of these infections: as a bactericidal agent against anaerobes, an inhibitor of toxin formation by certain anaerobes, an enhancer of the action of polymorphonuclear phagocytosis, and an agent to hyperoxygenate ischemic tissue preoperatively to clarify the line of demarcation between viable and nonviable tissue. Necrotizing fasciitis most commonly results from trauma (see Chapter 47). $HBO_2$ may not affect mortality, but it may facilitate early wound closure. $HBO_2$ should be instituted within 24 hours of diagnosis, if possible. If time allows, $HBO_2$ can be performed before surgery to stabilize the patient and the necrotizing process. Twice-daily treatments may be required until the infection is stabilized.

### 14. Does $HBO_2$ have a role in healing traumatic wounds?

Crush injuries cause tissue, bone, and vascular damage and may result in myonecrosis, shock, acidosis, hyperkalemia, and renal failure. $HBO_2$ mechanisms benefit traumatized tissue through hyperoxygenation, vasoconstriction, and protection from reperfusion injury. Indirect injuries that result in compartment syndrome may also benefit from $HBO_2$. Local tissue injury can result in edema, leading to a drop in $PO_2$, ischemia, and eventual tissue death. Compartment syndrome occurs when local pressure reaches 30–40 mmHg. Muscle fibers swell, and intracompartmental fluid accumulates. $HBO_2$ for traumatic wounds should be instituted as soon as possible after the patient is stabilized.

### 15. Does $HBO_2$ affect thermal wounds?

$HBO_2$ has been shown to have positive affects on frostbite and burn injuries. It may reduce the conversion of partial-thickness wounds to full-thickness wounds in thermal injuries as well as reduce edema and the need for skin grafting. As in all trauma situations, $HBO_2$ should be instituted as early as possible after diagnosis and stabilization of the patient. Treatment is ordered at 2 ATA twice daily for 90 minutes until healthy grafts cover the wounds.

### 16. Can $HBO_2$ be used to increase response to grafting?

Tissue flaps and grafts with signs of inadequate perfusion may benefit from $HBO_2$. At the earliest sign of circulatory compromise, accepted protocols warrant twice-daily $HBO_2$ therapy.

**17. Discuss the role of HBO₂ in healing diabetic foot wounds.**

$HBO_2$ is indicated for microvascular tissue ischemia in those who have failed, or are not candidates, for large vessel vascular bypass. Recalcitrant osteomyelitis that has failed to respond to surgical debridement and at least six weeks of antibiotics is an indication for adjunctive $HBO_2$. Leukocyte function that may be compromised due to hyperglycemia is enhanced with hyperoxygenation. Diabetic foot wounds require wide excision of wound and periwound callus and offloading of pressure areas.

**18. Does hyperbaric oxygen enhance topical growth factors?**

A tissue $PO_2$ less than 30 mmHg may not allow tissue response to growth factors or may lead to borderline results. Diabetic foot wounds that are mildly to moderately ischemic due to microvasculature changes typically respond well to $HBO_2$. However, $HBO_2$ and growth factors have not been studied together in randomized, controlled trials.

**19. Can irradiated tissue and bone respond to HBO₂?**

Progressive sclerosis of irradiated tissue can begin within 6 months of exposure to ionizing radiation or as late as 18 months and continues for the lifetime of the patient. Surgical or traumatic wounds in this hypoxic, fibrotic area may never heal to closure. If a procedure such as a flap, graft, or tooth extraction is planned for an irradiated area, pre- and postprocedural $HBO_2$ greatly improves the success rate and reduces the tissue loss affected by radionecrosis. For best results, an $HBO_2$ treatment plan calls for 20–30 preprocedural treatments and 10 postprocedural treatments, depending on the procedure and the underlying condition.

**20. What does the patient experience during HBO₂?**

$HBO_2$ is painless, although the patient may feel fullness in the ears similar to pressure changes experienced when a jet descends and lands. Valsalva maneuvers to gently clear the ears are performed. Breathing is normal.

Patients commonly spend their treatment time viewing a television situated outside the chamber. Some patients sleep through their treatment. Rarely, an antianxiety medication may be required to treat feelings of claustrophobia. The trained hyperbaric technician (e.g., EMT, RRT, RN, APRN, PA) is in constant attendance, communicating with the patient in the chamber via a telephone-like device.

Because of the presence of 100% oxygen in the chamber, safety is focused on elimination of fire risk. The patient dresses in 100% cotton clothing and takes nothing into the chamber, except a plastic drink bottle, to minimize risk of static electricity. Intravenous lines and ventilator equipment are specially adapted to prevent malfunction in the high-pressure environment. Overall, the patient's experience is uneventful; the time commitment is the most cumbersome aspect of $HBO_2$.

### BIBLIOGRAPHY

1. Elliott DC, Kufera JA, Myers RA: Necrotizing soft tissue infections: Risk factors for mortality and strategies for management. Ann Surg 224(5):672–683, 1996.
2. Kindwall EP: Uses of hyperbaric oxygen therapy in the 1990's. Cleve Clin J Med 59:517–528, 1992.
3. Kindwall EP: Contraindications and side effects to hyperbaric oxygen treatment. In Kindwall EP (ed): Hyperbaric Medicine Practice. Flagstaff, AZ, Best Publishing Company, 1995, pp 46–51.
4. Sheffield PJ, Workman WT: Noninvasive tissue oxygen measurements in patients administered normobaric and hyperbaric oxygen by mask. Hyperb Oxyg Rev 6:47–42, 1995.

# 33. ELECTRICAL STIMULATION

*Bonnie J. Sparks-DeFriese, PT, RN, CWS*

### 1. When should adjunctive therapies be initiated in wound care?

Adjunctive therapies should be initiated for chronic wounds or wounds that do not respond to optimal care.

### 2. How long has electricity been used as a medicinal treatment?

Electricity has been used to enhance healing for decades. Benjamin Franklin wrote about the use of "electrical shocks" for a frozen shoulder as early as 1757. Today electricity is used for diagnosis of human body functions (e.g., electrocardiography, electromyography) as well as for treatment of impaired body functions (e.g., to control pain, relax muscle spasms, decrease edema, enhance wound healing). When planning treatment, one may choose from different forms of electrical stimulation, including direct current, pulsed current, and alternating current. Monophasic (high-voltage) pulsed current is the preferred form for most therapists for all three phases of wound healing.

### 3. What is the connection between electrical stimulation and wound healing?

The body has been found to resemble a battery. Current can flow between parts of the skin if the circuit is complete. This concept is termed the *current of injury*. The outer layer of both human and animal skin is electronegative with respect to deeper skin layers. Kloth described electrical stimulation (ES) in wound healing with the human skin bioelectric system using the following concepts:

- Sodium ions ($Na^+$) are pumped to deeper epidermal and dermal cells.
- Skin surface has mean negative charge of $-23mV$ due to chloride ions ($Cl^-$)
- Wound tissue is positively charged.

ES mimics natural currents of injury, thereby correcting the damage to the human skin bioelectric system.

### 4. Where was the current of injury first demonstrated?

In a salamander amputee. Becker found that the salamander's regenerating limb produced a measurable current with a varying polarity during the regeneration process.

### 5. How is high-voltage pulsed current (HVPC) used in wound healing?

HVPC is the application of a pulsed, direct current to a wound. It works to release the body's natural endorphins. Depending on the electrode, it leaves a net charge—either positive or negative—in the wound. Research has shown that this net charge stimulates wound healing.

### 6. By what mechanism does HVPC help to heal wounds?

The monophasic current stimulates healing through angiogenesis, epithelial migration, and the electrical charge/battery system. Research has shown that the monophasic current can use these properties to enhance wound healing. In 1994, the Agency for Health Care Policy and Research Guideline for the Treatment of Pressures Ulcers stated: "at this time electrical stimulation is the only adjunctive therapy with sufficient supporting evidence to warrant recommendation by the panel." The other adjunctive therapies considered by the panel included hyperbaric oxygen; infrared, ultraviolet and low-energy laser irradiation; ultrasound; miscellaneous topical agents (including cytokine growth factors); and systemic drugs other than antibiotics. Although research has since supported these other modalities, ES is the earliest adjunctive method to be supported by both fiscal approval from third-party payors and well-established science.

### 7. What equipment is needed to use HVPC?

You need a stimulator that produces a high-voltage current. This current is the safest choice available for depositing a net charge in the wound, based on its polarity. It is also helpful to have multiple channels so that it is possible to treat more than one wound at a time. The device should also have adjustable pulse rates. Its output can be read in either volts or milliamps.

**8. What outcomes are seen with the different poles?**

Monophasic waves have one negative and one positive pole that remain constant during the treatment unless changed by the clinician. The table below compares several outcomes from each pole.

*Effects of Electrical Stimulation Polarity*

| ACTION | ANODE (POSITIVE POLE) | CATHODE (NEGATIVE POLE) |
|---|---|---|
| Attracts | Oxygen and acids | Alkalines |
| Repels | Alkalines | Acids |
| Tissue changes | Hardens | Softens |
| Vasomotor | Vasoconstriction | Vasodilation |
| Bleeding | Stops | Produces |
| Edema | Increases | Decreases |
| Germicidal effect | More | Less |

**9. How is HVPC applied?**

Two primary methods of application of HVPC may be used. In **monopolar application**, the active electrode, chosen from either the anode or cathode, varies from facility to facility based on individual protocols. Most clinicians prefer a custom-made electrode created for each patient because of infection control issues. The electrode can be a piece of aluminum foil encased inside a saline-soaked or hydrogel-impregnated gauze placed inside the wound. One also may use saline-soaked gauze placed under a traditional carbon electrode. The electrode is attached to a disposable, insulated alligator clip at the end of a lead wire, which is attached to the ES machine.

In **bipolar application**, one places two electrodes on opposite sides of the wound or four bifurcated dispersive leads connected to electrodes around the wound so that current will flow through the wound from two or four sides at once. The closer the electrodes are to each other, the more superficial the effect. This aspect makes bipolar application appropriate for partial-thickness wounds. The electrode size also makes a difference. The smaller the electrode, the more concentrated the current.

**10. What protocols are available for ES treatment?**

Several protocols are available to the clinician, each with its own unique characteristics. For example, some clinicians recommend that the polarity be changed on a particular given day of treatment, whereas others change the polarity when healing plateaus. Three sample protocols are included; each is listed with the name of the commonly associated clinician. The differences typically have to do with when to change polarity. Assessment of the wound-healing stage is the identified criterion for making such a decision. Each protocol starts with the same procedure

1. Position the patient for comfort. Explain the procedure.

2. Gently cleanse the wound with a noncytotoxic solution, such as normal saline or nonionic surfactant, to remove topical residuals such as bacteria, metal ions (e.g., povidone-iodine, zinc, silver sulfadiazine), or residual wound dressings without traumatizing the wound bed

3. Pat dry the surrounding skin.

**Example A (Sparks)**

1. Place the dispersive (second) electrode:
   • For an extremity wound, place the electrode on a large muscle group or an acupuncture point on the same side of the body proximal to the wound.
   • For a trunk wound, place the electrode on an acupuncture point in close proximity to the wound.

2. Fill the wound bed with a conductive dressing, such as saline-soaked gauze, conductive hydrogel-impregnated gauze, or hydrogel.

3. Attach an insulated alligator clip to the above dressing.

4. Cover the entire area with gauze and tape or a plastic film (e.g., Saran Wrap) to ensure no movement of electrode with subsequent damage to surrounding skin.

5. Determine wound-healing phase and begin treatment.

| HEALING PHASE | POLE | PULSE RATE | INTENSITY | DURATION | FREQUENCY |
|---|---|---|---|---|---|
| Inflammation | (–) | 100 pps | 150–200 V | 60 min | Daily, 5–7 times/wk |
| Proliferative | (–) until plateau; then (+) | 100 pps | Subsensory or sensory | 60 min | Daily, 3–5 times/wk |
| Remodeling | (+) | 80 pps | Subsensory or sensory | 60 min | Daily, 3 times/wk |

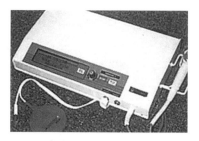

Rich-mar stimulator. (Courtesy of Rich-mar Corporation.)

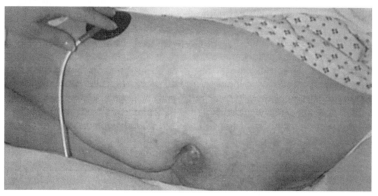

Dispersive/second active electrode placement. On an extremity: place on a large muscle group or an acupuncture point on the same side of the body proximal to the wound. On the trunk: place on an acupuncture point in close proximity (based on size of electrode) to the wound.

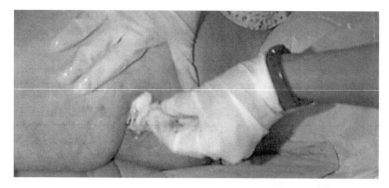

Fill wound bed with conductive dressing: saline-soaked gauze, conductive hyrdogel dressing, or hydrogel.

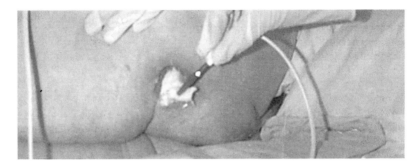

Attach an insulated alligator clipto the above dressing.

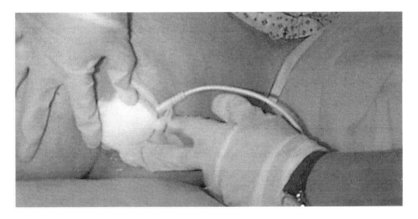

Cover entire area to ensure no movement of electrode and no damage to surrounding skin.

## Example B (Gogia)

| POLARITY | PULSE RATE | INTENSITY | DURATION | FREQUENCY |
|---|---|---|---|---|
| Negative for infected or inflamed wound and positive if not infected or inflamed. If chronically infected and inflamed, use negative for the first 3–4 days, alternating to positive polarity. | 50–120 pps | Subthreshold muscle contraction | 45–60 min | Daily, 5 times/wk |

## Example C (Sussman)

| HEALING PHASE | POLE | PULSE RATE | INTENSITY | DURATION | FREQUENCY |
|---|---|---|---|---|---|
| Inflammation | (–) | 30 pps | 100–150 V | 60 min | Daily, 5–7 times/wk |
| Proliferative | Alternate –/+ every 3 days | 100–128 pps | 100–150 V | 60 min | Daily, 5–7 times/wk |
| Remodeling | Alternate daily | 60–64 pps | 100–150 V | 60 min | Daily, 3 times/wk |

## 11. When should ES be considered in wound management?

- For patients who have not responded to optimal wound care
- If the clinician's goal is to stimulate angiogenesis (defined by the Food and Drug Administration as "increasing local blood circulation")
- Pain control
- Maintaining or increasing range of motion

## 12. What are the contraindications to ES?

- Use over or in close proximity to a malignancy
- Use over an electrical implant or demand cardiac pacemaker
- Use over a pregnant uterus
- Presence of active osteomyelitis
- Use over metal ions (e.g., iodine, zinc, or silver)
- Use over upper chest and anterior neck due to the presence of reflex centers and vital organs (e.g., carotid sinus, heart, parasympathetic nerves, ganglion, laryngeal muscles, phrenic nerve)

## 13. How dangerous is ES? Can I get electrocuted when using ES for wound healing?

No. ES protocols for wound healing produce a small amount of voltage. One good reason to choose HVPC is its demonstrated safety.

## 14. Can a staff nurse apply ES for wound healing?

No. ES is not within a nurse's scope of practice. ES is within the scope of practice for physical and occupational therapists. But nurses can and are encouraged to consider ES for patients with non-healing wounds. Ask for orders from the medical provider, or refer patients to rehabilitation services (physical or occupational therapy). The importance of the multidisciplinary approach cannot be overemphasized in wound care.

## 15. Does it matter what machine is used?

Various machines are available on the market. Questions that you should ask include the following:

- What safety features are included?
- What is the reliability of current delivery?
- Can the machine perform other treatment modalities? Do I need other modalities, such as ultrasound?
- What type of current does it provide?
- What is the history of the company and manufacturer?
- What type of service can be expected from the company and manufacturer?

## 16. What controversies are associated with ES?

Current controversies relate to suitability of ES therapy and the selection of protocols.

## 17. What issues should be considered in relation to suitability?

When considering the use of ES, ask yourself the following questions:

- Is it appropriate to use ES?
- Have I tried proper wound management?

Proper management includes debridement of nonviable tissue, moist healing techniques, assessment and treatment of dietary issues, enhancement of circulation to the involved area, control of infection, treatment of concurrent medical illness, and contributing risk factors. Many clinicians do not believe in adding adjunctive therapies, even though the research supports this practice.

## 18. What issues should be considered in relation to the ES protocol?

The frequency and polarity protocol components are not consistent from researcher to researcher. The frequency varies from 30 to 129 pps, and polarity recommendations vary from "no change" to "change from negative to positive every 3 days" or "change the pole when the healing plateaus." Relevant questions include the following:

- Does the frequency (pulses per second) really have an effect on the healing outcome?
- Does the changing of polarity really have an effect?
- Do we know the answer to either of these questions?

## BIBLIOGRAPHY

1. Becker R: The electrical control of growth processes. Med Times 95:657–669, 1967.
2. Becker R: The Body Electric: Electromagnetism and the Foundations of Life. New York, William Morrow, 1985.
3. Brown M, et al: Polarity effects on wound healing using electric stimulation in rabbits. Arch Phys Med Rehabil 70:623–627, 1989.
4. Frantz R: Electrical stimulation in acute and chronic wounds. In Bryant RA (ed): Acute and Chronic Wounds:: Nursing Management. St. Louis, Mosby, 1992, pp 308–311.
5. Gogia P: Physical therapy intervention in wound management. In Krasner D, Kane D (eds): Chronic Wound Care: A Clinical Source Book for Healthcare Professionals, 2nd ed. Wayne, PA, Health Management Publications, 1997, pp 252–253.
6. Griffin JW, et al: Efficacy of high voltage pulsed current for healing of pressure ulcers in patients with spinal cord injury. Phys Ther 71(6):433–442, 1991.
7. Kloth L, Feedar J: Acceleration of wound healing with high voltage, monophasic, pulsed current. Phys Ther 68(4):503–508, 1988.
8. McCulloch J, Kloth L, Feedar J (eds): Wound Healing: Alternatives in Management, 2nd ed. Philadelphia, F.A. Davis, 1995.
9. Sparks B: Physical therapy and wound care: What's the connection? Ostomy Wound Manage 40(4):22–29, 1994.
10. Sussman C, Byl N: Electrical stimulation for wound healing. In Sussman C, Bates-Jensen BM (eds) Wound Care: A Collaborative Practice Manual for Physical Therapists and Nurses. Gaithersburg, MD, Aspen, 1998, pp 357–388.

# 34. ULTRASOUND IN WOUND CARE

*Teresa A. Conner-Kerr, PhD, PT, CWS(D)*

### 1. What is ultrasound?

Ultrasound is acoustic energy or mechanical pressure waves transmitted at a frequency above 20 KHz. This frequency is inaudible to humans and is used in health care for both diagnostic and therapeutic applications.

### 2. How do therapeutic and diagnostic ultrasound differ?

**Therapeutic ultrasound** is delivered at a lower frequency, typically 1–3 MHz, whereas **diagnostic ultrasound** is delivered at higher frequencies, such as 5–8 MHz. Both approaches, however, depend on the differential absorption and reflection of acoustic energy by varying tissue types. Typically, tissues high in protein, such as tendons and ligaments, absorb ultrasound very well compared with fatty tissues, which allow almost complete transmission of ultrasound to deeper tissues.

### 3. What specific ultrasound diagnostic tools are available for examining wound depth and tissue involvement?

A relatively new diagnostic ultrasound technology aimed at visualizing skin and its components has become available in the United States. The Longport Diagnostic US Scanner, developed by Dyson and colleagues from United Medical and Dental Schools of Guy's and St. Thomas's Hospitals in London, can be used to detect injurious changes in soft tissues. This scanner can differentiate between the epidermal and dermal layers of skin. It can also distinguish between the papillary and reticular layers of the dermis and among structures such as blood vessels, tendons, and ligaments. The Longport Diagnostic US Scanner has been used successfully to detect deleterious changes resulting from excessive pressure to human tissues. This technology may prove useful in predicting persons and tissues at risk for breakdown and for monitoring effects of therapy.

### 4. What effects does therapeutic ultrasound have on wound healing?

Low intensity (0.2–0.5 W/cm$^2$) MHz (1 or 3) ultrasound has been shown to facilitate wound healing by enhancing fibroblastic, endothelial and white cell recruitment and activity during the inflammatory and proliferative phases of healing. Ultrasound appears to be particularly effective when applied shortly after tissue injury. Early application enhances the rate of progression of the treated tissue through the three phases of healing (inflammation, proliferation, and remodeling).

### 5. By what mechanisms does ultrasound achieve its effects?

One of the proposed mechanisms by which therapeutic ultrasound facilitates advancement through these stages is by enhancing the release of factors involved in the inflammatory and early proliferative phase of wound healing. Increased levels of mitogenic growth factors that intensify fibroblast proliferation have been detected when macrophage-like cells are exposed to low-intensity therapeutic ultrasound. Increased recruitment of mast cells, platelets, and macrophages also has been observed after treatment. Elevated numbers of these cells, which play critical roles in wound healing, are consistent with the findings of increased levels of fibroplasia and rates of wound contraction in ultrasound-treated wounds.

Low-intensity therapeutic ultrasound (0.1 W/cm$^2$) has also been shown to enhance the mechanical properties of scar tissue. Scar tissue from wounds treated with ultrasound has been shown to be stronger and more elastic. This increased strength is thought to be associated with the increased numbers of fibroblasts observed after treatment with MHz ultrasound. It may also be related to the histologic findings that tissues treated with MHz ultrasound have increased levels of collagen synthesis and demonstrate a more organized collagen pattern in the wound bed.

**6. At what stage of wound healing is therapeutic ultrasound indicated?**

Early intervention during the inflammatory and initial proliferative phases of wound healing appears to be most effective.

**7. What are the treatment parameters for therapeutic ultrasound usage in wound healing?**

Low-intensity parameters ($< 0.5$ W/cm$^2$) and short treatment times (about 5 minutes for small wounds using a 3-MHz generator) are recommended. The 3-Mhz generator is preferred over the 1-MHz generator because the acoustic energy is preferentially absorbed in the wound bed rather than transmitted to deeper tissues, as with the 1 MHz generator.

**8. How is ultrasound applied to the wound?**

MHz ultrasound can be applied to the periwound area via sonation over a hydrogel pad or with an amorphous hydrogel. Ultrasound may also be applied directly over the wound bed by placing a hydrogel pad or thin film dressing over the wound bed and sonating over the moistened dressing. If the wound has a significant cavity, the cavity may be filled with amorphous hydrogel or sterile normal saline and then covered by the hydrogel pad or thin film dressing to increase ultrasonic transmission. Ultrasound travels best through solid mediums and is attenuated by air; therefore, significant cavities should be filled with a conductive medium to replace the air interface. As with any wound treatment, the periwound skin and wound should be thoroughly cleansed before treatment.

**9. Summarize the relative ultrasound transmission rates through various wound dressings.**

Ultrasound transmission rates through common wound dressings were recently examined. Both hydrogels and thin film dressings were included. Two of the hydrogels exhibited the greatest rates of transmission: Nu-Gel (~77%) and ClearSite (~72%), followed by the thin film dressings CarraSmart Film (~61%), Bioclusive (~53%), and Tegaderm (~47%). This study suggests that Nu-Gel of ClearSite hydrogels should be used to optimize transmission of ultrasound energy to wound tissues during treatment.

**10. What are the common contraindications for MHz ultrasound treatment of a wound?**
- Precancerous or cancerous lesions
- Areas prone to hemorrhage
- Epiphyseal plates of children
- Pregnant uterus
- Gonads, eyes, cranium or spinal cord
- Deep venous thrombosis
- Devitalized/irradiated tissue
- Acute infections

Acute infections of localized tissues or high numbers of bacteria may not be a contraindication for treatment with several new ultrasound technologies that use a KHz frequency (30–50 KHz), which appears to disinfect (Hydrosound, Arjo, Roselle, IL) or to have bactericidal action (Mist Ultrasound Transport Therapy, Celleration, Eden Prairie, MN) when applied to human tissues.

**11. How can therapeutic ultrasound be used to deliver drugs?**

Delivery of medications via ultrasound is termed *phonophoresis*. Medications are pushed through the skin surface by the mechanical pressure waves that constitute ultrasound. Ultrasound has been shown to be effective in delivering dexamethasone transdermally in adult men when continuous-mode ultrasound is used at a thermal setting with a 1-MHz generator. Phonophoretic application of corticosteroids is commonly used by physical therapists to treat excessive levels of inflammation.

**12. Describe the new advances in therapeutic ultrasound.**

A new ultrasound technology, Mist Ultrasound Transport Therapy, uses a novel mechanism for the delivery of KHz ultrasound to the body surface. Ultrasound is transmitted to the body surface via a noncontact method that uses a carrier mist and a KHz rather than MHz frequency. Early studies indicate that this new technology is effective in killing bacteria such as *Pseudomonas* and *Staphylococcus* species as well as in promoting increased perfusion and granulation tissue formation in various wounds, including neuropathic, venous, arterial, and pressure wounds. A laser Doppler study has demonstrated enhanced perfusion after treatment with this noncontact device. In addition, a study using a diabetic mouse model has demonstrated increased collagen synthesis.

## BIBLIOGRAPHY

1. Conner-Kerr T, Sullivan PK: Effects of noncontact mist ultrasound therapy (M.U.S.T.) on bacterial levels in a chronic wound bed. Presented at the 14th Annual Symposium on Advanced Wound Care and Medical Research Forum on Wound Repair, Las Vegas, NV, 2001.
2. Houghton PD: Effects of therapeutic modalities on wound healing: A conservative approach to wound management. Phys Ther Rev 4(3):167–182, 1999.
3. Houghton PE, Campbell KE: Choosing an adjunctive therapy for the treatment of chronic wounds. Ostomy Wound Manage 45(8):43–52, 1999.
4. Klucinec B, Scheidler M, Denegar C, et al: Effectiveness of wound care products in the transmission of acoustic energy. Phys Ther 86(5):469–476, 2000.
5. Sullivan PK, Connor-Kerr T: Effects of noncontact mist ultrasound therapy (M.U.S.T.) in removal of *Pseudomonas aeruginosa* in vitro. Presented at the 14th Annual Symposium on Advanced Wound Care and Medical Research Forum on Wound Repair. Las Vegas, NV, 2001.
6. Sussman C, Dyson M: Therapeutic and diagnostic ultrasound. In: Sussman C, Bates-Jensen BM (eds): Wound Care: A Collaborative Practice Manual for Physical Therapists and Nurses. Gaithersburg, MD, Aspen, 1998, pp 427–445.
7. Wagner SA, Vetter E, Cockerill FR, Kavros SJ: The effect of mist ultrasonic transport therapy on common bacterial wound pathogens. Poster presentation at the Symposium on Advanced Wound Care and Medical Research Forum on Wound Repair, Las Vegas, NV, 2001.

# 35. SHORTWAVE DIATHERMY

James E.Tracy, MS, PT, CDP, MLD

### 1. What is electromagnetic radiation?

Electromagnetic radiation is composed of electrical and magnetic fields that are oriented perpendicular to each other. Unlike ultrasound, which needs a medium to propagate, electromagnetic radiation can propagate in a vacuum. All electromagnetic radiation travels at the speed of light or $3.0 \times 10^8$ m/sec. Electromagnetic radiation is traditionally categorized according to its frequency and wavelength, which are inversely proportional to each other. The entire electromagnetic spectrum includes low-frequency electrical currents, shortwaves, microwaves, infrared radiation, visible light, ultraviolet light, and higher-frequency radiation, such as x-rays and gamma rays.

### 2. What is shortwave diathermy (SWD)? How does it fit into the electromagnetic spectrum?

SWD is a nonionizing electromagnetic radiation with a frequency range of 10–100 MHz and a wavelength of 3–30 m. This frequency is found between low-frequency electrical currents and microwaves on the electromagnetic spectrum. To avoid interference with other radio signals, the Federal Communications Commission (FCC) has designated SWD to be used at frequencies of 13.56 MHz, 27.12 MHz, and 40.68 MHz for medical purposes. Almost all SWD in use in the United States operates at a frequency of 27.12 MHz, which corresponds to a wavelength of 11 m.

### 3. Differentiate between the thermal and nonthermal effects of SWD.

The therapist can manipulate the parameters of a typical SWD unit to create either thermal or nonthermal effects by altering the frequency and intensity controls that regulate the wattage or output of the machine. For example, if the therapist uses continuous SWD, almost all patients feel a heating effect, provided that the intensity is sufficient (> about 80 watts). Continuous SWD allows no time between pulses (interpulse interval) for the heat to dissipate. Pulsed SWD (PSWD) usually includes many different frequency options from 1 to 7,000 Hz. The pulse duration in most machines is set at 65 μsec. Therefore, the interpulse interval varies, depending on the frequency selected. If a frequency of 1 Hz is selected, the pulse-on time is only 65 μsec and the off time is 999,935 μsec. If the interpulse interval is long enough, there is adequate time to dissipate the heat, assuming that the patient has adequate local circulation. As a result, usually little, if any, heating effect is felt by the patient. The patient can still feel a thermal effect even with PSWD if the average wattage approaches 80 watts.

### 4. What beneficial physiologic effects can be attributed to treatment at a thermal level?

Local application of SWD causes vasodilatation and allows increased blood flow, thus creating a potential tissue temperature rise of 5°C. This effect enhances local circulation and oxygen delivery, both of which are important in all phases of healing. Increased blood flow also benefits wound healing by facilitating autolytic debridement of necrotic tissue, delivering critically needed oxygen and nutrients, and removing metabolites. Infection rates can also be reduced because they are inversely proportional to blood flow. Thermal effects also elevate the pain threshold, accelerate enzymatic activity, and increase soft tissue extensibility.

### 5. What beneficial physiologic effects can be attributed to treatment at a nonthermal level?

Research has shown that diathermy treatments, which are purely nonthermal, can have beneficial effects on wound healing. However, no evidence shows that these effects occur during PSWD when a thermal effect is produced. Among the proposed nonthermal physiologic effects are increases in microvascular perfusion, modulation of calcium binding, stimulation of cell proliferation, modulation of cell membrane diffusion and/or permeability, increase in plasma protein removal via lymphatic capillaries, and reactivation of the sodium pump so that the cell's normal ionic balance can be restored. Results of research have shown nonthermal effects to be helpful in treating edema, hematoma absorption, and pain (leading to an earlier return to functional activities compared with controls).

**6. How do I know which frequency to use for a thermal vs. nonthermal effect?**

Thermal or nonthermal effects depend on frequency and intensity. Typically, when the average output of the diathermy unit, whether it be continuous or pulsed, exceeds approximately 80 watts, a thermal effect is produced. In general, treating at 200 Hz or greater causes a vigorous heating effect, 90–200 Hz causes a mild heating effect, and treating below 90 Hz is usually nonthermal. Diathermy treatment doses are not precisely controlled, and the amount of heat that a patient receives cannot be accurately prescribed or directly measured. It is always best to ask patients what they feel as you increase intensity or change the frequency. Heating occurs in proportion to the square of the current density and in direct proportion to the resistance of the tissue.

$$\text{Heating} = \text{current density}^2 \times \text{resistance}$$

**7. What is meant by capacitive and induction techniques?**

When using SWD, the therapist has a choice of two different techniques depending on the desired effects. The **capacitive technique** involves placing two air-spaced electrodes over the area to be treated. This technique produces predominantly an electric field with current flowing between the two electrodes in body tissues. An oscillating current flows between the electrodes through the patient and, provided that the output is sufficient, heat is generated. Because of the greater proportion of electric field components generated with the capacitive technique, it heats the superficial tissue to a greater degree.

The **induction technique** uses a coiled electrode housed in an air-spaced drum (drum electrode) placed over the area to be treated. Electrical current flows through the coiled electrode, producing a large magnetic field that influences surrounding tissue and, in turn, produces secondary currents in the tissue. This magnetic field component has been shown to pass through superficial skin and fat. It creates a deeper heating effect in the targeted tissues.

**8. What is the difference between continuous and pulsed SWD?**

Continuous SWD flows without interruption at a designated frequency of 27.12 MHz, which is also called the carrier frequency. PSWD maintains the same carrier frequency but is modulated or interrupted at various intervals to create a pulsatile effect. Another way to look at the pulsatile effect is to think of it as the rate in which the carrier frequency is turned on and off.

**9. Why is PSWD used to treat a wound?**

PSWD involves using air-spaced electrodes that do not contact the skin. It allows treatment over areas with bandages and dressings, decreasing the possibility of infection. The stimulation at the skin level is not sufficient to depolarize pain nerve endings and is not painful to the patient. The penetration of the magnetic field into the tissues is not restricted by impedance from intervening structures such as skin, bone, or plaster. The therapist adjusts parameters to take advantage of the thermal and nonthermal physiological effects to augment wound healing.

**10. What are the contraindications and precautions for the use of PSWD?**

PSWD should be avoided over areas with compromised circulation, tendency to hemorrhage, any type of metallic implants, suspected metastasis, immature bone, abdomen or low back during pregnancy, any anesthetized area, eyes, and testes. Use caution when treating patients with heat sensitivity.

## BIBLIOGRAPHY

1. Cameron MH, Perez D, Otano-Lata S: Electromagnetic radiation. In Cameron MH: Physical Agents in Rehabilitation. Philadelphia, W.B. Saunders, 1999, pp 303–307, 321–344.
2. Kloth LC, Ziskin MC: Diathermy and pulsed electromagnetic fields. In Michlovitz SC (ed): Thermal Agents in Rehabilitation, 2nd ed. Philadelphia, F.A. Davis, 1990, pp 170–199.
3. Prentice WE, Draper DO: Shortwave and microwave diathermy. In Prentice WE (ed): Modalities for the Allied Health Professional. New York, McGraw-Hill, 1998, pp 169–197.
4. Sussman C: Pulsed short wave diathermy and pulsed radio frequency stimulation. In Sussman C, Bates-Jensen BM (eds): Wound Healing. Gaithersburg, MD, Aspen, 1998, pp 405–426.
5. Verrier M, Falconer K, Crawford JS: A comparison of tissue temperature following two shortwave diathermy techniques. Physiother Can 29:21–25, 1977.

# 36.  CELL PROLIFERATION INDUCTION

*Mary Beth Canham, RNC, Ruth Gallegos, RN, WOCN, and Mary C. Ritz, PhD*

### 1.  What is cell proliferation induction?

Cell proliferation induction (CPI) is based on the mitogenic (i.e., cell cycle-stimulating) properties of a specific radiofrequency signal that induces natural growth and proliferation in human soft
tissue cells, such as fibroblasts and epithelial cells. Laboratory results have shown that treatment
with CPI promotes the release of endogenous growth factors and increases the number of cells entering and progressing through the normal cell cycle from the resting phase (termed G0). In turn, this
triggers, in a physiologically normal and complete manner, the full cascade of second-messenger
events necessary for cell growth and proliferation, thus leading to wound closure. The net effect of
this "energy-to-molecule" transduction is observed as a significant increase in the rate of DNA synthesis, cell growth, cell division, and cell proliferation.

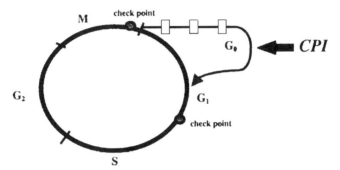

The cell division cycle.

### 2.  How does CPI influence the healing process?

Three distinct phases are associated with the process of wound healing: the inflammatory, proliferative, and remodeling phases. In the inflammatory phase, platelets aggregate to deposit granules,
which promote fibrin deposition, and to stimulate the release of growth factors. In the proliferative
phase, granulation tissue forms and epithelialization begins. Fibroblasts must proliferate and synthesize collagen to fill the wound and provide a strong matrix on which epithelial cells will grow. In the
differentiation or tissue-remodeling phase, the collagen in the scar undergoes repeated degradation
and resynthesis. During this final phase, the tensile strength of the newly formed skin increases.

The Provant Wound Closure System (Regenesis Biomedical, Scottsdale, AZ) induces the proliferation of cells critical to wound-healing: fibroblasts and epithelial cells. Fibroblast stimulation and growth
are critical to initiate wound healing and trigger the complex cascade of biochemical events leading to
granulation in the wound bed and overall healing. Epithelial cell growth is critical to completing the
wound-healing and closure process. Thus, Provant interacts with all phases of the wound-healing process.

Laboratory research has shown that a single dose of the CPI signal results in twice the number of
fibroblasts and a 50% increase in epithelial cells in the 24-hour period after treatment compared with
the number of matched untreated control cells. Part of the clinical effect of CPI on chronic wounds of
various causes relates to its ability to transform dormant cells, caught in the G0 resting phase of the cell

The authors hereby disclose their employment by Regenesis Biomedical, Inc., the manufacturer of the
Provant Wound Closure System discussed in this chapter.

cycle, into normally proliferating cells in the wound bed. These cells may include fibroblast, epithelial, vascular, and muscle cells. However, the signal used in CPI has been shown to maximally enhance the proliferation of fibroblast and epithelial cells. Thus, CPI actively facilitates the movement of a wound from the inflammatory phase of wound healing, through the granulation phase, and to the final re-epithelialization of the wound to full closure. In addition, other laboratory studies show that CPI causes cells to secrete soluble growth factors, via a calcium-mediated process, that signal neighboring cells. These newly released growth factors also provide powerful endogenous stimuli related to the removal of necrotic tissue from the wound bed and the formulation of new blood supply to the area via angiogenesis.

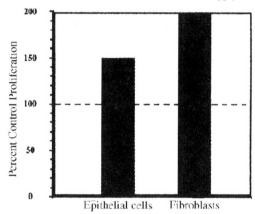

CPI enhancement of epithelial cell and fibroblast proliferation.

### 3. Is the cellular activity induced by CPI beneficial to all types of wounds?

Although many types of wounds and chronic ulcers are caused in part by various underlying diseases and trauma, most wounds must ultimately heal through similar cellular processes. CPI actively induces the release of growth factors, stimulating the regeneration of new tissue. The Provant system penetrates nearly 8 cm deep, inducing a complex cascade of events in the healing process throughout the entire wound, not just on the surface. To the extent that factors which caused the wound or inhibit the healing process may not be alleviated, CPI, like all wound treatments, is likely to produce somewhat less rapid healing in the presence of physiologic problems. Likewise, wounds related to specific disease processes may have a slower response to CPI than would be expected in the absence of such factors.

### 4. Describe the unique clinical effects of CPI on wound healing.

In some diabetic foot ulcers, an exaggeration in callus development may occur. This effect is not harmful and accompanies the formation of visible granulation of the wound as the depth decreases.

The CPI signal travels 7–8 cm through the wound dressing to penetrate all damaged tissue layers. It can penetrate through necrotic tissue and eschar. Necrotic ulcers often develop granulation buds below the eschar. This process becomes evident when granulation buds are seen as necrotic tissue is debrided. By the time autolytic debridement of the necrotic tissue is complete, granulation tissue has partially filled the wound bed.

Positive effects of CPI are related both to the induction of cell proliferation and the release of soluble growth factors during treatment, which over time lead to the formation of new blood vessels and capillaries. The clinical effect of angiogenesis is increased blood flow to the wound site, often observed as bleeding or serosanguinous drainage or via transcutaneous oxygen measurements.

After several weeks of treatment with CPI, venous stasis and diabetic ulcers often exhibit an increase in bleeding at the wound site during debridement due to angiogenesis and the new capillary formation at the wound site. In extreme cases, wounds that have not been observed to bleed for years have shown this effect after CPI treatment. Finally, there have also been some patient and physician reports of decreases in pain at the wound site.

## 5. Have clinical studies of the efficacy of CPI been performed?

Two major studies have been completed on the clinical effectiveness of CPI for treatment of chronic wounds in elderly residents of long-term care centers. A research protocol developed by physicians at a major burn center describing the first placebo-controlled trial of CPI for the accelerated healing of tissue graft sites in burn victims has recently been approved. As described below, these clinical studies show that CPI can reduce wound healing time by 50%, even for wounds that have not responded to other treatments. CPI appears to enhance the rate of wound healing across all phases of the process.

## 6. Describe the major scientific findings using CPI therapy.

In 1997, Bates-Jensen reported the results of the Open Trial of the Provant Wound Closure System for the Treatment of Pressure Wounds. This multisite study assessed the clinical effect of CPI on the rate of wound closure for stage II, III, and IV pressure ulcers. The frequency and rate of wound closure in CPI-treated patients were collected over 12 weeks of treatment and compared with previously published data related to the healing of pressure ulcers in a U.S. patient population. Bates-Jensen used the Pressure Sore Status Tool (PSST) to characterize wound-healing progress in over 990 patients across 13 healthcare facilities. Of a total of 1,870 wounds, 718 were pressure ulcers.

CPI was administered twice daily as an adjunct to standard care in high- or moderate-risk patients (mean Norton Scale Score = $13.6 \pm 0.6$) with severe, chronic wounds (mean PSST score = $37.5 \pm 1.3$, mean wound surface area = $12.5 \pm 2.6$ cm$^2$). Nearly half of the wounds were > 6 months old at the start of treatment. All wounds treated with CPI responded positively. Despite their large size and severity, 53% of the wounds progressed to full closure within the 12-week treatment period compared with a population average of only 15.7%. The results suggest that CPI treatment of pressure ulcers effectively accelerates wound closure compared with population norms.

| STAGE | MEAN AGE | MEAN NORTON SCORE | WOUNDS > 6 MO | PSST AT ENTRY | PSST AT 12 WK | INITIAL SURFACE AREA (cm$^2$) | CLOSURE RATE (mm$^2$/day) | PERCENT CLOSURE | | |
|---|---|---|---|---|---|---|---|---|---|---|
| | | | | | | | | > 50 | > 90 | 100 |
| II | 59.2 | 15 | 4/5 | 33.6±2.6 | 13.2±0.2 | 6.4±3. | 16.8 | — | — | 5/5 |
| III | 58.2 | 14 | 2/4 | 36.5±1.2 | 14.8±1.7 | 7.2+3.9 | 21.9 | — | 1/4 | 3/4 |
| IV | 65.3 | 13.5 | 4/8 | 40.4±2.2 | 28.4±2.9 | 19.0+4.6 | 23.7 | 4/8 | — | 1/8 |

The Controlled Trial of the Provant Wound Closure System for the Treatment of Pressure Wounds was the first placebo-controlled trial of any medical device used for the treatment of wounds. This randomized, placebo-controlled, double-blinded study investigated the clinical efficacy of CPI for the treatment of pressure wounds in elderly residents of long-term care facilities. The study design allowed a direct comparison of CPI with placebo and standard wound care protocols. Randomization and double-blinding ensured that the results were not confounded by rater biases or uncontrolled treatment effects.

Forty-nine elderly residents of nine Arizona long-term care facilities with stage II and III pressure ulcers met the criteria for entry into the trial. These patients were characterized by multiple significant diagnoses influencing their overall health. The most common diagnoses were diabetes (n = 19); coronary vascular disease (n = 11); respiratory dysfunction (n = 10); hemiplegia (n = 10); congestive heart failure (n = 13); chronic obstructive pulmonary disease (n = 7); paraplegia (n = 5); and quadriplegia (n = 7). In general, the patients were characterized as having high or moderate risk for skin breakdown with complex, chronic wounds. Sixty percent of the wounds were > 6 months old.

Treatment group patients received CPI twice daily as adjunct therapy to standard protocol. Control patients received standard wound treatment and twice-daily treatments with a placebo device (a CPI system modified to administer no treatment. Neither patients nor caregivers had knowledge of which patients were assigned to placebo control or active treatment. Overall, CPI produced a 50% faster healing rate in the treatment groups compared with placebo groups. Most importantly, CPI induced significantly more wound closures than placebo treatment. Full closure was achieved in all treated patients with stage II pressure ulcers, whereas in the placebo group only 36% of stage II ulcers reached full closure at 6 weeks. By the end of 12 weeks, only 64% of the control group had reached closure. On average, the treated stage II group healed at a 60% faster rate (26 days) than the stage II control group (66 days). In the treated group with stage III pressure ulcers, 50% of wounds reached full closure at 12 weeks; on average, the wounds reached an 87% reduction in surface areas toward full closure. In the control group, 14% of wounds were closed at 12 weeks; on average, the wounds had reached only a 56% reduction in surface areas toward full closure. This study indicates that CPI is an effective means of treating pressure wounds in elderly nursing home residents, even wounds unresponsive to standard treatment protocols.

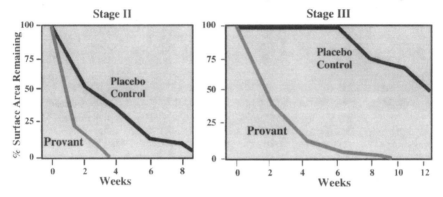

Comparison of CPI and placebo in treatment of stage II and stage III ulcers.

### 7. How does CPI differ from electrical stimulation devices, warming devices, vacuum-assisted devices, and ultrasound devices?

Electrical stimulation involves the transfer of electric current across the surface of a wound through applied electrodes placed in the wound bed or on the skin some distance away. A highly trained caregiver must determine and set the parameters for the electrodes, type of current, polarity, dose, duration, and timing. Vacuum-assisted devices assist wound closure by applying continuous localized negative pressure through a specialized dressing to draw the edges of the wound to the center and to help remove excess drainage. Therapies that apply heat to the wound or to the air space above a wound are designed to increase blood flow to the wound area via the dilation of blood vessels. Ultrasound devices are used to visualize tissue, even below the surface of the wound. Some research has suggested that ultrasound may enhance wound healing via antimicrobial effects of the ultrasound energy.

### 8. How does the demonstrated efficacy of CPI compare with efficacy studies of other devices?

Overall, there are few well-designed efficacy studies of wound care devices. In comparison with the efficacy studies of other wound care devices, the CPI studies show that therapy can reduce wound healing time by 50%, even for wounds that have not responded to other treatments. CPI also appears to enhance the rate of wound healing across all phases of healing to full closure in comparison with standard care. Clinical trials comparing CPI with other medical devices have not yet been initiated.

### 9. Describe the Provant Wound Closure System.

The Provant Wound Closure System is made up of two major components, both of which are contained inside a portable protective case measuring 14 by 10.6 by 6 inches and weighing 10 lb. The base unit houses the power source and the CPI signal generator. This console is connected to an electrical outlet by a grounded three-prong UL/CSA-approved 6-foot electrical cord of standard medical grade that connects the power source to a standard electrical outlet in the patient's room or home. The second component, the treatment applicator pad is connected to the base unit by an 8-foot cable. Both components are housed neatly inside the carrying case for easy transport. The single-use disposable treatment applicator pad cover is manufactured of two materials: a clear plastic front portion and a thin metallic back section. The two materials are sealed around three sides of the treatment pad; a fastener seals the open end of the cover. In addition to acting as a barrier for infection control, this disposable cover also enhances the dosage regulation circuitry, ensuring the most accurate dosing of the wound site.

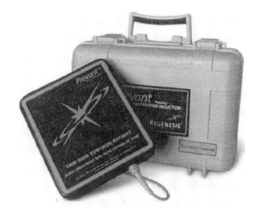

The Provant Wound Closure System.

**10. Are there any other special dressings or supplies needed to administer CPI treatment?**

No special dressings are required for the use of the Provant Wound Closure System in addition to those prescribed as most appropriate for optimal wound-healing potential.

**11. How is CPI treatment administered?**

A single-use disposable cover is placed over the treatment applicator pad before each 30-minute application. The treatment applicator pad is then placed adjacent to any standard wound dressing prescribed for protection of the wound area. The start/stop button is depressed on the base unit to initiate a visible 30-minute countdown timer and running LED light in the base unit, which certify that the system is working properly. A preset therapeutic dose is then delivered automatically to the treatment area through the cable and treatment applicator pad. The length of treatment is 30 minutes twice daily, with approximately 8–12 hours between treatments. An internal countdown timer in the base unit automatically turns off the system when the dosing is completed. After each 30-minute treatment is completed, the disposable treatment applicator pad cover is removed and discarded.

**12. Are any settings or adjustments needed to administer treatment?**

No adjustments by the patient or caregiver are necessary or possible. All preset dosing parameters are programmed to maximize the proliferation of fibroblasts and epithelial cells.

**13. Can two treatments be given less than 8 hours apart?**

Yes. No toxicity is associated with multiple treatments over a shorter period than that recommended by the manufacturer. However, maximal CPI effects are observed when treatments are administered *at least* 8 hours apart because slow-growing or dormant cells that have been induced to proliferate will not respond to CPI signals again while they are proceeding through the cell cycle.

**14. Is it necessary to remove dressings before treatment?**

No. The 7.5 × 8.5-inch treatment pad is placed against or adjacent to the existing dressing. The CPI treatment signal penetrates through dressings and into damaged tissue layers.

**15. Can CPI treatment be used with all commercially available wound dressings?**

Yes. Treatment may be used with all wound dressings currently on the market without adverse effects, including antimicrobial dressings containing silver.

**16. What are the contraindications to CPI treatment?**

Pacemakers may be a contraindication, although most newer models are immune to radiofrequency signals such as the CPI signals from the Provant Wound Closure System. Such patients should discuss wound treatment options with healthcare providers before using CPI. Children under age 18 and women who are or may be pregnant should not undergo CPI therapy. Finally, CPI therapy is contraindicated in the immediate area of a metal fixture.

**17. Can CPI be used in proximity to other medical equipment or monitors?**

Yes, in almost every case.Provant uses the FCC-approved frequency at which most electronic medical devices and monitors operate. In addition, manufacturers of newer devices are required to show proof that their devices are immune to interference from other medical devices. However, some older medical equipment still in use may be susceptible to minor interference from other electronic devices, including Provant. The Provant device has passed all facility-based biomedical department device reviews. If in doubt about the use of Provant with specific medical equipment, test the equipment first if possible.

**18. Are there any risks to the wound or patient during use of CPI?**

No. Over the past 3 years, Provant has been used extensively in patients with wounds due to a broad range of causes without adverse effects. Furthermore, the Provant treatment dose produces no sensation of tingling, pain, or heat.

**19. Are infected wounds contraindicated for treatment with CPI?**

No. CPI does not interact with antimicrobial medications or dressings. Adherence to clinical practice guidelines for the treatment of infection is recommended.

**20. How is the spread of infection controlled when CPI is used on multiple patients?**

The treatment applicator pad cover serves as an infection control barrier and as an additional shield that aids in directing the dosage to the wound site. The cover is designed to be changed each time treatment is administered. In addition, the treatment applicator pad surface is waterproof, bacteria-resistant, and designed to be placed directly adjacent to the top of any standard dressing.

**21. Is it necessary to debride necrotic wounds before applying CPI treatment?**

A novel observation in clinical practice with CPI is that, as necrotic tissue rapidly detaches, large granulation buds were already formed underneath the necrotic surface without sharp debridement. This observation suggests that it may not be necessary to debride necrosis from the wound before prescribing and administering CPI treatment.

**22. Who can administer CPI treatment?**

In hospitals and long-term care facilities, healthcare providers with prescriptive authority typically prescribe CPI, and the nursing staff associated with maintaining and administering facility wound care protocols administer the therapy. Physical therapists also administer treatment. In outpatient wound care settings, physicians typically prescribe CPI for administration in the home environment. Nursing staff may visit the home to educate and assist the patient with overall wound care. However, the patient or a caregiver typically administers the CPI treatment twice daily.

## BIBLIOGRAPHY

1. Bates-Jensen BM: The pressure sore status tool a few thousand assessments later. Adv Wound Care 10(5): 65–73, 1997.
2. Evans D, et al: Topical negative pressure for treating chronic wounds: A systematic review. Br J Plast Surg 54(3):228–242, 2001.
3. Gallegos R, et al: Cell proliferation induction (CPI) treatment of a chronic pressure ulcer in a prosthetic patient: A case study. Ostomy Wound Manage 2002 [in press].
4. Gallegos R, et al: Cell proliferation induction (CPI) treatment of a complicated post-surgical wound: A case study. Ostomy Wound Manage 2002 [in press].
5. George FR, et al: Clinical results of the Provant® Wound Closure System: A novel bioactive treatment for accelerated healing of pressure wounds to closure. Wounds 2002 [in press].
6. George FR, et al: In vitro mechanisms of cell proliferation nduction (PROVANT®): A novel bioactive treatment for accelerating wound healing. Wounds 14:107–115, 2002.
7. Joseph E, et al: A prospective randomized trial of vacuum assisted closure versus standard therapy of chronic nonhealing wounds. Wounds 12:60–67, 2000.
8. McCallon SK, et al: Vacuum-assisted closure versus saline-moistened gauze in the healing of postoperative diabetic foot wounds. Ostomy Wound Manage 46(8):28–32, 34, 2000.
9. Ritz MC, et al: Provant Wound Closure System accelerates closure of pressure wounds in a randomized, double-blind, placebo-controlled trial. Ann N Y Acad Sci 2002 [in press].

# 37. DIFFERENTIATING LOWER EXTREMITY ULCERATIONS

*Patricia Krawiec Bozeman*, RN, MSN, CVN

**1. How do I differentiate among venous, arterial, and neuropathic ulcers?**

First you must assess for risk factors and do a complete physical evaluation of the patient. Next determine the location and appearance of the ulcer, the appearance of the surrounding tissue, and the cause of the ulcer. The table below compares findings in arterial, venous, and neuropathic ulcers.

| | ARTERIAL ULCERS | NEUROPATHIC ULCERS | VENOUS ULCERS |
|---|---|---|---|
| Predisposing factors | Peripheral vascular disease<br>Diabetes mellitus<br>Advanced age | Diabetic patient with peripheral neuropathy<br>Long-term uncontrolled or poorly controlled diabetes | Valve incompetence in perforating veins<br>History of deep vein thrombophlebitis and thrombosis<br>History of previous ulcers<br>Obesity<br>Advanced age |
| Anatomic location | Between toes or tips of toes<br>Over phalangeal head<br>Around lateral malleolus<br>At sites subjected to trauma or rubbing | On plantar aspect of foot<br>Over metatarsal heads<br>Under heel | On medial lower leg and ankle<br>On malleolar area |
| Patient assessment | Thin, shiny, dry skin<br>Hair loss on foot<br>Thickened toenails<br>Pallor on elevation<br>Cyanosis<br>Decreased temperature<br>Absent or diminished pulses<br>Abnormal ABI | Diminished or absent sensation in foot<br>Foot deformities<br>Palpable pulses<br>Warm foot<br>ABI unreliable | Firm edema<br>Superficial veins<br>Dry, thin, scaly skin<br>Evidence of healed ulcers<br>Leg hyperpigmentation<br>Dermatitis<br>Normal ABI |
| Wound characteristics | Even wound margins<br>Gangrene or necrosis<br>Deep, pale wound bed<br>Blanched or purpuric periwound tissue<br>Severe pain<br>Cellulitis<br>Minimal exudate | Even wound margins<br>Deep wound bed<br>Cellulitis or osteomyelitis<br>Low-to-moderate drainage | Irregular wound margins<br>Superficial wound<br>Ruddy, granular tissue<br>Usually minimal-to-moderate pain<br>Frequently moderate-to-heavy exudate |
| Essential components of treatment | Restore circulation | Offload foot | Compression |

ABI = ankle/brachial index.

**2. What are the significant findings of the lower extremity perfusion exam?**
- Decreased skin temperature
- Delayed capillary refill (> 3 seconds)
- Color changes: pallor on elevation; rubor on dependence

- Paresthesias
- Diminished or absent peripheral pulses (dorsalis pedis and/ posterior tibial)
- Atrophy of subcutaneous tissue
- Shiny, taut, thin, dry skin
- Hair loss

### 3. List the various types of noninvasive diagnostic testing used to determine the severity of peripheral vascular disease (PVD).

When physical assessment reveals significant findings, it is important to consider the influence of PVD and its severity on the development of the ulcer as well as its effect on healing potential. Test results often assist the clinician in diagnosis of the wound etiology (arterial, venous, or mixed arterial-venous) and in determining options for treatment. Noninvasive tests include the following:

- Segmental pressure readings
- Ultrasonic Doppler waveforms
- Pulse volume recording (PVR)
- Transcutaneous oxygen tension
- Skin perfusion pressure
- Toe pressures
- Magnetic resonance angiography

### 4. When are these tests used?

*Noninvasive Vascular Testing*

| TEST | PROCEDURE | RESULTS | COMMENTS |
|------|-----------|---------|----------|
| Segmental pressures | Systolic blood pressure obtained with cuffs and Doppler at ankle, calf, thigh, arm<br>Calculate ABI as screening tool | Checks pressure gradient between cuffs to determine level of arterial disease<br>Ankle pressure > 40 mmHg associated with resting pain | Systolic blood pressure may be elevated due to calcification (e.g., diabetes) |
| Doppler waveform analysis | Doppler probe over femoral, popliteal, dorsalis pedis, posterior tibial arteries | Waveform analysis:<br>Monophasic = obstructed flow<br>Biphasic = decreased flow<br>Triphasic = normal flow | Not affected by calcification |
| Color duplex scanning | Ultrasound technology provides anatomic and physiologic data<br>Transducer held over vessels | Evaluates changes in peak systolic velocity near stenotic lesions | Long exam time |
| Transcutaneous oxygen ($T_C PO_2$) | Sensor placed on skin is warmed to produce local vasodilation<br>Oxygen level at skin is measured | $T_C PO_2 < 40$ mmHg is associated with impaired wound healing | Used to assess tissue perfusion in nonhealing ulcers<br>Used to determine potential response to hyperbaric oxygen |
| Skin perfusion pressure (SPP) | Cuff with laser Doppler sensor placed around toe, foot, ankle, calf, thigh<br>Sensor notes point at which flow resumes with deflation | SPP < 30 mmHg predictive of failure to heal | Accuracy not affected by edema; reproducible |
| Toe pressure (TP) | Cuff and photoelectrode on toe<br>Records systolic blood pressure as first return of waveform | TP < 30 mmHg indicates ischemia | Useful to detect arterial disease in foot<br>Digital vessels less likely to be calcified |

*Table continued on following page*

*Noninvasive Vascular Testing(Continued)*

| TEST | PROCEDURE | RESULTS | COMMENTS |
|------|-----------|---------|----------|
| Magnetic resonance angiography | Contrast dye ingested Scanning done | Sensitive and specific Very good images | Eliminates need for intra- vascular access Expensive Limited availability Contraindicated in patients with metallic implants |

### 5. What is the ankle/brachial Index (ABI)?

The ABI is one of the many tests that can be used to indirectly assess lower extremity arterial circulation and determine the amount of compression that can be safely applied in patients with venous ulcerations and mixed arterial-venous disease. Reliability is reported to be high, and the test is relatively simple.

### 6. How is the ABI test performed?

The ABI test can be performed in the clinic, nursing home, or home care setting with the use of a blood pressure cuff and a hand-held Doppler.
1. Place the patient in a supine position.
2. Apply a blood pressure cuff around the patient's upper arm.
3. Apply ultrasonic gel.
4. Listen with the Doppler, and inflate the cuff until the signal disappears.
5. Slowly deflate the cuff until a signal is heard. This sound is the systolic brachial pressure.
6. Obtain brachial pressures in both arms. For calculating purposes, use the higher pressure.
7. For ankle pressure, place the cuff on the lower extremity above the ankle.
8. Apply ultrasonic gel to the dorsalis pedis or posterior tibial artery.
9. Listen with the Doppler, and inflate the cuff unit the signal disappears.
10. Slowly deflate the cuff until a signal is heard. This sound is the ankle pressure.

### 7. How is the ABI calculated after the test is performed?

ABI = ankle pressure/systolic brachial pressure
Example: 60/120 = 0.5

### 8. How is the ABI interpreted?

| | |
|---|---|
| ≥ 1.2 | Calcification of vessels |
| 0.9–1.0 | Normal arterial reading |
| 0.8–0.9 | Mild arterial disease |
| 0.5–0.8 | Moderate arterial disease |
| < 0.5 | Severe arterial disease |

### 9. Are there any contraindications to using the ABI?

The ABI is not accurate in persons with diabetes. The reading will be falsely elevated because of a phenomenon called noncompressible vessels. This phenomenon is due to the calcification of the inner layer of the artery. Inflating the blood pressure cuff will not compress the vessel; therefore, the signal you hear will be inaccurate.

### 10. Is there an alternative noninvasive test for patients with diabetes?

Because digital vessels are less likely to be affected by medial calcification, evaluation of toe pressures (TP) in persons with diabetes is an alternative test. A TP < 30 mmHg is indicative of PVD.

**11. Describe the procedure for measuring toe pressures.**

Specialized equipment is necessary. It is best to follow the specific manufacturer's instructions that accompany the machine.

**12. Can the ABI be used as a predictor of wound healing?**

Yes. Wounds will heal if the ABI is $\geq 0.8$. An ABI of $0.5-0.8$ means that the wound is at high risk for nonhealing and revascularization will probably need to take place in order to heal the wound. Periodic measurements of the ABI are indicated for nonhealing leg wounds. In patients with PVD the ABI should be checked periodically because it may decrease over time.

### BIBLIOGRAPHY

1. Donayre CE: Diagnosis and management of vascular ulcers. In Sussman C, Bates-Jensen B: Wound Care: A Collaborative Practice Manual for Physical Therapists and Nurses. Gaithersburg, MD, Aspen Press, 1998, pp 301–313.
2. Doughty D, Waldrop J, Ramundo J: Lower extremity ulcers of vascular etiology. In Bryant R (ed): Acute and Chronic Wounds: Nursing Management. St. Louis, Mosby, 2000, pp 265–298.
3. Feigelson H, Criqui M, Aronek A, et al: Screening for peripheral arterial disease: Sensitivity, specificity and predictive value of non-invasive tests for a defined population. Am J Epidemiol 140:526–534, 1994.
4. Harris AH, Brown-Etris M, Troyer-Caudle J: Managing vascular leg ulcers. Part 1: Treatment. Am J Nurs 96(1):38–43, 1996.

# 38. VENOUS ULCERS

*Lisa Q. Corbett, APRN, MSN, CWOCN, CS, and Patricia E. Burns, RN, MSN, CWOCN*

**1. How common are venous leg ulcers?**

Approximately 3.2 million people in the U.S. (1/800) are afflicted with leg ulcers, 70–80% of which are caused by chronic venous insufficiency. Venous ulceration is most common in the elderly.

**2. Describe the pathogenesis of venous ulceration.**

The venous system of the legs contains deep veins (located adjacent to the arteries) and superficial veins (located in the subcutaneous tissue). Superficial veins empty into the deep veins through connecting perforator veins. In the normal venous system, blood flow through superficial and deep veins is unidirectional because of competent valves that prevent backflow. The action of the calf muscles helps to pump blood returning to the heart, overcoming high hydrostatic pressures.

In chronic venous insufficiency, the one-way valves fail within the perforating veins and allow backflow into the venous system. In addition, failure of the calf muscle pump to improve venous return complicates the venous hypertension. Over time the backflow into superficial veins causes capillary distention, increased permeability of large molecules into the interstitium, fluid extravasation, tissue ischemia, and eventually, ulceration. Associated pericapillary fibrin cuffing and white blood cell trapping contribute to decreased delivery of oxygen and nutrients to the skin, resulting in ulceration.

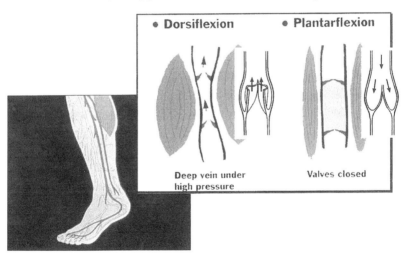

Normal venous return.

**3. List the risk factors for development of venous insufficiency.**

- Obesity
- Deep vein thrombophlebitis
- Postphlebitic syndrome
- Pregnancy
- Incompetent valves
- Congestive heart failure
- Muscle weakness

**4. Some people have venous insufficiency but do not develop ulceration. What additional risk factors may increase chances of venous ulceration?**

Trauma, smoking, malnutrition, and immobility.

**5. Describe the clinical findings of the leg exam in chronic venous insufficiency.**
- Edema: ranges from pitting to nonpitting, tight edema; tender to palpation; venous ooze, weeping
- Palpable peripheral pulses: may be masked by edema; may have to use Doppler with edema
- Lipodermatosclerosis: induration and woody fibrosis of dermis and subcutaneous tissue
- Hemosiderin pigment: chronic brown discoloration from extravasation of red blood cells (red cell lysis and iron pigment deposition)
- Ankle flare: intense pain, erythema, scaling, tenderness, and warmth above malleolus due to presence of microvaricosities in and around the ankle area
- Venous stasis dermatitis: dry, itchy, eczematous skin; due to sensitization to components of topical applications
- Atrophy blanche: patches of atrophic skin with white sclerotic plaques
- Varicose veins: palpable dilated subcutaneous veins, usually larger than 4 mm$^2$
- Moist shallow ulcers (see question 8)

**6. What are common locations for venous ulceration?**
- Medial aspect of lower leg and ankle
- Superior to medial malleolus

Seldom, if ever, do they occur on the foot or above the knee. (See Chapter 37 for differentiating characteristics of venous, arterial, and neuropathic ulcers.)

**7. Describe the pain associated with venous ulceration.**

In contrast to arterial ulceration, pain due to venous ulceration tends to improve with elevation of the leg. Instead of burning or ischemic-type pain, venous pain tends to be described as aching and fatigue. The degree of pain varies greatly from painless to extremely painful.

**8. Describe the typical characteristics of a venous ulcer**

In accordance with their pathophysiology, venous ulcers are characteristically moist, wet, highly exudative, and sometimes dripping with serous drainage.
- Size: small to circumferential, shallow or partial thickness, irregular wound margins
- Wound bed: ruddy base, granulation or fibrinous tissue, yellow slough common; small gray or black necrotic areas may be present
- Drainage: clear serous or bloody exudate; moderate-to-large amount
- Odor: sweet, putrid, or offensive due to large amount exudate
- Surrounding skin: scaling, pruritic, weepy

**9. The skin changes associated with venous insufficiency look like cellulitis. Should the patient be put on antibiotics?**

The change in the appearance and texture of the skin may be mistaken for cellulitis, but in fact it indicates a chronic inflammatory condition. Most venous ulcers are colonized with organisms as opposed to showing signs of acute infection. Sometimes the ulcers become heavily colonized and require the application of a broad-spectrum topical antimicrobial agent. Systemic antibiotics should be reserved for treating signs and symptoms of infection that extend beyond the wound margins. However, constant antibiotic treatment during venous ulcer care is not needed.

Patients with chronic venous insufficiency are prone to dermatitis, which can be difficult to differentiate from cellulitis. In general, the redness associated with dermatitis remains stable and does not advance as with cellulitis. Patients with bilateral chronic venous insufficiency probably have bilateral dermatitis, whereas cellulitis usually affects a single leg. Dermatitis does not tend to be as warm or as tender to palpitation as cellulitis. Differentiating between the two is important because dermatitis is treated with topical steroids and cellulitis is treated with antibiotics. In a time when overuse of antibiotics is a public health concern, differentiating dermatitis from cellulitis is particularly important.

**10. What are the typical pathogens in venous ulcers?**

*Staphylococcus aureus* and *Streptococcus* species can be indigenous flora in patients with venous ulcer changes.

### 11. What is venous stasis dermatitis?

In long-standing venous disease, fibrin accumulates in edematous tissues, and a chronic inflammatory process is set up. The skin becomes dry and scaly; pruritus is a common symptom. Venous stasis dermatitis can be treated with saline soaks and a mid-potency topical steroid when it is acute or weepy. Avoid long periods of topical steroids, which may cause epidermal atrophy, striae, and pigmentation changes. Moisturizing ointments with low sensitization potential should be used for dry, scaly skin. Avoid use of lanolin-, fragrance-, and dye-containing topicals. Bland emollients (such as petrolatum jelly) can be used to lubricate skin. Check the feet to assess for yeast or fungal growth. Topical application of over-the-counter antifungal agents may minimize the chronic flare of venous stasis and pruritus.

### 12. What diagnostic tests are appropriate for the evaluation of venous insufficiency?

Determining the underlying cause of a leg ulcer is crucial because treatment depends on causative pathology. It is critical to rule out arterial disease, both primary and coexisting. This step determines the appropriateness of compression therapy, the cornerstone of venous ulcer treatment.

The ankle-brachial index (ABI) and toe pressures are two noninvasive studies commonly performed to rule out arterial disease (see Chapter 37). An ABI $\geq 0.8$ indicates adequate arterial supply. Its clinical significance is the ability to safely compress the leg for treatment of venous disease.

### 13. Are laboratory tests appropriate for the evaluation of venous ulceration?

Assessment of systemic conditions such as diabetes, anemia, nutrition or infection through complete blood count, fasting glucose, and albumin analysis may be helpful as a general indicator of status. When the clinical picture is unclear, more studies may be necessary. For example, a high erythrocyte sedimentation rate may indicate vasculitis or osteomyelitis.

### 14. What are the main principles for management of venous ulceration?

They can easily be remembered as the **CORE** principles of venous management:.

**C** = **C**ompression
**O** = **O**ptimize the local wound environment
**R** = **R**eview contributing factors
**E** = **E**stablish a maintenance plan

### 15. What are the goals of compression therapy?

Compression therapy improves the efficiency of the calf pump, enhances valve function, reverses the capillary leak, reduces the pressure differential, and controls edema. Compression is used *only* for patients with an ABI $\geq 0.8$. Arterial ulcers have a low ABI. Compression therapy is contraindicated in patients with an ABI below 0.6. Many patients have mixed arterial and venous disease. Mixed arterial and venous disease results in an ABI between 0.6 and 0.8. Compression therapy is still needed in mixed disease to improve the venous condition, but only light compression can be used.

*Compression Guidelines*

| | | |
|---|---|---|
| Very light | 10–15 mmHg | More severe mixed arterial/venous disease |
| Light | 15–20 mmHg | Mixed arterial/venous disease |
| Moderate | 20–40 mmHg | Venous edema |
| High | > 40 mmHg | Woody fibrosis, lymphedema |

### 16. What are the options for compression therapy?

Almost every dressing manufacturer makes some type of compression wrap, stocking, boot, or garment. The modalities vary in amount of compression, stretch and elasticity, application, wear time, and ability to absorb. In choosing a product, considerations include the following:

- ABI results
- Wound status, wound drainage, and frequency of topical dressing changes
- Cost-effectiveness, insurance coverage
- Application ease
- Tolerance of compression modality
- Bathing preferences

*Compression Options*

| PRODUCT | ADVANTAGES | DISADVANTAGES |
| --- | --- | --- |
| Stockings | Removal for bathing, sleep<br>Washable, reusable<br>Appropriate for maintenance phase<br>("stockings for life") | Can be hard to put on<br>Compression reduces as edema resolves<br>Elasticity value decreases over time<br>Costly<br>Difficulty to use with open wounds<br>Hard to fit bariatric sizes |
| Multilayer compression bandages | Maintain pressure for up to 1 week<br>Stay in place<br>Some components reusable<br>Absorbs exudate | Limit bathing<br>Variable application instructions (read package insert) |
| Medicated wraps (Unna's type paste boot) | Low cost<br>Stay in place for up to 1 week | Limit bathing<br>May be rigid, uncomfortable<br>Little absorption ability |
| Pneumatic compression devices | Easy to use<br>Effective when edema is severe or refractory<br>Lymphedema control | Usage guidelines variable<br>Expensive |

**17. How do I decide which option is best for a particular patient?**

**Example 1:** A home care patient with two large venous ulcers in the gaiter area of the left leg, both of which drain large amounts of exudate and require daily changes of gauze dressing wrap. The right leg has no distinct ulceration but is weepy; both legs have +4 edema. The ABI = 0.9 on the left and 0.8 on the right. A good compression choice may be a multilayer compression wrap that can handle the exudate, provide consistent compression over several days, and firmly reverse the edema.

**Example 2:** An elderly patient with mixed venous/arterial disease and an ABI of 0.7 in whom a leg ulcer has just healed. Mild compression is needed for maintenance. A good choice may be a 10–15 mmHg stocking.

**18. How do I determine the best way to wrap the compression wraps?**

Each product comes with specific instructions in the package insert. Follow directions closely. Proper bandaging technique is critical to getting the therapeutic degree of pressure gradient. Some products use the 50% stretch (50% overlap technique), some use spiral or figure-of-eight bandages, and others use a combination of wrap techniques.

**19. How do I decide the frequency of compression wrap changes?**

Most products are approved for 7 days of therapy. Read the package inserts. However, wear time must be individualized according to clinical findings. The first few days of compression therapy often produce an increase in exudate from open wounds under the compression wrap. Venous ulcers are prone to becoming heavily colonized, and frequency of changing the compression wrap should be titrated based on the ulcer assessment.

**20. How do I optimize the local wound environment?**

Once compression therapy is determined, the topical care of venous ulcers follows the same basic management strategies for any wound:

- Remove devitalized tissue (see Chapter 12)
- Maintain moist wound bed
- Absorb excess exudate
- Protect surrounding skin

**21. What is included in the review of factors that can adversely affect healing?**
**Local factors**

- Sensitivity to wound products and topical ingredients such as lanolin, neomycin, and parabens. Because almost anything can cause skin sensitization, keep chemicals to a minimum.

- Local tissue hypoxia
- Heavy bacterial colonization or infection
- Edema
- Wound dehydration

**Systemic factors**

- Smoking
- Obesity
- Nutritional deficiencies
- Diabetes
- Cardiovascular disease
- Collagen vascular disease
- Inactivity

**22. What are important aspects of establishing a maintenance plan for venous disease?**

Long-term management and prevention of ulceration can be a challenge. The reoccurrence rate for venous ulcers has been described as 50–70%. Aspects of the maintenance program include:

- **Compression for life.** Once the acute phase of venous ulcer care is complete, the patient must wear some type of compression hose, wrap, or garment for life. Because stockings loose elasticity over time, patients should be taught to replace stockings on a routine basis (approximately every 6–12 months).
- **Avoid trauma.** Simple trauma, such as a bruise from bumping into small furniture, a fingernail catch, or skin tear, can begin the process of venous ulceration.
- **Skin care.** Maintenance of supple skin with nonsensitizing moisturizers and treatment of fungal infections of feet/nails.
- **Knowledge of disease process and chronicity.** Patients should know what steps to take to seek early intervention with reoccurrence. Routine follow-up care to evaluate disease process and progression is essential.

**23. Stockings are so hard for the elderly to put on. What aids are available?**

Stocking assist devices include cages and "donners," which allow the patient to step into a stretched stocking. These devices are available through medical suppliers. It is often helpful for an occupational or physical therapist to teach stocking application before the patient is discharged from supervised care. Some stockings come in a zippered form or a two-layer system that makes the second higher compression stocking easier to apply. Bariatric patients or patients with lymphedematous legs may use the Velcro-tabbed "boot" stocking (CircAid, Coloplast, Marietta, GA.)

**24. Describe the surgical management of chronic venous insufficiency and venous ulcers.**

Subfascial endoscopic perforator surgery (SEPS) is a procedure to bypass the faulty one-way valves in the perforator veins of the lower extremities. Perforator incompetence is determined by means of a duplex scan, and sites of problem perforators are mapped preoperatively. Research shows favorable ulcer healing rates with this procedure.

BIBLIOGRAPHY

1. Russell T: Subfascial endoscopic perforator surgery: A surgical approach to halting venous ulceration. J Wound Ostomy Contin Nurs 29(1):33–36, 2002.
2. Reichardt L: Venous ulceration: Compression as the mainstay therapy. J Wound Ostomy Contin Nurs 26(1):39–47, 1999.
3. Capeheart J: Chronic venous insufficiency: A focus on prevention of venous ulceration. J Wound Ostomy Contin Nurs 23(5):227–234, 1996.
4. Kunimoto BT: Management and prevention of venous leg ulcers: A literature guided approach. Ostomy Wound Manage 47(1):36–49, 2001.
5. Kunimoto BT: Assessment of venous leg ulcers: An in-depth discussion of a literature guided approach. Ostomy Wound Manage 47(5):38–53, 2001.
6. McGuckin M, Williams L, Brooks J, Cherry G: Guidelines in practice: The effect on healing of venous ulcers. Adv Skin Wound Care 14(1):33–36, 2001.
7. McGuckin M, Stineman MG, Goin JE, Williams SV: Venous Leg Ulcer Guideline. Philadelphia, University of Pennsylvania, 1997.
8. Hess CT: Management of a venous ulcer: A case study approach. Adv Skin Wound Care 14(3):148–149, 2001.

# 39. ARTERIAL ULCERS

*Patricia Krawiec Bozeman*, RN, MSN, CVN

**1. What is the number-one factor that predisposes to arterial ulceration?**
Peripheral arterial disease (PAD), lower extremity arterial disease, and peripheral arterial occlusive disease are commonly used to describe the chronic condition caused primarily by atherosclerosis, which results in progressive narrowing and eventual occlusion of the artery. Arterial occlusion leads to ischemic tissue and eventual ulceration.

**2. List the risk factors for PAD.**
- Smoking history
- Cardiovascular disease/
  cardiovascular surgeries
- Hypertension
- Dyslipidemia
- Diabetes
- Family history of PAD
- Advanced age
- Obesity
- Sickle cell anemia

**3. What is the most common clinical manifestation of PAD?**
Pain in the lower extremities is the most common clinical manifestation. A careful history of pain and associated activity is essential to the evaluation.

**Progression of pain in peripheral arterial disease**

Intermittent claudication $\rightarrow$ Nocturnal pain and/or positional pain $\rightarrow$ Resting pain

**4. Describe intermittent claudication.**
Intermittent claudication is characterized by a cramping in the lower extremity during activity. This pain begins with activity and disappears after approximately 10 minutes of rest. It is sometimes defined as cramping muscle pain brought on by walking a predictable distance and relieved by brief periods of rest. The pain can be experienced in the thigh area as well as the calf.

**5. Describe rest pain.**
As arterial occlusive disease progresses, continuous pain persists. First, the pain occurs only with predictable walking distance, then limits walking distance and activity tolerance. Next, the patient may experience pain with elevation of the legs, commonly noticed at night. When patients are positioned with elevated extremities, they complain of chronic throbbing pain, usually located on the top of the foot,across the metatarsal head. With elevation the foot becomes pale. Pallor with elevation occurs because the blood cannot be pumped into the capillary system against the gravity of the arterial blockages. People with elevational pain must hang their foot in a dependent position to get relief from the pain. In a dependent position the foot becomes red. This dependent rubor results from blood pooling in the arterioles. Eventually the patient experiences pain even with legs in the dependent "rest" position. Rest pain usually indicates a hemodynamically significant arterial blockage. If the blockages that cause rest pain are not corrected, tissue necrosis and gangrene are likely to develop, often leading to amputation.

**6. What type of invasive vascular testing is usually performed to determine severity of PAD?**
Angiography is the gold standard to determine exact location of the diseased segment of artery. Angiography is performed after a complete history and physical exam are completed and noninvasive diagnostic testing (see Chapter 37) has confirmed the presence of occlusion or diseased artery. The angiogram gives the vascular surgeon a road map to determine the best surgical procedure for the patient.

**7. What are the nursing considerations in caring for patients before and after angiography?**
The angiogram is performed by means of introducing a sheath and catheter into the common femoral artery. A dye is infused, and serial x-rays are taken of the target arteries. The catheter is then

removed, and pressure is applied to the common femoral artery. Most angiography is performed on an outpatient basis. Before the procedure the patient avoids oral ingestion or drinks only clear liquids after midnight on the day of the exam. This precaution is taken in case the patient needs to go to the operating room emergently. At the time of the exam an IV line is started to hydrate the patient for ease of dye flow and to minimize dye toxicity to the kidneys. Baseline blood urea nitrogen (BUN) and creatinine levels should be taken before the exam because of possible toxicity.

After angiography the patient must lie with the affected extremity straight. The hip on the affected side should not be flexed for approximately 6 hours. Gentle hydration continues. Nursing considerations include assessing for hematoma, bleeding, or increased ecchymosis at the puncture site (common femoral artery) every 15 minutes for the first hour, then every 30 minutes for 2 hours, and finally every hour for the remainder of the recovery period. If a patient is at high risk for renal insufficiency or renal failure, serum BUN and creatinine levels should be checked after the procedure.

**8. Will an arterial ulcer heal without adequate circulation in the leg?**

No. A wound must have adequate circulation in order to heal. In the absence of minimal arterial blood supply, no topical wound treatment is effective.

**9. List the major indicators of critical limb ischemia.**
- Rest pain requiring analgesia > 2 weeks
- Ankle pressure < 40 mmHg
- Toe pressure < 30 mmHg
- Tissue loss ulceration or gangrene

**10. What types of interventional procedures are available to increase perfusion to a patient with PAD and arterial ulceration?**

Angioplasty and stenting. Lower extremity bypass procedures are surgical options.

**11. What type of patient is a candidate for an interventional procedure such as angioplasty?**

Percutaneous transluminal angioplasty (PTA) is a nonoperative treatment option for patients with localized occlusions or patients with a number of comorbidities who are at great surgical risk.

**12. What types of bypass procedures are available to increase perfusion to the lower extremity?**

The superficial femoral artery and the popliteal artery are the most common sites for obstructions or lesions. A bypass is performed by taking a vein or synthetic material and creating an alternative route around the obstruction or lesion for distal flow of arterial blood. Femoral popliteal bypass is usually done for patients with claudication in whom angioplasty or stenting has been unsuccessful. Femoral tibial/peroneal bypass is usually done for patients with rest pain and critical limb ischemia.

**13. Describe the various bypass graft materials used.**

Veins can either be reversed and used as a bypass or left in situ (in their native bed). After the valves are rendered incompetent, they are anastomosed proximal and distal to the occlusion or lesion. Synthetic material may also be used as bypass material.

**14. Is skin grafting a good option for healing arterial ulcers?**

Once the ulcer has adequate blood supply through surgery, stenting, or medications, it may support a skin graft or tissue-engineered graft. Insufficient evidence supports the use of skin grafts in unreconstructed arterial disease.

**15. What medications are helpful in arterial disease?**

Cilostazol (Pletal) has been shown to improve walking distances, ankle/brachial index, and patient perception of improvement in physical function. It is a phosphodiesterase inhibitor that suppresses platelet aggregation and acts as a direct arterial vasodilator.

**16. Where are arterial ulcers usually located?**
- Between toes (web spaces)
- Tips of toes
- Over phalangeal heads
- Over lateral malleolus
- Areas exposed to repetitive trauma or rubbing of footwear
- Mid-tibia

**17. Describe the appearance of an arterial ulcer.**
- Ulcer margins are rounded and smooth, with a "punched-out" appearance
- Dry, pale, or necrotic ulcer base
- Minimal granulation tissue
- Wound size usually small
- Minimal exudate
- Gangrene (wet or dry); necrosis is common
- Clinical signs of infection surround the wound

**18. What is dry gangrene?**
Dry gangrene is dark brown or black nonviable tissue that eventually forms a hard mass. It is a result of tissue hypoxia and anoxia. Eventually, without treatment, the tissue may separate and autodebride.

**19. Describe wet gangrene.**
Wet gangrene is usually a result of an infection. The dry gangrene becomes soft and boggy or moist. Fluid may be drawn out in the form of pus. Treatment includes antibiotics, debridement, and addressing of the underlying cause.

**20. What is the treatment of a dry black eschar on the heel?**
Dry, stable black eschars in distal locations (heels, toes) should not be debrided until perfusion status can be done. If the eschar is "fused" at the margins and nonsuppurative, the appropriate treatment is to remove any offending pressure, friction, or shear factors and to allow the wound to dry and possibly re-epithelialize under the eschar. A suppurative wound, which is "mushy" or fluctuant to palpation, indicates a possible pocket of wet necrosis under the eschar. If the eschar becomes separated, suppurative, or draining or shows signs of infection, the necrotic tissue must be removed.

**21. What rules of thumb to determine the likelihood of healing can be based on vascular testing results?**

| ABI | INTERPRETATION | LIKELIHOOD OF HEALING AND MANAGEMENT |
|---|---|---|
| 0.9–1.0 | Normal | Blood flow adequate for healing |
| 0.8–0.9 | Mild occlusion | Trial of conservative wound care<br>Pressure relief<br>Nutrition<br>Wound management principles |
| 0.5–0.8 | Moderate occlusion | Vascular referral<br>Frequent monitoring of wound. |
| < 0.5 | Severe occlusion | Vascular referral<br>Maintain dry, stable eschar |
| < 0.4 | Critical occlusion: limb threatened | Urgent vascular referral |

ABI = ankle/brachial index.

**22. A 95-year-old patient has an ABI of 0.6, is not a surgical candidate, and has an eschar on the great toe tip that is just starting to lift at the margins. What is the best treatment?**
Preserve the eschar as a "physiologic dressing" by painting it with an antimicrobial drying agent such as povidone-iodine or alcohol, as in a skin preparation pad. This technique inhibits bacteria from entering under the eschar and keeps the eschar dry. Such a daily dressing also forces an assessment of

the wound so that caregivers will notice if it becomes suppurative and requires other interventions. In addition, pressure from bedclothes or shoewear should be avoided.

**23. A patient has wet gangrene of the heel and is not a surgical candidate. How should the wound be treated?**

1. Remove any necrotic tissue.
2. Treat or prevent wound infections.
3. Remove all sources of pressure.
4. Maximize distal arterial flow through medications and positioning.
5. Maintain a moist wound environment.

Depending on the patient's situation, a variety of wound care products may be used. These wounds often "re-necrose" after debridement because of limited blood supply for healing. In such cases, follow guidelines for maintaining a dry black eschar (see question 20).

**24. How can I detect infection in an arterial wound?**

Clinical signs of infection may be subtle because of reduced blood flow in PAD. Signs may include the following:

- No change in wound size for > 2 weeks
- Increase in wound size
- Increased drainage
- Purulence
- Odor
- Increase in necrotic tissue

**25. Should topical antibiotics be used on arterial ulcers?**

Topical antibiotics should not be used as the sole treatment infected ischemic wounds. Suspicious arterial wounds require culture and systemic antibiotics. Wounds treated with topical antibiotics may develop resistant organisms and/or sensitivity reactions.

**26. A patient had an ankle wound that would not heal because of poor arterial supply. After surgery for revascularization, he has a warm foot and palpable pulses ,and the wound is newly debrided to a clean, beefy red base. The surgeon has ordered a saline wet-to-dry dressing to be changed 3 times/day. Is this dressing appropriate?**

No. A wet-to-dry dressing is intended for debridement of devitalized tissue, and the patient's wound does not need further debridement. A more appropriate dressing might be a hydrogel to maintain a constant moist wound environment and support granulation.

**27. What type of follow-up is appropriate once the wound begins to heal?**

The patient should continue to receive nursing care and assessment in some type of environment, whether it is acute care, home care, or an extended-care facility. Dressings appropriate to the wound should continue until it is healed. Assessment for infection and perfusion to the lower extremity should continue. Follow-up with the physician should occur on a regular basis.

**28. List the most important patient/family education topics related to PAD and arterial ulcers.**

- Smoking cessation
- Chronic disease management (diabetes and hypertension)
- Diet control (low cholesterol, low fat) and good nutrition
- Medication compliance
- Avoidance of chemical, thermal, and mechanical trauma (e.g., heating pads, hot soaks, leg crossing, constrictive clothing)
- Routine professional care for toenails, corns, calluses
- Reasonable exercise
- Lower extremity/foot care and inspection on a daily basis
- Recognition of signs and symptoms of infection
- Recognition of signs and symptoms of graft failure (postoperative bypass)
- Regular follow-up with a healthcare provider

## BIBLIOGRAPHY

1. Dawson DL, et al: Cilostazol has beneficial effects in treatment of intermittent claudication: Results from a multicenter, randomized, prospective, double blinded trial. Circulation 98:678–686, 1998.
2. Donayre, Carlos E: Diagnosis and management of vascular ulcers. In Sussman C, Bates-Jensen B: Wound Care: A Collaborative Practice Manual for Physical Therapists and Nurses. Gaithersburg, MD, , Aspen Press, 1998, pp 301–313.
3. Doughty D, Waldrop J, Ramundo J: Lower extremity ulcers of vascular etiology. In Bryant R (ed): Acute and Chronic Wounds: Nursing Management. St. Louis, Mosby, 2000, pp 265–298.
4. Fahey VA., McCarthy WJ: Arterial reconstruction of the lower extremity. In Fahey V: Vascular Nursing, 2nd ed. Philadelphia, WB Saunders, 1994, pp 291–321.
5. Fry DE, Marek J, Langsfeld M: Infection in the ischemic lower extremity. Surg Clin North Am 78:465–479, 1998.
6. Hafner J, et al: Leg ulcers in peripheral arterial disease: Impaired wound healing above the threshold of chronic critical limb ischemia. J Am Acad Dermatol 43:1001–1008, 2000.
7. Harris AH, Brown-Etris M, Troyer-Caudle J: Managing vascular leg ulcers. Part 2: Treatment. Am J Nurs 96(2):40–46, 1996.
8. Holloway GA: Arterial ulcers: Assessment, classification, and management. In Krasner D, Rodeheaver G, Sibbald RG (eds): Chronic Wound Care: A Clinical Sourcebook for Healthcare Professionals. Wayne, PA, HMP Communications, 2001, pp 495–503.
9. Kupecz D: Intermittent claudication treatment. Nurse Pract 25(5):112–115, 2000.
10. Sussman G: Management of the wound environment. In Sussman C, Bates-Jensen B: Wound Care: A Collaborative Practice Manual for Physical Therapists and Nurses. Gaithersburg, MD, Aspen Press, 1998, pp 201–212.
11. Zink M, Rousseau P, Holloway GA: Lower extremity ulcers. In Bryant R: Acute and Chronic Wounds: Nursing Management. St. Louis, Mosby, 1992, pp 164–204.

# 40. MIXED VENOUS AND ARTERIAL DISEASE

*Patricia A. Slachta, PhD, RN, CS, CWOCN,*
*and Patricia E. Burns, MSN, RN, CWOCN*

### 1. Describe the typical patient with mixed venous and arterial disease.

Usually the patient presents with symptoms of venous disease (leg edema and/or exudating ulcer) and signs of vascular compromise (see Chapters 38 and 39). The correct diagnosis is most likely to lead to the correct treatment.

### 2. How often do patients present with mixed disease?

Up to 26% of patients with chronic venous insufficiency have an arterial component to the disease process. Patients with decreased arterial flow are slower to heal and more complicated to manage clinically.

### 3. What assessment data should be collected to determine whether a patient has mixed disease?

A careful and accurate assessment of patients with lower extremity ulcers is the first step. Patients often present with the clinical picture of venous disease. The patient assessment should include a review of the signs and symptoms associated with arterial and venous disease. The physical examination includes palpating the peripheral pulses, inspecting the skin, identifying the ulcer characteristics, and noting the presence or absence of hair. Ascertaining the ankle-brachial index (ABI) is an important, noninvasive bedside diagnostic test.

### 4. What clinical signs and symptoms are suggestive of mixed disease?

Because patients have components of venous and arterial disease, signs and symptoms may be varied. The patient may present with edema and hyperpigmentation of the lower extremity and the presence of a venous ulcer. Frequently, the clinical clue for associated arterial disease is an ankle-brachial index between 0.5 and 0.8. Other signs may include impaired healing and ulcer characteristics that are not consistent with venous disease—specifically, full-thickness tissue depth with or without the presence of black necrotic tissue.

### 5. Do patients with mixed disease complain of pain?

Pain depends mostly on the severity of the arterial disease. The arterially compromised patient may have intermittent claudication (pain on exercise), pain on elevation of the extremity, or pain at night when resting.

### 6. What tests help to confirm mixed disease?

In addition to palpation of distal pulses, the nurse should assess the ABI. Noninvasive studies identified for arterial disease are often necessary, including Doppler ultrasonography, duplex imaging, or photoplethysmography. The arteriogram, an invasive test, may also be performed.

### 7. How is the ABI interpreted?

| ABI result | Interpretation |
| --- | --- |
| > 0.8 | Venous disease |
| 0.5–0.8 | Mixed disease |
| < 0.5 | Arterial disease |

*Note:* ABI measurement is not reliable in diabetic patients with calcified vessels that cannot be compressed.

**8. Can compression therapy be used with mixed disease?**

Compression therapy remains the mainstay of treatment for the patient with chronic venous insufficiency and ulcerations with mixed disease. Only those patients with ABI results of >0.5 should use compression therapy. Patients with ABI results of 0.5-0.8 are best treated with light compression as compromised circulation may be aggravated by standard compression therapy. If your examination reveals an ABI of <0.5, you should refer this patient to a vascular surgeon.

**9. What is a "light" compression wrap?**

Light compression bandages have a pressure of 20–30 mmHg at the ankle. They are applied carefully and monitored closely. The goal is to apply an extraluminal pressure that is greater than the intraluminal pressure without compromising arterial circulation. Single-layer elastic bandages have low pressures and may be used for light compression. The four-layer bandage system may also be used. Apply only layers 1, 2, and 4. Avoid layer 3, which is the major compression bandage. Intermittent pneumatic compression pumps at low pressures may also be beneficial in selected patients.

**10. If the patient's condition starts to deteriorate, how should the assessment change?**

Patients need to watch for any numbness, tingling, increased pain, or signs of vascular compromise with cold, dusky erythema of toes when light compression bandages or compression pumps are used. If any of these signs appear, the patient should be instructed to call the care provider and to remove the bandage or pump if an immediate visit is not possible.

**11. If deterioration is noted at an ankle pressure of 20–30 mmHg, can less pressure be tried?**

Yes. Therapeutic compression stockings and socks are available in the range of 8–15 mmHg range and 15–20 mmHg. One product type, available in a roll form that is cut to the proper length, provides 10 mmHg. It should fit over the patient's leg from the base of the toes to the tibial tuberosity. These products (Tubigrip by ConvaTec and Tubifast by Smith and Nephew) need to be sized correctly by obtaining calf measurements.

**12. What is the prognosis for patients with mixed disease?**

Patients need frequent monitoring but may benefit from treatment for both the arterial and venous components of lower extremity disease. Their prognosis for healing depends on the severity of the arterial disease and the ability of medical or surgical management to have positive effects on the arterial circulation. In literature reports, 45% of patients with low ABI readings experienced healing with light compression therapy. Like traditional venous insufficiency management, treating edema of the lower extremity is also the mainstay therapy of mixed venous-arterial ulcerations.

## BIBLIOGRAPHY

1. Bowering DK: Use of layered compression bandages in diabetic patients. Adv Wound Care 11:129–135, 1998.
2. Bryant RA: Acute and Chronic Wounds: Nursing Management, 2nd ed. St. Louis, Mosby, 2000, pp 145–148.
3. Kunimoto BT: Management and prevention of venous leg ulcers: A literature-guided approach. Ostomy Wound Manage 47:36–49, 2001.
4. O'Brien SP, et al: Epidemiology, risk factors, and management of peripheral vascular disease. Ostomy Wound Manage 44:68–75, 1998.
5. Rudolph DM: Pathophysiology and management of venous ulcers. J Wound Ostomy Contin Nurs 25:248–254, 1998.
6. Sibbald RG: An approach to leg and foot ulcers: A brief overview. Ostomy Wound Manage 44:28–35, 1998.
7. Sibbald RG: Venous leg ulcers. Ostomy Wound Manage 44:52–64, 1998.
8. Sibbald RG, et al: Venous leg ulcers. In Krasner D, Rodeheaver G, Sibbald G (eds): Chronic Wound Care: A Clinical Source Book for the Healthcare Professional, 3rd ed. Wayne, PA, HMP Communications, 2001, pp 483–494.

# 41. NEUROPATHIC FOOT ULCERS

*Joyce G. Genna*, RNC, BSN, CDE

**1. What factors predispose diabetic patients to the development of foot ulcers?**
- Peripheral neuropathy
- Peripheral arterial disease
- Infection
- Pressure

**2. Define peripheral neuropathy.**
Peripheral neuropathy is a chronic complication of diabetes in which the nerves have been damaged so that the patient's foot is primarily insensate and does not feel pressure, injuries, or infection.

**3. Describe the three types of peripheral neuropathy that contribute to the development of a neuropathic ulcer.**
1. **Sensory neuropathy.** A diminished perception of sensation can lead to an unperceived injury. This loss of protective sensation is the most critical problem in the diabetic foot. It can also occur in patients with alcohol abuse and is commonly observed in leprosy.
2. **Autonomic neuropathy.** Damage to the nerves leads to decreased perspiration with dry, cracked skin. The resulting fissures are an avenue for bacterial entry.
3. **Motor neuropathy.** Muscle atrophy changes the pads in the forefoot and heel and prominent metatarsal heads on the dorsal foot. The result is increased pressure over the bony structures as well as changes in gait and mechanical stress points during ambulation. The changes in foot structure contribute to the development of calluses, blisters, and open wounds.

**4. How does peripheral arterial disease contribute to the development of neuropathic ulcers?**
The incidence of peripheral arterial disease is four times greater in people with diabetes than in the nondiabetic population. Inadequate blood flow caused by occlusion in the peripheral arterial circulation contributes to decreased delivery of oxygen, antibiotics, nutrients, and growth factors in both macrovascular (large arteries) and microvascular (capillaries) circulation. This ischemia results in reduced amounts of essential components and impaired healing. In addition, capillary basement membrane thickening further impairs diffusion of essential resources needed to maintain skin integrity and promote healing.

**5. What external factors contribute to the deadly cascade of a neuropathic ulcer?**
**Infection.** Loss of skin integrity from wounds, fissures, and cracks provides an area of entry for bacteria that can result in infection. This infectious process may not be perceived because of neuropathy; thus it can become quite advanced before recognition. Poor glucose control in diabetic patients leads to impairment of leukocyte function and the ability to fight infection. Ongoing infection causes reduced wound healing. Ultimately, gangrene of the tissue can occur.

**Pressure.** The motor changes that can occur in the foot cause increased pressure over the metatarsal heads. Repetitive plantar pressure over these bony prominence can result from walking or running with shoes that are not cushioned and have no other type of pressure relief. The person also may have limited joint mobility in the ankle or toes, causing a biomechanical change that leads to increased pressure. Lack of sensation may cause the person to wear improper footwear, causing blisters or increased pressure and ultimately wounds.

**6. How serious is a neuropathic ulcer?**
Diabetes is the leading cause of nontraumatic amputations in the United States. Patients with an amputation are at high risk of a second amputation within 2–3 years. Fifty percent of people having one amputation lose the other limb within 5 years.

### 7. What are the most common causes of amputations?

- Ulceration (84%)
- Faulty wound healing (81%)
- Initial motor trauma (81%)
- Neuropathy (61%)
- Infection (59%)
- Gangrene (55%)
- Ischemia (46%)

This information lends credence to the importance of healing neuropathic wounds as quickly as possible to prevent amputation. In addition, the literature identifies the sequence of events that most commonly precipitates an amputation (see below). Whenever any of these components in the progression is stopped, an amputation is prevented.

$$\text{Neuropathy} \rightarrow \text{minor trauma} \rightarrow \text{ulceration} \rightarrow \text{faulty healing} \rightarrow$$
$$\text{infection} \rightarrow \text{gangrene} \rightarrow \text{amputation}$$

### 8. Why do neuropathic wounds fail to heal?

In clinical studies, fewer than 25% of ulcers heal after 12 weeks of aggressive wound management. Causes may be systemic, cellular, or related to health care practices.

### 9. What are the systemic causes of nonhealing?

**Inadequate perfusion.** Healing requires adequate blood flow to the wound so that oxygen and nutrients are available for cellular growth. People with diabetes have a higher incidence of peripheral vascular disease, which causes inadequate perfusion to the lower leg and foot (distally). Atherosclerosis causes narrowing of the arteries. In diabetic patients, the occlusions that cause reduced blood flow are commonly located in the trifurcation area, just below the knee. At this location, the larger femoral artery branches into three smaller arteries: the anterior tibial, popliteal, and peroneal arteries. Although blood flow is reduced in this area, the smaller arteries in the ankle and foot may be spared from occlusion.

**Infection.** Infection in the wound area, the surrounding tissue, the foot or limb, or the underlying bone can cause reduced wound healing. Besides obvious infection, infection in the underlying bone, called osteomyelitis, is often unrecognized and untreated. The deeper infection delays or prevents healing.

**Edema.** Infection may cause edema or swelling in the wound area, which also can slow healing. In addition, the diabetic patient may have another chronic problem, called venous insufficiency, that also causes edema in the lower leg and retards wound healing.

**Inadequate nutrition.** When patients are not adequately nourished, they do not have sufficient nutrients for cellular growth. This problem also retards healing. Uncontrolled glucose can also result from inadequate nutrition caused by poor compliance with dietary regimens.

### 10. What are the cellular causes of nonhealing?

**Fibroblast senescence.** Fibroblasts are the primary components of connective tissue. They produce collagen, fibronectin, and other matrix proteins to form granulation tissue needed for wound closure. The fibroblasts are thought to have early senescence. They die early so that they are not available to the wound to facilitate normally occurring mechanisms.

**Keratinocyte migration inhibition.** Keratinocytes are the primary cell of the epidermis. They do not detach from the site of origin, which is the wound edge. If they do not migrate across the wound bed, they cannot reattach and complete epithelialization.

**Lack of growth factors.** Growth factors affect cell growth, reproduction, movement, or function. The availability of receptors is reduced in people with diabetes. They also have a reduced amount of growth factors. As a result, cellular migration and proliferation are not stimulated.

**Wound fluid inhibition of fibroblast growth.** The chronic wound fluid environment has components that inhibit cellular growth. Fibroblast growth is delayed. Enzymes called proteases chew up protein and growth factors. The extracellular matrix contains an extensive amount of protein. The proteases in the chronic wound fluid are constantly degrading growth factors, causing reduced healing capacity.

**Impaired healing process.** The healing process is stunted in patients with diabetes. For example, the dermis in patients with diabetes lacks normal collagen, glycosaminoglycans, and fibroblasts.

**11. How do health care practices cause nonhealing?**

**Inadequate assessment.** The skill of the health care team caring for the wound patient is important. If inadequate assessments are performed, underlying systemic problems or local wound problems may not be identified and addressed appropriately. Examples of inadequate assessment include undetected perfusion deficit, undiagnosed underlying infection or osteomyelitis, poor glucose control, undiscovered pressure problems, incorrect diagnosis of the wound type, and underappreciated loss of protective sensation.

**Inadequate debridement.** Current approaches to healing chronic wounds include aggressive sharp debridement of infected, nonviable, keratotic tissue. If debridement is not performed, healing is prevented or delayed.

**Dry wound environment.** Studies have documented that moist wound healing is better than dry wound healing. Epithelial cells can traverse the open wound faster when the wound bed is moist. Hardened eschar slows epithelial migration and thus delays wound healing.

**Use of cytotoxic agents.** Numerous products (discussed in previous chapters) have been proved to be cytotoxic to newly forming fibroblasts. These products should not be placed in the wound since they may delay healing.

**Inadequate financial resources.** Lack of financial support for care or local wound care products can delay healing. A social work referral can be helpful. Many wound care companies make products available to indigent patients.

## BIBLIOGRAPHY

1. American Diabetes Association: Diabetes Facts and Figures. Alexandria, VA, American Diabetes Association, 2000.
2. Margolis DJ, Kantor J, Berlin JA: Healing of diabetic neuropathic foot ulcers receiving standard treatment: A meta analysis. Diabetes Care 22:692–695, 1999.
3. Pecoraro RE, Reiber GE, Burgess EM: Pathways to diabetic limb amputation: Basis for prevention. Diabetes Care 13:13–21, 1990.
4. Steed DL, Donohoe D, Webster MW, Lindsley L: Diabetic Ulcer Study Group. Effect of extensive debridement and treatment on the healing of diabetic foot ulcers. J Am Coll Surg 183:61–64, 1996.
5. Sternberg M, Cohen Furterre L, Peyroux J: Connective tissue in diabetes mellitus: Biochemical alterations of the intercellular matrix of special reference to proteoglycans. Diabetes Metab 11:27–50, 1985.

# 42. PREVENTION AND TREATMENT STRATEGIES FOR DIABETIC NEUROPATHIC FOOT ULCERS

*Joan Halpin-Landry, RN, MS, CWCN, and*
*Catherine T. Milne, APRN, MSN, CWOCN, CS, ANP*

**1. What percentage of people with diabetes develop a foot or leg ulcer during the course of the disease?**
Approximately 15%.

**2. What percentage of nontraumatic lower extremity amputations in the United States occurs in people with diabetes?**
Fifty percent.

**3. Name the best treatment for diabetic neuropathic foot ulcers.**
The best treatment by far is prevention. It is also the cheapest; the cost of treating an ulcer is in excess of $35,000.

**4. Can diabetes-related lower extremity amputations be prevented?**
The United States Public Health Service estimates that up to 50% of all diabetes lower extremity amputations can be prevented through aggressive treatment and educational programs. Assuming an annual incidence of 80 amputations per 10,000 people, the American Diabetes Association projects that 15,000 amputations per year can be prevented, and the associated rates of morbidity, mortality, and disability can be markedly reduced.

**5. What percentage of diabetics is affected by sensory neuropathy?**
Twenty to 50% of people who have had the disease for more than 10 years experience distal sensory neuropathy, resulting in progressive distal-to-proximal loss of sensation in both lower extremities. Upper extremities also may be affected.

**6. Describe the physical assessment of the foot at risk for ulceration.**
The foot at risk is associated with diabetes or peripheral neuropathy from other causes. A comprehensive assessment has been shown to reduce the incidence of ulceration and amputation. A multifaceted assessment is based on identified best practices (see figure at top of following page). Risk level can be assigned after completing the in-depth assessment. In assessing the foot it is important to examine for deformities, including hammer toes and bunions, callus formation, hyperkeratotic nails, skin fissures, edema, areas of dry skin, skin redness or irritation, evidence of muscle atrophy, and evidence of current or previous skin injury or ulceration.

**7. Describe the history component of assessing the foot at risk.**
To determine risk levels, it is important to obtain the following information:
- Any subjective symptoms of neuropathy, such as burning, tingling, or pain
- Duration of the diabetes
- Medications
- Frequency of comprehensive foot exam by health care professional
- Any symptoms of claudication
- History of sores, surgery, or traumatic injury to the feet

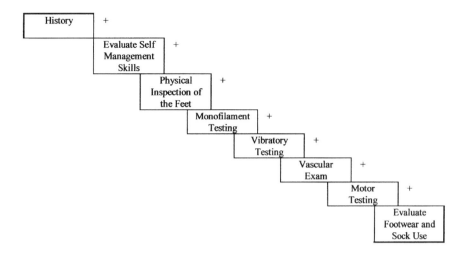

Best practices for a multifaceted assessment of the foot at risk for neuropathic ulcers.

**8. What questions should the clinician ask to determine how well patients participate in the self-care skills needed to manage their diabetes?**

Open-ended questions work best:
- How often do you see a doctor or podiatrist?
- How often is a self-fingerstick blood glucose test performed?
- What was the last reading?
- When was it last taken?
- Describe foot care regimens.

**9. Why is a callus significant?**

A callus is a sign of high pressure and repetitive mechanical stress on the affected area of the foot. Plantar ulcers typically begin as a callus, which is formed when structural deformities on the foot's plantar surface sustain excessive pressure. In a person with diabetic neuropathy, continued walking on calluses often results in underlying hemorrhages, abscess formation, and eventual ulceration on the dorsal plantar and distal aspects of the toes.

**10. What is a monofilament test?**

The Semmes-Weinstein monofilament is a thin nylon rod available in different weights. The monofilament is imbedded into an applicator. Some monofilaments are available in a set of three, with a 1-gm, 10-gm, and 75-gm monofilament on one applicator. Research has shown that protective sensation is perceived at the weight of 10 gm. In other words, a person would feel a blister forming or a small pebble in the shoe. If a 10-gm monofilament is applied for 1.5 seconds to the foot and the person can feel it, protective sensation is intact. When the monofilament is not felt, protective sensation is absent, placing the person at risk for the development of a neuropathic ulcer. Application of a 75-gm monofilament without any perception or feeling indicates that the patient has an insensate foot.

**11. How is the monofilament test performed?**

Ask the patient to close his or her eyes. Hold the 10-gm monofilament perpendicular to the area to be tested. Press the monofilament until it bends, and hold for 1.5 seconds; then quickly remove it. Ask the patient if he or she felt anything and where. Repeat in all designated areas (see figures at top of following page). Testing sites include the mid-dorsal foot; plantar surfaces of the first, third, and fifth toes; first, third, and fifth metatarsal heads; midfoot; and heel. Each area is recorded as "positive" when the 10-gm monofilament is felt by the patient or "negative" when it is not.

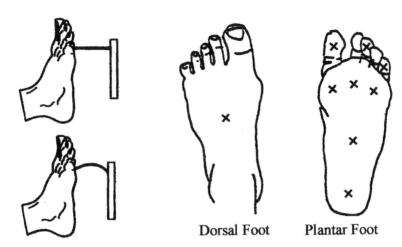

**Dorsal Foot    Plantar Foot**

*Left,* Application of monofilament. *Right,* Monofilament testing sites.

### 12. Can monofilament testing produce false results?

Yes. If the monofilament is applied over a callused area, the patient may not feel the monofilament because the hyperkeratotic epidermis is insensate. Avoid callused areas. Some patients "feel" the monofilament even when it is not applied or report sensation in a location that is not being tested. This problem frequently results from a previous surgical procedure or traumatic injury that disrupted the normal nervous innervation. It may also be a result of neuropathy. Some patients are simply anxious that they have or will develop neuropathy and "will themselves" to feel everything.

### 13. Can monofilament testing detect a predictable pattern to neuropathy?

Neuropathy usually starts in the first and third toes and progresses to the first and third metatarsal heads. It is likely that these areas will be the first to have negative results with 10-gm monofilament testing. Repeated monofilament testing, at least annually and more often if loss of protective sensation is present, can vividly demonstrate to patient and clinician the progression of disease.

### 14. What is a vibratory test?

A tuning fork is placed on the distal joint of the great toe, and the patient is asked when the vibration is no longer perceived. The clinician can verify the presence or absence of vibration by placing the index finger on the plantar surface of the toe beneath the joint as the vibration is transmitted through soft tissue and bone. Results are recorded as follows:

| RESULT | PATIENT FEELS VIBRATION | CLINICIAN FEELS VIBRATION | PATIENT AND CLINICIAN AGREE ON TIME WHEN VIBRATION STOPS |
|---|---|---|---|
| Normal | + | + | + |
| Diminished | + | + | − |
| Absent | − | + | − |

### 15. Discuss the components of the vascular assessment during a comprehensive foot evaluation.

Full discussion of this subject is found elsewhere in this text. In brief, palpation of dorsalis pedis and posterior tibial pulses, capillary refill time, skin color, nail condition, and the absence or presence of hair should be evaluated.

### 16. How is motor function evaluated?

Muscle strength, deep tendon reflexes, and spatial perception with passive movement are assessed. Place your hands against the plantar surface of each foot. Ask the patient to "step on the gas" and push downward to extend the foot. Repeat the process by placing your hands on the dorsal foot and asking the patient to dorsiflex both feet simultaneously. The clinician should feel equal and strong movement against the hand.

Both knee and ankle reflexes should be tested with a reflex hammer. To test spatial perception with passive movement, ask the patient to close his or her eyes. Move the great toe up, down, or sideways. Ask the patient to tell you where the toe was moved. Patients with neuropathy are unable to correctly describe passive toe motion.

**17. Describe the evaluation of footwear.**

The ideal shoe should have a thick but flexible non-skid sole. The shoe should have no uneven patterns on the heel. Look for uneven wear patterns in the shoe. They usually can be found at toe tips, on the side or heel, or inside the shoe. In many cases they look like denuded areas. The shoe should have ample width and be soft and flexible as well as have a toe box (the front of the shoe) that is large enough vertically to prevent the tops of the toe from rubbing or coming in contact with the inside of the shoe. Ask patients if the shoes that they wear at the examination are worn at least 3 days per week. Many patients wear the "Sunday best" to a foot exam, giving the clinician the wrong visual clues. Also look at the patient's socks or foot garb for fabric type, stain patterns, presence of holes from uneven wearing, or absence of a foot sock or foot covering altogether.

**18. Are there any hidden benefits to an annual comprehensive foot exam in patients with normal findings?**

Besides early detection of the foot at risk, the ultimate goal is to prevent an amputation. The repetition of the exam emphasizes several points to the patient:
- The importance of a foot exam
- A visible mechanism to monitor the disease
- An opportunity for the clinician to convey the value of self-management skills, such as daily foot and nail care and how to select proper footwear, which is done by both teaching and reinforcing skills on a repetitive basis.

**19. After the complete assessment is finished, how is risk determined? Why is risk stratification important?**

Risk stratification guides the frequency of repeated comprehensive foot evaluation.

*Risk Stratification*

| RISK | DESCRIPTION | SUGGESTED FREQUENCY OF EVALUATION |
|---|---|---|
| Low | Normal findings | Annually |
| Medium | Areas of high pressure (callus, corns) or visible deformity or loss of protective sensation with negative history and normal vascular exam | Every 6 mo |
| High | Loss of protective sensation with history of ulcer, amputation; severe deformity; absent pedal pulses | Every 3 mo |

**20. What are the essential elements to teach a patient about self care of the foot?**

A number of salient points should be emphasized. Because most patients do not readily absorb all of the information, written and visual teaching aids should be provided for later reference. Reinforce this information at each visit:
- Avoidance of tobacco
- Control of blood glucose
- Daily exercise
- Weight control (to reduce outward pressure on the feet)
- Avoidance of "home surgery" for calluses and corns

- Daily change of socks
- Use of white socks only (they show blood or fluid stains from a wound that may not be felt)
- Avoidance of socks with seams
- When trimming toenails, cut to match the shape of the toe and avoid cutting into the corners
- Avoidance of walking barefoot (even for short periods, such as in trips to the bathroom in the middle of the night)
- Testing of bath water temperature with the elbow before bathing
- If an open area or sore is found, call your health care provider immediately

**21. What information about foot-care regimens should be taught to patients?**

1. The patient should be taught to inspect each foot daily to look for blisters, drainage, dry skin, changes in skin color, redness, scratches, odor, injury, calluses, and corns. Check in the toe web spaces for moisture or fissures. A mirror may be used to visualize the bottom of the foot. Patients who are unable to do so should enlist the help of a significant other.

2. The feet should be washed with a mild soap daily and dried thoroughly, with special attention to areas between the toes. Avoid soaking the feet.

3. After washing, apply a moisturizer that can be massaged into the skin.

4. Look into the shoe for pebbles, rough worn areas, and other abnormalities. Follow the visual inspection with a hand sweep of the shoe to verify. This process should be done each time footwear is worn.

**22. What general advice should be given to patients about buying shoes?**

1. If a foot deformity is present, an orthotist or podiatrist should be consulted for proper fit.

2. Buy leather shoes. Sneakers, of course, are the exception to this rule.

3. Shoes should be bought at the end of the day when feet are largest.

4. Avoid shoes with straps between toes or across the top of the foot. Likewise, avoid shoes that have inside seams.

5. Buy more than one pair. Alternate pairs daily. Break in a pair of shoes by wearing them a few hours a day and gradually increase the time.

6. Buy a shoe with the correct width. To determine correct width, trace an outline of your foot on a piece of paper. Place the shoe on this outline. If the shoe is not the correct width, the outline of the foot will be visible. Do this procedure for both feet.

**23. What is Charcot foot?**

Charcot foot is a form of diabetic osteoarthropathy that affects one in every 700 people with diabetes. It is usually limited to people with moderate-to-severe neuropathy and is believed to be triggered by incidental trauma, such as an unnoticed bone fracture, misstep, or twist of the foot, that leads to damage to the ligaments of the foot and supporting arch. As the bones disintegrate, foot deformity results. The arch of the foot collapses, leading to blistering, ulceration, and infection. The loss of bone density, due to autonomic dysfunction and neuropathy, is the underlying pathophysiologic process.

**24. What are the symptoms of Charcot foot?**

The foot may appear swollen, slightly red, and warm to the touch with bounding pedal pulses. There may be crepitus when the joints are put through passive range of motion. The process is usually unilateral. It is often initially confused with an infectious process, such as cellulitis. The presence of these symptoms, along with plain radiographs showing bony degradation with intact skin, indicates the diagnosis of Charcot foot.

**25. How is Charcot foot managed medically?**

Rest is the primary treatment. No weight should be placed on the foot for 8–12 weeks (if not longer). To monitor healing, documentation should note a reduction in local skin temperature, edema, and crepitus and improvement in radiographic results. Resumption of weight-bearing is gradual. A permanent foot orthosis is required to prevent recurrence.

### 26. Describe the appearance of neuropathic ulcers.

Neuropathic ulcers are characteristically covered by hyperkeratotic tissue. If ischemia is present, the ulcer may be atrophic in appearance with full-thickness loss of the skin down to the ulcer base, and the base itself may be necrotic, fibrous, or granular in appearance. If the ulcer is covered by hyperkeratotic tissue, debridement is indicated.

### 27. How do foot infections develop?

Infections develop as the neuropathy and vascular disease associated with diabetes create opportunities for significant microbial invasion. Infections are usually polymicrobial, reflecting the normal flora of the foot. In a patient with diabetes, the usual inflammatory response may be blunted with diminished erythema, induration, and edema.

### 28. What are the most accurate methods for identifying pathogens that cause foot infection?

Curettage of the ulcer base and deep tissue and/or bone biopsy culture is the most reliable method for identifying tissue pathogens.

### 29. Should antibiotic therapy be initiated for foot infections?

Yes. Once culture and sensitivity results are available, antibiotic therapy should be targeted at the specific pathogens so that long-term use of broad-spectrum antibiotics can be avoided.

### 30. Which foot infections are considered non–limb-threatening?

Superficial foot cellulitis infected with staphylococci or streptococci usually is not limb-threatening. Such infections may be treated with oral antibiotics, good local wound care, offloading, and glucose control measures on an outpatient basis.

### 31. What defines a limb-threatening foot infection?

Diabetic ulcers with exposure of tendon, muscle, or bone carry a higher probability for deep infections and delayed healing times. Deeper ulcers with polymicrobial, mixed gram-positive and gram-negative infections extending into subcutaneous tissue are limb-threatening. In addition, patients who have been on prior broad-spectrum antibiotic therapy and develop resistant gram-negative bacilli infections are at risk for limb amputation. Treatment focuses on the standard measures used in the non–limb-threatening ulcer, with aggressive surgical debridement and parenteral antibiotics, which usually are initiated in an acute care facility.

### 32. Is osteomyelitis common once a foot infection develops?

Yes. If a callus, blister, or open wound is present, a metal probe may be inserted into the wound. If the probe touches bone, osteomyelitis can be assumed with an 85% probability (see Chapter 20 for a discussion of treatment).

### 33. What is included in the assessment of a neuropathic ulcer?

Ulcer assessment includes evaluating a number of factors: location, size, and depth of the ulcer; length of time that the ulcer has been present; condition of the periwound skin; presence of cellulitis and/or crepitus; type and amount of drainage; presence or absence of odor, tenderness, and/or pain (assessed with an analog scale); condition of the ulcer base and wound edges (including the percentage of viable and nonviable tissue in the wound base); presence of sinus tracts; and visible or palpable bone. A comprehensive foot exam, performed as during the foot-at-risk phase, should be done. The ulcer is then categorized by the University of Texas Diabetic Wound Classification System.

### 34. Describe the University of Texas Diabetic Wound Classification System.

| STAGE | GRADE 0 | GRADE I | GRADE II | GRADE III |
|---|---|---|---|---|
| A | Pre- or postulcerative lesion completely epithelialized | Superficial wound not involving tendon capsule, or bone | Wound penetrating to tendon or capsule | Wound penetrating to bone or joint |

*Table continued on following page*

| STAGE | GRADE 0 | GRADE I | GRADE II | GRADE III |
|-------|---------|---------|----------|-----------|
| B | Pre- or postulcerative lesion completely epithelialized with infection | Superficial wound not involving tendon, capsule, or bone with infection | Wound penetrating to tendon or capsule with infection | Wound penetrating to bone and joint with infection |
| C | Pre- or postulcerative lesion completely epithelialized with ischemia | Superficial wound not involving tendon, capsule, or bone with ischemia | Wound penetrating to tendon or capsule with ischemia | Wound penetrating to bone and joint with ischemia |
| D | Pre- or postulcerative lesion completely epithelialized with infection and ischemia | Superficial wound not involving tendon, capsule, or bone with infection and ischemia | Wound penetrating to tendon or capsule with infection and ischemia | Wound penetrating to bone and joint with infection and ischemia |

## 35. How is the neuropathic ulcer managed?

Management of the ulcerated foot is multifaceted and multidisciplinary:

1. Complete rest for the injured part via an offloading device (see Chapter 43) until the wound heals. (Walking on an ulcer without adequate pressure relief may enlarge the ulcer and potentially force bacteria deeper into the foot.)

2. Aggressive instrumental or surgical debridement of necrotic tissue or bone. (Wound healing is optimized and the potential for infection is decreased when necrotic tissue is removed.)

3. Appropriate moist wound therapy and follow-up foot care. The ideal wound dressing should protect and insulate the wound, maintain a moist wound environment, and absorb wound exudate. Choose a dressing that will not desiccate a wound bed on removal. Topical gel with platelet-derived growth factors have shown potential in resolving neuropathic ulcers when combined with aggressive wound debridement.

4. Patient education about local wound care, offloading, and glucose control are essential.

5. Concurrent medical conditions, such as hyperglycemia, renal failure, and nutritional deficits, must be controlled during wound management. Significant hyperglycemia and renal insufficiency have been associated with impaired wound healing, decreased granulation tissue, and poor tensile strength of the wound tissue.

6. Patients presenting with ischemic rest pain and tissue loss who meet the surgical selection criteria should be treated promptly and aggressively with appropriate arterial reconstruction to restore adequate arterial circulation, relieve disabling ischemic pain, and restore tissue integrity. Surgery can result in the preservation or restoration of limb function.

7. Drug therapy may include pentoxifylline to improve microcirculation status, gamma linoleic acid and tricyclic antidepressants for subjective neuropathic pain symptom relief, and supplementation with L-arginine to improve nitric oxide production in the capillary bed.

## BIBLIOGRAPHY

1. American Diabetes Association: Consensus development conference on diabetic foot wound care. Diabetes Care 22(1):1354–1360, 1999.
2. Inlow S, Orsted H, Sibbald RG: Best practices for the prevention, diagnosis and treatment of diabetic foot ulcers. Ostomy Wound Manage 46(11):55–68, 2000.
3. Mulder GD: Evaluating and managing the diabetic foot: An overview. Adv Wound Care 13(1):33–36, 2000.
4. Steed DL: Diabetic wounds: Assessment, classification, and management. In Krasner D, Kane D (eds): Chronic Wound Care. A Clinical Source Book for Health Care Professionals, 2nd ed. Wayne, PA, Health Management Publications, 1997, pp 172–177.
5. Zangaro GA, Hull MM: Diabetic neuropathy: Pathophysiology and prevention of foot ulcers. Clin Nurse Spec 13(2):57–66, 1999.

# 43. OFFLOADING THE NEUROPATHIC FOOT

*Teresa A. Conner-Kerr, PhD, PT, CWS(D)*

### 1. What is offloading?

Offloading or pressure downloading of tissue is the cornerstone of both prevention and treatment of diabetic neuropathic ulcers. It is an appropriate preventive strategy for people at moderate-to-high risk for ulcer development. The underlying principle of this approach is the control, limitation, or removal of both intrinsic and extrinsic risk factors.

### 2. What are intrinsic risk factors for neuropathic ulceration?

Intrinsic risk factors for neuropathic ulceration include faulty biomechanics of the foot and the presence of a bony deformity.

### 3. What are extrinsic risk factors for neuropathic ulceration?

Trauma, ill-fitting shoes, and prolonged positioning in a posture conducive to pressure development, such as lying supine in bed or maintaining the heel against the leg-rest, are examples of extrinsic risk factors for neuropathic ulceration.

### 4. What types of forces contribute to neuropathic ulceration?

Pressure, friction, and shear. Pressure-induced injuries have been identified in several different situations:
- Low force over an extended time period (such as a heel on a bed or wheelchair)
- High force in a short period of time (acute trauma)
- Repeated low-to-moderate forces over time (walking in tight shoes also involves pressure)

Shearing occurs when surface tissues move in a direction opposite to that of deeper tissues; for example, when a sweaty foot slides forward in a shoe that is too large. Frictional injuries are produced by a scrubbing effect, such as a shoe that is too tight across the dorsal surfaces of the foot or the lower Achilles tendon area.

### 5. Why is offloading an essential component of the diabetic neuropathic wound management program?

Offloading the plantar tissue surfaces is key to plantar ulcer prevention and treatment because of sensory loss and the inability of diabetic patients to detect the potential for tissue harm. By offloading tissues, offensive forces are decreased or eliminated in at-risk tissue, thus preventing or limiting tissue damage that results in ulcer onset.

### 6. What approaches are available for offloading tissue?

Offloading approaches can be categorized into nonsurgical and surgical interventions. Nonsurgical interventions include therapeutic footwear, rocker soles, custom orthotics, and walking casts. Surgical pressure downloading includes surgical dissection of the wound bed and offending bony tissue deformities.

*OFFLOADING APPROACHES*

| | LOWEST RISK | | | HIGHEST RISK | |
|---|---|---|---|---|---|
| | 0 | 1 | 2 | 3 | 4 |
| Nonsurgical downloading | Screen yearly | Screen 2 ×/yr | Screen 4 ×/yr | Screen every 1–3 mo | See as needed for wound care |

*Table continued on following page*

*OFFLOADING APPROACHES (Continued)*

| | LOWEST RISK | | | | HIGHEST RISK |
|---|---|---|---|---|---|
| | 0 | 1 | 2 | 3 | 4 |
| Footwear | Suggest slippers with firm soles | Professionally fitted from now on | Extra-depth modified, or custom-made | Extra-depth, modified, or custom-made | Extra-depth, modified, or custom-made |
| Rocker sole | No | Perhaps if foot shows forefoot pressures | Yes, with stiff joints or deformity distal to meta-tarsal heads | Yes, if forefoot pressures not relieved by orthotics | Perhaps, if ulcer is distal to meta-tarsal heads |
| Custom orthotic | If needed bio-mechanically | Yes: accommo-dative, using medium-to-soft density material | Yes, using soft density material | As in 2, but line with Spenco (or similar) material with long-lasting "memory" | Heat-molded foot bed if removable walker is used |
| Walking casts | No | No | Perhaps, if deformity shows pre-ulcerative signs | If at high risk for recurrent ulceration | Total-contact cast, neuropathic walker or other custom ankle-foot orthosis, if avail-able; otherwise, removable walker for mid and fore-foot ulcers |
| Surgical pressure downloading | *Elective* genetic bun-ions or other deformities | *Elective* hammer toes, bunions, hallux limitus | *Elective* as in 1, plus other deformities causing plantar pres-sure problems | *Urgent* if recur-rence of ulcer imminent and nonsurgical attempts are ineffective | *Urgent and emergent* as Wagner scale increases; limb and life are threatened |

Adapted from Inlow S, Kalla TP, Rahman J: Downloading plantar pressures in the diabetic patient. Ostomy Wound Manage 45(10):28–34, 1999, with permission.

## 7. Discuss the design features of therapeutic footwear and custom orthotics.

A wide range of **therapeutic footwear** is possible, from a well-designed tennis shoe for people with no loss of protective sensation to extra-depth shoes for people with mild-to-moderate foot de-formities and custom-molded shoes for people with a history of ulceration and severe foot deformi-ties. Common design features of therapeutic footwear include soft, breathable leather that is able to conform to foot deformities; high tops for ankle stability; rocker soles/bottoms for pressure/pain relief across the plantar metatarsal heads; extra-depth toe box for deformities such as claw and hammer toes; extra-width shoes to accommodate deformities such as hallux valgus; and flared lat-eral soles to control varus instability.

**Custom orthotics** typically are made of plastazote and Poron for relief of pressure and shear, shock absorption, and accommodation of foot deformities.

## 8. What types of walking casts are available?

Total-contact casts or healing casts are made by clinicians for individual clients and consist of proper padding for areas at risk for breakdown, followed by a plaster shell that is reinforced with plaster splints and a walking heel for ambulation. The final component of the cast includes fiber-glass reinforcement. The cast is molded for a snug fit, which decreases the shearing forces over the plantar surface of the foot by limiting any sliding of the foot in the cast. Pressure is relieved by the distribution of forces across the entire casted extremity and the placement of the walking heel for weight-bearing in areas removed from the ulceration.

### 9. Discuss the design of splints and walkers.

Several designs are available for offloading the ulcerated limb. Advantages include the ability to modify cast design as the client's limb changes as well as the ability to view the ulceration daily. The disadvantages are that splints and walkers do not provide the same degree of pressure and shear relief. They are also more dependent on client adherence to the treatment program because they can be removed. Splints and walkers have removable plastazote/Aliplast inserts with an outer shell of fiberglass that is bivalved for removal in the Orthotic Dynamic System Splint (ODSS) and an outer copolymer shell with Velcro straps for adjustment in the Neuropathic Walker.

### 10. What about special socks for people with diabetes?

White cotton socks allow early detection of any bloody exudate from a wound if the sweating response is absent. On the other hand, a sock that has moisture-wicking properties is preferred for people with an intact sweat response. Socks should also be nonconstricting and seamless over bony prominences. Technologically advanced socks utilize silicone and other materials for cushioning protection and shear protection.

### 11. Can total-contact casting be used with an infected neuropathic ulcer?

No. Total-contact casting is contraindicated for use in the management of infected ulcers because of the inability to view the wound site and to provide daily treatment for reduction of microorganisms.

### 12. Are there any other options for offloading in patients with an infected neuropathic ulcer?

Yes. The Orthotic Dynamic System Splint (ODS) is an option for offloading the foot with an infected neuropathic ulcer (Fig. 1). It is similar to the total-contact cast but allows for daily foot inspections and treatment in addition to removable and modifiable inserts and reliefs. The Neuropathic Walker also allows inspection of the plantar surface of the foot (Fig. 2)

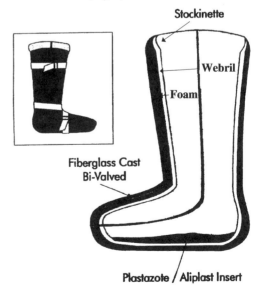

**FIGURE 1.** The Orthotic Dynamic Splint. (From Chambers RB, Elftman N: Orthotic Management of the neuropathic and dysvascular patient. In Goldberg B, Hsu JD (eds):Atlas of Orthoses and Assistive Devices, 3rd ed. St. Louis, Mosby, 1997, p 441, with permission.)

### 13. How do offloading devices affect balance?

The literature demonstrates increased postural sway with decreased postural stability in the standing position when the total-contact cast with walking heel is compared with the removable cast walkers.

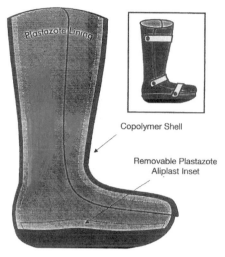

Copolymer Shell

Removable Plastazote
Aliplast Inset

Rocker Sole

**FIGURE 2.** The Neuropathic Walker. (From Chambers RB, Elftman N: Orthotic management of the neuropathic and dysvascular patient. In Goldberg B, Hsu JD (eds):Atlas of Orthoses and Assistive Devices, 3rd ed. St. Louis, Mosby, 1997, p 448, with permission.)

### 14. Are people with diabetic neuropathy who use these devices at risk for falling?

Recent data from a pilot study indicate that people with type II diabetes are at risk for falling even when they do not have protective sensation loss in the lower extremities because of the high numbers of comorbidities, medications, and other risk factors common to the geriatric population. Together with the information about increased sway/postural stability in static standing when various offloading devices are worn and multiple balance studies that demonstrate increased sway in people with diabetes, a good case can be made for increased risk for falling. In addition, particular offloading devices may present a greater risk than others (total-contact cast vs. removable cast walker). Fall prevention education should be part of diabetes self-care training, especially when the plan of care includes offloading devices.

### BIBLIOGRAPHY

1. Bergin PS, Bronstein AM, Murray NMF, et al: Body sway and vibration perception thresholds in normal aging and in patients with polyneuropathy. J Neurol Neurosurg Psychiatry 58:335–340, 1995.
2. Cavanagh PR, Derr JA, Ulbrech RE, et al: Problems with gait and posture in neuropathic patients with insulin-dependent diabetes mellitus. Diabetic Med 9:469–474, 1992.
3. Courtemanche R, Teasdale N, Boucher P, et al: Gait problems in diabetic neuropathic patients. Arch Phys Med Rehabil 77:849–855, 1996.
4. Elftman N: Management of the neuropathic foot. In Sussman C, Bates-Jensen BM (eds): Wound Care: A Collaborative Practice Manual for Physical Therapists and Nurses. Gaithersburg, MD, Aspen, 1998, pp 315–343.
5. Granek E, Baker SP, Abbe H, et al: Medication and diagnoses in relation to falls in a long-term care facility. J Am Geriatric Soc. 35:503–511, 1987.
6. Inlow S, Kalla TP, Rahman J: Downloading plantar foot pressures in the diabetic patient. Ostomy Wound Manage 45(10):28–38, 1999.
7. Inlow S, Orsted H, Sibbald RG: Best practices for the prevention, diagnosis and treatment of diabetic foot ulcers. Ostomy Wound Manage 46(11):55–68, 2000.
8. Lavery LA, Fleishli JG, Laughlin TJ, et al: Is postural instability exacerbated by off-loading devices in high risk diabetics with foot ulcers? Ostomy Wound Manage 44(1):26–34, 1998.
9. Ojala JM, Matikainen E, Groop L: Body sway in diabetic neuropathy. J Neurol 232:188, 1985.
10. Skyler JS: Diabetes mellitus: Old assumptions and new realities. In Bowker JH, Pfeifer MA (eds): Levin and O'Neal's The Diabetic Foot, 6th ed. St. Louis, Mosby, 2001 pp 3–12.
11. Tinetti ME, Williams TF, Mayewski R: Fall risk index for elderly patients based on number of chronic disabilities. Am J Med 80:429–434, 1986.
12. Inlow S, Kalla TP, Rahman J: Downloading plantar pressures in the diabetic patient. Ostomy Wound Manage 45(10):28–34, 1999.
13. Chambers RB, Elftman N: Orthotic management of the neuropathic and dysvascular patient. In Goldberg B, Hsu, JD (eds): Atlas of Orthoses and Assistive Devices, 3rd ed. St. Louis, Mosby, 1997, pp 441 and 448.

# 44. PRESSURE ULCERS OF THE HEEL

*Teresa A. Conner-Kerr, PhD, PT, CWS(D)*

### 1. What makes pressure ulcers on the heel different from other ulcers?

Pressure ulcers on the heels result from detrimental levels of tissue ischemia due to excessive external pressure. Compromised perfusion and the resultant lack of oxygenation and critical tissue constituents lead to tissue necrosis. Excessive forces may be delivered to the tissue via a low force applied over an extended period (e.g., heel on bed or wheelchair), high force in a short period (trauma), or repeated low-to-moderate forces over time (walking in tight shoes). The bone to tissue ratio is 1:1, permitting even small shifts in pressure to affect interface pressure. The microcirculation in the heel is anatomically different from that in other parts of the body. Aging redistributes fat padding and reduces its cushioning effect over the heel.

### 2. How frequently do heel pressure ulcers occur?

The heel has been identified as the second most common site for pressure ulcer development. One study reported an incidence of 32% in patients without preventive interventions. A second study found the incidence of heel pressure ulcers to be 19% in a community hospital. In the past decade, an increasing prevalence of pressure ulcers has been documented. According to the National Pressure Ulcer Prevalence Surveys, the prevalence of heel pressure ulcers rose from 19% to 30% in 5 years. Although the prevalence of pressure ulcers at some sites has remained constant or decreased, the overall prevalence of heel pressure ulcers has continued to increase.

### 3. What factors contribute to the development of heel pressure ulcers?

A study of the factors that contribute to the development of heel pressure ulcers in the hospitalized client found that incontinence and the Braden Moisture Item were two statistically significant variables in the prediction of heel pressure ulcers. Although moisture is not thought to be a direct predictor of heel pressure ulcers, it has been suggested that the precipitating factors for incontinence may be similar to those for the development of heel pressure ulcers. A second study also identified moisture (incontinence) as a risk factor for the development of heel pressure wounds. Other common factors include age, altered mental status, decreased activity level, and a diagnosis of diabetes.

### 4. How is the risk for heel pressure ulcers assessed?

The Braden Scale appears to have some utility in the risk assessment for heel pressure ulcers. A predictive relationship has been identified with the Braden Moisture Item. However, because the Braden Scale appears to have a limited potential for risk prediction of heel pressure ulcers compared with other types of pressure ulcers, an alternative tool is needed. Early data indicate that the Heel Pressure Ulcer Risk Assessment Tool (HPURAT) may be useful; it appears to be accurate in the prediction of heel pressure ulcer risk. After implementation of the HPURAT at the medical center where it was developed by a multidisciplinary team, the prevalence of nosocomial heel pressure ulcers dropped from a high of 23% to 2%.

### 5. How is the HPURAT used?

The HPURAT is summarized below. Clients are assessed for the following risk factors: age, diabetes, mental status, and activity. Activity or mobility level is then ranked on a scale of 0 to > 3.

*Heel Pressure Ulcer Risk Assessment Tool*

1. Assess for the following risk factors (count total):
   - Age > 70 yr
   - Diabetes
   - Mental status changes: agitated, confused, stuporous, and/or unresponsive
   - Lack of movement in any lower extremity

*Table continued on following page*

*Heel Pressure Ulcer Risk Assessment Tool (Continued)*

2. Total number of risk factors
3. Assess activity level and treat according to risk factor level:

| | TOTAL = 0 | TOTAL = 1 | TOTAL = 2 | TOTAL = 3 |
|---|---|---|---|---|
| Ambulatory | Universal | Universal | Universal | Universal |
| Walks with assistance | Universal | Universal | Preventive | Strict |
| Confined to wheelchair or bedridden | Universal | Preventive | Strict | Strict |

*Heel Precaution Guidelines*

| UNIVERSAL HEEL PRECAUTIONS (FOR ALL PATIENTS) | PREVENTIVE HEEL PRECAUTIONS (FOR PATIENTS IDENTIFIED ON RISK ASSESSMENT TOOLS} | STRICT HEEL PRECAUTIONS (FOR PATIENTS IDENTIFIED ON RISK ASSESSMENT TOOLS} |
|---|---|---|
| 1. Assessment of feet and documentation each day<br>• Skin integrity<br>• Pulses DP/PT<br>• Edema<br>• Document level of precautions initiated<br>2. Daily skin care (no massage to bony prominences) Apply cream or lotion to heels each day for patients who need assistance for daily skin care.<br>3. Turn or assist with turn every 2 hours if patient is unable to turn self. Remind patient to turn if necessary.<br>4. Place on standard hospital pressure reduction mattress. Use therapeutic surface algorithm for determining additional surface.<br>5. Mobilize patient out of bed as soon as possible; minimum of 3 times/day.<br>6. Teach alert patients active range of motion exercises for ankle; patient should do exercises every hour while awake. | **Includes all universal precautions plus:**<br>1. Assessment of feet twice daily<br>2. To reduce friction, choose one or two of following (choose c or d when patient has continuous friction on heels):<br>  a. Apply cream/lotion to heels twice daily<br>  b. Encourage patient to wear socks or, if ordered, support hose.<br>  c. Apply transparent film to heels and change weekly<br>  d. Apply hydrocolloid to heels and change weekly.<br>3. To reduce pressure, choose one or two of the following (to maintain heels off bed):<br>  • Pillow supporting lower extremity to maintain heels off bed<br>  • Bath blanket roll under ankle<br>  • Apply heel cushion<br>4. Turn every 2 hr with proper repositioning of heels/feet for all patients who need assistance with turns.<br>5. Mobilize patient out of bed as soon as possible twice daily.<br>6. Perform ankle passive range of motion exercises twice daily with morning and afternoon care for patients who need assistance.<br>7. Consult physical and/or occupational therapists if unable to range ankle easily into neutral. | **Includes all universal and preventive precautions plus:**<br>1. Assessment of feet 3 ×/day<br>2. Apply cream/lotion to feet 3 ×/day<br>3. Choose one of the following forms of heel protection. While waiting for heel product to arrive, elevate heels off bed with bath blanket roll under calf.<br>  a. Apply heel lift if heels reddened or with breakdown.<br>  b. Apply heel cushion if skin is intact.<br>  c. Apply transparent film to heels of patients who are actively moving lower extremity and showing continual friction on heels.<br>4. Mobilize patient out of bed as soon as possible each day. |

From Blaszczyk J, Majenski M, Sato F: Make a difference: Standardize your heel care practices. Ostomy Wound Manage 44(5):35, 1998, with permission.

6. **What are some common prevention strategies for heel pressure ulcers?**

The key to preventing pressure ulcers begins with removing the external agents or events that cause excessive pressure. If excessive pressure is the result of immobility, several strategies can be used. The appropriate strategy for remobilization depends on the patient's physical status (intact upper body strength vs. generalized debilitation), cognition, and motivation. The patient should assist as much as possible with any mobilization procedures. Adaptive equipment is available, including leg straps for use with moving the legs in patients with lower extremity paralysis but functional upper body and extremity strength. Caregivers also should be encouraged to help with motivation or to assist in mobilization procedures if assistance is required.

Mobilizing or repositioning the dependent client should be done as frequently as possible with use of pressure-reduction or, preferably, pressure-relief equipment, for the heels. Pressure relief can be obtained easily by inserting pillows (long-way) under the lower legs while leaving the feet freely suspended in air. Care also should be taken to position the rest of the body appropriately. Various foam cuffs are available with cutouts for relief of pressure, and inflatable air devices can be used for pressure reduction. Various splints and boots that provide protection by freely suspending the heel in space are also available.

7. **Do heel protectors made of fluffed cotton or sheep skin help reduce pressure on the heel?**

Careful examination of these products demonstrates that few tissue interface numbers are available from the manufacturers. As with other pressure-reduction surfaces, evaluation of tissue interface pressures before purchasing the product is prudent. A minimum of 4–6 inches of high-quality, high-density foam is needed to reduce pressure—a quality not seen in the cotton, quilted, or synthetic sheepskin products. When using these products, always ask the manufacturer for pressure-reduction data. Then evaluate the integrity and scientific rigor of the data. A good product has good data.

8. **How are heel pressure ulcers staged?**

Although different classification systems are available for staging pressure ulcers, the system currently recommended by the Agency for Healthcare Policy and Research (AHCPR) guidelines and the National Pressure Ulcer Advisory Panel (NPUAP) is outlined in question 5.

9. **Do heel pressure ulcers go through a distinct identifiable progression?**

It appears so. Anecdotally, stage I ulcerations initially feel boggy and soft with or without accompanying erythema. Erythema, usually with tenderness on palpation, follows. In stage II, a partial-thickness open wound or an intact, fluid-filled blister appears. The clear fluid undergoes a hemorrhagic stage, in which the blister is replaced with purple or red-purple hemorrhagic fluid. This fluid is reabsorbed into the tissue, leaving a dry, black, eschar-like wound. The eschar peels off after several months, leaving pink epithelial tissue. Stage III and IV ulcers present as described in NPUAP definitions.

10. **Discuss the treatment of heel pressure ulcers.**

Consensus among clinicians and practice guidelines suggest leaving the eschar intact if blood flow is impaired and the area has no edema, erythema, or drainage. The natural covering is considered protective. Debridement is required only if the heel becomes suppurative, erythematous, fluctuant, or tender or begins to drain. To summarize, the goal of heel pressure ulcer management is to keep the area dry, black, and intact.

11. **When should a heel pressure ulcer be debrided.**

Circulation status should be established in the lower extremity before debridement. Initially, the dorsalis pedis pulses should be palpated. Approximately 5% of people lack a posterior tibial artery, and 14% lack a dorsalis pedis artery. These vessels may also take aberrant courses or may be difficult to palpate because of edema. A hand-held Doppler may prove useful in obtaining a pulse. The presence and character of the pulse should be documented. Further noninvasive vascular testing that may be conducted at the bedside by most clinicians includes assessment of the ankle/brachial index (ABI). A dry, intact eschar over a heel pressure ulcer should not be debrided unless blood flow to the limb is adequate because the ulcer will be at risk for invasive sepsis. In this situation, the stable, dry eschar should be protected from trauma and moisture. Calcification of the peripheral arteries in diabetes leads to errors in the calculation of the ABI; as a result, blood flow may appear aberrantly high. Use of the ABI in this population is discouraged.

**12. Why are pressure ulcers at the heel so difficult to heal?**

Posterior pressure ulcers of the heel tend to be difficult to heal because of their location in an end-tree territory for blood supply. An end-tree territory is an area of tissue that receives blood flow from one major supply vessel and lacks significant collateral blood flow from other vessels. The medial side of the heel receives blood supply from the posterior tibial vessels. The lateral side of the heel receives blood supply from the peroneal vessels. Blockage in either vessel leads to significant tissue ischemia and eventually necrosis. People with diabetes are at particular risk for developing heel ulcers because of atherosclerosis of peripheral blood vessels and the compromised perfusion that results from these fatty plaques. In addition, basement membrane thickening reduces oxygen and nutrient diffusion to the tissues.

**13. How are clinical outcomes for heel ulcers different in diabetic vs. nondiabetic populations?**

Although the mortality is high in people with and without diabetes, a recent study indicates that people with diabetes undergo a higher number of interventions and have greater rates of amputation as well as an increased mortality rate. For example, the rate of surgical intervention in the diabetic group was 97% compared with 85% in the nondiabetic group. Similarly, the amputation rate was 71% in the diabetic group vs. 63% in the nondiabetic group.

**14. Can occlusive bandages be used on heel pressure ulcers as a method of debridement?**

Yes. Occlusive bandages provide protection from frictional trauma as well as maintain a moist wound bed for healing and promote autolytic removal of necrosis. They also may offer moisture and bacterial control. Pain is also decreased with moist wound therapy and as a result may provide increased comfort. However, they should not be placed on a dry, intact eschar if the limb is ischemic because they will cause the eschar to become moist and detach from the wound bed. "Dry, black, and intact" is the mantra.

**15. Discuss the role of exercise therapy in the plan of care.**

If the client is ambulatory or semiambulatory, a program of graded exercise may be started with medical clearance to promote collateralization if the wound is ischemic. This goal can be accomplished via a rehabilitation program that incorporates endurance training through daily graded activities such as ambulation or cycle ergometry. For patients with a wound, the cycle ergometer may be modified to prevent weight-bearing. If this approach is not possible, referral to physical therapy for rehabilitation is appropriate once healing has occurred and a protective device is in place. Patients with rest pain are not candidates for these programs. Patients with no evidence of ischemia benefit from mobility and endurance exercises to decrease the risk for pressure ulcer damage associated with immobility.

## BIBLIOGRAPHY

1. Bergstrom N, Braden BJ, Laguzza A, Holman B: The Braden Scale for predicting pressure ulcer risk. Nurs Res 36(4):205–210, 1987.
2. Blaszczyk J, Majewski M, Sato F: Make a difference: Standardize your heel care practice. Ostomy Wound Manage 44(5):32–40, 1998.
3. Cavanagh PR, Ulbrecht JS: Biomechanics of the foot in diabetes mellitus. In Levin ME, O'Neal LW (eds): The Diabetic Foot, 5th ed. St. Louis, Mosby, 1993, pp 199–232.
4. Gosnell DJ, Johannsen J, Ayers M: Pressure ulcer incidence and severity in a community hospital. Decubitus 5(5):56–62, 1992.
5. Jacobs TS, Kerstein MD: Is there a difference in outcome of heel ulcers in diabetic and non-diabetic patients? Wounds 12(4):96–101, 2000.
6. Kosiak M: An effective method of preventing decubitus ulcers. Arch Physical Med Rehabil 47:724–729, 1966.
7. Meehan M: National pressure ulcer prevalence survey. Adv Wound Care 7(3):27–38, 1994.
8. Tourtual DM, Riesenberg LA, Korutz CJ, et al: Predictors of hospital acquired heel pressure ulcers. Ostomy Wound Manage 43(9):24–40,1997.

# 45. INFLAMMATORY ULCERATIONS

Patricia A. Slachta, PhD, RN, CS, CWOCN, and
Patricia E. Burns, MSN, RN, CWOCN

**1. Can every leg wound be attributed to arterial disease, venous insufficiency, or a combination of the two?**

No. The essential key to the differential diagnosis of lower extremity ulcers is a thorough history and physical examination.

**2. If the ulcer is neither venous nor arterial, what else can it be?**

Pyoderma gangrenosum and vasculitis may cause painful, difficult-to-heal wounds referred to as inflammatory ulcers. Other common causes of leg ulcerations include the following:

- Epidermal carcinomas
- Lipodermatosclerosis
- Sickle cell disease
- Microthrombotic disorders
- Calciphylaxis
- Atrophie blanche
- Necrobiosis lipoidica diabeticorum

**3. What information in the medical history should raise suspicion that a leg ulcer may be inflammatory?**

Inflammatory ulcerations are frequently related to chronic, systemic diseases or hypersensitivities. The table below offers an overview of inflammatory ulcerations and related systemic diseases. The cause is unknown in 50% of patients with pyoderma gangrenosum, and the ulcers are considered idiopathic. The clinician's questions should focus on systemic health as well as specific information about the development of the ulcers.

*Inflammatory Ulcerations and Associated Systemic Diseases.*

| INFLAMMATORY CLASSIFICATION | ASSOCIATED SYSTEMIC DISEASES, SYNDROMES, CAUSES |
| --- | --- |
| Pyoderma gangrenosum | Inflammatory bowel disease (Crohn's disease, ulcerative colitis) |
| | Rheumatoid disease (rheumatoid or osteoarthritis) |
| | Immunologic abnormalities (systemic lupus erythematosus, AIDS) |
| | Inflammatory diseases (sarcoidosis) |
| | Hematologic abnormalities (polycythemia vera, leukemia) |
| | Chronic active hepatitis |
| Vasculitis | Hypersensitivity reactions (medications; viral, fungal, or parasitic infections) |
| | Connective tissue diseases (systemic lupus erythematosus, rheumatoid arthritis) |
| | Primary syndromes (polyarteritis nodosa, Wegener's syndrome, Churg-Strauss syndrome) |

**4. What is pyoderma gangrenosum (PG)?**

PG is a rare, chronic inflammatory disease of unknown etiology that results in painful skin ulcers that may appear anywhere on the body but are most common on the trunk and lower extremities.

**5. What does PG have to do with leg ulcers? Is it a complication of inflammatory bowel disease (IBD)?**

PF is an uncommon disease linked to IBD, but it also has been associated with several other chronic diseases (see question 3). Pyoderma is a neutrophilic inflammatory disease. The name is misleading because PG is not infectious and does not produce gangrene.

## 6. Who is most likely to develop PG?

PG most typically affects men and women between the ages of 40 and 60 years. Approximately one-half of patients have some chronic systemic disease process in addition to PG.

## 7. Why does the pyoderma lesion form?

PG is often associated with other diseases, but it does occur in isolation. The pathophysiology of the development of PG lesions is unknown. Histologic exam reveals a dense neutrophilic infiltrate in the dermis. PG is classified into four different variants: ulcerative, pustular, bullous, and vegetative. A distinct characteristic of PG is the phenomenon known as pathergy, the development of a lesion in an area of local tissue trauma. Ascertain any recent history of leg trauma from accidents, falls, or bumps. Pathergy may explain the development of lesions around a stoma site, considered a surgical trauma.

## 8. Which diagnostic tests should be ordered?

No specific histologic or serologic tests are available for PG. It is a diagnosis of exclusion. Clinical and laboratory tests are done to rule out other possible causes. These tests may include complete blood count, blood chemistry, antinuclear antibodies, rheumatoid factor, hepatitis profile, and urinalysis. In selected cases, biopsy of wound margins may be done and sent for histology and culture. Although the histologic findings are not specific for PG, the biopsy results help to exclude other causes such as ulcerative and neoplastic disease. The patient's history is extremely useful in diagnosing PG. There is, however, some controversy regarding biopsies. Many clinicians resist obtaining a biopsy, unless it is a last resort. The trauma caused by the biopsy instrument can enlarge the ulcer as pathergic forces take over.

## 9. Describe the pyoderma ulcer.

The ulcer has a different appearance depending on the variant. Look for irregular, jagged, raised wound margins; undermined edges; and violaceous appearance

*Characteristics of PG Variants.*

| | |
|---|---|
| Ulcerative PG | Small, discrete pustules surrounded by an inflammatory halo. |
| Pustular PG | Lesions also have a halo of erythema and may or may not progress to ulcerative PG. IBD is often present. |
| Bullous PG | Painful, inflammatory bullae that may occur in patients with leukemia or other myeloproliferative diseases. |
| Vegetative or superficial granulomatous PG | Lesions are limited and nonaggressive, chronic, and superficial. The borders are less violaceous than in ulcerative PG. |

An established PG ulcer may look like other ulcers, but the key to successful treatment is an ever-present suspicion for inflammatory ulcerations. The ulcer often begins as a pustule or bulla and subsequently extends to a full-thickness and often necrotic, wound. Again, thorough wound assessment and patient history are important.

## 10. If the lesion is draining and necrotic, does treatment begin with the cleansing and debriding that is done for most wounds?

Cleansing is a necessary part of all good wound care. Gentle cleansing should be done for PG lesions. For debridement, however, the answer is often no. If necrotic tissue is present, a gentle approach is to use autolytic debridement. The local tissue trauma, even if minor, may be part of the pathophysiology.

## 11. How is the PG ulcer treated?

There is no specific treatment for PG, but the plan of care should focus first on control of any underlying chronic diseases. The goals for the patient with PG are the same as for all wound patients: wound healing, pain control, and prevention of complications. The treatment plan should focus on good local wound care, prevention of trauma, medications, and/or systemic treatments. Some patients require long-term therapy because PG may be chronic and recurrent.

### 12. What is the best local wound care?

The goals for local wound care are exudate management, maintenance of a moist wound environment, and prevention of trauma to the wound bed and surrounding skin. Because of the extreme pain associated with these lesions and the tendency toward pathergy, wound care needs to be provided in a gentle manner. Nonadherent dressings are preferred. The table below identifies objectives for local wound care as well as appropriate interventions and products.

*Topical Wound Management*

| OBJECTIVE | INTERVENTION/PRODUCT |
| --- | --- |
| Cleanse wound | Gently irrigate wound with normal saline solution. |
| Manage exudate | Use products that are nonadherent and absorptive (foams, alginates, acrylic strands) |
| Maintain moist wound environment | Monitor level of wound exudate. |
| | When wound drainage has decreased, use products that add or maintain moisture on the wound surface (amorphous hydrogels, hydrogel sheets, hydrogel-impregnated gauze). |
| Protect surrounding skin | Use skin protection wipes. |
| | Avoid adhesives. Use stockinette, roll gauze or self-adhesive elastic wraps to secure primary dressing. |

### 13. Discuss the role of corticosteroids in the treatment of systemic immune diseases.

Corticosteroids are often used with systemic immune diseases and may be administered orally, intravenously, or in pulsed therapy. Immunosuppressive agents may also be given in addition to corticosteroids for patients with severe PG and underlying systemic disease. Systemic corticosteroids have proved to be the most successful agents for treating PG. However, use of systemic steroids may be limited by the significant side effects.

### 14. When are topical steroids used?

With milder forms or smaller ulcers, intralesional corticosteroids have been effective. They may be used alone or in conjunction with intermittent does of oral steroids. Topical steroids are usually ineffective.

### 15. What other systemic and local treatments are available for PG?

Systemic treatments may consist of hyperbaric oxygen, administration of thalidomide, or use of granulocyte-macrophage colony-stimulating factor. Skin grafting with cultured allograft may decrease pain at the ulcer site. These therapies have been used with varying degrees of success.

### 16. How does a PG ulcer respond to treatment?

Response to therapy varies significantly. Unfortunately, it is not unusual for the ulcer to respond poorly or slowly.

### 17. What other care should be provided?

One of the nurse's responsibilities is to provide adequate rest time for the patient. In addition, patient referrals to the pain management team or nurse specialists for counseling are appropriate. Depression and the need to learn coping mechanisms are common.

### 18. Define vasculitis.

Vasculitis is defined as inflammation and necrosis of the blood vessel wall.

### 19. What causes inflammation of the blood vessels?

Vasculitis is a frequent manifestation of collagen vascular diseases. It may occur as a primary or secondary syndrome, as seen in hypersensitivity vasculitis. Because collagen is the most significant part of connective tissue, any disease, genetic defect, or other problem that affects collagen can cause a wide range of clinical manifestation.

*Primary Syndromes of Necrotic vasculitis*

| | |
|---|---|
| Polyarteritis nodosa (PAN) | Affects medium and small vessels, especially at bifurcation points |
| Wegener's syndrome | Affects medium and small vessels of lungs, kidneys, and other organs |
| Churg-Strauss syndrome | Rare, systemic vasculitis affecting multiple systems |

Hypersensitivity vasculitis may be a reaction to medication; viral, fungal, or parasitic exposure; or a manifestation of an immune disorder.

## 20. Why does the vessel become inflamed or necrotic in vasculitis?

The pathology is not known, but it is believed that the disease process allows immune complexes to be deposited on vessel walls. Leukocytes then infiltrate these areas of deposit and release enzymes. The enzyme release precipitates destruction of the vessel wall, leading to inflammation and possible necrosis at the site.

## 21. Where do vasculitic ulcers occur?

Vasculitis can affect vessels of any size anywhere in the body. Internal organs may be affected. The skin may have ulcerations. However, skin ulcers associated with vasculitis are frequently located on the lower extremity, often near the malleoli, which is also a frequent site of venous ulcers. Vasculitic ulcers may come and go at regular intervals or appear only once. Scarring at the site of the ulcer is common.

## 22. How are the vasculitic ulcers different in appearance from other types of ulcers?

The cutaneous manifestations of vasculitis vary depending on the disease or syndrome. The most common presentation is palpable purpura. Palpable purpura is a raised, nonblanchable erythema that results from the extravasation of red cells out of the blood vessels into the skin. The lesions can vary in presentation, making diagnosis difficult. Clinical presentation may include red macules, wheals, papules, nodules, vesicles, and blisters. Pain and itching may also be present.

## 23. Describe the typical history of the patient with vasculitis.

Patients may relate signs and symptoms that indicate systemic, immune diseases. Vague symptoms are often present in patients with systemic immune diseases, including general malaise, fever, aching, and weight loss. Other symptoms depend on the organs involved in the systemic disease.

## 24. How is vasculitis diagnosed?

In addition to the signs and symptoms described in the history and assessment of the ulcers, a wound biopsy is helpful. The history establishes the diagnosis by revealing the typical histologic features of cutaneous vasculitis and may aid in identifying the underlying systemic disease. An array of laboratory tests can be used to determine possible immune/hypersensitivity issues (see table below).

*Common Laboratory Tests for Vasculitis*

| TEST | RESULT |
|---|---|
| Complete blood count | Leukocytosis<br>Thrombocytotosis |
| Chemistry panel | Elevated blood urea nitrogen, liver function studies, creatine phosphokinase with renal, liver, or muscle involvement |
| Erythrocyte sedimentation rate | Elevated with inflammatory processes |
| Urinalysis | Microscopic hematuria, proteinuria present with renal damage |
| Serology | Rheumatoid factor,[*†] cytoplasmic-pattern antineutrophil cytoplasmic autoantibodies (C-ANCA),[*] perinuclear-pattern antineutrophil cytoplasmic autoantibodies (P-ANCA),[†‡] hepatitis tests,[†] antinuclear antibodies (ANA)[§] |

[*] Positive with Wegener's, [†] positive with PAN, [‡] positive with Churg-Strauss syndrome, [§] positive with systemic collagen diseases.

**25. Describe the treatment for vasculitic ulcers.**

If the patient has secondary syndrome vasculitis, treatment of the underlying disease or hypersensitivity is appropriate. Clinical interventions aimed at the immune disorder or systemic infection or withdrawal of the offending medication is essential. Depending on the severity of the disease process, regardless of primary or secondary causation, immunosuppressive and corticosteroid therapies are used. For localized or mild disease, antihistamines, colchicines, or dapsone may be useful. If ulcers are located on the lower leg, compression and leg elevation are helpful. In more severe cases, plasmapheresis may be necessary to remove the circulating immune complexes.

**26. Which topical dressings are appropriate to use with vasculitic ulcers?**

As with other inflammatory ulcers, the goals for local wound care are exudate management, maintenance of a moist wound environment, and prevention of trauma to the wound bed and surrounding skin (see question 12).

## BIBLIOGRAPHY

1. Bryant RA: Acute and Chronic Wounds: Nursing Management, 2nd ed. St. Louis, Mosby, 2000, pp 145–148.
2. Choucair MM, Fivenson DP: Pyoderma gangrenosum: A review of the disease and treatment options. Wounds 13:119–122, 2001.
3. De Araujo TS, Kirsner RS: Vasculitis. Wounds 13:99–110, 2001.
4. Dockery GL, Crawford ME: Cutaneous Disorders of the Lower Extremity. Philadelphia, W.B. Saunders, 1997, pp 190–194.
5. Ehrlich MR: Vasculitic ulcers: A complication of collagen-vascular disorders. Ostomy Wound Manage 39:12–25, 1993.
6. Kerdel FA: Inflammatory ulcers. J Dermatol Surg Oncol 19:772–778, 1993.
7. Kerstein MD: The non healing leg ulcer: Peripheral vascular disease, chronic venous insufficiency, and ischemic vasculitis. Ostomy Wound Manage 42:19S–35S, 1996.
8. Margolis DJ: Management of unusual causes of ulcers of lower extremities. J Wound Ostomy Contin Nurs 22:89–94, 1995.
9. Powell FC, et al: Pyoderma gangrenosum: Classification and management. J Am Acad Dermatol 34:395–412, 1996.
10. Powell FC, Collins S: Pyoderma gangrenosum. Clin Dermatol 18:283–293, 2000.
11. Rubano JJ, Kerstein MD: Arterial insufficiency and vasculitides. J Wound Ostomy Contin Nurs 25:147-157, 1998.
12. Seaman S: Considerations for the global assessment and treatment of patients with recalcitrant wounds. Ostomy Wound Manage 46:10S–29S, 2000.
13. Trent JT, Kirsner RS: Unusual wounds. Adv Skin Wound Care 14:151–153, 2001.

# 46. THE KENNEDY TERMINAL ULCER

*Karen Lou Kennedy*, RN, CS, FNP

**1. Define the Kennedy terminal ulcer.**

A Kennedy terminal ulcer is a pressure ulcer that some people develop as they are dying.

**2. Describe a Kennedy terminal ulcer.**

- It is can be shaped like a pear.
- It is usually on the sacrum.
- It can include the colors red, yellow, and black.
- The borders of the ulcer are usually irregular.

**3. What is its trademark presentation?**

It has a sudden onset. You may hear one of the following statements:

- "Oh, my gosh, it was not there yesterday."
- "I worked Friday, it was not there then. I was off the weekend. When I came back on Monday, there it was."

**4. What is meant by the 3:30 syndrome?**

The 3:30 syndrome describes the surprisingly sudden onset of the Kennedy terminal ulcer. In the author's experience at the Byron Health Center, which has been shared by many nurses around the country, the lesion tends to develop quickly, sometimes in a matter of hours. It often appears as little black spots. The spots tend to look like a speck of dirt or dried bowel movement. When caregivers try to wash it away, they find that it is under the skin rather than on the skin. As the hours progress, the lesion becomes larger. In several hours it may become almost the size of a quarter. Rapid progression leads to an appearance of several quarters lined up in a row. The lesion may look like someone colored the skin with a permanent marker.

In the usual scenario, the skin is observed to be intact, with no discoloration, when the patient gets up in the morning. At 3:30 PM, when patients are placed back in bed for a nap, the skin shows a blackened discoloration. Asked why the lesion was not reported before, caregivers explain that the ulcer was not there when the patient awoke. Most patients die within 8–24 hours, but some live for up to 2 weeks.

**5. How does a Kennedy terminal ulcer progress?**

It usually starts as a blister (stage II) and rapidly progresses to stage III or IV. In the beginning it almost looks as if someone dragged the patient's bottom over a black top driveway. It can look much like an abrasion. The lesion becomes deeper, and the color starts to change. As a rule, the lesion starts as a red area, then turns to yellow and progresses to black.

**6. How are Kennedy terminal ulcers different from other pressure ulcers?**

They start out larger than other pressure ulcers, are usually initially more superficial, and develop rapidly in size and depth.

**7. When was a Kennedy Terminal Ulcer first described?**

In March of 1989, the National Pressure Ulcer Advisory Panel met in Washington, D.C., to determine the prevalence of pressure ulcers and to formulate guidelines for predicting who was at risk. During her talk about the prevalence of pressure ulcers in a long-term care facility, Karen Lou Kennedy gave the first description of the Kennedy terminal ulcer.

---

The Kennedy terminal ulcer is named for the author, who first described it as a distinct clinical entity.

**8. In what age group is the ulcer most common?**

The Kennedy terminal ulcer tends to be a geriatric issue. It does not seem to be prominent in pediatrics. It is reported frequently in hospice patients.

**9. What causes a Kennedy terminal ulcer?**

Further research needs to be done. According to one theory, the cause may be a perfusion problem exacerbated by the dying process. The skin is the largest of the body organs and is the only organ on the outside of the body that reflects what is happening inside. As people approach the dying process, the internal organs may begin to slow down and go into multisystem organ failure. No particular symptoms may be detected except that the skin over bony prominences starts to show the effect of pressure in a very short period of time. This is true skin failure.

**10. How is the Kennedy terminal ulcer treated?**

The treatment of a Kennedy terminal ulcer is the same as for any other pressure ulcer. When it is in the blanchable or nonblanchable intact skin stage, the major goal is to relieve the pressure. When it becomes a stage II or partial-thickness ulcer, a thin film, hydrocolloid, foam, or gel could be used. For a stage III or IV full-thickness wound, depending on the amount of drainage, a hydrocolloid, foam, gel, or calcium alginate may be appropriate. Usually, these ulcers do not have a lot of drainage. If slough (yellow tissue) or necrotic tissue (black eschar) is present, you may consider removal of nonviable tissue with an enzymatic debriding agent, autolysis, or mechanical debridement. If the patient is clearly terminally ill, containment of odor and pain control rather than aggressive debridement,is the goal.

**11. Can a Kennedy terminal ulcer improve?**

Most do not. However, reversal has been demonstrated on occasions in terminally ill patients whose family suddenly want aggressive life-saving interventions.

**12. Why should clinicians know about the Kennedy terminal ulcer?**

Some staff, families, physicians, other healthcare providers, and lawyers believe that all pressure ulcers are preventable. When the blame starts, it is nice to have an explanation, along with literature sources, that accounts for the rapid decline in skin integrity.

## BIBLIOGRAPHY

1. Agency for Health Care Policy and Research: Treatment of Pressure Ulcers Clinical Practice Guideline Number 15. Rockville MD, U.S. Department of Health and Human Services, Publication No. G5-0652.
2. Kennedy KL: Gaymar Pictorial Guide to Pressure Ulcer Assessment. Orchard Park, NY, Gaymar Industries, 1997.
3. Kennedy KL:The prevalence of pressure ulcers in an intermediate care facility. Decubitus 2(2):44–45, 1989.
4. Kozier B, Erb G, Olivieri: Fundamentals of Nursing, 4th ed. Boston, Addison-Wesley, 1991.
5. Krasner DL, Rodeheaver, Sibbald RG: Chronic Wound Care: A Clinical Source Book for Healthcare Professionals, 3rd ed. Wayne, PA, Health Management Publications, 2001.

# 47. RARE BUT THERE: NECROTIZING SOFT TISSUE INFECTION

*Ovleto William Ciccarelli*, MD, FACS

**1. What are necrotizing soft tissue infections (NSTs)?**

NSTs spread quickly and silently, and can be lethal. They arrive under the level of radar as deep, progressive bacterial infections.

**2. List other common names for NST.**
- Necrotizing fasciitis
- Streptococcal gangrene
- Gas gangrene
- Bacterial synergistic gangrene
- Clostridial myonecrosis
- Fournier's gangrene
- Synergistic necrotizing cellulitis
- Many more names and eponyms

**3. What can be infected?**

Think layers:
- Skin
- Fat
- Fascia
- Muscle

The common mnemonic is **S**kinny's **f**latus is **f**airly **m**usical.

**4. Can just one layer of connective tissue be infected?**

Solitary levels of fascia can be involved with sparing of adjacent layers. Exceptions do occur. After all, the bubonic plague did not kill everyone.

**5. Can multiple layers be infected simultaneously?**

Yes. Bacteria are not diplomats and do not recognize the borders between soft tissue layers. Necrotizing fascitis can involve muscle, and myonecrosis can involve fascia.

**6. How do NSTs develop?**

NSTs can result from horrible, overt trauma, perforation of internal organs, or seemingly trivial injury, such as a minor scratch or abrasion. However, the difficult cases of NST usually have no evidence of epidermal violation.

**7. Who gets these nasty infections?**

Older patients, patients with heavily contaminated wounds, and obese or diabetic patients. Also at risk are patients with ischemic extremities, immunocompromised state, cirrhosis, cancer (with corticosteroid treatment), or an underlying illness such as renal failure. In brief, almost all of your patients or anyone in your own household may be a candidate.

**8. What bugs are involved with NST?**
- Group A streptococci (GAS)
- *Staphylococcus aureus*
- *Clostridium perfringens* and other species of *Clostridium*
- Mixed infections with a variety of gram-negative rods, both aerobic and anaerobic organisms

The closer the infection is to the torso, perineum, or a surgical wound, the more likely it is to be a mixed infection. Think of gram-negative rods. If you do not think of gram-negative rods, you cannot treat gram-negative rods. You will soon have a dead patient as evidence. Be aware, and be prepared.

**9. What are the symptoms of NST?**

Pain, often out of proportion to physical findings, is noted early. A confused, agitated, or toxic patient is a grave sign of advanced infection.

**10. What are the signs of NST?**

Often no signs are noted. This is the major difficulty with NST. The following clinical signs are helpful but not mandatory to make a diagnosis:

- Swelling
- Edema
- Ecchymosis
- Erythema
- Bullae or vesicles
- Gas in tissue (crepitus)
- Induration
- Thrombosed cutaneous vessels
- Fever
- Tachycardia
- Tachypnea

**11. Are laboratory tests helpful in making the diagnosis of NST?**

No. An elevated white blood cell count, a depressed white blood cell count, or a shift to the left with a preponderance of juvenile white blood cells (the so called left shift) will give you dyspepsia and be a cause for concern. These laboratory tests are of little help in making a decision to treat the patient.

**12. What radiologic tests are helpful in making the diagnosis of NST?**

Ultrasonography may reveal a deep abscess. Computed tomography may note edema, loss of distinction between tissue planes, or gas in soft tissues. Occasionally, magnetic resonance imaging can be of assistance in determining inflammation of tissue planes.

**13. True or false: Gas in soft tissues means that a clostridial infection is present.**

False. Gas in soft tissues may be due to a perforation of a gas-containing organ, such as a large bowel perforation into the soft tissues, or to a nonclostridial, gas-producing bacteria in the soft tissues. The metabolic activity of bacteria produces hydrogen, nitrogen, and methane. Do not light up and smoke.

**14. Are *Clostridium* species the most common gas-forming bacteria in "gassy" infections?**

No. *Clostridium perfringens* and other *Clostridium* species may produce the most extensive and dramatic infections, but streptococcal species are probably the more common pathogens involved in the production of gas in soft tissues.

**15. Can staphylococci cause NST?**

Uncommon, but not unheard of. Staphylococci can cause deep, spreading infections. Staphylococcal infections associated with a foreign body, such as an open, gauze-packed wound or a tampon, can also cause toxic shock syndrome, which can be confused with NST.

**16. What should I do if I see blisters, bullae, or vesicles?**

Aspirate the fluid in the blister and send it for culture as well as Gram stain.

**17. What is the significance of hypotension at the time of admission?**

Hypotension at admission is a grave sign of an advanced septic state. Emergency treatment is needed. The patient goes to the front of the triage line—pronto.

**18. What is the significance of dark urine at the time of admission?**

The patient may have hemoconcentration or myoglobinuria. This sign demands attention and treatment.

**19. What should I do if I see dark urine?**

Send a urine specimen for routine analysis and culture. Send blood studies for myoglobin, serum creatine phosphokinase, and serum lactate dehydrogenase.

**20. What is the significance of dark urine due to myoglobinuria?**

Myoglobinuria is due to the presence of myoglobin in the urine. Myoglobin is an oxygen-carrying compound found in striated muscle. It is released into the blood stream after skeletal muscle gangrene, necrosis, and cell death. Myoglobin is filtered by the kidney and excreted in the urine. Myoglobinuria can be a contributing factor in the development of acute renal failure. It may be due to clostridial myonecrosis. It is a grave clinical sign.

**21. What is Fournier's gangrene?**

Fournier's gangrene is an NST of the soft tissues of the perianal area, external genitalia, or perineum. It is seen in association with diabetes mellitus.

**22. What is "dishwater pus"?**

Dishwater pus is an often talked about, but seldom seen, phenomenon. It is a thin, gray, inflammatory exudate that may be found at the site of an injury. It may signify a clostridial infection.

**23. How are NSTs diagnosed?**

- Think infection. You cannot diagnose something unless you consider the possibility of its existence.
- History: recent surgery or recent trauma.
- Patient complaints: pain, fever, chills, pain, and more pain. Often the pain is out of proportion to the visible injury or wound.
- Physical examination: check all orifices, wounds, skin folds, interdigital spaces, nooks, and crannies.

**24. Is vague pain around a recent incision or stoma worrisome?**

It may mean that a deep infection is beginning to burrow along a muscle or fascial path.

**25. What is the meaning of ankle pain associated with a puncture wound on the bottom of the foot?**

A deep infection is tracking along the deep plantar space and fascia. It has left the foot and is surfacing at the ankle. This condition is seen in patients with neuropathy affecting the feet.

**26. Does the presence or absence of odor mean anything?**

Any odor equals trouble—cell death. Absence of odor can mean any of the following:
- Nothing
- Early infection without cell death
- Absence of function in the olfactory fibers in your first cranial nerve

**27. How are NSTs treated?**

1. Initial resuscitation: A, B, C (airway, breathing, circulation)
2. Be prepared to treat all aspects of shock.
3. After adequate airway and breathing are assured, circulatory support becomes paramount. Aggressive fluid resuscitation is mandatory with two large-caliber intravenous lines utilizing Ringer's lactate solution.
4. Perform blood studies for complete blood count, coagulation profile, complete metabolic profile (including all enzymes), and blood cultures.
5. Perform urinary studies with urinary catheter.
6. A chest x-ray is appropriate.
7. Examine all orifices, wounds, skin folds, nail beds, intertrigal areas, and interdigital spaces. Do not forget to look for carious teeth. Use pain localization to focus your examination.
8. Begin empirical antibiotics with combination therapy.

**28. Is operative treatment needed?**

Almost invariably. Areas should be opened if tender, red, edematous, or otherwise clinically suspicious.

**29. Can wounds or injuries be adequately evaluated under local anesthesia or in an ambulatory setting?**

No. Exploration of an area in question needs to be done in an operating room where wide debridement can be performed.

**30. Are limited explorations adequate?**

No. A wide exposure is needed. Expect to see a big, open wound postoperatively. Cheating on the initial debridement almost invariably leads to failure.

**31. How big is a "big" wound?**

The surgeon passes a clamp along the interface between the fascia and the muscle. Viable tissue is noted when resistance to the passage of a clamp is felt. All necrotic tissue is removed and pus is drained. Non-bleeding muscle is resected. Cut muscle that bleeds and contracts is a sign of life. Extremities may need to be amputated. Communicating infections into the pelvic and abdominal cavities need to be filleted wide open and left open postoperatively. Expect to see an open, bloody wound with previously unseen viscera greeting your eyes. This is the sign of an adequate debridement. Bleeding is a sign of life.

**32. Is a clostridial polyvalent antitoxin useful?**

No. It is useless.

**33. Does hyperbaric oxygen have a role in the treatment of NST?**

Yes (see Chapter 32).

**34. Is there a single best choice of antibiotics ?**

No. Definitive treatment requires specific information determined by culture. An acceptable regimen covers gram-positive and gram-negative organisms along with anaerobic bacteria. An aminoglycoside with a penicillin and an antianaerobic agent is appropriate. Triple antibiotic treatment is often prudent until specific culture data are received.

**35. Can you summarize everything in one paragraph so a neophyte can make sense of it?**

- Think deep and hard to find infections.
- Pain points the way to the problem.
- Damaged skin of any sort is a potential infective site.
- Forget arbitrary and lengthy classifications of these infections. All of these patients are sick and need resuscitation, prompt surgery, and wide-spectrum antibiotic treatment. Let the professors sort out the trivia!

**36. Any other clinical pearls?**

Try not to think of NST the next time you personally get a scrape. You will drive yourself mad.

BIBLIOGRAPHY

1. Stone D, Gorbach S: Atlas of Infectious Diseases. Philadelphia, W.B. Saunders, pp. 138–139, 2000.
2. Swartz M: Cellulitis and subcutaneous tissue infections. In Mandell GL, et al (eds): Principles and Practice of Infectious Disease, 5th ed. New York, Churchill Livingstone, 1999, pp 1050–1057.
3. Stevens DL: Infections of the Skin, Muscle and Soft Tissues. In Fauci AS, et al (eds): Harrison's Principles of Emergency Medicine, 14th ed. New York, McGraw Hill, 1998, pp 827–830.
4. Fry DE: Necrotizing skin and soft tissue infections. In Rakel, Bope (eds): Conn's Current Therapy 2001, 53rd ed. Philadelphia, W.B. Saunders, 2001, pp 138–139.
5. Jimenez MF, Marshall JE: Source control in the management of sepsis. Intens Care Med 27 (Suppl 1):S49–S62, 2001.
6. Howard RJ: Surgical infections. In Schwartz SI, et al (eds): Principles of Surgery, 7th ed. New York, McGraw-Hill, 1999, pp 123–153.

# 48. RARE BUT THERE: OTHER LOWER EXTREMITY WOUNDS

*Catherine T. Milne, APRN, MSN, CWOCN, CS, ANP, and Lisa Q. Corbett, APRN, MSN, CWOCN, CS*

**1. Various ulcerations not attributed to venous insufficiency, arterial disease, or an inflammatory process occur on the lower extremity. What are they?**

Although they are rare, clinical suspicion should always be lurking for wounds not caused by an inflammatory, venous, or arterial disease, including::

- Bowen's disease
- Calciphylaxis
- Necrobiosis lipoidica
- Kaposi's sarcoma
- Squamous, basal cell carcinoma
- Malignant melanoma
- Bullous diseases
- Infectious lesions

**2. What clinical clues should prompt a clinician to consider an atypical ulceration?**

Three hallmarks of an atypical ulcer are as follows:

1. Unusual presentation (if you think it looks "odd," it probably is)

2. Unusual location (if it looks venous in origin but is located on the knee, it is something else)

3. No improvement (failed attempts with multiple treatment regimen are a clue that one should step back and examine possible explanations of a nonhealing wound [see Chapter 49])

**3. What is Bowen's disease?**

Bowen's disease is intraepithelial squamous cell carcinoma. It appears on the lower extremity, usually on the shin, as a light pink or reddish lesion. Its color is uniform, and some lesions may be slightly scaly. It can be confused with psoriasis or an early venous insufficiency lesion because the border can be irregularly shaped and crusting may occur.

**4. How is Bowen's disease diagnosed and treated?**

Biopsy of the area confirms the diagnosis and assists in determining treatment. Management varies from topical chemotherapeutic agents to cryotherapy to surgical excision. Referral to a dermatologist or oncologist is paramount. Bowen's disease is usually in situ but can progress to an invasive form.

**5. Who is at risk for developing calciphylaxis?**

Calciphylaxis almost diagnoses itself, if you are aware of its existence. Calciphylaxis is seen exclusively in end-stage renal disease and hyperparathyroidism. Biopsy is confirmatory.

**6. What causes calciphylaxis?**

Cutaneous necrosis occurs as excessive calcium is deposited in the microvascular system, causing painful necrotic lesions.

**7. How do these lesions present?**

Often they start as a painful purple lesion that progresses to black areas. Early appearance is round. Eventually, because of ischemia and gangrene, the affected areas slough off, leaving erosions that extend into the subcutaneous tissue. Secondary infection is common, as is lesion enlargement. It also is seen on the fingers, abdomen, buttocks, and penis.

**8. What is the treatment for calciphylaxis?**

Treatment of the underlying cause—renal failure or hyperparathyroidism—is essential. Reducing serum calcium levels, aggressive debridement, and treatment of infection in addition to standard wound care are essential. Because these lesions are very painful, except in cases of severe neuropathy, aggressive pain management is essential. Unfortunately, most patients die from multi-system organ failure. Like the Kennedy terminal ulcer, calciphylaxis is an example of "skin failure."

**9. Do necrobiosis lipoidica lesions have a characteristic presentation?**
Early lesions are plaque-like with a well-defined irregular edge. They may be yellow, red, or brown. The diagnostic clues are a shiny epidermis and visible dermal blood vessels. As lesions evolve, ulceration occurs in the plaque. Ulcerations frequently appear necrotic.

**10. When should suspicion be high for necrobiosis lipoidica?**
Two-thirds of these slowly evolving lesions occur in patients with long-standing diabetes. In addition, patients may have a history of trauma to the site. Lesions are frequently seen on the shins or bony areas of the feet.

**11. How is necrobiosis lipoidica diagnosed?**
These lesions are distinct because of the visible dermal blood vessels in the plaque; biopsy is usually not necessary. However, there will always be someone who argues that the lesion is a venous stasis ulcer and that the plaque is stasis dermatitis. Settle the discussion by suggesting a biopsy.

**12. How is necrobiosis lipoidica treated?**
Necrobiosis responds to topical or intralesional corticosteroids. Most lesions heal with good wound care.

**13. Can one assume that HIV is present in a patient with Kaposi's sarcoma (KS)?**
No. Although KS has seen a resurgence because of HIV-associated immunosuppression, elderly eastern Europeans, patients receiving chemotherapy, and transplant recipients are also affected.

**14. What does KS look like?**
KS starts as a dark purple macule or nodule. A number of lesions close together may coalesce into a large area. Deep involvement initiates lymphedema. The telling difference between ecchymosis and KS lesions can be found at your fingertips—KS is palpable, ecchymosis is not. KS lesions can be found anywhere on the body, including the oral cavity. They may progress to a plaque or nodular appearance.

**15. Is biopsy the standard of care for diagnosis?**
Yes.

**16. Name the different types of KS.**
Classic KS, African-endemic KS, immunosuppresive drug-associated KS and HIV-associated KS. Despite the different etiologies, KS remains a cutaneous malignancy that may also involve the pulmonary, gastrointestinal, urogenital, and neurologic systems.

**17. How is KS treated?**
Because there is no cure, the goal of therapy is to control symptoms. Classic KS responds to radiation therapy. African-endemic KS is best treated with systemic chemotherapy. Drug-induced KS abates when the offending agent is withdrawn. A number of treatments are available for HIV-associated KS, including radiation, cyrosurgery, laser surgery, local excision, and intralesional chemotherapy.

**18. How can squamous cell and basal cell cancers be described?**
Basal cell carcinoma is the most common type of skin cancer. First presenting as a pearly pink papule or nodule, it may have a depressed center and a rolled border. Lesions of squamous cell carcinoma appear as red ulcerated nodules, with or without crusting, that resemble granulation tissue. Biopsies are confirmational and guide treatment decisions.

**19. If a patient presents with an ulcer in a scarred area due to a burn, what should be your first and second thoughts?**
**First thought:** Squamous cell cancer is a strong possibility. You need to prepare the patient for this possibility. In such cases, squamous cell cancer carries a 20% metastatic rate.

**Second thought:** Who is a good dermatologist or surgeon? Who will see the patient as soon as possible?

**20. How is basal cell carcinoma treated?**
Surgical excision and cryosurgery are usually performed.

**21. How is squamous cell carcinoma treated?**
Topical chemotherapeutic agents, excisional surgery, and cryosurgery are the options, depending on lesion size, dermal infiltration, and location.

**22. What is the most important intervention nurses can do to reduce the incidence of basal cell and squamous cell carcinoma?**
Teach patients how and when to use sunscreen, to avoid the most intense sunlight hours between 10 AM and 2 PM., to wear a hat, and to cover exposed skin when possible. There is an association between sun exposure in younger years and the later development of skin cancer.

**23. Is malignant melanoma caused by sun exposure?**
Although sun exposure plays a definite role in the development of malignant melanoma, a positive family history of the disease suggests a genetic predisposition to its development.

**24. Name the five cardinal signs of malignant melanoma.**
Use the **ABCDE** method to identify patients who need referral to the dermatologist:
**A**symmetry: The lesion is irregularly shaped. If cut in half, one side would not resemble the other.
**B**order: Look at the edges of the lesion. Abnormal borders are scalloped and irregular.
**C**olor: The color of the lesion is not uniform. Black, gray, pink, tan, and/or brown hues may be present and appear to be randomly placed.
**D**iameter: Usually greater than a pencil eraser.
**E**nlargement and **e**levation: Increasing size above the surface level of the surrounding skin.

**25. Is biopsy the diagnostic test of choice?**
Yes. As in all of the previously described lesions, a skin biopsy is necessary to confirm the clinician's suspicion and determine appropriate treatment. Sentinel node dissection is also recommended if the lesion is thicker than 1.0 mm.

**26. How is malignant melanoma treated?**
Complete excision is warranted. Additional management strategies depend on the depth and presence of positive nodes at the time of excision or biopsy. Two percent of all cancer deaths annually are attributed to malignant melanoma. It is the third leading cause of cancer mortality.

**27. What about bullous and infectious diseases?**
Bullous diseases (llesions with fluid-filled blisters) may or may not be infectious, depending on the cause. Not all infectious skin alterations start with blisters.

**28. What are the most common bullous and infectious lesions on the lower extremities?**
Herpes virus, bullous pemphigus, fungal infections, and bacterial and mycobacterial lesions. Although discussion of these lesions beyond the scope of this book, consideration of the tenets of lower extremity assessment and high suspicion for lesions that "don't look normal" will lead to the appropriate work-up, correct diagnosis, and proper treatment.

## BIBLIOGRAPHY

1. Elgart GW: Biopsy of cutaneous ulcers: When it is helpful. Dermatol Ther 30(Suppl):30-S, 1999.
2. Falanga V, Eaglstein WH: Leg and Foot Ulcers: A Clinician's Guide. St. Louis, Mosby, 1995.
3. Falanga V, Phillips T, Harding K, et al: Text Atlas of Wound Management. London, Martin Dunitz, 2000.
4. Fitzpatrick T, Johnson RA, Wolff K, et al: Color Atlas and Synopsis of Clinical Dermatology, 3rd ed. New York, McGraw-Hill, 1997.

# 49. COMMON PITFALLS IN WOUND HEALING

*Catherine T. Milne, APRN, MSN, CS, CWOCN, ANP,
and Lisa Q. Corbett, APRN, MSN, CS, CWOCN*

**1. What is the definition of the nonhealing wound?**

The literature varies. The following definitions have been reported:

- No improvement in 14 days.
- No improvement in 4 weeks (considered a chronic or nonhealing wound).
- The components of wound fluids change over time, leading to the accepted definition by the Wound Healing Society as a wound that "fails to proceed through an orderly and timely process to produce anatomical and functional integrity or proceeded through the repair process without establishing a sustained anatomic and functional result."
- An imbalance between the matrix metalloproteinases (MMPs) and the tissue inhibitors of the matrix metalloproteinases (TIMPs) is one example of the disruption that occurs. Chronic wound fluid has been shown to degrade growth factors. No time frame is placed on this process, but an examination of fluid from a 12-week-old wound is different from that of a 4-week-old wound. Anyway you look at it, the common theme is this: the wound is *not* getting better.

**2. Describe a framework that can help the clinician determine why a wound fails to heal.**

Many factors impact wound healing. If the wound is not healing or deteriorating, it is best that the clinician step back from the situation and analyze a number of different factors to determine the causes. In many cases, the causes are multifactorial. Consider going through the following list in its entirety. Finding one explanation does not necessarily mean that it is the only one.

*Top Ten Reasons for Failure to Heal*

10. **Failure to appreciate the real cause**
    - Is the real cause a squamous cell cancer? Necrobiosis lipodica? Pyoderma gangrenosum? Parasitic infection? Pressure? Factitious?
    - Solution: Consider cultures and wound biopsy. Refer the patient, if necessary.

9. **Failure to modify the physical environment**
    - Is shear controlled? Is pressure reduction adequate? Is it available all the time? Many clinicians use a support surface on the bed but neglect to consider all possible surfaces (e.g, the favorite lounge chair, park bench, and even the commode).
    - Solution: Play detective. Find out what extrinsic mechanical forces are contributing factors and reduce them. Obtain offloading devices if the wound is located in the plantar surface of the foot. Use moisture barriers to protect the skin from moisture and wound drainage.

8. **Failure to debride**
    - If the wound bed is not clear of nonviable tissue, all of the expensive wound growth factors in the world will not help it.
    - Solution: Initiate debridement therapy. Mechanical, enzymatic, surgical, autolytic, conservative, biotherapy, or sharp debridement are options. Be aggressive.

7. **Failure to recognize when the goal of therapy is not to heal the wound**
    - A cachetic, terminally ill patient with metastatic disease may have "skin failure" as part of the dying process.
    - Solution: Be clear about the ultimate goal of wound care at all times. The goal for some patients may start out to be healing-oriented but change as time passes. It is not a failure of the clinician, the setting in which the patient is treated, the caregivers, or the local dressing. The patient is dying. Keep the patient comfortable, manage pain appropriately, and readjust wound-healing goals accordingly.

*Table continued on following page*

*Top Ten Reasons for Failure to Heal (Continued)*

6. **Failure to view the wound as the window to the patient's condition**
   - A wound that has been healing suddenly gets worse despite no change in therapy, setting, care-givers, extrinsic forces, nutritional status, or other factors. This situation may herald the onset of an acute illness, such as an upper respiratory infection, urinary tract infection, or exacerbation of chronic obstructive pulmonary disease or congestive heart failure, by 3–5 days.
   - Solution: Unfortunately, until the patient exhibits a problem, there is not much that you can do. But at least you can take comfort in knowing that it was not anyone's fault. Possible causes include an increase in metabolic needs without adequate reserve or perhaps a "shunting" of nutrients and white blood cells to the newest insult to the body. This cause can usually be ruled out if no signs of illness are seen within 7 days of sudden wound deterioration.

5. **Failure to appreciate the role of nutrition in wound healing**
   - Inadequate protein and caloric intake slow wound healing. The reasons for such problems are too numerous to be listed here.
   - Solution: Enlist a dietitian's assistance to determine nutritional needs for healing. A comprehensive assessment and initiation of the recommendations can improve outcomes. Obtain nutritional labs to evaluate current status.

4. **Failure to appreciate host factors**
   - A vast number of issues can be listed here. Several of the overlooked areas include the patient's pain, depression, inability to afford expensive wound-healing modalities, or inadequate control of blood sugar.
   - Solution. This area is perhaps the most time-consuming, because many issues require a coordinated effort among many disciplines. Nurses are adept in the art of coordination and facilitation. Often, the art of wound care is getting the multitude of specialists along with the primary care physician to agree to and stick with a plan of care with which the patient and significant other can comply.

3. **Failure to get patients to take ownership of the wound**
   - Patients come to us with preconceived ideas. Many times it is the perception that the wound will heal "in a week" or that their mother always told them to keep the wound open and dry, to soak it in ocean water, or to stuff it with shark cartilage, molasses, or raw honey. Smoking cigarettes helps; so does smoking pot. Nurses have heard these perceptions—and more—in their practice. Some day time we may tell you about the caregiver who had the dog clean the wound one day.
   - Solution: Start patient and caregiver education early in the relationship. Teach them anatomy and physiology of wound healing in terms that they can understand. Educate them about what makes wounds better and what can make them worse. Dispel myths and discuss science—the sooner the better.

2. **Failure to check the simple things**
   - Is there adequate circulation to the wound? Is edema controlled? Was the initial assessment comprehensive? Is bone exposed?
   - Solution: Retrace your steps. Check skin perfusion pressures, toe pressures, and ankle brachial indexes, if not previously done. Start the work-up to rule out or confirm osteomyelitis if it was not already done.

1. **Failure to appreciate and reduce bioburden in a clean-looking wound bed**
   - The wound characteristics of an over-bioburdened wound include:
     a. Friability: a friable wound bleeds easily when touched lightly on the surface.
     b. Change in the amount of drainage: increasing drainage, with or without an odor, can indicate increased bioburden.
     c. Hypergranulation tissue: "proud flesh" syndrome is typically associated with a colonized wound. Puffy, pink, or red granulation tissue usually protrudes above the surface of the surrounding skin.
     d. Abnormal discoloration of granulation tissue: tissue that is dull, pale, or ruddy may indicate an increase in microorganisms.
   - Solution: Adequate wound cleansing significantly reduces bioburden. Use the right solution, in sufficient volume and at the correct pressure. Topical antimicrobial agents can significantly improve wound healing in the over-bioburdened wound. Use them accordingly. Consider obtaining a tissue culture to identify causative organisms.

*Table continued on following page*

*Top Ten Reasons for Failure to Heal (Continued)*

---

• Although the controversy of sterile vs. clean technique has not yet been definitively decided, observation of the wound-dressing change technique can sometimes be of assistance. Look for the most obvious factors. Are the caregivers washing hands? Are the tips of cream and ointment tubes touching fingers or skin at the time of application? What about open jars of petrolatum? Has this jar been open and used for other purposes, such as reducing hemorrhoidal discomfort or treatment of a dry, pruritic skin patch on the cat? These last two examples are from our own practice. Perhaps the next edition of this book should have a truth is stranger than fiction chapter.

---

### BIBLIOGRAPHY

1. Krasner DL: How to prepare the wound bed. Ostomy Wound Manage 47(4):59, 61, 2001.
2. Lazarus GS, Cooper DM, Knighton DM: Definitions and guidelines for assessment of wounds and evaluation of healing. Arch Dermatol 130:489–493, 1994.
3. Seaman S: Considerations for the global assessment and treatment of patients with recalcitrant wounds. Ostomy Wound Manage 46(Suppl 1A):10S–29S, 2000.
4. Siegel DM: Contact sensitivity and recalcitrant wounds. Ostomy Wound Manage 46(Supp 1A):65S–74S, 2000.
5. Yager DR, Chen SM, Ward SI, et al: Ability of chronic wound fluids to degrade peptide growth actors is associated with increased levels of elastase activity and diminished levels of proteinase inhibitors. Wound Repair Regen 5:23–32, 1997.

# 50. OPTIONS IN TISSUE CLOSURE

*Joseph J. Robles, MD*

## 1. Explain closure by primary intention.

The classic example of healing by primary intention is a surgical incision with little or no loss of tissue. The wound edges are approximated with staples, sutures, or adhesive skin closure strips, and the wound heals by connective tissue deposition.

## 2. When is primary closure appropriate?

- Clean wounds less than 6 hours old with no tissue loss
- Linear incisions
- Surgically created incisions
- Incisions without tension

## 3. Explain closure by secondary intention.

In healing by secondary intention, the wound edges remain open and healing occurs by the formation of granulation tissue in the dead space as well as contraction of the wound margins. The wound heals from the bottom up and from the edges toward the center by means of granulation, contraction. and re-epithelialization. A decubitus ulcer healing on its own without skin graft or flap closure is an example.

## 4. When is healing by secondary intention appropriate?

- In grossly contaminated traumatic wounds (e.g., dirt in the wound)
- Infected postoperative wounds (e.g., debridement of necrotizing fasciitis)
- Wounds highly suspicious for infection if closed primarily (e.g., stoma site wound after reversal of the colostomy)
- Wounds too large to close when skin grafting and flaps are inappropriate (e.g.. decubitus ulcer)

## 5. Explain delayed primary closure.

Delayed primary wound closure may be used for wounds with a high index of suspicion for infection immediately after surgery, as in the case of a ruptured appendix. Once the patient is afebrile for 24 hours and no local signs or symptoms of infection are present, a wound packed open at the time of surgery can be closed primarily with well-spaced stitches. Although this approach decreases the likelihood of wound infection, there should be a low threshold to open the wound if signs and symptoms of wound infection appear.

## 6. What are the options for wound closure by primary intention?

- Sutures
- Staples
- Adhesive strips
- Tissue adhesives

## 7. When are sutures used for closure of a wound?

- Small incisions from surgical procedures
- Incisions on the face
- Incisions from skin lesion excisions
- Incisions requiring multiple layers of closure

## 8. How is suture material chosen for various types of wound?

See table on following page.

| WOUND CLOSURE MATERIAL | INDICATIONS/COMMENTS |
|---|---|
| **Sutures** | |
| Nonabsorbable | |
|   Braided (silk) | Ligation of deep vessels |
| | Anchoring of drain tubes and catheters to the skin |
| | Usually not used in skin closures |
|   Monofilament (nylon) | Uncomplicated skin closure |
| | Needs to be removed |
| | Permanent fascial closure in patients at high risk for stress and disruption (e.g., patients who are malnourished or taking steroids) |
| Absorbable | |
|   Braided (Vicryl) | Ligation of deep or superficial vessels |
| | Buried stitches and knots in layered closure |
| | Tissue at low risk for stress and disruption (e.g., deep layer of multi-layered closure) |
|   Monofilament (PDS) | Running fascial closure of abdomen |
| | Longer half-life than Vicryl |
|   Monofilament (Monocryl) | Cosmetic subcuticular closures |
| | Dermal closures |
| | Fewer stitch granulomas than braided stitch |
|   Chromic (catgut) | Shortest lasting absorbable material |
| | Used on peritoneum or sometimes on skin minimum tension setting |
| **Adhesive skin closure strips** | Used to reinforce subcutaneous skin closures |
| | Skin preps (e.g., benzoin) may increase adhesion |
| | Superficial nonbleeding skin tears |
| **Staples** | Used to close large incisions in a timely manner |
| | Useful in scalp lacerations |
| | Require special staple remover |
| **Tissue adhesive** | Used in clean, dry linear incisions or lacerations 6–8 cm in length |
| | May be preferable to stitches in children since no needles are used |
| | No follow-up is necessary in uncomplicated incisions or lacerations |

### 9. Does the age of the wound influence the approach to skin closure?

Dirty, contaminated wounds open for longer than 6 hours should be irrigated and left to close by secondary intention (e.g., dog bite with tissue loss more than 6 hours old). Fresh incisions and traumatic wounds can almost always be closed within 6 hours of presentation.

### 10. Does wound location influence the type of material chosen for closure?

- Small or shallow incisions and those in cosmetically significant areas can be closed with stitch, adhesive strips, or tissue adhesives.
- Moderate-sized incisions and incisions across joints should be closed with stitch or staples. They may also require a buried layer of absorbable stitch.
- Large incisions are most often closed with staples with or without buried layers of absorbable stitch.

### 11. Outline the recommended postprocedural care for a wound closed by primary intention.

- Stitches and staples may be dressed with antibiotic ointment and dry gauze initially
- Adhesive strips and tissue adhesives should be kept dry for the first 48 hours.
- Avoid use of alcohol, iodine, and peroxide, which are cytotoxic and may prevent wound healing.
- After 48 hours, incisions can be cleansed with mild soap and water.
- Dry gauze dressing and paper tape can be placed if there is a small amount of drainage or friction from clothing.
- When there is no drainage or chance of friction on suture line, leave open to air.

**12. How do you dress a wound closed by primary intention?**
1. If adhesive strips or tissue adhesives are used: Leave dressing in place for 48 hours. After 48 hours, uncover; the patient may shower.
2. If staples or sutures are used: Bacteriostatic moist environment should be maintained for 48 hours (e.g,. with antibiotic ointment/impregnated gauze). After 48 hours, open to air; the patient may shower.

**13. How long do sutures remain in place before removal?**
- Face: 3–5 days
- Trunk, arms, legs, scalp: 7 days
- Hands, feet, over joints, back: 10–14 days

**14. What patient characteristics influence the choice of closure material?**
1. Patients at risk for poor tissue healing (e.g., malnutrition, steroid use) usually require stitches or staples that should be left in place for approximately 14 days.
2. Patients who are unlikely to return for follow-up (e.g., homeless people, migrant workers, uninsured people) benefit from buried absorbable stitch closure when appropriate.
3. Children may benefit from closure with tissue adhesives because fewer needles are required.

**15. What is a tissue adhesive?**
Tissue adhesives are gaining popularity for simple laceration closures, especially in emergency departments. Cyanoacrylates are a group of chemicals that polymerize when exposed to tissue and then form a strong bond. Proponents state that adhesive closure is faster, less painful, and more economic than traditional stitch closure. They also state that the cosmetic results are equal and in some cases superior.

**16. On what types of wounds should a tissue adhesive used?**
- Simple linear incisions without significant tissue loss that are less the 6–8 cm in length
- Incisions that are tension-free
- Incisions in dry areas of the body

**17. List the contraindications to using a tissue adhesive.**
- Across joints or areas of increased mobility
- In moist areas (e.g., groin, axilla) or on mucous membranes
- In areas subjected to frequent washing (e.g., hands of health care providers)
- In patients with poor tissue healing potential (e.g., vascular disease, steroid use, malnutrition)

**18. How is a tissue adhesive applied?**
Tissue adhesives are applied across an incision or laceration that is easily approximated, clean, and dry. Local anesthesia and deep absorbable stitches are used as needed. The skin edges are everted, and the adhesive is painted on as a film across the wound and at least 0.5 cm beyond the skin edge on either side. The skin should be held in place until the adhesive dries (about 1 minute). The flexible film forms its own sterile dressing, and no dressing is required, but a sterile dressing can be placed as necessary once the adhesive is completely dry. Adhesive strips are not necessary. Tissue adhesives should be applied only to the skin surface, because cyanoacrylate in a wound can cause a foreign body reaction and may prevent proper epithelialization.

**19. Summarize the postprocedural care for wounds treated with tissue adhesive.**
Creams and ointments should not be used, because they may weaken the adhesive. The film should be kept dry for the first 24 hours. Showering is then allowed, but prolonged soaking or swimming should be avoided. The film falls off naturally after 1–2 weeks, and follow-up visits are not always necessary.

### BIBLIOGRAPHY

1. King ME, Kinney AY: Tissue adhesives: A new method of wound repair. Nurse Pract 24(10):66–73, 1999.
2. Gordon CA: Reducing needlestick injuries with the use of 2-octyl cyanoacrylates for laceration repair. J Am Acad Nurse Pract 13(1):10–12, 2001.

# 51.  THE NONHEALING SURGICAL WOUND

*Daniel J. Scoppetta, MD*

### 1.  What causes a surgical wound to open?

A surgical wound will open if sutures or staples are removed too early. Surgical wound sutures or staples typically remain in place for 7–10 days in patients with anticipated normal wound healing. Wounds may reopen because of the development of an abscess, hematoma, or seroma.

### 2.  What factors place patients at risk for developing a nonhealing surgical wound?

- Diabetes mellitus
- Poor nutrition
- Prolonged hospitalization
- Poor arterial circulation (especially in the legs)
- Surgical procedures of long duration
- Peritonitis as cause of surgical procedure
- Prior radiation therapy near surgical site
- Chronic steroid use

### 3.  Are some wounds more apt to develop infection?

Surgical wound sites can be categorized into four types:

1.  In clean wounds, no viscus is entered and no breaks in sterile technique occur.

2.  Clean-contaminated wounds are virtually the same except that a viscus is entered.

3.  Contaminated wounds have minor spillage of infected material or result traumatically from a clean source.

4.  Dirty-infected wounds have gross spillage of infected material or involve trauma from a contaminated source. Infection rates vary accordingly.

| TYPE | EXAMPLE | INFECTION RATE (%) |
|------|---------|--------------------|
| Clean | Hernia repair | 2.1 |
| Clean-contaminated | Elective cholecystectomy | 3.3 |
| Contaminated | Appendectomy | 6.4 |
| Dirty-infected | Repaired diverticula with colectomy | 12 |

### 4.  What can be done to prevent or minimize the chance of a nonhealing wound?

- Adherence to guidelines for skin preparation immediately preoperatively
- Use of prophylactic perioperative antibiotics
- Attention to gentle handling of tissues and careful hemostasis intraoperatively

### 5.  How are patients assessed for a nonhealing surgical wound?

A surgical wound should be inspected regularly and palpated, especially if new or atypical pain or discomfort develops. The signs of infection should be excluded: redness, pain, swelling, or drainage.

### 6.  When the skin around an incision is pressed and the incision line oozes, does this mean that the incision will open?

Wound drainage can be the first sign of a significant wound problem. Small amounts of bloody drainage are usual after any operation. However, persistent or new drainage is often a sign of a wound problem. Opening of the wound spontaneously or deliberately may be necessary for complete healing.

### 7.  What is the purpose of retention sutures?

Retention sutures in abdominal wounds prevent evisceration and complete dehiscence, which are more common in obese patients, patients with history of radiation to affected area, and chronic steroid-dependent patients.

**8. When should retention sutures be removed?**

Retention sutures are usually removed after 2–3 weeks once the risks of evisceration have diminished and any cause of increased intra-abdominal pressure has resolved (e.g., prolonged postoperative ileus with distention or severe coughing).

**9. When the wound is open, what is the best way to treat it?**

Open wound management should be individualized. Certain principles of wound care should be incorporated into the management:
- Maintain a moist barrier between the wound surface and dressing.
- Promote approximation of the wound edges by not overpacking the wound.
- Avoid wound contamination from other sources.
- Avoid accumulation of excessive fluid or nonviable tissue within the healing wound

These principles can be achieve by:
- Irrigation with normal saline at dressing change
- Use of advanced wound care products, such as hydrogels and alginates
- Selective sharp wound debridement and/or use of chemical debridement agents
- Application of closed-vacuum suction system

**10. What is challenging about healing wounds with visible mesh?**

Absorbable or nonabsorbable mesh is used in wounds with a large surface area that requires granulation tissue to cover and envelop. The challenge arises in developing a local wound environment that promotes steady healing and contracture of the wound toward closure by secondary intention or with the help of skin grafting for closure.

**11. Why is it problematic when vascular grafts are visible in an open wound?**

This situation places the graft at great risk to infection. If vascular graft infection develops, several scenarios are likely:
- Need for further surgical intervention
- Excision of the graft and additional surgery for re-vascularization
- Threat of loss of limb
- Threat of life-threatening hemorrhage

**12. Why is it problematic when orthopedic hardware is exposed in an open wound?**

The threat of infection of the foreign material (i.e., hardware) is a possibility and may lead to bone or joint infection that can compromise the successful healing of the bony injury or repair.

**13. What is a fistula?**

A fistula is an abnormal communication between two areas. Fistulas can result from abnormal healing or ongoing inflammation. Crohn's disease is an example of a fistula-prone condition because of its repetitive inflammatory and infectious nature. Anal fistulas result from incomplete or faulty healing of a perirectal abscess.

**14. How are fistulas named?**

Fistulas are named by the two areas that they connect. For example, an enterocutaneous fistula connects the small bowel and the skin.

**15. How are fistulas managed?**

Management should be individualized. The principles of treatment for intestinal fistulas include:
- Avoidance of ongoing abscess or infection around the intestine when the fistula arises internally. This can be evaluated by a computed tomography scan or fistulogram.
- Avoidance of distal obstruction within the intestines beyond the site of the fistula.
- Control of output of fistula by suction or drainage collection to avoid skin excoriation. Continuous low suction can be used to control and collect fistula output. Wound vacuum/closed suction systems have been successfully used to treat fistulas in anecdotal reports.

- Low-output fistulas are more likely to heal than high-output fistulae. The risk or electrolyte and metabolic disturbances should be considered for high-output intestinal fistulas.
- Adequate nutritional support is necessary for healing of intestinal fistulas. Sometimes this require complete bowel rest and central venous hyperalimentation.

**16. What is every surgeon's nightmare when it comes to a surgical wound?**
Whenever a serious wound infection arises, it is disconcerting for a surgeon. The morbidity, patient discomfort, and distress are usually substantial. Particularly difficult surgical wound problems include:
- Incisions containing vascular prostheses. Infection usually means excision and replacement through healthy, noninfected routes. The extremity distal to wound site is at risk.
- Incisions containing prosthetics, such as abdominal wall hernia with mesh repair. Infection may require removal of mesh, and the residual abdominal wall defect can pose a challenge for closure. Additional operations of increasing complexity and risk may be necessary.

## CONTROVERSIES

**17. What are alternatives to wet-to-dry dressings, changed 4 times/day, for a surgical wound?**
To promote wound healing, an optimal local environment at the wound surface is essential. Often because of the shape, contour, depth, or location of the wound, wet-to-dry gauze coverage is not maintained because of slippage or nonadherence, and the critical surface contact fails. Hydrogels have a superior ability to coat and cover, maintain surface contact and adhere to the wound bed. In addition, the hydrogel does not dry out, causing unintended harm to the granulating wound bed on removal. In highly exudative surgical wounds, an alginate or foam can provide the absorption needed to maintain the critical moist surface contact, while avoiding maceration to periwound skin.

The frequency of wound care treatment is another consideration that favors advanced wound care products. Typically wet-to-dry gauze treatments are required every 4–6 hours to maintain a moist environment. This necessitates an inpatient level of wound care. The use of hydrogel or absorptive products permits a daily schedule that allows ambulatory care.

**18. How do you convince a physician to change from wet-to-dry to an advanced wound care product?**
- Use objective data to justify the treatment change: drainage amount, pain, nonhealing dimensions.
- Match the physical properties of the wound dressing to desired wound characteristics. Choose by category and dressing performance, not just by advocating your favorite name brand.
- Set realistic goals for reevaluation of wound and report changes with comparison dimensions. Do not promise that the new wound dressing will make overnight improvement. Depending on the therapy used, it may take up to 14 days to see an improvement.
- Have supporting literature on hand. Send copies of product inserts or high-quality studies (randomized, controlled studies) to support the use of the dressing. Avoid the "happy-ending" case study, which is not science!
- If you are treating bilateral lower extremities or multiple wound sites, suggest a trial of one site with the advance wound product for comparison.

* Work off the surgeon's current likes and dislikes:

| SURGEON LIKES | SUGGEST |
| --- | --- |
| Saline wet-to-dry dressings | Saline gel dressings |
| Povidone-iodine | Cadexomer iodine |
| Silver sulfadiazine (clean wound) | Nanocrystalline or ionic silver |
| Silver sulfadiazine (wound with necrotic material) | Chemical debridement with or without pulsatile lavage |

• Choose the right patient to introduce new concepts. Do not choose Mrs. Jones, who has un-controlled diabetes with blood glucose levels ranging over 400, smokes 3 packs of cigarettes per day, takes steroids for chronic obstructive pulmonary disease, and has an unintended weight loss of 5% in the past month with a dropping hemoglobin. Instead, choose Mrs. Smith, who has all of her comorbidities well under control but calls the office 4 times a week, asking what can be done to help her heal faster.

• Make rounds with the physician. Although this strategy may sound a bit old-fashioned, it does not mean that you carry the chart or give up your chair. It means that you and the physician see the same thing at the same time and hear what is being said between the physician and the pa-tient. Most patients do not absorb all of the information, and you can later use this opportunity to teach and clarify information.

## BIBLIOGRAPHY

1. Briggs M: Principles of closed surgical wound care. J Wound Care 6(6):288–292, 1997.
2. Harken AH: Acute abdomen. In Harken AH, Moore EH (eds): Abernathy's Surgical Secrets, 4th ed. Philadelphia, Hanley & Belfus, 2000.
3. Hunt TK, Hopf HW: Wound healing and infection: What surgeons and anesthesiologists can do. Surg Clin North Am 77:587–607, 1997.
4. Partridge C: Influential factors in surgical wound healing. J Wound Care 7(7):350–353, 1998.
5. Peterson SL: Surgical wound Infection. In Harken AH, Moore EH (eds): Abernathy's Surgical Secrets, 4th ed. Philadelphia, Hanley & Belfus, 2000.

# 52. MEETING THE NEEDS OF OBESE PATIENTS

*Liz Lemiska, CWOCN, BSN, RN*

### 1. Define obesity, bariatrics, and morbid obesity.

**Obesity** is a state of excessive adipose tissue mass. Adipose tissue is a normal constituent of the human body that serves the important function of storing energy as fat for mobilization in response to metabolic needs. Excessive body fat is a result of an imbalance between energy intake and expenditure. The causes of obesity in the United States are complex and multifactorial. Although its etiology is not firmly established, genetic, metabolic, biochemical, cultural, and psychosocial factors contribute to obesity. **Bariatrics** is defined as the field of medicine that focuses on the treatment and control of obesity and diseases associated with obesity. **Morbid obesity** is defined as an excess of body fat that threatens normal body functions. It is a chronic disease.

### 2. What is the body mass index (BMI)?

BMI is the most universally accepted formula for determining morbid obesity. The formula for calculating BMI is weight in pounds, divided by height in inches, and multiplied by 703. Fortunately, a quick and easy table has been developed.

## Body Mass Index (BMI) Table

| BMI | 19 | 20 | 21 | 22 | 23 | 24 | 25 | 26 | 27 | 28 | 29 | 30 | 31 | 32 | 33 | 34 | 35 |
|---|---|---|---|---|---|---|---|---|---|---|---|---|---|---|---|---|---|
| *Height* | | | | | | | | | *Weight (in pounds)* | | | | | | | | |
| 4'10" (58") | 91 | 96 | 100 | 105 | 110 | 115 | 119 | 124 | 129 | 134 | 138 | 143 | 148 | 153 | 158 | 162 | 167 |
| 4'11" (59") | 94 | 99 | 104 | 109 | 114 | 119 | 124 | 128 | 133 | 138 | 143 | 148 | 153 | 158 | 163 | 168 | 173 |
| 5' (60") | 97 | 102 | 107 | 112 | 118 | 123 | 128 | 133 | 138 | 143 | 148 | 153 | 158 | 163 | 168 | 174 | 179 |
| 5'1" (61") | 100 | 106 | 111 | 116 | 122 | 127 | 132 | 137 | 143 | 148 | 153 | 158 | 164 | 169 | 174 | 180 | 185 |
| 5'2" (62") | 104 | 109 | 115 | 120 | 126 | 131 | 136 | 142 | 147 | 153 | 158 | 164 | 169 | 175 | 180 | 186 | 191 |
| 5'3" (63") | 107 | 113 | 118 | 124 | 130 | 135 | 141 | 146 | 152 | 158 | 163 | 169 | 175 | 180 | 186 | 191 | 197 |
| 5'4" (64") | 110 | 116 | 122 | 128 | 134 | 140 | 145 | 151 | 157 | 163 | 169 | 174 | 180 | 186 | 192 | 197 | 204 |
| 5'5" (65") | 114 | 120 | 126 | 132 | 138 | 144 | 150 | 156 | 162 | 168 | 174 | 180 | 186 | 192 | 198 | 204 | 210 |
| 5'6" (66") | 118 | 124 | 130 | 136 | 142 | 148 | 155 | 161 | 167 | 173 | 179 | 186 | 192 | 198 | 204 | 210 | 216 |
| 5'7" (67") | 121 | 127 | 134 | 140 | 146 | 153 | 159 | 166 | 172 | 178 | 185 | 191 | 198 | 204 | 211 | 217 | 223 |
| 5'8" (68") | 125 | 131 | 138 | 144 | 151 | 158 | 164 | 171 | 177 | 184 | 190 | 197 | 203 | 210 | 216 | 223 | 230 |
| 5'9" (69") | 128 | 135 | 142 | 149 | 155 | 162 | 169 | 176 | 182 | 189 | 196 | 203 | 209 | 216 | 223 | 230 | 236 |
| 5'10" (70") | 132 | 139 | 146 | 153 | 160 | 167 | 174 | 181 | 188 | 195 | 202 | 209 | 216 | 222 | 229 | 236 | 243 |
| 5'11" (71") | 136 | 143 | 150 | 157 | 165 | 172 | 179 | 186 | 193 | 200 | 208 | 215 | 222 | 229 | 236 | 243 | 250 |
| 6' (72") | 140 | 147 | 154 | 162 | 169 | 177 | 184 | 191 | 199 | 206 | 213 | 221 | 228 | 235 | 242 | 250 | 258 |
| 6'1" (73") | 144 | 151 | 159 | 166 | 174 | 182 | 189 | 197 | 204 | 212 | 219 | 227 | 235 | 242 | 250 | 257 | 265 |
| 6'2" (74") | 148 | 155 | 163 | 171 | 179 | 186 | 194 | 202 | 210 | 218 | 225 | 233 | 241 | 249 | 256 | 264 | 272 |
| 6'3" (75") | 152 | 160 | 168 | 176 | 184 | 192 | 200 | 208 | 216 | 224 | 232 | 240 | 248 | 256 | 264 | 272 | 279 |

### 3. How is BMI used to classify obesity?

The following BMI classifications are based on the World Health Organization 1997 recommendations: 18.5–24.9 is considered normal for an adult; 25–29.9 is considered overweight; 30–40 is considered obese; and > 40 is considered extremely obese. Some experts refer to people with a BMI in excess of 50 as the supermorbid obese.

#### 4. Why is obesity a concern in wound healing?

Many patients with wounds meet the criteria for obesity. In addition, obesity can be attributed to the development of certain wounds, such as venous stasis ulcers. Obese patients have slower healing times, are more apt to have surgical dehiscence, and are predisposed to surgical wound infections.

Obesity now affects 25% of the U.S. population, and it is estimated that 12 million Americans are morbidly obese by BMI definition. Obesity is considered epidemic by the Centers for Disease Control and Prevention (CDC). Of special concern, the obesity prevalence rate for children in the U.S. is also rising. Given this major public health problem, acute care hospitals can expect that 1–3% of the daily inpatient census will be morbidly obese.

Severe obesity can lead to a multitude of health- and life-threatening disorders, including hypertension, diabetes mellitus, hypoventilation syndrome, sleep apnea syndrome, degenerative osteoarthritis, cholelithiasis, gastroesophageal reflux, mental disorders, infertility, and severe psychosocial problems. These issues also affect wound healing. Obesity in males is also associated with higher mortality rates from colon, rectal, and prostate cancer. In obese females, cancer of the gallbladder, bile ducts, breast, endometrium, cervix and ovaries occurs more frequently than in non-obese counterparts.

Mortality rates increase significantly in adults with a BMI > 40, and death occurs 10–15 years earlier. The financial burden to society is significant. It is estimated that 150 billion U.S. dollars are spent annually as a direct result of this chronic disease. Americans trying to lose weight spend approximately 30 billion dollars each year. Obesity is an expensive, epidemic problem and is second only to motor vehicle accidents as a preventable cause of death.

Nurses cannot ignore chronic disease states in patients with a wound, because successful management of this disease improves wound outcome. Unfortunately, many health care providers, perhaps out of bias or ignorance, do not view morbid obesity as a clinical entity and place the patient at risk for impaired or failed wound healing.

#### 5. What is the medical treatment for obesity and extreme obesity?

Conservative measures, such as dieting, exercise, behavior modification, and pharmaceuticals, are the current first-line treatment for the obese and morbidly obese. Permanent weight loss with any one method or combination of methods is often unsuccessful. Temporary success in weight loss may be followed by regaining even more pounds. A medical cure is not in the near future because of the complexity of this chronic disease. Aggressive attempts to lose weight during the wound-healing process may be counterproductive except in the case of venous ulcerations, although data in this area are lacking.

#### 6. Describe the surgical treatment for extreme obesity.

Surgical intervention for obesity began in the 1950s. Techniques and results have greatly improved since. Surgery is an option when conservative treatment has repeatedly failed or the patient is at high risk for obesity-related morbidity and mortality. The most common surgical approaches to morbid obesity are the vertical-banded gastroplasty and the gastric bypass, also known as the Roux-en-Y. Studies have demonstrated that surgery is overwhelmingly better than conservative management in improving quality of life, controlling high blood pressure, reducing atheroma, improving rates of employment, and decreasing health care costs. Additional data indicate that surgical intervention improves adverse lipid profiles, sleep apnea, joint problems, gastroesophageal reflux, urinary incontinence, and asthma. Health care providers can expect to see an increasing number of severely obese people who choose this treatment. Few scientific data support or reject surgical options in morbidly obese patients with a wound.

#### 7. What is the outcome of surgical treatment? What does it involve?

Bariatric surgery appears to have better long-term outcomes in keeping the patient's weight down than nonsurgical therapies. It is best delivered in a multidisciplinary environment with a bariatric team. A well-devised plan of care and good communication among disciplines are critical for a successful patient outcome. The team consists of a bariatric surgeon, psychologist, primary care physician, registered dietitian, and trained nursing staff. Numerous others in the health care system are also needed to support this therapy, such as physical therapists, operating room staff, pharmacists, material management personnel, and wound, ostomy, and continence nurses. Lifelong follow-up is required for patients who undergo this therapy.

**8. How is health-seeking behavior affected by obesity or morbid obesity?**

The problems of obesity and morbid obesity can affect anyone, regardless of race, ethnic group, gender, age, or socioeconomic status. In fact, many believe that discrimination against obese people is the last socially acceptable prejudice in America. Extreme obesity is a barrier to equal opportunities for employment, education, travel, recreation, and health care, despite laws and government regulations. Our society's fear of "fatism" does indeed drive this bias.

One result is that morbidly obese people often postpone seeking health care until a crisis occurs. Once in crisis, they tend to deteriorate quickly, setting off a cascade of negative events. Many find that they cannot cooperate or access treatment simply because they are too large. Physicians' offices, outpatient facilities, and laboratories often do not even have a suitable chair for them to sit in. Diagnostic testing may be next to impossible because current technologic devices cannot accommodate or perform at peak accuracy because of the patient's massive bulk.

Health care providers may lack the knowledge, training, and sensitivity for interaction with the obese population. Staff often appear reluctant to care for the obese and overwhelmed by the prospect of caring for the morbidly obese. They may convey this message unconsciously and, on occasion, intentionally, both verbally and nonverbally. Care providers may blame obese patients by viewing them as lazy, overindulgent, lacking self-control, unemployable, physically repulsive, and impossible to diagnose and treat. Obese patients feel ridiculed, out of control, powerless, and vulnerable to physical and emotional hurt when they interact with health care providers. They fear that they may unintentionally harm others because of their extreme size. Patients and families become embarrassed.

The patient often withdraws emotionally from shame, humility, and indignity. Clinical depression is common. Eighty-nine percent of morbidly obese patients require treatment for depression. As their size grows larger, their world grows smaller.

**9. What barriers to health care exist in the community environment for the morbidly obese?**

When morbidly obese people become homebound, they often suffer from social isolation. Transportation often is difficult. If an adequate-sized vehicle is not available, it is impossible for them to attend appointments. Even in the face of crisis, ambulance services can be challenging. Transporting the morbidly obese patient requires additional assistance from the community. Staff and equipment from the local fire department may be required to ensure both patient and care provider safety. Outpatient treatment, hospitalization, and transportation can be facilitated by planning, training, and proper resources. Training, education of staff, and appropriate equipment that meets the needs of this patient population are often lacking. In all settings, caring for the severely obese is challenging but not impossible.

**10. What is needed for the hospital room environment?**

Whether the patient is a surgical or medical admission, the need for adequate equipment cannot be overemphasized. An extra-large sphygmomanometer cuff is essential for accurate blood pressure readings. Bariatric wheelchairs, chairs, commodes, walkers, mechanical lifts, stretchers, and beds are necessary for patient and staff safety and comfort. Bariatric equipment may be rented or purchased from several manufactures and retailers:

- Hill-Rom (www.hill-rom.com)
- Plexus Medical (www.plexusmed.com)
- KCI (www.kci1.com)
- Kendall Company (www.kendallnq.com)
- Dale (www.dalemed.com
- ERGO-IKE (www.phil-e-slide.com)
- Size-wise (www.sizewiserentals.com)

A means of weighing the patient accurately, safely, discretely, and respectfully needs to be considered. Most bariatric beds have a built-in scale to ease this task. Floor and stretcher scales need to accommodate larger weights.

All equipment needs to be fully explained to the patient and family before it is used to reduce apprehension, reassure the patient, and encourage cooperation. The linen department should have sufficient quantities of 10XL-sized patient gowns. It is helpful if these gowns are of a different color from the standard facility patient gown for easy identification by staff. A box fan placed in the patient's room serves several purposes: it keeps the patient cooler, provides the perception of relief from respiratory distress, and helps dry the skin during bathing, especially in skin folds. Even when the patient is ambulatory, a bariatric commode is recommended instead of the standard toilet. It is safer, usually higher, and often more easily accessed. Bed-panning an obese patient is difficult and should be avoided if possible. When required, obese walkers are preferred to canes and crutches, because they are more stable and durable. Of course, not all obese or even morbidly obese patients require special oversized equipment, but often they do. Be prepared!

**11. Give specific examples of bariatric equipment.**

**Bariatric beds** are available in differing widths. Be sure that the facility's doorways will accommodate the extra width! Many of these beds convert to a recliner chair mode, which can be helpful because the physical space of a typical hospital room is taken up by special equipment. An over-bed trapeze can assist the patient in moving in and out of bed. For bigger and taller patients, the bed may need to be extended to accommodate height.

The 24-hour availability of a **bariatric hoyer or mechanical lift** is an absolute necessity. When investigating these devices for facility use, first determine whether the leg base of the mechanical lift can fit under all of the bed frames, including rental beds. The lift should also have the ability to lower to the floor in case it is needed to facilitate retrieving a morbidly obese patient (e.g., in the case of an accidental fall).

A newer piece of equipment that works on the principle of sliding instead of lifting the patient is the PHIL-E-SLIDE. These **low-friction slide sheets** are portable, durable, and nonabsorbent. They can be helpful in moving the obese patient to another surface. The manufacturer recommends a mechanical lift if the patient is actually wider than the slide sheets or exceeds the recommended weight limits.

**12. What equipment is available in the long-term care or home health setting?**

Check with the distributor for a environmental evaluation before accepting delivery in the home setting. This evaluation should determine what equipment is best suited for the home setting without jeopardizing the safety of the physical structure or the patient.

**13. What about intravenous access?**

Intravenous access is often difficult because of obtuse anatomic landmarks and increased body bulk. The typical technique to cannulate a vein may not work. If two or three unsuccessful attempts are made for an intravenous line, a peripheral-inserted central catheter (PICC) may be the best choice, particularly for long-term access. Short-term preoperative intravenous access for the gastric bypass patient is best done in the operating room by the anesthesiologist; peripheral vasodilatation by some anesthetic agents can be helpful in locating a suitable site.

**14. What about respiratory support?**

Airway management also can be difficult. Morbidly obese people have decreased vital capacity of the lungs, increased work of breathing, and cardiac insufficiency. Periods of rest between activities are necessary. Sleep apnea is common and can be defined as five or more episodes of apnea per hour of sleep. Continuous positive airway pressure (CPAP) may be required; usually the device is worn only at night but occasionally is used during the day as well. The mask used for delivery must fit snugly, or the machine will alarm, annoying both patient and staff. Staff should be alert to monitor for signs of tissue breakdown under the mask due to overly zealous tightening of the mask or facial edema.

In the event of respiratory arrest, endotracheal intubation is difficult because of the large amount of fatty tissue around the neck. An extra-long endotracheal tube may be required as well as a fiberoptic scope for successful intubation. If tracheostomy is required, extra-long tubes may be required. Having several in stock and readily available is paramount when airway crisis occurs.

Often the tracheotomy wound is larger than average, and postoperative site care is more complex because of increased wound drainage. Advanced wound dressings, such as nonadhesive foams, absorb well and can be cut to fit around the tracheotomy tube without risk of introducing gauze fibers into the wound. Tracheostomy tube ties need to be longer and wider to avoid undue trauma, pressure, and friction to neck fat folds, which can result in tissue necrosis. Manufacturers of tube-stabilizing devices offer extra-wide and longer devices. Nursing staff should bear in mind that the position for optimal respiratory function is a semi-Fowler's position.

### 15. What equipment is needed for the operating room?

A table that is designed to accommodate the bariatric patient is essential. Extra-depth surgical instruments are also needed. Two safety belts with cotton cast padding are recommended below and above the knees for adequate stabilization of obese patients. To reduce the risk of lower extremity blood clot formation, extra-large sequential compression devices (SCDs), lower leg wraps, or intermittent plantar venous compression therapy foot pads (A-V impulse system foot pump) with extra-large knee length antiembolism stockings or Ace wraps to the lower extremity are recommended.

Thorough nursing assessment of the skin and pressure points should be done before and after surgery, along with careful positioning to prevent injury. A common myth is that extremely obese patients have more padding and can therefore better tolerate the forces of friction, pressure, and shear. Not so. Operating room staff and surgeons need to be alert to excessive and prolonged leaning into the patient's body mass during surgery, which may cause soft tissue injury. Step stools may be needed to ease access to the abdomen when the patient is in the supine position. Unless an extra large stretcher is available, a bariatric bed is needed to transfer the patient from the operating table. Coordination of care cannot be overemphasized.

After surgery, staff need to be aware that, because anesthetic agents are stored in body fat, morbidly obese patients may experience the effects of anesthesia longer than average-sized patients. Sedation may recur 8–9 hours after surgery. If an abdominal binder is needed postoperatively, an extra-large size that fits up to 94 inches is manufactured by Dale.

### 16. How are patient mobility and transport affected?

Maintaining and encouraging physical activity within the limits of the patient's condition are important. A physical therapy referral may be warranted. Obese patients are at high risk for venous thrombosis due to factors such as prolonged operating time, decreased mobility, polycythemia, and increased intra-abdominal pressure. Extra-large antiembolism devices for the lower leg, subcutaneous heparin therapy, encouragement to move, deep breathing, and leg exercises are critical to the plan of care. If patients must be transported to other departments and cannot go by an oversized wheelchair, it is best to move them in the bariatric bed or on a bariatric stretcher. Communication with other departments to facilitate the process is invaluable. A simple phone call to alert staff in the other department that the patient has bariatric needs helps ensure that adequate staff and equipment are in place to manage the situation safely, guarding both staff and patient from injury. The element of surprise is in no way beneficial.

### 17. Why are the morbidly obese at risk for surgical wound dehiscence and infection?

Surgical patients with extraordinary body size spend more time on the operating table. Obviously they require greater degrees of retraction during an operation, thus increasing the risk of more soft tissue injury. Postoperatively the incision is stressed and pulled by the forces of gravity and the increased weight of the surrounding tissues. Adipose has less of a blood supply than other tissues and heals more slowly. Wound healing is further compromised when the patient has underlying respiratory problems. Some research suggests that abdominal infection rates are higher with underlying obesity. A severely obese patient may not appear malnourished but certainly may be so. Poor nutritional status equals poor wound healing.

### 18. Are obese and morbidly obese patients more susceptible to tissue breakdown?

The health care team is hard pressed to provide the usual preventive measures for complications such as pneumonia, thrombophlebitis, pressure ulcers, muscle wasting, and incontinence because of high intra-abdominal pressures. Severely obese patients are at risk for incontinence. Poor personal hygiene practices can result in skin rashes, infections, and breakdown. Morbidly obese patients are subject to pressure ulcer development from the same risk factors as average-sized patients. Obese patients are more prone to mobility problems. They may develop pressure ulcers in atypical locations, such as deep fat folds, from tubes and other medical equipment in direct contact with the body.

### 19. Which areas of the body are at increased risk?

A particularly problematic location is the posterior waist skin fold or lumbar shelf. When the patient is in the supine position for extended periods, the extra bulk of the buttocks is flattened and pushed upward against the fatty bulk of the lower back, causing fat necrosis from excessive interface pressures in this deep intertriginous area. Another unusual presentation is bilateral trochanter pressure ulcers due to the forces of pressure, friction, and shear from getting in and out of as well as sitting in a chair that is far too small. Both locations are difficult. If the patient with these types of breakdown is confined to bed, a bariatric pressure-relieving mattresses is required. Bariatric pressure-relieving mattresses in low air loss or gel mediums can be rented or purchased. Tubes, such as Foley catheters, telemetry lines, and chest tubes, need to be repositioned frequently to avoid pressure-related tissue necrosis.

## 20. How are lower extremity wounds managed?

The cause of the lower extremity wounds determines the management. Chronic venous insufficiency is common in obese and morbidly obese people. Compression is the mainstay of therapy. When ulcers develop, they can be difficult to manage. Traditional Unna boot therapy or layer compression wrap dressings can be used but may take more than the average amount of supplies because of leg circumference and drainage. Drainage from large wounds may require additional use of advanced wound dressing and/or more frequent dressing changes. New advanced topical dressings that address the issue of heavy bioburden may be quite helpful at preventing acute cellulitis. Cellulitis of the lower extremity is a frequent cause for hospitalization if conservative outpatient management fails. Some patients can be accommodated with an extra-large, zippered compression knee-high stocking. If the ulceration is small and can be managed with a hydrocolloid dressing, the therapeutic stocking or a rigid strapping device can be used and has the advantage of removal for daily showering. Chronic lower extremity ulceration is difficult to treat and resolve in obese patients. Weight reduction is the key to overall improvement.

## 21. Why is lower extremity cellulitis a frequent complication in obese patients?

Venous insufficiency and edema compound the above problems. Adipose tissue is thicker in the lower extremity of obese patients. Patients unable to perform self foot care may have extensive tinea pedis (athlete's foot). Microfissuring of the epidermis allows entry of bacteria and subsequent cellulitis.

## 22. How does skin care differ in the obese population?

Maintaining clean, dry skin can be a challenge for the nursing staff. The extreme body mass results in increased energy expenditure at rest and with physical exertion. To control body temperature, increased perspiration occurs, resulting in offensive body odors. Cotton clothing and a room fan are helpful. Personal hygiene is important. If the patient is ambulatory, showering is preferred. A hand-held shower-head makes attention to skin folds easier.

Urge or stress incontinence is 2–3 times more common in obese women. The subsequent hygiene-related problems require vigilant management to avoid adverse skin conditions. Intertriginous areas need careful management to minimize the risk of yeast or bacterial infections. Absorptive, but not bulky, padding can help keep deep skin folds dry and reduce skin friction injury. Padding must be changed routinely. Avoid tugging and pulling during removal.

## 23. What other dermatologic conditions are seen in morbidly obese patients?

When performing a skin assessment, do not mistake pseudo-acanthosis nigricans as dirt from poor hygiene practices. This condition can be a complication of obesity and is more common in patients with darker pigmentation. Pseudo-acanthosis nigricans is a diffuse, velvety thickening and hyperpigmentation of the skin, usually found in the axilla, groin, neck fold, and upper inner thigh. The cause is not fully understood and may be related to insulin resistance. Lipomatosis dolorosa can also occur. This disorder is characterized by the abnormal accumulation of painful, tender fat deposits.

## 24. Are nutritional needs different in the obese population?

Care providers may mistakenly assume that excessive body fat supports a nutritionally compromised patient through a health crisis. Social bias in dealing with obesity can cloud the issue of nutritional support. While patients are in the hospital, they may feel embarrassed eating in front of staff, drastically restricting their intake. Reducing dietary intake to very low levels can result in lethargy, depression, and impaired wound healing, which can affect recovery. Obese patients have increased fluid requirements because of larger insensible losses.

Registered dietitians are invaluable in assessing and treating patients at nutritional risk, including the severely obese. In the pre-, intra-, and postoperative management as well as outpatient care of obese patients—especially gastric-bypass patients—the dietitian plays a key role in the success of therapy. Both chronic and acute wounds require careful dietary recommendations for optimal support of the body in the healing process. Some patients refuse to have their eating habit closely scrutinized and may be more receptive after discharge. All obese or morbidly obese patients should be given the opportunity for referral to the dietitian for assessment and advice.

### 25. Is wound pain management affected by morbid obesity?

If the pain medication—or in fact any medication—is to be administrated intramuscularly, a needle longer than the traditional 1.5 inches is required. Some pain medications are absorbed into adipose tissue, and some are not. Consultation with a pharmacist helps determine whether metabolism is affected and how best to administer the medication.

### 26. If urinary catheterization in morbidly obese women is needed to prevent contamination of the wound bed, what is the best approach?

If catheterization is necessary in morbidly obese women to prevent wound contamination, the posterior approach may be the best option. Usually the patient cannot tolerate lowering the head of the bed < 45% for any length of time for a procedure because the tremendous abdominal weight shifts to the middle and upper chest cause respiratory distress. If the patient is unable to help, the traditional anterior approach requires a minimum of five staff members, two on either side of the bed to hold up the abdominal pannus, two to abduct the legs, and the fifth person to perform the catheterization. The logistics of this procedure are obviously difficult, uncomfortable, and embarrassing not only for the patient but also for the staff. An invasive procedure becomes even more invasive.

### 27. How is the posterior approach performed?

The posterior approach is usually best done with the patient in a side-lying, modified knee-chest position, because the urinary meatus is more easily visualized. The risk of accidental catheter contamination is less, which may also reduce the risk of catheter-related urinary tract infection. Fewer people are needed to perform the procedure. Of course, an adequately sized bed that accommodates the patient in side-lying position is essential. A direct beam of light on the perineum is essential—that old goose-neck lamp really comes in handy! An extra pair of hands holding a good flashlight works, too. The assigned nurse should approach the patient before catheterization and explain the procedure, describing the technique to be used and who will be in the room assisting with the procedure. Patient privacy and dignity need to be preserved as much as possible. The nurse should also explain the plan for a safe and sensitive procedure to her assistants. Each member's task should be determined before entering the patient's room. This approach keeps bedside chatter and comments to a minimum.

### 28. What about male catheterization?

In male patients, nurses obviously are faced with different geography. The penis is often retracted and the urinary meatus is difficult to access. Again, the nursing staff needs to explain the procedure and proceed with respect and sensitivity. If the patient can cooperate, ask him to abduct his legs and lift his pannus to facilitate access to the perineum. If the patient cannot assist, two staff members are needed to lift the large abdominal pannus, while the third staff member performs the catheterization. Good lighting is vital for visualizing the urinary meatus to reduce the risk of contamination and possible introduction of bacteria to the urinary tract.

### 29. What about sexuality in obese and morbidly obese people?

Sexuality is as much about being a man or woman as it is about physical sexual expression related to genitalia or their functioning. Feelings of self-worth, body image, and ego are part of sexuality. Providing dignity, privacy, and emotional support acknowledges that the morbidly obese person is an individual. Efforts to help maintain the patient's sense of personal identity are important, and the bigger patient is no exception. Negative attitudes toward morbidly obese patients can hinder their care.

**30. What special issues affect discharge planning for morbidly obese patients with a wound?**

The care of morbidly obese patients is more complex and time-consuming. It is always best to involve the discharge planner as soon as possible, particularly if an extremely obese patient is going to need skilled nursing home placement. Some facilities cannot or will not accept the patient because of inadequate staffing and equipment resources. Coordination for continuity of care is imperative for a smooth transition. Sharing the plan of care and modifying it to the patient's setting will streamline case management. Home care arrangements can also be challenging, especially when the patient requires additional equipment. Reimbursement issues can be colossal barriers for obtaining needed resources in long-term care, rehabilitative care, and home care. A social work consultation can be of tremendous value as well as communication with a durable medical equipment specialist.

**31. What special issues are involved when the morbidly obese patient dies?**

There is most certainly a gap in the medical and nursing literature about end-of life-issues for morbidly obese patients. The untimely death of a loved one is devastating to family and complicated by the mere size of the patient. Simple issues such as a shroud that is too small make the usual methods for caring for the body difficult. Medical manufacturers do make shrouds in an extra-large size.

To avoid injuries, staff should not attempt to transfer the corpse to a standard stretcher for transport to the morgue. A mortician and funeral home that can handle extremely obese patients should be determined as soon as possible. An extremely obese corpse probably needs to be removed and stored in a refrigeration unit that only the mortician can provide. Embalming needs to be quick and can be quite difficult for the mortician, because it is challenging to locate the necessary blood vessels. Oversized caskets are available but increase the cost of burial. The weight limit for cremation is about 700 pounds.

**32. What resources for obesity are available on the web?**

Journals, conferences, textbooks, and inservices are helpful, but at times a clinician needs information quickly. Although some of sites below do not discuss wound care specifically, a holistic approach to the wound patient who happens to be obese is essential to facilitating wound healing.

http://www.obesityhelp.com  
http://www.asbs.org  
http://www.obesitysurgery.com/  
http://wwwnhlbi.nih.gov/guidelines/obesity/ob.home.htm  
http://www.cdc.gov/nccdphp/dnpa/bmi/bmi-adult.htm  
http://www.niddk.nih.gov/health/nutrit/pubs/statobes.htm  

http://www.obesity.org  
http://www.obesityresearch.org/  
http://shapeup.org

## BIBLIOGRAPHY

1. Baxter J: Obesity surgery—another unmet need. Br Med J 32:523, 2000.
2. Gallagher S: Bariatric issues across the continuum. Presented at the WOCN 33rd Annual Wound, Ostomy, Continence Conference. Portland, OR, June 2–6, 2001.
3. Gallagher S: Morbid obesity: A chronic disease with an impact on wounds and related problems. Ostomy Wound Manage 43(5):18–27, 1997.
4. Gallagher S: Needs of the homebound morbidly obese patient: A descriptive survey of home health nurses. Ostomy Wound Manage 44(4):33–42, 1998.
5. Goldberg S, et al: Vertical banded gastroplasty: A treatment for morbid obesity. AORN J 72(6):998–1010, 2000.
6. Green SM, Gillett A: Caring for patients with morbid obesity in hospital. Br J Nurs 7(13):785–791, 1998.
7. Health Implications of Obesity. NIH Consensus Statement. 1985, Feb 11–13. 31 March 2001, 5(9):1–7. <http://text.nlm.nih.gov/nih/cdc/www/49txt.htm>.
8. Lyznicki J, et al: Obesity: Assessment and management in primary care. Am Fam Physician 63(11):2185–2196, 2001.
9. Martin J: Bariatric weight loss surgery: Implications for WOCN nurses. Presented at the WOCN 33rd Annual Wound, Ostomy, Continence Conference. Portland, OR, June 2–6, 2001.
10. Mohrlein W: Aurora-McCarthy Funeral Home. Personnel interview. 13 June 2001.
11. Murphy K, Gallagher S: Care of an obese patient with a pressure ulcer. J Wound Ostomy Contin Nurs 28(3):171–176, 2001.
12. Rotkoff N: Care of the morbidly obese patient in a long-term care facility. Geriatr Nurs 20(6):309–313, 1999.

# 53. SUPPORT SURFACES: CLASSIFICATION AND SELECTION CRITERIA

*Rebecca E. McBride*, RN, BSN, CWOCN

### 1. What is a support surface?

A support surface is a bed, mattress, or chair cushion that provides the ability to lower tissue interface pressure. Some, but not all, surfaces are designed to reduce the mechanical forces of friction and shear and the effect of moisture on a wound or surgical site. Hundreds of different support surface products are available on the market.

### 2. What standard terms are used to select the best surface for a particular patient?

- **Tissue interface pressure:** the amount of pressure that the skin-resting surface exerts over a bony prominence (measured in mmHg).
- **Capillary closing pressure:** the external pressure needed to collapse blood capillaries (measured in mmHg).
- **Density:** related only to foam products, density refers to how much air space is interspersed between the foam cells. It is reported in cubic feet.
- **Indentation load deflection:** the stiffness of a foam product (measured in reported number of pounds).
- **Static:** products without a motor. Although the term describes some air, foam, water, and gel surfaces, it usually refers to a surface that incorporates air only.
- **Dynamic:** support surfaces that oscillate, turn, pulsate, or alternate.

In recent years the market has become saturated with various products. All claim to reduce tissue interface pressure. These specialty products are designed to reduce pressure, friction, and shear by redistributing body mass over a large area while maximizing surface contact. They are categorized by their physical characteristics such as overlays, mattress replacement systems, or full-bed systems, and by composition, such as foams, gels, or low air-loss. They can be static or dynamic.

### 3. How do overlays and mattress replacement systems differ?

**Overlays** are placed on top of the standard mattress and are intended as an adjunct to relieve pressure. **Mattress replacement systems** are designed to replace the standard mattress while decreasing interface pressures. Full-framed specialty beds are integrated bed systems, consisting of a pressure-relief mattress and bed frame designed to replace the existing bed during wound treatment.

These specialty products are further classified according to their prevention and treatment functions. Construction is designed to address issues of friction by utilizing a low-friction exterior surface covering; pressure, shear, and moisture issues are addressed with a foam, gel, air, or water interior. Because of the variety of choices on the market, restrictions set by a specific facility or agency and criteria set by a third-party payor such as Medicare are generally used. It is helpful to follow a systematic approach in choosing a support surface.

### 4. What are the characteristics of an overlay mattress?

Overlays are made from foam, gel, water, air, or a combination thereof. The overlays can also be static or dynamic. The static overlays are usually single-patient use items purchased by the facility, although reuse has been reported. For reimbursement, static overlays are termed group I surfaces.

### 5. Describe foam overlays.

With static foam overlays, such as egg crate foam, pressure reduction depends on the base height as well as the density of the foam. To offer pressure reduction, foam height must exceed 4 inches from the base to the point where the convolutions begin. Foam less than 3 inches is considered a comfort mattress. The efficacy of a foam overlay also depends on density and indentation load deflection (ILD), which are available from the manufacturers. Ask manufacturers to provide body weight guidelines and recommended length of use, which vary from product to product. The features to look for in a therapeutic foam include the following:

- Base height of 4 inches
- 25% ILD of 30 pounds
- Density of 1.3–1.6 pounds per cubic foot

Even the best foams have a limited life, which can be shortened by repeated episodes of incontinence. They are hot and trap moisture, and most do not address issues of friction, shear, and moisture. They are inexpensive and can provide a first-line strategy for prevention.

### 6. What about water overlays?

Water overlays can significantly lower interface pressures compared with standard hospital mattresses. Disadvantages in hospitals, long-term care, and home health settings include the possibility of leaks, maintenance issues, and proper filling concerns. They can be heavy and cumbersome.

### 7. How do gel overlays work?

Gel overlays are constructed with silicone elastomer, silicone, or polyvinyl chloride. The gel overlays provide first-line pressure reduction and can be used for single or multiple patients. They can be purchased or rented, are easy to clean, and require little maintenance. Gel overlays are heavy and control friction and shear. They do not address the problem of moisture. If the patient is kept in a semi-Fowler or high Fowler position for an extended period, the gel becomes displaced, creating folds or creases. This dramatically increases tissue interface pressures. Because gels relieve pressure and shearing forces, they are a good choice for patients in traction, who tend to stay better-positioned on a gel surface than on an air surface. The thicker the better—immersion into the gel material is the key principle that reduces pressure.

### 8. Describe static overlays.

Static overlays are constructed with interconnected bulbous cells, which are inflated with an air blower or hand pump. They can be used for single or multiple patients. Successful use as a prevention and early intervention device for partial-thickness wounds has been reported. They are durable and low maintenance but can lose air over time and require frequent monitoring to ensure proper inflation. Some products have a 1-year warranty.

### 9. What are dynamic overlays?

Dynamic overlaps, termed group II surfaces for reimbursement purposes, are reserved for patients who have not responded to a group I surface or have full -thickness wounds. An alternating dynamic or a low air-loss dynamic style is available. Dynamic overlays contain air-filled chambers or cylinders into which air is pumped at periodic intervals for inflation and deflation. This process creates high-pressure and low-pressure areas to decrease tissue pressures in the deflated cells at rhythmic intervals. The inflation/deflation cycle may create a bothersome sensation for some patients. The blower type pump may be noisy. Easy to clean and to deflate for emergencies, the dynamic air overlays can be purchased or rented for multipatient use.

Like their dynamic counterparts, the low air-loss overlays have a low-friction, air-permeable, waterproof, and bacteria-impermeable covering that allows air to flow over the skin while keeping incontinence and bacteria from penetrating the overlay. Advantages of low air-loss overlays include the ability to treat moisture, friction, and shear problems and to maintain a constant inflation and ease of use. They can be purchased or rented for multipatient use.

### 10. How do mattress replacement systems differ from an overlay mattress?

Mattress replacement systems are designed to reduce interface pressures and replace the standard hospital mattress. They are constructed of foam, gel, air, or a combination thereof, with a bacteriostatic, low-friction cover. They can be purchased or rented. Mattress replacements can be a cost-effective prevention alternative for patients at risk for breakdown. Many facilities are beginning to replace standard hospital mattresses with these products, most of which are constructed of foam.

As seen with the foam overlays, mattress replacement systems have a limited wear time of 3–5 years. It is best to inspect the integrity of the foam yearly for density loss, cracks, splits, and creases, all of which markedly reduce the pressure-reduction capability.

Gel alternating dynamic and low air-loss products are also available as mattress replacement systems. These products are advantageous in that they provide the pressure reduction of an overlay without increasing the height of the sleeping surface. This characteristic allows easier transfers and decreases the risk for falls. Usually rental items, they are used to treat full-thickness wounds and are considered group II surfaces. They can reduce tissue interface pressures significantly.

### 11. What are the characteristics of a full-bed system? When is it used?

Whereas mattress replacement systems substitute one type of mattress for another on an existing bed frame, a full-bed system requires removal of the entire bed from the patient's room. The full-bed system replaces the bed. Specialty bed systems are available in both high air-loss (also known as air-fluidized) and low air-loss formats. They are indicated for the treatment of patients with limited turning surfaces because of wounds or injuries. Low air-loss systems are categorized as group II surfaces, whereas high air-loss systems are considered group III surfaces. A group III surface provides the maximal amount of tissue interface pressure reduction.

Some of the low air-loss beds provide pulsation and rotation, which may improve cutaneous blood flow and reduce edema. Rotation has been shown to improve outcomes in patients with acute respiratory distress. These full-bed systems, usually rental items, are expensive. They are constructed of an air-permeable, waterproof, low-friction cover and eliminate friction, shear, and moisture problems.

The air-fluidized system consists of a bed frame and air-permeable cover containing silicone-coated beads. The beads are "fluidized" by a high airflow, which causes them to behave like a liquid. The patient is suspended on the sheet while partially immersed in the warm, dry beads. The beads are sand-like in texture and made of sodium lime. When in contact with body fluids, they clump together and release sodium ions that increases the pH. The high pH creates a bacteriostatic environment. The high airflow and warm, dry environment can decrease the effects of incontinence and high wound exudate. On the downside, it can also cause dehydration and hypernatremia. The high air-loss beds are high maintenance and expensive. The height of the bed can make some nursing care difficult. They are not recommended for ambulatory patients because transfers out of the bed are difficult. Current recommendations suggest limiting their use to postoperative musculocutaneous flap patients or patients with multiple full-thickness wounds on more than one turning surface with no improvement after 30-days use of a group II surface in conjunction with a comprehensive treatment plan.

### 12. Do patients on specialty beds need to be turned?

The patient should still be turned to facilitate mobilization of body fluids and decrease the incidence of atelectasis and pneumonia.

### 13. Are patients on speciality beds at risk for calcaneous breakdown?

Some evidence indicates that high and low air-loss beds may not sufficiently reduce interface pressures in the occipital and calcaneous areas. The low air-loss beds can be adjusted to reduce the amount of air in the pillows at the head or heel zones, but the patient should be closely monitored. Other pressure-relieving interventions are usually required to prevent breakdown.

### 14. What does it mean when a patient "bottoms out"? How do I check for this problem?

Bottoming out refers to patients whose body weight is no longer supported on the surface but rests directly on the surface beneath the overlay or on the bed frame, if a mattress replacement or full bed system is used. Patients should be checked frequently, because some overlays lose air over time and no longer provide adequate support or pressure relief. Slide your hand, palm facing upward, under the overlay or at the bed frame surface. You should be able to get your fingers all the way under all bony prominences. Because different positions affect both force and surface area (pressure = force/area), bottoming out should also be checked with the patient in a semi-Fowler position. Patients may be adequately supported while flat but bottom out in a more upright position, which puts more body weight in the center of the mattress.

### 15. How do I determine the best support surface for my patients?

Familiarize yourself with the goals of therapy, what is available at your agency, and what reimbursement options are available. Follow certain basic principles to make the correct choice to meet patient needs, which may change over the duration of therapy, thereby requiring a change in support surface. By determining the correct surface for the patient in a timely manner, you reduce costs and improve patient outcomes. Always match the bed to the patient, not the patient to the bed.

### 16. What basic principles will assist me in the appropriate selection of a support surface?

1. **What is the overall goal: prevention or healing?** Determine whether the purpose is to prevent skin breakdown or to treat an existing pressure ulcer or wound. If the goal is prevention, choose a less aggressive therapy, such as foam, water, gel, or static air overlay or a group I mattress replacement. If the goal is treatment of an existing wound, you need a more aggressive approach. Choose a dynamic bed system, mattress replacement system, or overlay. Keep in mind that most small partial-thickness wounds can improve on static air overlays.

2. **How many turning surfaces are affected?** If three surfaces are affected by the wound, a group II surface is generally needed to ensure pressure relief on all areas. Aggressive therapy is also needed for patients with a posterior wound who are unable to turn, reposition, or keep the head of bed at < 30°.

3. **Are safety considerations involved because of altered mental status?** Patients who are restless or confused may be at risk for falls. An overlay mattress with a high profile may place the sleeping surface too high. In this case, a low-profile mattress replacement system will be determined by prevention or treatment indicators. Some are available with bumpers to reduce falls.

4. **What is the patient's body type?** Most manufacturers specify weight limits for overlays mattress replacement and bed systems. Along with weight specifications, consider how the weight is distributed. Tissue interface pressure varies, depending on the patient's weight and body build. If the patient is apple-shaped, weight is concentrated around the center of the body. Such patients may need a deeper support surface to provide the necessary pressure relief in this area.

5. **What factors contribute to skin breakdown?** If skin breakdown is related to moisture from profuse perspiration, a low air-loss bed may be appropriate to decrease maceration and control skin surface temperature. If skin breakdown is related to friction and shear, a cover designed to reduce these effects is necessary. Hemodynamically unstable patients who cannot be turned and repositioned may need a full specialty bed. If they are able to be turned, you should determine whether an overlay will provide adequate support. Rotation therapy has been shown to improve outcomes in patients with early acute respiratory distress syndrome.

6. **What scientific evidence supports the product?** Some research may be required to answer this question. Do not rely solely on product inserts.

7. **How is the product reimbursed?** Reimbursement varies from setting to setting. Acute care absorbs the cost of the special mattress, whereas reimbursement options may be available for extended care and home care through Medicaid, Medicare, and health maintenance organizations. Often reimbursement is not available for prevention but only for treatment of an existing pressure ulcer. The only exception is in the home care setting.

*Support Surface Reimbursement by Setting*

| | | | HOME | | SNF | | | |
|---|---|---|---|---|---|---|---|---|
| GROUP TYPE | | INDICATIONS | MCR | MCD | MCR | MCD | MNG | HOSP |
| I  Static: | Air<br>Foam<br>Gel<br>Water | Prevention<br>Treatment of partial-<br>  thickness and stage<br>  I/II wounds | C | P | F | FP | F | F |
| II Dynamic: | Alternating pressure<br>Low air-loss | Multi stage II<br>Stage III/IV on trunk,<br>  pelvis | C | P | PPS | FP | P | F |

*Table continued on following page*

*Support Surface Reimbursement by Setting (Continued)*

| | | HOME | | SNF | | | |
|---|---|---|---|---|---|---|---|
| GROUP TYPE | INDICATIONS | MCR | MCD | MCR | MCD | MNG | HOSP |
| III   Air-fluidized | Group II failure<br>Trained caregiver<br> needed<br>Comprehensive plan<br> in place | C | P | PPS | FP | P | F |

SNF = skilled nursing facility, HOSP = hospital, C = covered under Medicare B DMERC Guidelines, P = prior approval required, PPS = 100 days comprehensive, F = facility discretion/facility-owned, Mcr = Medicare, Mcd = Medicaid, Mng = managed care.

*Reimbursement Criteria: Support Surface for Pressure Reduction/Relief*

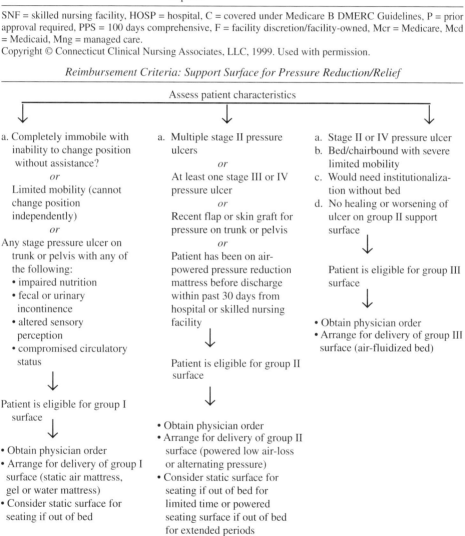

Assess patient characteristics

a. Completely immobile with inability to change position without assistance?
*or*
Limited mobility (cannot change position independently)
*or*
Any stage pressure ulcer on trunk or pelvis with any of the following:
• impaired nutrition
• fecal or urinary incontinence
• altered sensory perception
• compromised circulatory status

Patient is eligible for group I surface

• Obtain physician order
• Arrange for delivery of group I surface (static air mattress, gel or water mattress)
• Consider static surface for seating if out of bed

a. Multiple stage II pressure ulcers
*or*
At least one stage III or IV pressure ulcer
*or*
Recent flap or skin graft for pressure on trunk or pelvis
*or*
Patient has been on air-powered pressure reduction mattress before discharge within past 30 days from hospital or skilled nursing facility

Patient is eligible for group II surface

• Obtain physician order
• Arrange for delivery of group II surface (powered low air-loss or alternating pressure)
• Consider static surface for seating if out of bed for limited time or powered seating surface if out of bed for extended periods

a. Stage II or IV pressure ulcer
b. Bed/chairbound with severe limited mobility
c. Would need institutionalization without bed
d. No healing or worsening of ulcer on group II support surface

Patient is eligible for group III surface

• Obtain physician order
• Arrange for delivery of group III surface (air-fluidized bed)

## 17. What about seating surfaces?

Ischial tuberosity pressures often exceed 200 mmHg and can be as high as 300 mmHg. If a patient requires a support surface for a bed, it naturally follows that one will be needed where they sit! Unfortunately, many clinicians overlook this aspect, resulting in subsequent skin alterations.

**18. What kind of seating surfaces are available?**

Lower-end seating surfaces use foam, water, gel, and static air. They are similar to group I bed support surfaces, and the same principles used for mattress support surfaces can be applied.

**19. Do powered seating surfaces provide a high-end alternative?**

Yes. A few powered alternating air and low air-loss seating surfaces are available. They should be used for patients who would normally qualify for a group II surface. Most have a battery pack so that the patient can have some mobility in a wheelchair.

**20. What specific issues should be kept in mind in considering a seating surface?**

Always consider tissue interface pressures. If possible, consultation with a seating specialist who performs tissue interface mapping studies with the patient on several types of seating surfaces should be obtained—particularly if the patient is deemed high risk for breakdown and spends a lot of time sitting (e.g., paraplegic office worker).

**21. What about reimbursement for seating items?**

Unfortunately, unless the seating surface is part of a customized wheelchair covered by an insurance policy, Medicare, or Medicaid, seating surfaces are rarely covered.

## BIBLIOGRAPHY

1. Agency for Health Care Policy Research: Pressure Ulcers in Adults: Prediction and Prevention. In AHCPR Clinical Practice Guidelines. Rockville, MD, Agency for Health Care Policy Research, Public Health Service, U.S. Department of Health and Human Services, 1992.
2. Bryant RA, Shannon ML, Pieper B, et al: Pressure ulcers. Acute and Chronic Wounds—Nursing Management. St. Louis, Mosby, 1992, pp 105–152.
3. Day AL: Seeking quality care for patients with pressure ulcers. Decubitis 6:32–43, 1993.
4. Hednick-Thompson J, Haloran T, Strader MK, McSweeney M: Pressure reduction products: Making appropriate choices. J Enterostom Ther 20:239–244, 1993.
5. Holzapfel S, Lyons NJ: Support surfaces and their use in the prevention and treatment of pressure ulcers. J Enterostom Ther 20:251–260, 1993.
6. Milne CT, Corbett LQ: A two-phase program at a community hospital to reduce mattress costs. Presented at the Symposium on Advanced Wound Care and Medical Research Forum on Wound Repair, Las Vegas, NV, 2001.
7. Whittemore R: Pressure-reduction support surfaces: A review of the literature. J Wound Ostomy Contin Nurs Soc 25:6–25, 2000.

# 54. METASTATIC SKIN LESIONS

*Carole Bauer*, BSN, RN, OCN, CWOCN

**1. What are the most common malignancies associated with metastatic skin lesions?**

The most common malignancies associated with metastatic skin lesions are breast, kidney, head and neck, lung, ovarian, colon, penis, and bladder cancers. They occur less commonly in lymphoma, leukemia, and melanoma. These lesions occur in 19–50% of all women with breast cancer. The most common occurrence in men is associated with bronchogenic carcinoma, with an incidence of 3-8%. Most metastatic lesions occur on the anterior trunk.

**2. How do metastatic skin lesions develop?**

Metastatic skin lesions develop as a direct extension to the skin from the primary tumor. They also can develop as a secondary tumor. Some lesions develop as a result of lymph nodes that are involved with the disease.

**3. What do the lesions look like?**

Initially the lesions appear as raised, flesh-colored nodules. They may eventually turn red or blue. The lesions quickly develop a necrotic core due to poor oxygenation, metabolite toxicity, or a combination of these factors. This necrotic core leads to the characteristic skin breakdown associated with metastatic lesions.

**4. How is wound healing altered in a metastatic skin lesion compared with the normal wound-healing process?**

Normal wound healing occurs in a series of events that lead to an orderly closure of the wound. In tumor wounds, the malignant cells take the place of platelets in the wound-healing cascade, resulting in a disruption of the wound-healing process. Substituting for platelets, the tumor cells express clotting factors and growth factors that damage normal cells. This causes the bleeding commonly seen in metastatic skin lesions. Tumor cells also produce a decrease in leukocytes in the wound bed, affecting the inflammatory phase of wound healing. Tumor wounds are also hyperpermeable to fibrinogen and plasma colloids. Vascular permeability factor (VPR), secreted by many tumor cells, is responsible for the large amounts of fibrous exudate in malignant wounds. VPR is ten thousand times more potent than histamine in increasing permeability. Tumor wounds also lack the ability to contract. Without contraction, there is a greater area to be filled with granulation tissue than in a normal wound.

**5. What is the first step in determining treatment of the metastatic skin lesion?**

Before determining the treatment of a metastatic skin lesion, the goal of treatment must be established. Most metastatic skin lesions occur at the end of life. These lesions are prognostic of a poor outcome. Once the goal of care has been determined jointly with the patient, the treatment plan phase can begin. Generally, nursing interventions are aimed at local care with attention to prevention and elimination of infection, maintenance of comfort, improvement in the patient's quality of life, and control of odor, drainage, and bleeding.

**6. Is it possible for metastatic lesions to resolve or heal?**

Metastatic wounds usually have a poor outcome. It is generally accepted that resolution is not the primary goal of care. However, if the goal of care is resolution of the wound, the cause of the wound must be controlled. Many different types of treatments have been used to either control or cure metastatic wounds. Treatment decisions are based on whether the disease is localized or has spread distally. If definitive treatment is the plan, usually it is achieved with surgery, radiation, and/or hyperthermia. If distant spread is present, management is usually attempted with hormonal manipulation, immunotherapy, and/or chemotherapy.

**7. Once the goal of care is identified, what other steps should be taken before the institution of a topical treatment plan?**

The need for systemic support and measures to reduce existing and potential cofactors must be assessed. The resources of patient and staff also need to be assessed. A cost-effective dressing with the least amount of caregiver burden should be used. Finally, the dressing must be acceptable to the patient.

**8. What variables are involved in caring for a metastatic skin lesion?**

A metastatic skin lesion requires the same assessment as any other wound. The appearance, size, drainage amount and character, presence of infection, periwound skin, and size and shape of the site need to be assessed and documented. Systemic factors, such as malnutrition, diabetes, use of steroids, and anemia, are addressed and corrected if this approach is congruent with the goal of care.

**9. Is pain a common problem with metastatic wounds?**

Pain is often associated with the trauma of changing the dressings. Nonadherent dressings are indicated, such as nonadherent gauze, gauze impregnated with a hydrogel or petrolatum, semipermeable foam, hydropolymers, and silicone-based dressings. The surrounding skin is fragile and friable. Dressings should also be secured in a nonadherent manner with the use of tubular stretch net dressings, tube tops, T-shirts, mesh panties, or other tapeless securing devices.

**10. What complications are associated with metastatic skin lesions?**
- Bleeding
- Foul odor
- Infection
- Copious drainage
- Altered quality of life

Systemic effects include anemia, electrolyte imbalances, and infection.

**11. How can bleeding be controlled in metastatic wounds?**

The best method of control is to prevent bleeding by providing nontraumatic dressing changes. The use of nonadherent dressings is also effective. If bleeding occurs, direct pressure to the wound is the first step. Absorbable hemostatic dressings and silver nitrate sticks may also be indicated if the bleeding is difficult to control. Alginates also demonstrate a hemostatic effect and may be indicated.

**12. The wound bed seems to have a large amount of yellow slough or necrotic tissue. Should the wound bed be debrided?**

Autolytic debridement is the only accepted method in metastatic lesions. Hydrogels are the best method for autolytic debridement. However, if the wound is highly exudative, a hydrogel is contraindicated. and a calcium alginate may be tried. Sharp and mechanical debridement methods are contraindicated because of the risk of bleeding.

**13. How is odor controlled?**

Foul odor is a common complaint with metastatic wounds. Many patients complain of odor when people around them smell nothing. In determining how to control odor, consider caregiver burden and cost. The first step is to decrease the bacterial load by copious irrigation with saline or by having the patient take a shower. Topical and oral metronidazole have been documented to decrease anaerobic bacteria and the odor associated with metastatic wounds. Metronidazole tablets can be crushed and sprinkled onto the wound bed. The recommended amount of metronidazole is enough crushed tablets to provide a sparse coating over the wound. Either 250-mg or 500-mg tablets can be used. Metronidazole tablets can also be mixed with a hydrogel and applied to the wound bed. One such product is available commercially as MetroGel (Galderma, Fort Worth TX).

Charcoal dressings applied in the top layer of the dressing can also be used to control odor. To work effectively, they must be changed if wet. The use of gauze saturated with a quarter strength sodium hypochlorite solution (Dakin's solution) can also be used. Dressings should be removed with care so that they do not stick to the wound bed.

**14. Are yogurt and buttermilk good ways to control odor?**

Yogurt and buttermilk historically have been used to control odor in wounds when no other products were available. Although most reports about the care of metastatic skin lesions are anecdotal, little in the literature supports the use of yogurt or buttermilk for odor control. The theory behind the use of these products is that the low pH of the lactobacilli inhibits the growth of odor-producing bacteria. This treatment is messy, does not improve quality of life, and does not adequately control odor.

**15. What other old-fashioned remedies are recommended for odor control?**
- Placing a sliced onion under the bed
- Using kitty litter in the dressing or the room
- Charcoal briquettes under the bed
- Pet deodorizers
- Spirits of peppermint

Although many clinicians in desperation may attempt these methods, the best way to control the odor is to eliminate the causative factors: anaerobes in the wound bed, devitalized tissue, and infection.

**16. How can infection be managed?**

Infection is indicated by redness of the periwound skin, increased drainage, increased pain, and change in the character of the wound drainage. Offending organisms frequently identified in malignant wounds are *Escherichia coli, Pseudomonas aeruginosa,* and strains of *Staphylococcus, Proteus,* and *Klebsiella* species. If infection is identified in the wound, a systemic antibiotic may be tried. Topical antibiotics and antimicrobials may be more effective because of the decreased vascular supply to the wound bed and the presence of necrotic tissue in the wound.

**17. How is increased drainage managed?**

Various products to control drainage are available at varying costs. The least costly and time-consuming product should be initiated. Bulky dressings, alginates, foam dressing, absorptive powders, and wound drainage pouches may be used to identify the best product for the wound.

**18. How do metastatic skin lesions affect the patient and family psychosocially?**

Metastatic skin lesions have a major impact on the patient and family. They represent a constant, visible reminder of cancer. In addition, the patient and family have to cope with many changing roles as a result of the lesions. Some patients confine themselves to their home and give up traditional roles because of odor, drainage, and the social stigma that a draining wound represents. The patient also has to meet the financial burden of purchasing dressings. The family may also have to cope with the loss of a wage earner because metastatic lesions occur at the end stage of the disease process.

**19. Do metastatic wounds require a sterile dressing?**

Metastatic skin lesions typically are colonized with bacteria even if an active infection is not noted. Thus, a clean dressing change is indicated. Nonsterile dressings are a useful way to decrease the cost of the dressings.

**20. Why is there so little in the literature about metastatic skin lesions?**

Because they occur at the end of life, limited research has addressed this topic. In addition, when practitioners define a standard treatment that will improve quality of life, few find it ethical to perform a double-blind study when one arm of the group is unable to benefit.

## BIBLIOGRAPHY

1. Bauer C, Gerlach MA: Care of metastatic skin lesions. J Wound Ostomy Contin Nurs 27:247–251, 2000.
2. Bryant RA: Acute and Chronic Wounds: Nursing Management, 2nd ed. St. Louis, Mosby, 2000.
3. Finaly IG, Bowszyc J, Ramlau C, Gwiezdzinski Z: The effect of topical 0.75% metronidazole gel on malodorous cutaneous ulcers. J Pain Symptom Manage 11:158–162, 1996.
4. Goodman M, Ladd LA, Purl S: Integumentary and mucous membrane alterations. In Groenwald SL, Frogg MH, Goodman M, Yarbro CH (eds): Cancer Nursing Principles and Practice, 3rd ed. Boston, Jones & Bartlett, 1993, pp 734–799.
5. McDonald AE: Skin ulceration. I: Groenwald SL, Frogge MH, Yarbro CH (eds): Cancer Symptom Management. Boston, Jones & Bartlett, 1996, pp 364–381.

# 55. BURN WOUND CARE

*Pamela A. Wiebelhaus, RN, BSN, and Sean L. Hansen, BS, CRA*

**1. What are the initial priorities in treatment of the burn patient?**

Stop the burning process, and promptly remove every article of clothing or jewelry that may retain heat. Rings are especially important to remove before swelling begins because they act as a tourniquet.

As with any trauma, use the ABCDEs of assessment (airway, breathing, circulation, disability, and exposure). Carefully examine the face, nares, mouth, and neck for signs of an inhalation injury. The circulation must be assessed regularly, paying specific attention to burns on the extremities and about the thorax. Circumferential burns in these areas can quickly become tight from edema, impeding blood flow into the extremities or constricting the chest to the point that air exchange is severely compromised.

Document the presence or absence of pulses in the extremities initially, and monitor the adequacy of capillary filling in the digits. Watch for labored or limited ventilatory excursions when major burns encompass the entire chest. Large-bore IV access should be obtained in an unburned extremity, if possible. If no unburned site is available, IVs are placed directly through the burn.

Continue the primary survey by looking for obvious disabilities, and assess any changes in level of consciousness. Keep the patient warm. Hypothermia can result in failure to resuscitate the patient. After the primary survey has been accomplished, a thorough head-to-toe "trauma physical" of both sides of the patient should be carried out. Do not let the appearance of the burn injury distract you from the secondary survey.

**2. How is the depth of a burn wound classified?**

The depth of a burn injury is described as superficial, partial-thickness, or full-thickness. A **superficial burn** affects only the outermost layer of skin, the epidermis, and appears reddened. It can be painful to touch. Sunburn is an example of a superficial burn.

A **partial-thickness burn** penetrates the full thickness of the epidermis and varying degrees of the dermal layer. As the depth of injury progresses, a partial-thickness burn shows redness and signs of tissue destruction with blistering. Severe pain is characteristic. On occasion, blistering does not appear in the first 24–48 hours after the burn injury was sustained. A partial-thickness burn blanches when pressure is applied, as with a finger, and quickly returns to red once pressure is removed. As the depth of the burn injury increases into the dermis, the pain may begin to decrease somewhat due to damage to the nerve endings. Some whitish mottling may be seen interspersed with the redness.

A **full–thickness burn** involves destruction of both epidermal and dermal layers. These deep burns typically have a more firm, leathery texture, often appearing tan or white. Severe burns may even be charred and blackened. They do not blanch when pressure is applied because of the loss of circulation to the burned tissue. Unlike superficial and partial-thickness burns, full-thickness burns are essentially painless. Nerve-ending destruction leaves the skin insensate. Pain may be appreciated around the edges of the full-thickness burn where partial-thickness injury persists. Often some areas interspersed in a large full thickness burn retain sensation, which can be confusing.

*Characteristics of Burns of Different Depths*

| CLASSIFICATION | DEPTH OF BURN | COLOR AND APPEARANCE | CAPILLARY REFILL* | PINPRICK SENSIBILITY[†] | RECOVERY |
|---|---|---|---|---|---|
| First-degree | Epidermis | Red or pink | Yes | Yes | 5–7 days |
| Second-degree Superficial partial | Epidermis, with extension into dermis | Red, possibly blistered | Yes | Yes | 7–15 days |

*Table continued on following page*

## Characteristics of Burns of Different Depths

| CLASSIFICATION | DEPTH OF BURN | COLOR AND APPEARANCE | CAPILLARY REFILL* | PINPRICK SENSIBILITY[†] | RECOVERY |
|---|---|---|---|---|---|
| Second-degree Deep partial | Epidermis with deeper extension into dermis | Red to marbled white | Possibly | Possibly | 15–30 days |
| Third-degree Full thickness | Extends into subcutaneous tissue | Charred and leathery, often depressed | No | Possibly | > 30 days |

* Capillary refill refers to blood supply. For an example, press in on your thumbnail. The nail will turn white but immediately becomes rosy again as the capillaries refill. This indicates a good blood supply.
[†] Pinprick sensibility: If a pinprick can be felt on the burned tissue, it indicates that all of the nerve endings have not been destroyed. A full-thickness burn has no sensitivity because the nerve endings have been destroyed.
Adapted from www.burnfree.com.

**3. How do you determine the extent of a burn injury?**

The extent of the burn injury may be calculated relatively quickly by using the "rule of nines," which gives a useful approximation of body surface area and allows rapid and reproducible estimation of the extent of the burn. Some modification of this rule is required in children because of the difference between the shape of adults and children. A child's head is proportionally larger than the rest of the body, and the legs are proportionally shorter (see figure and table on following page). Another effective method for smaller burns is to use the "rule of palm." This principle states that the patient's palm (not including the fingers) represents 1% of total body surface area. By comparing the palm to the extent of the burn and using 1% as a guide, a fair estimate of the extent of the burn can be made.

**4. What common topical antimicrobial agents are used on burn wounds?**

**Silver sulfadiazine** (Silvadene cream 1%) is a broad-spectrum antibiotic used in the treatment of partial- and full-thickness burns. Patients find application to be cool and soothing. Penetration of eschar is limited, and cross reactivity may occur in patients who are allergic to sulfa drugs.

**Mafenide acetate** (Sulfamylon) exerts bacteriostatic action against many gram-negative and gram-positive organisms. It is used on deep partial-thickness and full-thickness burns, especially when an infection is suspected, because it effectively penetrates eschar.

**Petroleum-based products** (e.g., bacitracin) are typically used on superficial burns because of their limited antimicrobial activity.

**Nanocrystalline silver** (Acticoat) is a relatively new option in the management of partial thickness burns and an especially good choice for patients who are allergic to sulfa drugs. It provides infection control against more than 150 pathogens and can be left in place for up to 3 days.

**Silver nitrate solution** (0.5%), which has broad-spectrum activity against many miroorganisms, including fungi, is used on partial-and full-thickness burns.

**5. What type of burns should be refereed to a burn center for treatment?**

The American Burn Association has identified the following injuries as requiring referral to a burn center:
- Second degree burns involving > 10% total body surface area (TBSA)
- Burns involving the face, hands, feet, genitalia, perineum, and major joints
- Electrical burns, including lighting injury
- Third-degree burns in any age group
- Chemical burns
- Inhalation injuries.
- Burn injury in patients with preexisting medical disorders that may complicate management, prolong recovery, or affect mortality.
- Any patient with concomitant trauma (e.g., fractures) in which the burn injury poses the greatest risk of morbidity or mortality. In such cases, if the trauma poses the greater immediate risk,

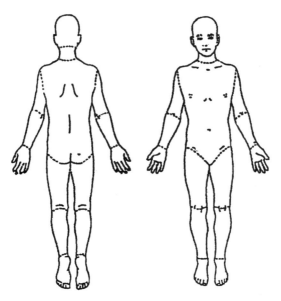

**AGE vs. AREA**

| AREA | BIRTH 1 Yr. | 1-4 Yrs. | 5-9 Yrs. | 10-14 Yrs. | 15 Yrs. | ADULTS |
|---|---|---|---|---|---|---|
| Head | 19 | 17 | 13 | 11 | 9 | 7 |
| Neck | 2 | 2 | 2 | 2 | 2 | 2 |
| Anterior Trunk | 13 | 13 | 13 | 13 | 13 | 13 |
| Posterior Trunk | 13 | 13 | 13 | 13 | 13 | 13 |
| Right Buttocks | 2-1/2 | 2-1/2 | 2-1/2 | 2-1/2 | 2-1/2 | 2-1/2 |
| Left Buttocks | 2-1/2 | 2-1/2 | 2-1/2 | 2-1/2 | 2-1/2 | 2-1/2 |
| Genitalia | 1 | 1 | 1 | 1 | 1 | 1 |
| Right Upper Arm | 4 | 4 | 4 | 4 | 4 | 4 |
| Left Upper Arm | 4 | 4 | 4 | 4 | 4 | 4 |
| Right Lower Arm | 3 | 3 | 3 | 3 | 3 | 3 |
| Left Lower Arm | 3 | 3 | 3 | 3 | 3 | 3 |
| Right Hand | 2-1/2 | 2-1/2 | 2-1/2 | 2-1/2 | 2-1/2 | 2-1/2 |
| Left Hand | 2-1/2 | 2-1/2 | 2-1/2 | 2-1/2 | 2-1/2 | 2-1/2 |
| Right Thigh | 5-1/2 | 6-1/2 | 8 | 8-1/2 | 9 | 9-1/2 |
| Left Thigh | 5-1/2 | 6-1/2 | 8 | 8-1/2 | 9 | 9-1/2 |
| Right Leg | 5 | 5 | 5-1/2 | 6 | 6-1/2 | 7 |
| Left Leg | 5 | 5 | 5-1/2 | 6 | 6-1/2 | 7 |
| Right Foot | 3-1/2 | 3-1/2 | 3-1/2 | 3-1/2 | 3-1/2 | 3-1/2 |
| Left Foot | 3-1/2 | 3-1/2 | 3-1/2 | 3-1/2 | 3-1/2 | 3-1/2 |

Rule of nines with area adjustments according to age.

the patient may be initially treated in a trauma center until stable before being transferred to a burn center. Physician judgment is necessary in such situations and should be in concert with the regional medical control plan and triage protocols.

• Hospitals without qualified personnel or equipment for the care of children should transfer children with burns to a burn unit with appropriate capabilities.

• Burn injury in patients who require special social, emotional, or long-term rehabilitative support, such as cases involving suspected child abuse and substance abuse.

**6. What technique is commonly used to cleanse the burn wound?**

Hydrotherapy is the standard of care by using a shower, spray table or immersion. Depending on local protocols, burn wounds are cleansed daily or B.I.D. using an antimicrobial soap such as chlorhexidine gluconate. Facial burns are cleansed with a mild soap since chlorhexidine gluconate is toxic to both the eyes and ears. Hair on areas surrounding the burn should be shaved clean to minimize the chance for infection to develop.

**7. What is an escharotomy?**

An escharotomy is a procedure used to reduce pressure in the burned area. The eschar is slit open with surgical scalpels.

**8. Why are escharotomies performed on the burn patient?**

The circulation to an extremity with a full-thickness circumferential burn may be impaired by tissue swelling. Circumferential full-thickness burns are inelastic and, when complicated by edema formation, can compromise circulation. Patients who present with such burns should be monitored closely for any changes in circulation or breathing patterns if the burn involves the torso. Indications for escharotomy include a progressive decline or absence of pulsatile flow during repeated examinations of circulation.

**9. Describe the initial management of a chemical burn.**

First brush any dry chemical off the patient, and then flush the affected area with copious amounts of water. Clothing should be removed as soon as possible to minimize contact with the caustic agent. If the patient has received a chemical burn to the face, ensure that he or she is not wearing contacts, then flush with water or saline, irrigating medial to lateral to avoid injury to the tear duct and other eye. Irrigation of chemical burns should be continued until the patient is transferred to a burn center. Identify the chemical and the concentration.

**10. How are chemical burns classified?**

**Acids** cause proteins to precipitate as dense, clot-like coagulum over the burn. Acid injuries can be caused by pool cleaners, rust removers ,and drain cleaners.

**Alkalis** dissolve fats and lipids in the cell membrane. They are commonly found in cement, paint removers, and fertilizers.

**Organics** break down lipids in the cell wall. They are commonly found in phenols and petroleum products.

**11. How is a tar burn treated?**

Tar needs to be cooled and removed as soon as possible to minimize tissue damage. Mineral oil, lard, vegetable shortening, or petroleum-based topical antimicrobial agents have been useful in removing tar. Wound cleansing is often slow and tedious, involving the repeated application of one or many of the above products to the surface of the tar and then wiping it away with a soft cloth.

**12. Describe the management of an electrical burn.**

As with any burn trauma, assess airway, breathing, and circulation; then look for and stabilize any associated trauma. Attach a cardiac monitor, and treat life-threatening dysrhythmias as necessary. Closely monitor distal pulses. Hyperkalemia is a potential complication. Electrical burns are often "tip-of-the-iceberg" injuries (what you see is not necessarily what you get). Internal damage can be extensive, necessitating observation for myoglobin. Examine the patient for entrance and exit wounds (contact points), which may be very small. Wound care is the same as for other types of burns.

**13. What are the early clinical signs of a burn wound infection?**

Pain around the burn, erythema, cellulitis, change in wound drainage, or change in wound appearance are early signs of burn wound infection.

**14. What type of burn requires surgical intervention?**

Full-thickness burns require surgical intervention for optimal healing. In addition, some deep partial-thickness burns may require surgery if they take longer than 21 days to heal. Surgical intervention is aimed at debridement and skin grafting. Skin grafting and skin substitutes are discussed in Chapters 26 and 28, respectively.

**15. Can scars be completely prevented in a burn patient?**

No. However, scars can be minimized with the use of a variety of techniques. The use of custom fitted pressure garments is common in many burn centers. Patients typically are required to wear their pressure garments for 23 hours a day for up to one year. Pressure applied to healed wounds do not prevent scars, it only flattens them. Silicone gel sheeting underneath pressure garments has also been used to help control scaring in smaller areas where adequate pressure can not be obtained. It is not well understood why the above techniques prove to be effective. Vitamin E application has not been shown to improve cosmesis.

**16. Should blisters be removed during wound care?**

To remove or not to remove: this has been a controversy in burn care since 1969. Removing blisters during wound cleansing allows the clinician an accurate view of the wound bed and thus facilitates classification of the degree of burn. In addition, after blisters are removed, a topical antimicrobial agent is more successful in preventing infection because it has direct access to the burn. Some clinicians believe that blisters are a clear sign of a superficial injury that will heal on its own if left undisturbed. There is also the practice of draining the fluid from the blister to decrease pain and leaving the overlying skin to cover the wound.

## BIBLIOGRAPHY

1. Baxter CR: Management of burn wounds. Dermatol Clin 11:709–714, 1993.
2. Heimbach D, Mann R, Engrav L: Evaluation of the burn wound, management decisions. In Herndon DN (ed): Total Burn Care. Philadelphia, W.B. Saunders, 1996, pp 81–87.
3. Monafo WW: Initial management of burns. N Engl J Med 335:1581–1586, 1996.
4. Morgan EM, Bledsoe SC, Barker J: Ambulatory management of burns. Am Fam Physician 62:2015–2026, 2000.
5. Mozingo DW, Barillo DJ, Pruitt BA Jr: Acute resuscitation and transfer management of burned and electrically injured patients. Trauma Q 11(2):94–113, 1994.
6. Nebraska Burn Institute: Advanced Burn Life Support Manual. Lincoln, Nebraska Burn Institute, 1994.
7. Quinn KJ, Evans JH, Courtney JM, Gaylor JDS: Non-pressure treatment of hypertrophic scars. Burns 12(2):102–108, 1985.
8. Sheridan RL, et al: Planimetry study of the percent of body surface represented by the hand and palm: sizing irregular burns is more accurately done using the palm. J Burn Care Rehabil 16:605–606, 1995.
9. Ward RS: Pressure therapy for the control of hypertrophic scar formation after burn injury: A history and review. J Burn Care Rehabil 12(3):257–262, 1991.
10. Winfree J, Barillo DJ: Nonthermal injuries. Nurs Clin North Am 32(2):275–296, 1997.

# 56. MANAGEMENT OF WOUND PAIN

*Lynn Wentland Batchelder,* ARNP, MSN

### 1. What is pain?

Pain is whatever the patients says it is. Pain is subjective. A caregiver should *always* listen to the patient. The accepted definition is an unpleasant sensory and emotional experience arising from actual or potential tissue damage or described in terms of such damage. If you have ever been in pain, you know that this definition is an understatement!

### 2. What effects does pain have on the body?

Pain is one response to trauma. Injured tissue releases substances that evoke stress hormone responses. These responses break down body tissue, increase the metabolic rate, promote blood clotting and water retention, impair immune function, and trigger autonomic features (the fight-or-flight reflex).

### 3. What else happens when pain is felt?

Pain also elicits negative emotions. Anxiety often coexists with acute pain, and depression is a common response to chronic pain. Assessment and treatment of these comorbid conditions are essential to successful management of pain. The literature shows that patients who do not have adequate pain management develop more complications and have a prolonged recovery time, which increases health care costs.

### 4. What is the difference between acute and chronic pain?

**Acute pain** has a sudden onset and is generally a protective mechanism. It is often self-limiting and readily corrected. Pain usually decreases as the damaged area heals. The typical response pattern includes visible signs and changes in vital signs associated with stimulation of the sympathetic nervous system, such as a rise in blood pressure, tachypnea, tachycardia, diaphoresis, and dilated pupils. The cause is often injury, trauma, spasm, or disease. Procedural pain, as in wound dressing changes, is considered acute pain.

**Chronic pain** is prolonged and defined as lasting more than 6 months. Chronic pain does not respond to usual therapy. This lack of response often leads to behavioral and psychological reactions as patient and family try to cope with chronic pain. Depression often occurs with chronic pain. Sources of chronic pain include the following:

- Cancer
- Chronic disease states
- Pain with unidentifiable source
- Pain that persists past the expected time after an acute cause

### 5. Do patients with wounds have pain?

Definitely. Studies of wound pain are limited, although clinicians are learning more about this area of care. Pain adversely affects quality of life in the patient with a wound. Dressing changes can be very painful (especially in the adolescent age group). Wound pain can be related to infection, osteomyelitis, surgical procedures, neuropathy, debridement, and wound therapies. Because investigation into wound pain and its management is still in its infancy, it is an exciting time to conduct nursing research in this area. Keeping abreast of new developments can be difficult. Periodic visits to websites and journals are probably the best way to learn the latest developments.

### 6. How is pain assessed?

Many assessment tools are available. An in-depth history during which you ask questions and listen to the patient is crucial. The **PQRST** approach is a comprehensive method to assess pain:

**P = P**ain. One site or several sites? Were there any precipitating factors or trauma before the onset of the pain? Is the wound causing pain? What does the patient think is the cause of pain?

**Q = Q**uality. Ask the patient to describe the pain. Is it burning, throbbing, stabbing, aching, squeezing, constant, intermittent, spasmodic, tender, or crushing? Does the quality seem out of proportion to the wound itself? If so, have you considered necrotizing fascists?

**R = R**egion. Where is the pain? Does it move or radiate to another site? Is it generalized or in a specific area?

**S = S**everity. How bad is the pain? Use research-validated scales such as the 0–10 numeric pain intensity scale or a visual analog scale. Ask the patient where the pain falls on a 0 (no pain) to 10 (severe or "dipped in hot oil" pain) or the Wong Baker Scale (happy to sad "faces"), which is often used with children and has shown validity in the elderly.

**T = T**emporal aspects. The patient should talk in greater depth about the characteristics of the pain. What makes it better or worse? Have you tried any treatment, and has it been effective? When does the pain occur? How has it affected the patient's life?

**7. Is the assessment of pain different for wounds?**

Essentially, no. It is important to assess acute and chronic pain associated with wound care.

**8. How do you differentiate the causes of chronic pain? How is it treated?**

Chronic pain is often differentiated based on location and defining characteristics. Often patients have a combination of types of pain.

*Types of Pain and Treatment*

| TYPE | SOURCE | DESCRIPTION | TREATMENT |
|---|---|---|---|
| Bone pain | Fractures (including compression fractures) Cancer Surgical interventions Joint pain: major and minor joints, including facet joints in back, sacroiliac joint | Sharp pain or "hard ache" Increased pain with movement of affected area | Medications: first NSAIDs, opioids Steroids: oral or injected into joints Acetylsalicylic acid (aspirin) |
| Centrally mediated pain syndrome | Pathophysiology is unclear Pain can be severe, may travel to one or more extremities, and causes sympathetic changes in affected extremities | Sympathetic changes: Color changes in skin due to vasoconstriction- (often pale to blue/gray) Decrease in perspiration, temperature, hair growth Constant burning, shooting, or stabbing pain | Medications: tricyclics, anticonvulsants (Neurontoin is commonly used in varying doses) Sympathetic nerve blocks, such as stellate ganglion blocks |
| Neurologic pain | Nerve pain along one or more dermatomes (e.g., postherpetic neuralgias, spinal cord impingement, including spinal stenosis) Damage to any nerve or nerve roots from trauma or surgical interventions Diabetic neuropathy | Burning, shooting, stabbing pain; feeling that area is hot or cold; lancinating pain Diabetic neuropathy: squeezing, burning, shooting pain in lower extremities from knee down (like tight knee-high stocking) Spinal stenosis: relief of pain with sitting or bending (as in leaning over shopping cart) | Medications: tricyclics, anticonvulsants (especially Neurontoin, mexetil for diabetic neuropathy) Reduction of cord compression by decreasing inflammation in cord with epidural steroid injections or surgery to remove whatever is compressing nerve Nerve block for shingles to prevent postherpetic neuralgias and decrease immediate pain |

*Table continued on following page*

*Types of Pain and Treatment (Continued)*

| TYPE | SOURCE | DESCRIPTION | TREATMENT |
|---|---|---|---|
| Somatic pain | Pain originating in muscle or connective tissue<br>Myofascial pain<br>Fibromyalgia | Aching, pulling, squeezing, sharp pain, often worse after use of affected muscle and at end of day; heat and hot showers make it better temporarily<br>Tension headaches | Medications: muscle relaxants, NSAIDs, sometimes anticonvulsants; opioids do not help much<br>Trigger point injections into affected areas<br>Botulism toxin injections<br>Stretching exercises<br>Heat, massage, ultrasound |
| Skin pain | Pain originating from dermal layers | Raw, burning, sharp, stabbing, pinching pain | Topical anesthetics such as EMLA and Lidoderm may help, but no evidence indicates that they promote healing of tissue |
| Vascular pain | Pain originating from vasculature<br>Migraine headaches<br>Peripheral vascular disease | Migraine headaches: throbbing, pulsating quality, unilateral; may have stabbing, lancinating qualities<br>Peripheral vascular disease symptoms vary depending on severity of disease | Medications: Imitrex causes vasodilation to reduce migraines; often gives immediate relief; migraines can be complex problem with various treatment modalities<br>Try to treat underlying problem; e.g., if circulation to a limb can be improved surgically<br>Sometimes sympathetic blockade can help with vasodilation to improve circulation to an extremity |
| Visceral pain | Pain originating from abdomen or thorax, including any organ contained in these areas | Varied symptoms; often difficult to assess due to nature of referral patterns of visceral organs | Mediations: opioids (if no risk in slowing bowel)<br>Treat underlying problem |

NSAIDs = nonsteroidal anti-inflammatory drugs, EMLA = eutectic mixture of local anesthetics.

**9. How do I know which medications to use?**

When you take a good history, you can identify the most likely type and source of pain and treat appropriately. Keep it simple is a golden rule. Use the least potent analgesic with the fewest side effects. Also use the least invasive method for delivering the medication. "If the gut works, use it." We do not need to complicate treatment. The World Health Organization (WHO) offers a three-step ladder approach designed for chronic cancer pain. However, it is used as a guide for all types of pain.

*Three Step Approach to Pain Management*

| STEP | MEDICATION | REGIMEN |
|---|---|---|
| Step 1 | Acetaminophen<br>Salicylates<br>NSAIDs | Nonopioid with or without adjuvant treatment |
| If pain persists, try different nonopioid, maximize dose, and add step 2 opioid. | | |
| Step 2 | Codeine<br>Hydrocodone<br>Oxycodone, 5 mg every 6 hr | Opioid for mild-to-moderate pain with or without nonopioid and/or adjuvant treatment |

*Table continued on following page*

*Three Step Approach to Pain Management (Continued)*

| STEP | MEDICATION | REGIMEN |
|------|-----------|---------|
| If pain persists, increase opioid or change to step 3 opioid | | |
| Step 3 | Morphine<br>Oxycodone, 7.5–10 mg every 6 hr<br>Hydromorphone<br>Fentanyl | Opioid for moderate-to-severe pain<br>with or without nonopioid and/or<br>adjuvant treatment |

Adapted from World Health Organization: Cancer pain relief and palliative care. Report of WHO Expert Committee. WHO Technological Report Service 804:1–73, 1990.

## 10. What guidelines about medication use are available?
- Use analgesics for an adequate period and in appropriately titrated doses.
- Use analgesics on an around-the-clock schedule and not on an as-needed schedule only.
- Use time-released medications when available, but always have medication for rescue dosing. The rescue or breakthrough doses range from 5% to 15% of a 24-hour dose.
- If pain relief is needed for a procedure, give the medication so that the analgesic effect peaks at the time of the procedure.
- Watch for side effects. A laxative protocol is often necessary to prevent constipation.
- Some medications have "ceiling effects"; that is, larger doses have no greater effect than lower doses and may have adverse/ toxic effects compared with smaller doses. Aspirin has a ceiling effect at 650 mg per dose, whereas acetaminophen (Tylenol) has a range of 560–1000 mg per dose (do not exceed 4-6 gm/day to prevent liver toxicity).

## 11. How do I know if the patient is getting enough medicine, especially when the route of delivery is switched from parenteral to oral?
When a patient is switched to a different type or form of opioid medication, it is important to calculate the appropriate equianalgesic dosing so that the patient gets an adequate amount of pain control.

*Opioid Equivalency Guidelines*

| DRUG | PARENTERAL EQUIVALENT DOSE (mg) | EQUIPOTENT ORAL DOSE (mg) | AVERAGE DURATION OF ACTION (hr)* |
|------|---------------------------------|---------------------------|----------------------------------|
| Morphine | 10 | 20 ( may be 30 mg in some patients) | 3–4 |
| Codeine | 120 | 180 | 3–4 |
| Oxycodone | N/A | 20 | 3–4 |
| Hydrocodone | N/A | 30 | 3-4 |
| Meperidine<br>Useful for brief courses of acute pain. Generally should not be used long term due to the toxic metabolite nor-meperidine | 100 | 300 | 2–3 |
| Methadone | 2.5<br>With chronic dosing, parenteral equivalent may be decreased | 5 | 4–8 |
| Hydromorphone (Dilaudid) | 2 | 8 | 3-4 |

*Table continued on following page*

## Opioid Equivalency Guidelines (Continued)

| DRUG | PARENTERAL EQUIVALENT DOSE (mg) | EQUIPOTENT ORAL DOSE (mg) | AVERAGE DURATION OF ACTION (hr)* |
|---|---|---|---|
| **Agonist-antagonist drugs** | | | |
| Butorphanol[†] (Stadol) | 2 | N/A | 3–4 |
| Pentazocine[†] (Talwin) | 60 | 150 | 3–4 |

\* Duration of actions are only averages. Some patients require more or less frequent dosing. Each patient should be titrated individually.
[†] Can cause withdrawal if given to patients on chronic pure agonists

## Morphine/Duragesic Equivalency*

| PARENTERAL 24-HR MORPHINE | DURAGESIC EQUIVALENT (mg/hr) |
|---|---|
| 30 | 25 |
| 60 | 50 |
| 90 | 75 |
| 120 | 100 |
| 150 | 125 |

• This dose equivalency chart is not the same as that in the Duragesic product insert.

### 12. What about addiction?

True addiction occurs in less than 1% of patients who take pain medication for chronic pain. It is important to understand several definitions:
- **Addiction** is a psychological dependence in which the patient exhibits drug- seeking behavior.
- **Pseudoaddiction** occurs when the patient is undermedicated and therefore shows drug-seeking behavior.
- **Physical dependence** withdrawal occurs when an opioid is abruptly stopped. The abstinence syndrome includes anxiety, irritability, chills, hot flashes, salivation, diaphoresis, nausea, vomiting, abdominal cramps, and insomnia. Many classes of drugs cannot be withdrawn abruptly without significant physical symptoms (e.g, tricyclics, antipsychotics, selective serotonin reuptake inhibitors [SSRIs]).
- **Tolerance** occurs when larger doses of opioids are required to maintain the original effect. The first sign of tolerance is a decrease in the duration of effectiveness of the opioid. When switching opioids, start at one-half of the equianalgesic dose.

### 13. Describe the available adjuvant therapies.

Adjuvant medications include tricyclics, SSRIS, caffeine, anticonvulsants, topical and injectable anesthetics, muscle relaxants, mexitil, corticosteroids, benzodiazepines, barbiturates, and botulism injections. Nerve blocks, joint, trigger point, and epidural injections with and without steroids can also be used. Many of these therapies have not been well researched in the wound pain area.

Nonpharmacologic adjuvant therapies include modalities such as meditation, relaxation, therapeutic touch, exercise, physical/occupational therapy, education, biofeedback, visual imagery, stress management, cutaneous treatments such as heat and cold, transcutaneous electrical nerve stimulators (TENS), acupuncture, acupressure, massage, surgery, and dorsal column stimulator implants.

Referral to a clinician experienced in pain management should be considered if pain is not well controlled or is affecting adherence to the wound treatment plan.

### 14. What are the traditional ways of treating wound pain?

As nurses, we were educated to assess for pain and pretreat it if necessary. Premedicating a patient before a potentially painful procedure is sound practice. Most of us learned the "trick" of using irrigation fluid to help remove dressings that may be stuck to the surface of the wound. Of course, nursing techniques such as distraction, patient education, and visual imagery also can be traditional methods.

Local dressings that promote moist wound healing go a long way to reduce pain at the time of dressing change. A moist wound bed naturally reduces tissue disturbance and pain. Pressure-relieving devices can also decrease pain.

Skin stripping from dressing adhesives and tape is reduced by using products designed to avoid such trauma. Frank discussion with a product representative about stratum corneum removal test results can often elicit information about the potential for a product to damage the skin. If tape must be used, the literature shows that paper tape is less detrimental to the skin on removal.

### 15. What are some more novel approaches?

The use of topical anesthetics such as EMLA or Lidoderm on the intact skin around the wound can be helpful for preprocedural treatment of anticipated acute pain for debridement or dressing changes. It is sometimes useful to apply these creams at each dressing change. Always consult the product insert for the correct dosage and application.

Neuropathic and reflex sympathetic dystrophy pain syndromes respond nicely to low-dose tricyclics and anticonvulsants. Treating the pain is the easy part; the accurate and detailed assessment of pain is paramount. If done correctly, it naturally leads to the correct treatment.

### 16. Where can I learn more about pain on the Internet?

- Arthritis foundation: www.arthritis.org
- American Chronic Pain Association: www.theACPA.org
- American Pain Society: www.ampainsoc.org
- American Occupational Therapy Association: www.aota.org
- American Physical Therapy Association: www.apta.org
- Department of Pain Medicine and Palliative Care at Beth Israel Medical Center: www.StopPain.org
- International Association for the Study of Pain: www.halcyon.com/iasp
- National Headache Foundation: www.headaches.org
- National Institute of Arthritis and Musculoskeletal and Skin Diseases: www.nih.gov/niams

### BIBLIOGRAPHY

1. Carr DB, Jacox AK, Chapman CR, et al: Acute Pain Management: Operative or Medical Procedures and Trauma. Clinical Practice Guideline No. 1. AHCPR Pub. No 92-0032. Rockville, MD, Agency for Health Care Policy and Research, Public Health Service, U.S. Department of Health and Human Services, 1992.
2. International Association for the Study of Pain: Pain terms: A list with definitions and notes in usage. Pain 6(3):249, 1979.
3. Jacox A, Carr DB, Payne R, et al: Management of Cancer Pain. Clinical Practice Guideline No. 9. AHCPR Publication No. 94-0592. Rockville MD, Agency for Health Care Policy and Research, U.S. Department of Health and Human Services, Public Health Service, 1994.
4. Krasner D, Rodeheaver G, Sibbald G: Chronic Wound Care: A Clinical Source Book for Healthcare Professionals, 3rd ed. Wayne, PA, HMP Communications, 2001.
5. Portenoy RK (moderator), Bennett GJ, Cruciani RA, Katz N: Enhancing opioid analgesia: Emerging mechanisms and treatment strategies. Program and abstracts of the American Pain Society 20th Annual Scientific Meeting, Symposium 112, Phoenix, AZ, April 20, 2001.
6. American Academy of Pain Medicine and the American Pain Society: The use of opioids for the treatment of chronic pain: A consensus statement. Clin J Pain 13:6–8, 1997.

# 57. LYMPHEDEMA MANAGEMENT

*Lynette Jamison, MOT, OTR/L, CDP*

### 1. Define lymphedema.

Lymphedema is a swelling that may arise when protein-rich fluid collects abnormally in the tissues as a result of compromise of the lymph drainage system. This ultrafiltrated fluid includes plasma proteins that attract water and further increase swelling. Most often the swelling occurs unilaterally in the legs, but it may occur in the torso or face. Even if both extremities are affected, obvious differences may be observed. Stagnant lymph fluids that have collected in the interstitial tissue spaces provide an environment rich for infection, placing the patient at risk for infections such as cellulitis. Lymphedema can affect more than one body part. In the case of inherited primary lymphedema, both legs are often involved.

### 2. How many people suffer from lymphedema?

According to the National Cancer Institute, more than 250,000 people in the United States suffer from secondary lymphedema. Currently, 25–30% of men and women who have breast cancer surgery with lymph node resection and radiation therapy develop lymphedema. It may also occur in men who have had prostate or testicular surgery, people who suffer from lymphoma, and others. The statistic of those suffering from lymphedema is unclear because it so often goes undiagnosed.

### 3. Describe the pathogenesis of lymphedema.

The underlying cause of lymphedema determines its pathophysiology. Non–cancer-related lymphedema can be caused by various conditions, such as obesity, chronic venous insufficiency, deep vein thrombosis (DVT), or harvesting/stripping of veins from the legs, which causes the lymphatic system to increase the amount of fluid transported through its vessels. This increased load can eventually overwhelm the lymphatic system, causing it simply to shut down. Typically, non–cancer-related lymphedema in the lower extremity develops so gradually on the dorsum of the foot and ankle that it is well established before it becomes apparent and then progresses proximally. Lymphedema caused by cancers of the pelvis, on the other hand, tend to begin proximally and progress distally. Edema can invade the trunk area, as well as the genitals, when the nodes in the groin area are damaged.

Radiation therapy, used in treating various cancers and some AIDS-related diseases (e.g., Kaposi's sarcoma) can damage otherwise healthy lymph nodes and vessels, causing lymphedema. Scar tissue forms in the radiated area to interrupt the normal flow of the lymphatic fluid. Radiation can also cause skin dermatitis or a burn similar to a sunburn.

### 4. What is the difference between edema and lymphedema?

Edema caused by trauma, injury, or surgery is a natural response to heal the assault. This form of edema is made up of natural body water and fluids and void of high levels of protein. Treatment for edema may be achieved with anti-inflammatory medications, elevation, and icing. These modes of treatment are not effective for lymphedema, which is best known for the high levels of protein. The protocol for treating lymphedema is manual lymph drainage, compression bandage/garments, and therapeutic exercise.

### 5. How does lymphedema affect wound healing?

Lymphedema presses on blood vessels to decrease circulation to the affected body part, affecting the delivery of oxygen and nutrients while inhibiting removal of waste products and causing local ischemia. Therefore, wounds tend to heal more slowly. Weeping lymph fluid may also slow the healing process as the wound area becomes macerated.

**6. What are the defining characteristics of an extremity wound with lymphedema?**

Wounds associated with lymphedema weep excessively and heal very slowly. Often they do not bleed. Their product is a clear, straw-colored fluid.

**7. What are the types and classifications of lymphedema?**

Lymphedema is classified as either primary or secondary. **Primary lymphedema** is a rare, inherited condition in which lymph nodes and vessels are absent or abnormal. **Secondary lymphedema** is caused when the lymphatic system is blocked or interrupted. The most common causes of secondary lymphedema are surgery involving the lymph nodes, radiation therapy, trauma, obesity, and cancer.

**8. When does secondary lymphedema occur?**

Secondary lymphedema may have its onset immediately after surgery, radiation therapy, illness, or injury to the lymph nodes or vessels, or the onset may be delayed for as long as 20 years. It is difficult to determine who will experience lymphedema.

**9. Describe the three stages of lymphedema.**

**Stage I** is characterized by edema that comes and goes without treatment. **Stage II** is characterized by pitting of the tissues underlying the epidermis. Pitting is the displacement of protein-rich fluids after pinching the edematous body part. Skin pitting may take as long as 15 minutes to resolve. **Stage III** is characterized by an orange-peel skin texture ("peau d'orange") and a hard, wood-like feeling called indurosis. Patients with stage III lymphedema have poor skin turgor, and pitting is absent. Foeld and Lerner believe that over 90% of people who have had surgery and/or radiation experience stage 0 lymphedema. **Stage 0** is a subclinical stage, in which no or minimal signs are observed, but lymph flow is impaired. A person can remain in stage 0 for many years before moving into stage I.

**10. How is indurosis different from fibrosis?**

Indurosis refers to firm tissue that normally would be soft. Indurosis is directly associated with stage II and III lymphedema. Fibrosis is irreversible hardening of normally soft tissue. Fibrosis is often associated with venous insufficiency in the lower legs ("woody leg syndrome").

**11. Describe the secondary effects of lymphedema.**

Reflex sympathetic dystrophy or complex regional pain syndrome, decreased sensation wounds, limited rage of motion (ROM), and limited function may be secondary effects of lymphedema. Management should include evaluation and treatment of lymphedema. It is also necessary to address wound care as simply as possible. Physical or occupational therapy is necessary for treating decreased ROM and limited function. Decreased sensation is often resolved with lymphedema treatment.

**12. What environmental conditions may exacerbate lymphedema?**

Anecdotal information suggests that extreme temperature changes, trauma, sunburn, infection, blood pressure cuffs on the affected limb, compressed air cabins (e.g., on commercial airplanes), psychological stress, lack of treatment, carrying heavy loads, and lack of exercise may exacerbate lymphedema. However, no conclusive research supports this information.

**13. Is pain associated with lymphedema?**

Lymphedema is generally a painless condition. In patients with lymphedema, pain is usually related to conditions such as reflex sympathetic dystrophy, cancer, or cellulitis.

**14. How is lymphedema diagnosed?**

Lymphedema can be diagnosed through medical history, family history, lymphangiography, and lymphoscintigraphy. Medical history may identify surgical removal of lymph nodes and vessels. Family history may reveal a generational tendency for primary lymphedema. Lymphangiography and lymphoscintigraphy are x-ray visualizations of the lymphatics and lymph nodes after injection of a contrast medium. Physical examination includes palpation to determine if pitting or indurosis is present. Skin color and texture and evidence of wet, weepy skin with or without wounds are also assessed.

**15. How accurate are the diagnostic methods?**

Lymphangiography and lymphoscintigraphy are extremely accurate for diagnosing lymphedema. Medical history, family history, and physical examination are not always accurate.

**16. How do you objectively measure the volume difference between the affected and unaffected limb or body part?**

Volumetric measurements, obtained by immersing each limb and capturing the displaced water, are taken to determine volume difference between sides. A second method for calculating volume difference is to take circumferential measurements of the affected and unaffected limb in 4-cm increments, squaring each number, taking the sum of the square, and dividing the sum by pi (3.14). The resulting number equals volume in milliliters.

**17. What is the focus of palpation in assessment of a limb?**

Attention is paid to temperature, skin texture, underlying tissue texture, skin turgor, and evidence of indurosis or pitting.

**18. Describe skin turgor.**

Skin turgor refers to the ability of the skin to stretch. When a patient suffers from lymphedema and their tissues are full, they often experience decreased skin turgor. During elevation, a comparison is made with the opposite side.

**19. Why should you not use the affected extremity for blood pressure measurement or placement of an IV line?**

Because lymph flow is responsible for removing bacteria from the host, any impediment to flow can result in bacterial proliferation in the protein-rich fluid. Placing an IV in the affected extremity may cause the onset of cellulitis because IV placement may introduce bacteria. Compression > 40 mmHg temporarily collapses the lymph vessel. Blood pressure cuffs are often inflated above 20 mmHg, potentially exacerbating or causing the onset of lymphedema.

**20. Does lymphedema resolve on its own?**

Damage to the lymph system is irreversible, but lymph fluid may find alternative pathways through anastomosis. Proper treatment can encourage alternate pathways, thereby decreasing lymphedema volume.

**21. Is lymphedema curable?**

No—but it is manageable. Patients are taught management techniques, including self-manual lymph drainage, compression bandaging, short-stretch bandages, and therapeutic exercises that assist in maintaining a reduced limb or body part. Stage I lymphedema is easily managed with self-manual lymph drainage, therapeutic exercise, and, on occasion, self-compression bandaging. Stages II and III require treatment for the reduction of indurosis, edema/girth size, and improvement of tissue health. Without treatment, patients are at risk for increased edema, decreased function, cellulitis, and loss of limb. Stages II and III are associated with permanent tissue changes, and all symptoms may not be possible to reverse.

**22. What is the treatment for lymphedema?**

Treatment for lymphedema includes the use of short-stretch compression bandages covering the edematous body part, manual lymph drainage, and therapeutic exercise. Once a limb or body part has reduced in girth size, patients are fitted for compression garments that maintain the girth reduction gained through therapy. Pneumatic intermittent compression pumps are used in extreme cases of stage III lymphedema, followed by manual lymph drainage, compression bandaging, and therapeutic exercise.

**23. Do you treat primary lymphedema differently from secondary lymphedema?**

For the most part, primary and secondary lymphedema are treated similarly. The manual lymph drainage methods may differ in pattern. Compression bandaging of a lower extremity with primary lymphedema uses 50 mmHg, whereas compression bandaging of a lower extremity with secondary lymphedema uses 30–40 mmHg.

### 24. What is manual lymph drainage?

Manual lymph drainage is the use of skin-stretching massage techniques to encourage lymph fluids to drain in a specific direction. Several schools offer instruction for manual lymph drainage techniques combined with the use of pneumatic intermittent compression pumps. Among the better known schools are the Doctor Vodder School of North America, Foeldi School, Casley-Smith School, Lerner Lymphedema Service Academy of Lymphatic Studies, and the Institute of Lymphatic Studies.

### 25. What is the rationale behind manual lymph treatment and compression bandaging?

Manual lymph drainage is a massage technique that encourages lymph fluids to flow in the direction of the massage. The direction is determined by preestablished patterns learned in training. The patterns of massage bypass the area of obstruction, using anastomotic connections. Correct use of a short-stretched compression bandage increases tissue pressure, thereby forcing absorption of excessive water and ultimately reducing the size of the affected body part.

### 26. When should a patient receive manual lymph treatment and compression bandaging?

A patient should be treated for lymphedema on diagnosis. Treatment in the early stages of lymphedema is more successful. Success is defined by fewer incidents of cellulitis, smaller girth size, and absence of indurosis with good skin turgor.

### 27. How do you know where to direct lymph flow with manual treatment?

In a healthy person, lymph fluid follows specified pathways. For example, lymph fluid from the feet drains to the backs of the knees, then to the groin via the inguinal lymph nodes, then to a lymph collection sack at the abdomen called sisterna Kailai, on to thoracic duct, and then into the left clavicle area, at which point it joins the circulatory system and is evacuated through the urine.

### 28. Can patients perform self-massage to facilitate the lymph drainage?

Patients are often instructed in self-manual lymph drainage for home management of lymphedema. Occasionally, patients are unable to reach parts of their bodies to complete a full manual lymph drainage pattern.

### 29. What else are patients taught for self-management of lymphedema?

Patients who have lymphedema are also instructed compression bandaging and therapeutic exercise. Skin care is also a vital part of managing lymphedema. Compression garments are worn during the day, and compression bandages are worn in bed. Patients are instructed to wear compression 20 of 24 hours a day. They are encouraged to exercise daily and apply manual lymph drainage as needed.

### 30. Do pharmacological treatments or oral medications, such as diuretics, help lymphedema?

No. Often physicians attempt to use diuretics for treatment of lymphedema. Reduction of edema may be observed initially, but the reduction is short-lived. Diuretics remove fluid, not protein. The fluid temporarily leaves after diuretic administration but returns as the remaining protein exerts an oncotic pull. Often cellulitis infections are associated with lymphedema. Penicillin is the favored antibiotic, but antibiotic choice is influenced by local resistance patterns, probable organisms involved, and patient-specific factors such as allergies. Anecdotal reports suggest that antioxidants and horse chestnut herbs are helpful in treating lymphedema, but no research supports this practice.

### 31. What exercises can be performed to prevent or maintain lymphedema?

Water exercise is an excellent activity. Immersion in water provides compression to the edematous body part while allowing full range of motion with resistance against water with movement. Casley-Smith published a series of exercises in two books, *Exercises for Patients with Lymphoedema of the Arm: A Guide to Self-Massage and Hydrotherapy Exercises* and *Exercises for Patients with Lymphoedema of the Leg: A Guide to Self-Massage and Hydrotherapy Exercises*. Each describes specific exercises for an edematous extremity.

**32. Why do you bandage extremities?**

Bandaging an extremity increases oncotic tissue pressure, forcing the bloodstream to absorb excessive water. The fluid collecting in the interstitial spaces is, in large part, plasma protein. This protein fluid attracts water, which makes up the majority of the total edema. Therefore, compression bandaging provides the single most successful mode of reduction of the edema.

**33. What types of bandages are used?**

Short-stretch bandages are the most effective in reducing lymphedema. Two German manufacture these bandages, Rosidal and Compriland. Compriland is distributed by Jobst, an American company. The Rosidal bandages are available through several American companies, including Bandages Plus and North American Rehabilitation.

**34. How are short-stretch bandages different from an Ace wrap?**

Ace bandages are considered long-stretch bandages and do not provide the proper compression necessary to reduce lymphedema. Ace bandages may increase from original size by 3 times, whereas the short-stretch bandages increase in size just enough to follow the contours of the wrapped limb.

**35. What results can you expect from manual lymph treatment and compression bandaging?**

The combination of manual lymph drainage and compression bandaging decreases girth size, and improves skin turgor and integrity by decreasing indurosis and pitting. Improved skin integrity decreases the incidence of cellulitis.

**36. Can compression bandaging be applied if the edema has resulted in decreased sensation?**

Decreased sensation often results from lymphedema. The edema presses on associated nerves, rendering them ineffective. The compression bandages relieve this pressure, thereby restoring sensation. It is vitally important to inspect the skin and surrounding tissue of a wrapped limb with decreased sensation. Edema reduction and time may or may not resolve decreased sensation.

**37. When the extremity is bandaged, does it need to be elevated?**

No. Elevating the extremity shifts water from one interstitial space to another. Conversely, compression bandaging forces the blood stream to absorb excessive water for ultimate elimination of the water. Elevation produces a temporary, yet short-lived, reduction.

**38. What is recommended for skin care under the bandage?**

Skin care with lymphedema can be accomplished with skin moisturizers such as Eucerin. Debridement is often necessary in the case of stage III lymphedema, in which the skin is callused, has an orange peel-texture, and appears to weep (see Chapter 58 for additional recommendations).

**39. Why can't the doctor just prescribe a compression garment on diagnosis?**

The function of a compression garment is to maintain current size and shape. Compression bandages are needed for reducing the lymphedema. If he patient uses only a compression garment, girth size will remain relatively unchanged. Treatment and instruction in a home program are necessary for the initial reduction of edema. Once the patient has reduced girth size by 50–70% or more, he or she is fitted for compression garments.

**40. What happens if lymph fluid weeps constantly through the compression bandages?**

If lymph fluid weeps through compression bandages, the compression bandages become wet and hold the fluid against the skin. After prolonged contact with this lymph fluid, skin breakdown may occur. Layers of absorbent dressings may be necessary for extremely weepy wounds. It is important to minimize the lymph fluid that leaks through the bandages. The bandages are washable.

**41. Can compression bandages be used over a bandaged wound?**

In most cases, a wound due to lymphedema heals best with compression. It is necessary to apply extra-absorbent products to the wound because of weeping lymph fluid. The absorbent products protect the short-stretch compression bandages from excessive fluid. Products containing zinc oxide facilitate the healing process of a lymphedema wound.

### 42. How often do you change lymphedema-related wound dressings?

Lymphedema-related wounds tend to be extremely weepy and require frequent dressing changes. Wound dressings may need changing as often as 2–3 times/day or as seldom as once every 3 days.

### 43. When do you use a figure-eight vs. a spiral wrap for applying compression bandages?

Patients are provided with a spiral wrap on initial visits to therapy. Spiral wrap is simple to apply and simple to learn. Figure-eight wrap is used for an irregularly shaped limb and stage II or III lymphedema.

### 44. When is a sequential intermittent pneumatic compression pump used to treat lymphedema?

Sequential, intermittent pneumatic compression pumps are used in extreme cases of stage III lymphedema, followed by manual lymph drainage and compression bandaging. The purpose of the pump is to soften indurotic tissue. The intermittent pneumatic compression pump has been used to a great extent in the United States as a substitute for manual lymph drainage and compression bandaging. This phenomenon is due, in large part, to a shortage of skilled practitioners and poor understanding of treatment possibilities. Other modalities may be used, including ultrasound and electrical stimulation, to soften indurotic tissue if a patient has no history of cancer.

### 45. When is treatment contraindicated for patients with lymphedema?

When patients are ill and/or infection is present in the affected body part.

### 46. Can secondary lymphedema be treated if cancer is malignant and the patient is not being treated for malignancy?

There are different theories about treating lymphedema when cancer is present. According to one theory, if a patient is receiving treatment for cancer, treatment is indicated for lymphedema. A second theory suggests that if cancer is present, lymphedema should not be treated under any circumstances for fear of spreading the cancer. A third theory proposes that if cancer is present and a patient has lost function and is uncomfortable due to lymphedema, treatment is indicated. The author believes that if patients are undergoing treatment for cancer with full understanding of possible outcomes for lymphedema treatment, treatment is indicated.

### 47. What signs and symptoms indicate infection?

Cellulitis infections are characterized by skin that is red, warm or hot, tender to touch, and associated with fever and chills. Often patients experience malaise and decreased appetite. Skin rashes may be associated with cellulitis.

### BIBLIOGRAPHY

1. Casley-Smith JR, Casley-Smith JR: Modern Treatment for Lymphoedema. Sydney, Lymphoedema Association of Australia, 1997.
2. Foeldi M, Foeldi E: Lymphoedema: Methods of Treatment and Control. A Guide for Patients and Therapists. Portland, OR, Medicina Biologica, 1991.
3. Guyton AC, Hall TE: Textbook of Medical Physiology. Philadelphia, W.B. Saunders, 1996.
4. Harris RH: The Vodder method: An introduction to manual lymph drainage. Massage Ther J 31:1, 1992.
5. Kasseroller R: Compendium of Dr. Vodder's Manual Lymph Drainage. city, Haug Verlage, 1998.
6. Leduc A, Caplan I, Leduc O: Lymphatic drainage of the upper limb: substitution lymphatic pathways. Eur J Lymphol 4:11–18, 1993.
7. Lerner R: Chronic lymphedema. In Chang JB (ed): Textbook of Angiology. New York, Springer-Verlag, 2000, 1227–1236.
8. Petrek J, Pressman PI, Smith RA: Results from a workshop on breast cancer treatment-related lymphedema and lymphedema resource guide. Cancer 83:2775–2890, 1998.
9. Weissleder H, Schuchhard C: Lymphedema: Diagnosis and Therapy. Viavital Publishers, 2001.

# 58. MANAGEMENT OF SKIN PROBLEMS ASSOCIATED WITH LYMPHEDEMA

*James E. Tracy, MS, PT, CDP, MLD,*
*and Teresa A. Conner-Kerr, PhD, PT, CWS(D)*

**1. How does lymphedema interfere with the normal physiological processes of the skin?**

Lymphedema increases the amount of fluid in the interstitial (extravascular) space that bathes individual cells. Normally, cells are in close approximation to capillary beds, thus allowing easy perfusion of oxygen and nutrients and concomitant elimination of metabolic by-products. The increased space between cells and capillary beds created by lymphedema severely limits oxygenation and nutrient delivery. Because of the accumulation of stagnant fluid and the interruption in normal metabolic processes, cellular necrosis occurs. In addition, lymphedema contains increased colloidal proteins that, over time, lead to stagnation of protein and fluid with the eventual fibrosis of connective tissue.

**2. What skin problems are commonly seen in patients with lymphedema?**

Common skin conditions include chronic dermatitis, cellulitis (skin inflammation and infection), hyperkeratosis (patches of roughened skin), and fibrosis (a brawny leathery appearance due to connective tissue scarring). The skin often becomes thickened, horny, or callused. Weeping of lymphatic fluid leads to a softening of the skin, thus creating an environment conducive to bacterial, yeast, and/or fungal infections. Cracks and fissures in the skin can provide a portal of entry for staphylococcal and streptococcal bacteria that thrive in the stagnant lymph fluid.

**3. How do these skin problems develop?**

When lymphatic vessels are obstructed or destroyed, they are unable to drain away microbes that colonize or penetrate the skin. The protein-rich, stagnant lymph fluid creates a perfect environment for bacteria to grow and flourish. In addition, a relative hypoxia develops in the tissues due to the increased time needed for oxygen and nutrients to perfuse across the expanded interstitial space to tissue cells.

**4. What topical applications assist in maintaining microbial balance?**

After thoroughly cleansing the skin with a mild soap or just warm water, depending on skin sensitivity, application of a nonfragrance moisturizing cream is recommended to readjust the pH of the skin and prevent overgeneration of bacteria and other microbes.

**5. What potential allergens may be contained in topical products such as moisturizing creams?**

Common skin allergens, especially in patients with swelling, include wool alcohols, balsam of Peru, fragrances, cetylsterol alcohol, parabens, benzocaine, propylene glycol, neomycin, framycetin, gentamicin, and chloramphenicol. Products containing these ingredients should be avoided if possible.

**6. How can the development of folliculitis be minimized when moisturizing creams are applied?**

Always apply the cream from proximal to distal in longitudinal strokes so that the cream follows the downward orientation of extremity hair. Avoid rubbing the cream into the skin using techniques such as circular motions. Circular motions can predispose hair follicles to irritation because the cream is rubbed into the follicular openings.

**7. Which cancerous conditions are associated with chronic lymphedema?**

Lymphangiosarcoma is a form of cancer that sometimes develops in patients with chronic lymphedema. It usually presents with the appearance of purple-red patches or bumps on the skin of the involved limb and is often fatal. Control of lymphedema and prevention of chronic tissue infections can help in the prevention of this fatal condition.

**8. How do I address treatment of lymphedema in patients with skin conditions related to radiation?**

Many patients with lymphedema have undergone or are undergoing radiation therapy while being treated for lymphedema. The skin effects are usually localized and depend on the area treated, the volume of tissue irradiated, and individual skin differences. Unstable scars after radiation therapy make the tissue ischemic, susceptible to injury, and prone to breakdown. Lymphedema treatment can continue in such patients, but caution should be used over areas that are fragile or hypersensitive. When treating with manual lymphatic drainage, the therapist should try to direct the lymph flow around the involved area. In doing so, the fragile skin is protected while lymphatic drainage is augmented. If at any time during the treatment, the patient complains of pain, treatment should be terminated.

**9. How does radiation affect the skin?**

Radiation not only targets cancer cells but is detrimental to highly proliferative normal skin cells in the lower strata of the epidermis. Ionizing radiation used in cancer treatments damages DNA in the actively replicating cells of the stratum basale and spinosum of the epidermis. Skin reactions to radiation include erythema, dry desquamation, and moist desquamation. Erythema is characterized by a reddening of the skin with increased temperatures. Erythematous reactions usually occur after an accumulated dose of 2,000 centiGrays (cGy) or after approximately 10 treatment sessions. However, a milder form of this reaction has been noted after 24 hours.

Dry desquamation is usually seen after 3–4 weeks of radiation therapy or a total dose of 4,000 cGy. This reaction is described as a drying of the skin with scaling and peeling of the epidermal layers. It often presents with significant pruritus that requires topical corticosteroid therapy with agents such as 0.1% triamcinolone acetonide (Kenalog). The skin becomes scaly and thickened in appearance if new skin cells are generated faster than older damaged cells can be shed. On the other hand, if new cells are not generated quickly enough to replace dying and damaged cells, the skin looks thin and atrophied.

Moist desquamation of the skin is a more severe reaction to radiation therapy and results in ulceration. The skin is erythematous with serous exudate. Moist desquamation usually appears after 5–6 weeks of radiation therapy or with a total exposure level of 5,000 cGy. Moist wound dressings are beneficial in preventing infection and facilitating healing.

**10. What interventions are commonly recommended for irradiated skin?**

*Moisturize, moisturize, and moisturize some more.* Maintaining skin integrity is important for patients who have undergone radiation therapy. Moisturizing is recommended for maintenance of skin health, pain relief, and prevention of infection. Moisturizers should be selected that do not contain metals, alcohols, deodorants, perfumes, or talcum powder. These agents can be irritating to the skin as well as slow the radioactive particles delivered during treatment, thus producing a more severe reaction in the skin. Alternative deodorant products are available for women receiving radiation therapy to the axilla that do not irritate the skin or interact with the radiation particles. These include herbal deodorants and deodorant stones.

**11. What particular moisturizing agents are recommended for irradiated skin?**

Hydrophilic or water-based lubricants are recommended such as Aquaphor, Eucerin, or Lubriderm. They can easily be washed off without causing excessive skin trauma and are readily absorbed by the skin. Hydrophobic products are not recommended because they are difficult to remove and may result in skin damage due to scrubbing. In addition, the residue left on the skin after using a hydrophobic agent may interfere with radiation treatment.

**12. What dressings are appropriate for irradiated skin lesions?**

As with other types of wounds or skin lesions, no one dressing is appropriate for every situation. Dry wounds benefit from hydrogel dressings, with care taken to prevent periwound maceration. Because of their associated lowering of skin temperature, hydrogel dressings are thought to relieve pain related to inflammation. Edematous wounds benefit from topical corticosteroids and absorptive dressings. Topical antibiotics such as silver sulfadiazine (SSD, Silvadene) have also been used for bacterial control.

**13. What other interventions are useful in decreasing trauma to irradiated skin?**
Patients who have undergone radiation therapy should be instructed to use gentle, mild soaps for bathing treated areas as well as to avoid scrubbing these areas during cleansing. The areas should be patted dry, not rubbed with a towel. Affected areas should not be shaved or exposed to excessive heat or cold. Ultraviolet protectants, loose clothing, and a hat prevent exposure to direct sunlight. Loose cotton clothing is recommended to prevent heat build-up, and bras should be avoided in women with open lesions.

## BIBLIOGRAPHY

1. Belcher AE, Selekof J: Skin care for the oncology patient. In Chronic Wound Care: A Clinical Source Book for Healthcare Professionals, 3rd ed. Wayne, PA, HMP Communications, 2001, pp 711–720.
2. Korinko A, Yurick, A: Maintaining skin integrity. Am J Nurs 97(2):40–44, 1997.
3. Macdonald JM: Wound healing and lymphedema: A new look at an old problem. Ostomy Wound Manage 47(4):52–57, 2001.
4. Sibbald RG, Cameron J: Dermatological aspects of wound care. In Krasner DL, Rodeheaver GT, Sibbald RG (eds): Chronic Wound Care: A Clinical Source Book for Healthcare Professionals, 3rd ed. Wayne, PA, HMP Communications, 2001, pp 273–285.
5. Swirsky J, Nannery DS: Coping with Lymphedema. Garden City Park, NY, Aspen, 1998, pp 14–16.

# 59. EVALUATING WOUND THERAPIES

*Catherine T. Milne, APRN, MSN, CS, CWOCN, ANP,*
*Heather R. Hamilton, MPT, and Ashley E. Webb, MPT*

### 1. How should we evaluate outcomes of wound therapies?

Unfortunately, the "outcome" by which we evaluate therapy has the tendency to be experiential rather than scientific. A wound therapy may work on one or two patients (experiential), but will it work for the next patient or the next 50 or 100 patients? Evaluation on this basis is scientific. In experiential wound therapy evaluation, how often do we try a wound care treatment on a second patient if it failed with the first? In scientific wound therapy evaluation, we are more likely to try again if the body of knowledge behind the therapy is theoretically sound, the studies are well designed, and outcomes are statistically significant.

After evaluating a wound therapy on the basis of science, address the "art," which includes the clinician decision to use a certain therapy based on individual patient assessment, intended goal of therapy, reimbursement challenges, availability of therapy, setting in which the therapy will be given, and the skill set of professional caregivers and significant others.

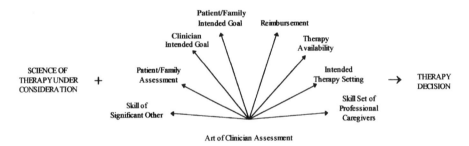

Decision elements in choosing wound therapy.

### 2. What is meant by the "science behind therapy"?

Science is the evidence that a therapy works.

### 3. Where can one find the scientific data?

Several sources should be consulted, including results from clinical trials, product inserts, clinical practice guidelines, material safety data sheets, and independent laboratory data.

### 4. Do the marketing materials in journals or distributed at trade shows or by sales representative summarize the scientific data?

Yes and no. Marketing materials are intended is to sell the product. Depending on the company, the product, and at whom the material is aimed, all unbiased scientific data may be promoted or none at all. Although most of this material is helpful, it should be examined with a critical eye. Ask the following questions:

1. How many patients were involved in the trials? Is this a case study of one patient, or did a large number of patients participate?

2. What were the characteristics of the patients? Was the therapy used on healthy 20 year olds or patients with characteristics similar to those for whom you are considering for this therapy? Did all patients have similar characteristics?

3. How long was the therapy used? Was it for 2 hours or 6 weeks?

4. How is outcome defined? If it is defined as "improved," what does improved mean? Ten percent healthy rate? One hundred percent healthy rate? How is healthy defined? As complete wound closure or decreased wound size?

5. Was the product evaluated in a randomized, double-blind trial, or is the evaluation a patient or clinician testimonial?

6. Besides the therapy in question, what other interventions were used at the same time? How do they confound results? Ask about nutrition, support surfaces, use of compression, and other therapies that may have contributed to the success or failure of the item in question.

7. Does the scientific theory make physiologic sense? Does the therapy support current knowledge of the physiology of wound healing? If so, in what stage? A good example of this concept is the old antacid and heat lamp treatment for an open wound. Although popular at one time, the practice fell out of favor when greater knowledge of wound healing physiology (moist wound healing) was disseminated.

8. What side effects were found? When is therapy be contraindicated?

9. How does the therapy affect pain? Activities of daily living? Does it have any hidden costs that may adversely affect financial status, such as electricity cost or need for building renovation?

### 5. Are you saying that marketing materials are unreliable?

Not at all. Let the buyer beware. It is amazing that the same healthcare professional who asks detailed questions, independently researches claims. and is the biggest skeptic when buying a used car or insurance chooses therapy for a patient based on the sales representative's pitch, the pens, doughnuts, or candy distributed, or glitzy marketing material. The same level of diligence should be applied to wound therapies.

### 6. So a case study with one patient is not good?

Science needs to start somewhere. A single case study is one way to develop a basis for further evaluation and perhaps lead to a new gold standard.

### 7. Are clinical practice guidelines (CPGs) helpful?

CPGs are based on levels of evidence to assist the professional in making clinical decisions. CPGs are developed through government initiatives and professional organizations. Typically, a review of the scientific literature and a consensus of expert opinion are the basis of CPG development. Most CPGs are presented by a graded recommendation:

**Level A:** Evidence supported by many (usually more than five) well-designed, randomized, controlled trials.

**Level B:** Evidence supported by some (usually less than five) well-designed, randomized, controlled trials.

**Level C:** No well-designed scientific studies support the recommendation, but it is advocated by expert opinion.

### 8. What is the value of a level C recommendation?

Many interventions cannot be studied in a randomized, controlled fashion; therefore, a level A grading can never be obtained. A good example is an intervention that does not allow access to pain medication. Another example is a study in which too many variables must be controlled, such as those contributing to tissue tolerance.

### 9. What are the limitations to CPGs?

CPGs are not static; they should change. New science is added daily that may change a level C recommendation to level A or a level A recommendation to a level C (or perhaps to a level that is no longer supported). When evaluating a CPG, determine when it was last updated.

### 10. What commonly accessed web sites are available to view CPGs?

By no means an exhaustive list, the following web sites are a great way to begin the search.
- www.update-software.com/cochrane/cochrane-frame.html
- www.guidelines.gov
- www.medmatrix.org/spages/practice_guidelines.asp

- www.wocn.org
- www.ncbi.nlm.nih.gov (Medline search)
- www.herts.ac.uk/lis/subjects/health/ebm.htm

**11. Summarize the hierarchy in the strength of evidence for evaluating a new or existing therapy.**
From least to most scientific, each level of the pyramid adds to the scientific base of a new or existing therapy.

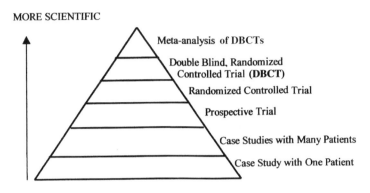

Hierarchy of evidence.

**12. How can this hierarchy can be applied in clinical practice?**
When approached by a vendor trying to sell you on a product, it becomes important to distinguish valid and useful products from products irrelevant to your immediate needs. Here are three tips to help rate the information that you hear and read.
- **Product information.** Check for important red flags, specific sources used by the company, and comparisons to see whether the information is objective and in accordance with other published data.

*Red Flags in Product Literature*

---

Claims of miraculous improvements over previous products
Nonscientific rationale for product development
No references cited from the literature
No anecdotal citations from the field
Limited company contact information
No consideration of troubleshooting assistance after purchase
No trial products or samples available
Warranties and guarantees that are not well defined or lacking altogether

---

- **Vendor oration.** Always have specific questions ready if this is a product that you think may be useful.
- **Technical assistance:** If you read the literature and are unsure of some treatment/product parameters, contacting technical assistance will put you in touch with someone who can answer your questions.

If you are familiar with the product and desire to try it out in your practice setting, be prepared with specific questions for the sales representative. This two-way dialog can be extremely informative. Even if you do not have access to the representative and have the product information in hand, technical assistance is readily available by phone, fax, or e-mail. If you are clueless about what is being presented, you may not know the right questions to ask. In such cases, it helps to know some general rules of thumb about the evaluation of research and the meaning of evidence-based practice.

### 13. Give an example of how to evaluate a new product.

Maura, an occupational therapist, has just been to a regional meeting and is intrigued by a new splinting product offered by a savvy vendor. She deals with pediatric burn patients on a regular basis but uses only the materials with which she was taught. Maura decides to be a diligent student again and spend the weekend in the library, finding out all the relevant information to pass along to her supervisor in the hope of incorporating this new splinting product into the clinic. What should be Maura's first strategy to locate good information? The library is the right place to be, but it can be daunting to initiate an extensive search, especially if you have logged few hours doing so. It is useful to start with general information to become oriented to the topic.

*Tip:* For general and broad topic information, use review articles and texts

Even though Maura has product information in hand, she may feel the need to brush up on basic information. In some cases, this step is unnecessary. However, if Maura were asked to assess a diabetic oral agent to control glucose metabolism and possessed little recall about the physiology of diabetes, she would have to investigate this information further before moving to specific science articles referenced in the product information. Maura now feels comfortable with the conceptual information about this topic but knows she must produce sound scientific evidence for its use to sell the physician in charge and also to confirm her basic knowledge of the subject. How does Maura best pursue the more specific and advanced scientific information about splinting materials she seeks? The next step in the process is to go to published basic science papers that ask a specific question about the topic and attempt to answer it in the laboratory through purely experimental means.

*Tip:* Use basic science articles for first-hand experimental data and discussion.

First Maura must have the product information in hand with specific references. She should look up these references to see how extensive the quoted literature is. Maura also needs to search for other published data. The best search engine of which the author is aware is the Pubmed database (www.ncbi.nlm.gov), which shows all abstracts matching the keyword search (e.g., hard plastic splinting material, wound healing). Now it is Maura's job to sort through what comes up and read each abstract thoroughly.

*How to Spot a Good Abstract*

---

Assess whether the topic is relevant to your interests with a quick scan.

Look for basic science (actual experiment) rather than a broad-scoped review articles.

Look to see that statistical analysis has been performed on the data.

At the end of the abstract, assess whether the authors' conclusions are logical.

---

Maura has now poured through many journals discussing the science involved in the splinting material that she would like to try. She lacks one piece of information: How did the plastic perform for patients before it was approved for clinical usage? Is there any information to answer Maura's question? How can Maura rate these papers so that she can incorporate this information into an evidence-based practice? Now Maura needs to investigate clinical trials of the product. At this point, it is most important to be able to weed out good scientific design. If the design is poor, the author can misinterpret or manipulate the study's results. Therefore, you should be able to critically rate the trial set-up, the measures used, the statistical interpretation and the logical discussion at the end of such an article.

*Tip:* Use clinical trial articles for information bridging scientific rationale with clinical efficacy of the treatment

*Criteria for Rating a Research Article*

---

Does the study have clinical relevance?

Is the background information well thought out, logical, relevant to the current study, and cited from reputable sources?

Are the purpose and hypotheses of the study clearly stated and logical?

---

*Table continued on following page*

*Criteria for Rating a Research Article (Continued)*

Is the experimental design of good quality?
• Appropriate sample number
• Statistical tools used
• Randomization

Have all parameters of the study been fully reported fully through statistical analysis?

Have the authors made logical conclusions from the reported data?

After listening to the speaker at the conference and conducting her own extensive literature review, Maura is encouraged about this treatment and wants to incorporate its use into the burn clinic at which she is employed. Maura now has to determine the most effective way to meet that goal.

**14.  What would be an effective means for introducing the splinting material into the clinic?**
The first option is to contact the company that markets the splinting material. Most companies have local contacts who will be eager to come to the clinic and give an inservice demonstration of their product. If that option is not available, you may want to consider formulating and conducting an inservice demonstration yourself. You can use the information offered at the conference and your own literature review.

**15.  What key considerations need to be addressed before successful incorporation of the product into the clinic?**
One factor is cost effectiveness. For a given patient population, this factor compares the current with the new treatment option. Furthermore, if the new treatment costs more for implementation, is the initial cost counterbalanced by shorter treatment times and more positive short-term and long-term outcomes vs. the current treatment for the same patient population?
Another factor is the specific guidelines for usage of the product. These guidelines should include appropriate patient population, contraindications, precautions, and potential side effects. Although these guidelines may already be established, health care providers will have to be educated about the rationale and maintenance of these guidelines. They will also need extensive training in the proper administration of the material. This point is extremely important, because improper usage can significantly alter the outcomes of treatment. A representative from the company marketing the new product would be extremely helpful at this stage to ensure proper education and training.

**16.  What about patient's rights?**
As with all treatments, current or new, every patient should be well informed. It is the patient's right to be aware of every aspect of treatment before it is initiated. Education should include appropriate patient population, contraindications, precautions, and side effects. Other areas to address, especially for a new treatment or product, are outcomes from clinical trials and references for the patient to read. Maura may even make copies of her own literature for the patient. Patient education ensures cooperation and compliance.

**17.  If the new product does not have the same positive findings reported in clinical research studies and the most current literature, what is the next step?**
Consider the possibility that inappropriate administration of the product may be the cause of the negative outcomes. Possible reasons include misinterpretation of guidelines for appropriate patient population, contraindications, and precautions. It is also possible that the administration instructions are not being appropriately followed. At this point it may be necessary to conduct another inservice demonstration to ensure that these issues are addressed. A sales representative should be present to address the current situation and to ensure correct and appropriate treatment.

**18. Despite re-education and correct administration of the material, the treatment still does not have a positive outcome. What should be done next?**

At this point consideration should be taken to the possibility that the treatment may not result in the same clinical outcomes demonstrated in clinical trials. It becomes your ethical responsibility to report your clinical findings through the appropriate channels and to the appropriate people. First of all, contact the specific company that markets the product and let them know of your findings. Consider creating your own literature report. If the correct documentation has been performed throughout the term that your patients received this therapy, you can compile the data needed to create such a report. After writing the article, submit it to an appropriate scientific journal. Considering the fact that this is a new treatment on the market, acceptance of professionally written, specific clinical outcome reports about its use should be readily accepted for publication, even if the outcomes of using the material are negative.

**19. If the treatment works well for the appropriate patient population, how can you become involved in promoting its use?**

The plan of action is similar for both situations. First, contact the company that markets the product and let them know of your success. The company may even request for specific data about your use of the product and use the information for its promotion. You can also write-up a case report, compiling the data obtained through patient notes and formulating this information into a report that can be submitted to a scientific journal. Finally, you can conduct inservice demonstrations for local clinics similar to the one at which you are employed, promoting the use of the specific treatment for the indicated patient population.

## BIBLIOGRAPHY

1. Bolton L: Clinical studies and product evaluation: How to maximize their value. Ostomy Wound Manage 41(7A Suppl):88S–95S, 1995.
2. Bolton L, Van Rijwijk L, Shiffer FA: Quality wound care equals cost-effective wound care: A clinical model. Adv Wound Care 10(4):33–38, 1997.
3. McSweeney M, Spies M, Cann CJ: Finding and evaluating clinical practice guidelines. Nurse Pract 26(9):30–47, 2001.
4. Ovington L: Wound care products: How to choose. Adv Skin Wound Care 14(5):259–264, 2001.
5. Roe B, Moore KN: Utilization of incontinence clinical practice guidelines. J Wound Ostomy Contin Nurs 28(6):297–304, 2001.

# 60. HAVING A WOUND: PATIENT AND CAREGIVER VIEWS

*Gail and Jim Fitzpatrick*

**1. After 18 months of wound care for several pressure ulcers that occurred after your car accident, what is most memorable to you?**

We had no idea how serious wounds could be. They can kill you. We also know that nurses can do a lot for you at home and that nurses are responsible for curing ulcers—through hands-on care, by teaching us about the wounds and good wound care, and by getting the other professionals whom we need, such as the dietitian, plastic surgeon, and physical therapist. When we needed another doctor, we asked the nurses' advice. They kept up with the new stuff and talked to the doctors to make it happen.

**2. Was there a lot of pain?**

Because of the paralysis, there was no pain. However, at each dressing change and each debridement we could see the muscle spasms, which were rather powerful.

**3. What treatment helped the most?**

The most important point that we learned is that a number of approaches worked. As the wound changed, we had to change wound care. We got fairly good at noticing changes, and the nurses would rework the wound care plan when the wound changed.

**4. Did the wound always change for the better?**

No. Sometimes the wounds got worse. They would become necrotic or get larger, or the drainage amount or characteristics would change, or the graft failed to take. It seemed that when a urinary tract infection or a respiratory tract infection happened, the wound got worse. In fact, the wound would get worse a few days before the illness was apparent. We learned to watch the wounds, which were a mirror of what was going on elsewhere.

**5. What treatments did you try?**

We first had an air-fluidized bed, but, despite what we were told, it didn't work. During the hot humid summer months, the beads would absorb the humidity and become solid—it was like sitting on a concrete slab! The nurses said that they had never seen anything like it. Eventually, we got a low air-loss bed. The wheel chair has a good pressure reduction seat. Physical therapy helped, too.

We also concentrated on eating properly. High protein, lots of calories, and vitamin C, zinc, and gulatamine/arginine supplementation. It seemed as if the appetite is almost nil when you need it most. The dietitian did calorie counts and gave us tips on how to get the right kinds of foods to heal the wounds. Through the home care agency, the following treatments were available: pulsatile lavage, debridement, negative pressure therapy, oxandrolone, pressure reduction, collagen—even skin grafting! We used both skin from the leg and bioengineered skin.

We were lucky. I rarely had to go to the hospital for my wounds—only for complications of the spinal cord injury. Between the plastic surgeon and all of the other health care providers, things just seemed to happen. The nurses coordinated everything.

It was strongly suggested that a diverting colostomy and muscle flap surgery be done to make the wounds heal faster. As someone who recently became paralyzed, I knew that I could not mentally deal with another insult to my body. Besides, I would have this reminder of the whole experience every time I looked at my belly. Although wound healing was not guaranteed either way, I opted for the slower way. The nurses and the doctors were very good about accepting my decision, and we really worked like a team to heal the wounds.

### 6. What do caregivers need to know?

First, I wanted to learn everything that I could. I also wanted to be an active partner in wound care, not a passive observer. I really felt that the nurses tried to teach me everything that they could. When I was overwhelmed, or tired, instructions were repeated so that I understood what was needed.

Second, I wanted to know more about wound care or that the wounds were in the early stages of getting worse or infected. Occasionally, a nurse simply would not listen to me. Caregivers should speak up and be advocates. Wound care can be learned.

Third, I was overwhelmed when Jim left the rehabilitation hospital and I had to learn so much. I did not appreciate how important it was to prevent the wounds from getting worse or how to do so, how to know what those signs and symptoms were and who to call. Within 48 hours of his being home, the wounds really got bad. I wish the rehabilitation nurses had prepared me for this.

### 7. What do patients need to know?

Probably the same things as a caregiver. The patient also should pick people who have a lot of experience in wound care. One would not go to an obstetrician to fix a broken bone. The same goes for wounds—get a team together with certified wound nurses, doctors, and physical therapists. I understand that dietitians, nurse aides, and others are not certified, but they should have some experience in these areas. New nurses or a nurses new to this area need to learn more; they should look around for a person who can train and develop them as well as read as much as possible about wounds. We learned a lot from the Internet.

### 8. What do nurses need to know?

Although Jim had no have wound pain, other people do. Pain can affect appetite, ability to turn, and ability to get better. A nurse should look for wound pain and make sure that it gets treated.

Teach...teach...teach. Treat the patient and the caregiver as you would treat your fellow nurses. We want what's best. Being treated like a partner helps a lot.

Respect our opinion. Sometimes we know more than you.

Advocate for us. Show us how to survive the maze of health care. It is a different system to us—like going to a foreign country. We don't know the language, we don't know or understand the forms that will show us the way, we have to eat different foods, we are in different beds and not sleeping well. Yes, we get cranky. We don't understand that when we want answers, the health care system seems to take forever to get them or doesn't have the answers at all. Please explain this alien environment and acknowledge how frustrating it can be.

Keep up to date with new developments. The wounds improved because the nurses knew how wounds healed and when to change the treatment. New treatments can help heal the wounds faster.

# 61. SPECIAL CONSIDERATIONS FOR HOME CARE

*Theresa M. Bachhuber,* BSN, RNC

### 1. How is the home health setting unique?

The once immediately available conveniences of code and IV teams, pharmacists and dietitians, physicians and social workers, food services and central supply, are left behind in the institution. The practitioner is left to his or her own resources and ability to improvise in the field (the patient's home). Cost containment in light of the prospective payment system (PPS) is of great concern to home care agencies, placing an added burden on the nurse to manage costs.

### 2. What is the PPS?

This method of reimbursement for patients on Medicare is similar to a diagnosis-related group (DRG) system. The home health agency receives a set amount of reimbursement for a 60-day care period to cover all agency expenses. The amount is determined by completion of an Outcome Assessment and Information Set (OASIS) form. These data place the patient in an acuity category called the Home Health Resource Group (HHRG). Fee-for-service visits no longer are the rule.

### 3. What places an agency at greater financial risk?

- High frequency of visits
- High supply use
- Use of costly supplies
- Inefficient use of staff time
- Poor clinical outcomes

### 4. List strategies that are helpful in maximizing financial and clinical outcomes with PPS.

* Code the OASIS correctly. To do so, one must understand the definitions of wound terms used in this document.
- Employ appropriate support surfaces to prevent and treat wounds.
- Develop a formulary that should cover 90% of the wound treatments used in the agency.
- Use protocols based on sound scientific practice guidelines.
- Do not be afraid to use adjunctive strategies or expensive dressings. Often the wound healing can be accomplished faster. Up-front costs are more, but savings are achieved through staff efficiency, fewer visits, and improved healing rates.
- Use wound-healing tools to monitor progress and identify outliers earlier rather than later.

### 5. Where can I find definitions for wound classification terms used in the OASIS document?

Until recently, there were no uniform definitions. However, the Wound, Ostomy, and Continence Nurses (WOCN) Society recently published a document, developed by a panel of experts, that outlines the following definitions for wounds:

- Pressure ulcer (all stages)
- Fully granulating wounds
- Early/partially granulating wounds
- Nonhealing Wounds
- Classification of surgical wounds healing by primary intention

A complete glossary is also included in this document and can be obtained through Wound, Ostomy and Continence Nurses Society, 1550 South Coast Highway, Suite 201, Laguna Beach, CA 92651, or www.wocn.org.

### 6. Why do physical therapists need to be concerned with the wound care OASIS questions?

In agencies where the therapist can stand alone, therapists must be very familiar with the OASIS data set wound and lesion questions, lest the agency be penalized financially or otherwise.

**7. What can be done to save on wound care supplies in the home?**

Many supplies are bundled together in the PPS rate, making it quite costly for agencies to provide care to patients with multiple needs or complex wounds. Aggressive measures need to be taken to identify the type of wound and the most appropriate type of treatment to ensure the most efficient healing. Consulting with WOCNs about complex wounds is a sound investment for home-care providers. WOCNs quickly identify products that will decrease the frequency of visits while providing expert advice and guidance to the primary care nurse.

*Role of a WOCN in Home Care*

---

- Train staff and physicians in complex wound treatment modalities
- Consult with and mentor home care nurses and supervisors
- Provide policies and procedures related to wound care management
- Establish formularies of wound care products and equipment
- Review, revise, and design forms for assessment and documentation
- Advise about equipment purchases (e.g., camera for documenting wound progress)
- Assist in quality improvement and outcomes measurement system

---

In addition, simple measures, such as teaching the patient how to make irrigation solutions for wound, ostomy, and continence care, should be promoted. Although Dakin's solution and acetic acid are cytotoxic to wounds, some physicians still order them and cannot be swayed. It is included here. Using clean supplies quickly adds significant savings.

*Preparation of Sterile Solution*

---

1. Assemble equipment needed: glass container of appropriate size with properly fitting cover, teaspoon or tablespoon, large pan with cover.
2. Place bottle, lid, and spoon in pan. (Do not put lid on bottle.)
3. Fill pan with enough water to cover equipment, and place cover on pan.
4. Boil for 20 minutes. (Start timing when the water starts to boil.) Allow to cool with the cover on the pan.
5. When the water is cool, pour off enough water from the pan to be able to remove the bottle. Pour remaining sterile water into bottle. *Do not touch the inside of the bottle.*
6. Pick up spoon by handle. *Do not touch the bowl of the spoon.*
7. Add proper amount of substance to make solution.
8. Apply lid without touching inner rim or lip of jar.
9. Shake to mix well.
10. Put label on container indicating type of solution and date prepared. Solution is stable for 24 hours from date of preparation.

| SOLUTION | INGREDIENTS |
|---|---|
| 0.9% Normal saline | 4 cups sterile water; 2 tsp salt (iodized or noniodized table salt) |
| 0.25% Acetic acid | 5 cups sterile water; 4 tbs white distilled vinegar |
| Dakin's solution | |
| Full strength (0.50) | 1 pint sterile water; 50 ml bleach |
| Half strength (0.25) | 1 pint sterile water; 25 ml bleach |

**8. How do I decrease the manpower and inventory of running a supply closet?**

Work with a local medical supply house to be your "supply closet." Clinicians complete a requisition for each patient as supplies are needed. Requisitions are faxed to the supplier, who packages the orders per patient and delivers them to the home-care office. The supplier bills the home-care agency monthly. The agency then bills the appropriate insurance. By implementing such an arrangement, inventory is minimized to basic supplies, manpower is decreased, and dollars are saved.

**9. Why is clean technique used in the home more often than sterile technique?**
1. In the home care setting, clean technique is the standard of care and can be used unless a fresh postoperative wound or severely immunocompromised patient is involved. The patient is exposed to his or her own flora.
2. Cost is the other factor. Sterile products are much more expensive than clean products.

**10. Is there a best way to irrigate a wound at home?**
Wound irrigating systems are ideal but not always available. A hand-held shower is an inexpensive and convenient means for irrigating a wound at home. Home centers sell hand-held showers at reasonable rates. Depending on the type of shower head and its proximity to the wound, it can provide a moderate psi of pressure.

**11. How do you irrigate a wound with a windowed cast around it without getting the entire cast wet?**
Using household wax paper, create a slide by tucking the wax paper into the window, allowing it to drape over the lower and side edges of the window. At the lower end of the wax paper, place a catch basin. The basin will contain the irrigant that comes down the slide. The interior of the cast will remain dry.

**12. How long are irrigation solutions good once they are opened?**
Although no study has addressed this issue in home care, most agencies discard unused, opened solution after 7 days.

**13. What is the recommended method for disposal of wound care supplies in the home?**

*Disposal Tips for Home Health Care*

| MATERIALS | DISPOSAL |
|---|---|
| Needles, syringes, lancets | 1. Collect in a hard plastic (nonrecyclable) or metal container with screw-on lid.<br>2. Reinforce lid with heavy-duty tape.<br>3. Label "not for recycling."<br>4. Discard with regular household trash, |
| Soiled bandages, disposable pads, medical gloves | 1. Place in securely fastened plastic bag.<br>2. If saturated with blood or bloody fluids, pour in one-fourth cup of 1:10 bleach solution and double bag.<br>3. Discard in regular household trash. |

**14. Is there any means of cleaning supplies other than boiling?**
Boiling may decrease the useful life of supplies and has become passé. In the patient's own home, washing equipment in warm, soapy water and allowing to air-dry with a loose covering (e.g., paper toweling) is most effective.

**15. What types of items should I stock in my car or bag to care for patients with wound, ostomy, or continence issues?**
Gloves, saline, gauze, stoma paste, underpads, catheters, tape, and a few dressings from each of the major advanced wound care categories: hydrocolloid, transparent film, foam, alginate, and hydrogel.

**16. What do you do if you run out of transparent film dressings in the home?**
A plastic wrap (e.g., Saran Wrap) contains drainage for a short period of time. Windowpane the wrap with tape to secure it.

**17. How do I keep patient's pets away from the treatment area?**
A patient's pets are part of the family and should be recognized as such. However, during wound care or other treatments it is essential that they be kept away from the area. Educating the patient

about the potential for infection and contamination will prevent hard feelings when you suggest that Fido or Fluffy be put in another room. Bringing treats for the furry friends goes a long way too!

### 18. What can be done if the air-fluidized or high air-loss bed is leaking?

A leaking air-fluidized or high air-loss bed is an emergency. With a leak or malfunction, this category of specialty bed will become hard, dangerously increasing tissue interface pressures over bony prominences. The patient should be removed from the bed to prevent breakdown, and frequent turning and repositioning should occur until the bed is repaired. A call to the bed representative should get an immediate response.

### 19. What is the best way to prevent episodes of urinary incontinence?

The single, most effective way to prevent these episodes is through bladder training. Instruct the patient to void on a regular schedule, whether or not the urge is felt. Begin with every 1 hour and progress to every 2 hours. By getting the bladder on a regular schedule, episodes of incontinence may be minimized or eliminated. Incontinence is one of the most frequent reasons for institutionalization. This simple nursing intervention will save the patient's skin as well as health care dollars.

### 20. Are there any options for incontinence pads when insurance coverage does not pay for them?

Improvise by doing the following: In a bed or chair, line the surface with economy trash bags and cover with a towel. The towel can be washed when soiled. The plastic can be discarded.

### 21. What is an economic way to increase protein for a patient whose wound is not healing?

Assuming that you have already had a nutritional consultation and that the patient needs more protein and not just a treatment change, an inexpensive means to boost protein is to supplement the patient's diet with a homemade nutritional supplement. This supplement contains the nutritional value of many prepackaged supplements.

*Nutritional Supplement*

- 1 package Carnation Instant Breakfast
- 1–2 scoops ice cream (any flavor)
- 4–8 oz. whole milk*
- 1–2 tbs chocolate or Karo syrup†
- Fresh fruit‡

Blend together. Serve.

* Less milk if patient has difficulty with swallowing.
† Karo syrup when supplement is fruit-flavored.
‡ If using fruit, use fruit-flavored ice cream.

### BIBLIOGRAPHY

1. Ovington LG: Wound care products: How to choose. Home Healthcare Nurse 19:224–231, 2001.
2. Schema KD: Payment strategies: Home health wound services under Medicare PPS. Adv Skin Wound Care 14:74–75, 2001.
3. United States Environmental Protection Agency: Solid Waste and Emergency Response (5305W). December, 1998. www.epa.gov/osw.
4. Wound, Ostomy and Continence Nurses Society: OASIS Guidance Document. WOCN Society, Laguna Beach, CA, 2001. www.wocn.org

# 62. SPECIAL CONSIDERATIONS FOR OUTPATIENT WOUND CARE CENTERS

*Patricia J. Conwell, RN, BS, CWCN, Lisa Mikulski, RN, BSN, and Catherine T. Milne, APRN, MSN, CWOCN, CS, ANP*

**1. What defines an outpatient wound care center?**

Wound care centers are outpatient treatment centers that provide interdisciplinary and comprehensive wound treatment programs that integrate the provision of growth factors, living skin equivalents, and other advanced wound techniques, products, and services. Patients are taught to care for their wounds at home and are educated about nutrition and exercises that may aid the healing process and prevent future wounds. Patients with nonhealing wounds are taught how to care for their wounds, use specialty devices, and prevent further wounds from developing. The patient is then taught when it may be necessary to return to the wound care center. Outpatient wound care centers vary in scope and availability of advanced wound care diagnostics, dressings, protocols, staff, and ownership.

**2. What makes outpatient centers so popular?**

Marketing to patients with nonhealing wounds is very attractive. People are desperate to return to their previous quality of life. Many patients have pain. Their life is centered on a big, draining, odorous, year-old wound with expensive dressings that has shown no improvement after seeing providers with little training and knowledge in wound care.

**3. What national standards must an outpatient wound care center meet?**

No professional organization has developed standard quality criteria for wound care centers. However, all hospital-owned wound care centers must meet criteria set up by Joint Commission on Accreditation of Hospital Organizations (JCAHO), local health codes, and clinical criteria identified in contracts with third-party payors. The literature supports the use of a multidisciplinary team in improving wound healing. Data comparing outcomes of wound centers with wound specialists or other provider groups are not available but would make an interesting topic for a well-designed research study.

**4. What resources are available at the ideal wound care center?**

- **Multidisciplinary staff.** Minimal requirements include a physician, registered nurse, physical therapist, and dietician, each certified in wound care. Access to a vascular surgeon, podiatrist, dermatologist, social worker, pain management specialist, and psychiatric nurse specialist is required.
- **Availability of wound care diagnostic equipment.** Noninvasive testing equipment for the assessment of lower extremities, wound culturing, biopsies by dermopathologists, ability to test for wound healing capability, access to magnetic resonance imaging, computed tomography, and radiology procedures are essential.
- **Variety of local topical dressings.** A center that evaluates the patient and matches the dressing to the wound and holistic patient needs is promoting advanced wound care knowledge. Avoid centers that use only one or two types of local care (e.g., using wet-to-dry saline or petrolatum-based dressings for the majority of patients).
- **Adjunctive technology and therapy.** Great strides in wound care knowledge over the past decade mandate the use of adjunctive therapy based on sound clinical research. Access to these therapies is critical. Again, matching the wound care modality to the patient and not the patient to the therapy is key. Not everyone should undergo hyperbaric treatment, electrical stimulation, manual lymph drainage, surgery, or negative pressure therapy.
- **Active quality improvement (QI) and outcomes monitoring program.** Team meetings should be held on a routine basis to review cases, plan care, examine outcomes, and initiate

steps to improve care. There is a saying, "In God we trust; all others must bring data." Without data, any QI program is useless. Continuing education of staff plays a significant role in improving quality.

- **Patient and significant other involvement.** Many outpatient wound care centers have patients sign a contract agreeing to compliance with a treatment plan. Others achieve this goal by negotiating or verbal goal setting. As in all aspects of health care and nursing, the establishment of a positive patient relationship, intensive individualized teaching, and patient empowerment lead to improved outcomes.
- **Participation in wound care clinical trials.** Because wound care knowledge is rapidly expanding, so is the development of new technology, dressings, and adjunctive therapies. Current care, some without a scientific research base and the "old wives' tale" method, are undergoing rigorous clinical trials to validate their use. Patients can often benefit by participating in such studies.

### 5. How many outpatient centers meet these criteria?

No national data are available. Outpatient wound care centers vary, based on owner philosophy, financial stability. and clinician expertise and savvy. Some companies provide consultation and management of outpatient wound care centers.

### 6. How is reimbursement different in these settings?

Hospital-owned centers get reimbursed under the APC system for Medicare patients. The patient is charged separately for a facility fee and a provider fee. The patient is responsible for a percentage of each.

### 7. What does the facility fee cover?

The facility fee covers routine supplies and care by non-Medicare providers, including non-physician staff employed by the hospital.

### 8. What does a provider fee cover?

The provider fee covers the costs of services by the health care provider. The provider may include the physician and non–hospital-employed providers, such as an advanced practice nurse.

### 9. What other methods of reimbursement are available at these centers?

Services may be reimbursed through Medicaid, health maintenance organizations (HMOs), and managed-care contracts. In non–hospital-owned centers, these methods are used in addition to traditional indemnity Medicare and self-pay methods.

### 10. Do wound care centers take over the patient's care?

No. Their goal is not to usurp the primary care provider's role. Typically, these centers take responsibility for the local and adjunctive wound care. Any adjustments in the medical regimen to enhance wound healing are frequently accomplished by discussing such needs with the primary care provider. Written updates to primary care providers are helpful, facilitate good will, and provide holistic health care.

### 11. What considerations are important when the patient also receives care in other settings?

A patient who receives care from an outpatient wound care center may also receive care from a home-health agency or skilled nursing facility. Communication and coordination of the treatment plan with these settings by the wound care center is essential to improve patient outcomes. This process is time-consuming but well worth the effort. For example, the home health nurse may not visit the patient on the day of a wound care center appointment, sparing the patient an extra dressing change. Comprehensive nutritional assessments may have already been completed in the skilled nursing facility. Thus, this work-up will not need to be repeated. Other considerations should be given to reimbursement of wound care modalities, dressings, and treatment frequencies available in these settings because of conflicting priorities and financial impediments to care.

**12. What types of wounds are treated at a wound care center?**

Nonhealing wounds of any origin, such as: diabetic ulcers, venous stasis ulcers, ischemic ulcers, pressure ulcers, collagen vascular ulcers, posttrauma wounds, postsurgical wounds, wound dehiscence, and other wounds that resist healing.

## BIBLIOGRAPHY

1. Granowitz EV, Szostek R, Burns P, et al: Etiologies and outcomes of wounds in an outpatient program. J Wound Care 7(8):378–380, 1998.
2. Keyser JG: Diabetic wound healing and limb salvage in an outpatient wound care program. South Med J 86(3):311–317, 1993.
3. Salcido R: A collaborative model of wound care. Adv Wound Care 12(2):56–57, 1999.
4. Valdes AM, Angderson C, Giner JJ: A multidisciplinary, therapy-based, team approach for efficient and effective wound healing: A retrospective study. Ostomy Wound Manage 45(6):30–36, 1999.

# 63. SPECIAL CONSIDERATIONS FOR SKILLED NURSING AND SUBACUTE FACILITIES

*Janice A. Lexton, RN, BC, BSN*

### 1. What sets long-term care apart from another care environment?

The long-term care environment has been undergoing changes over the past several years. Many changes in practice have been directed at creating an environment that is less institutionalized and more like home. Nursing homes have traditionally operated under a medical model of care. Many of us who have worked in long-term care have seen a new culture change that attempts to go beyond providing excellent care. The long-term care environment focuses on the resident's individuality and unique needs. The resident is the center of all decision-making.

### 2. What is PPS?

PPS refers to the prospective payment system, which is the payment method for Medicare Part A inpatient status. As the name implies, Medicare pays prospectively to care for its beneficiaries. Each resident is assessed on admission, day 5, day 14, day 30, day 60, and day 90. Each of these assessments groups the resident into a category based on individual needs. This grouping determines how much the facility will be reimbursed until the next assessment. The reimbursement category is an all-inclusive rate, regardless of what supplies or services the facility needs to provide for the resident. This system encourages efficiency and aggressive care while providing preventive services.

### 3. How does PPS affect wound management in long-term care (LTC)?

If a resident with a wound requires a lot of staff time, supplies, and equipment, the LTC facility receives a set rate between evaluation periods. If the patient is healed anytime during that period, the facility continues to receive the higher reimbursement through the end of the time frame. At the same time, if a facility is not efficient and the resident's condition worsens, the reimbursement level will be less than the actual spending involved. The facility will incur financial losses for the remainder of the time.

### 4. How is the LTC facility reimbursed for wound care under managed care?

Reimbursement is based on acuity. The facility is reimbursed at a higher rate for a medically complex resident than for a resident who requires less care. There is no separate or additional reimbursement based exclusively on the presence of a wound.

### 5. What must facilities know to provide wound management under managed care contracts?

PPSs do not provide separate reimbursement for wound care. The facility provides the wound management for the contracted price. To remain fiscally viable, facilities that provide wound care with a managed care contract must know their costs.

### 6. What is the standard of care for pressure ulcer management in LTC?

The Pressure Ulcer Guidelines released by the Agency for Health Care Policy and Research (AHCPR) represent the standard for pressure prevention and treatment. Even though they are almost 10 years old, state surveyors and lawyers refer to these guidelines as the gold standard.

### 7. How can these guidelines be used by staff in your facility?

The Pressure Ulcer Guidelines offer recommendations for staff who assess and treat residents who are at risk for or have pressure ulcers. Regulatory agencies use these recommendations as their guideline in evaluating the effectiveness of prevention programs and management of pressure ulcers in your facility.

**8. What is the National Pressure Ulcer Advisory Panel (NPUAP)?**
It is a nonprofit organization dedicated to the prevention of pressure ulcers.

**9. How has the NPUAP been instrumental in reducing pressure ulcers?**
The NPUAP has been involved in educational and legislative activities focused on quality pa-tient care and pressure ulcer management. The Centers for Medicare and Medicaid Services (for-merly the Health Care Financing Administration) use the standards developed by the NPUAP as a basis to measure facility quality during the survey process in relation to pressure ulcers.

**10. What can a facility do to prevent residents from developing a pressure ulcer?**
On admission residents must be assessed thoroughly to identify whether they are at risk for de-veloping an ulcer. If there is a change in condition, the risk assessment should be done again to iden-tify new issues that may affect the development of a wound.

**11. What factors put a resident at risk for developing a pressure ulcer?**
Lack of follow-through when a high-risk resident is identified, improper use or lack of pressure relieving devices, lack of departmental communication to address wounds, and lack of emphasis on inservicing staff.

**12. What does adequate preventive care for pressure ulcers include?**
Preventive care includes turning and positioning, incontinence management, application of pres-sure relief devices, good skin care, and adequate nutrition and hydration.

**13. Is there a uniform instrument in LTC to assess residents?**
Through the passage of the Omnibus Budget Reconciliation Act (OBRA), all residents in LTCs must be assessed with a resident assessment instrument (RAI).

**14. What is the RAI?**
The RAI has two components: the minimum data set (MDS) and resident assessment protocols (RAPs). The MDS is the assessment component, and the RAPs identify 18 clinical areas in the MDS that require a written plan of care to be initiated.

**15. What areas in the MDS are associated with pressure ulcers and risk for pressure ulcers?**
The content areas include noting the presence or absence of a pressure ulcer. In addition, the fol-lowing 14 pressure ulcer risk factors are examined: impaired transfer or bed mobility, bedfast, hemi-plegia, quadriplegia, urinary or bowel incontinence, peripheral vascular disease, diabetes mellitus, hip fracture, weight loss, history of pressure ulcers, impaired tactile sensory perception, use of an antipsychotic medication, restraints, and lack of a skin maintenance program.

**16. What is the objective of a pressure ulcer protocol in LTC?**
The objective of a pressure ulcer protocol is to ensure the adequacy of the facility's pressure sore prevention and implementation process. Identifying risk factors on assessment, addressing these factors in the care plan, and initiating interventions consistent with the care plan are the key concepts of the RAP for pressure ulcers.

**17. How is it determined whether your facility is in compliance with pressure ulcer protocols?**
The bottom line is whether the pressure ulcer is identified by the surveyor as an avoidable or un-avoidable clinical outcome.

**18. What does it mean to be avoidable or unavoidable?**
An outcome is clinically unavoidable only in the presence of accurate assessment, adequate care plan, implementation of the care plan, and periodic evaluation of interventions, with modifications in the care plan as needed based on the resident's response to previous interventions. A large mone-tary fine is assessed against a facility if a surveyor finds that an ulcer is "avoidable."

**19. What does a state surveyor look for in regard to preventing ulcers?**

Surveyors look for aggressive preventive care for residents at risk for developing ulcers. Also under scrutiny is the consistency between the interdisciplinary team's daily charting and the MDS and plan of care. There is nothing worse than one discipline documenting "ate 100%" and another charting "poor food and fluid intake."

**20. What factors does the surveyor consider in assessing a resident who developed a pressure ulcer after admission to the facility?**

Surveyors look at whether the facility identified the resident as being at risk, whether the facility provided appropriate measures to address the resident's specific risk factors, and whether preventive measures were implemented.

**21. What factors are considered for residents who have pressure ulcers at the time of the survey, including residents readmitted from the hospital with pressure sores?**

The surveyor is concerned with whether measures to assist in healing and prevent infection were implemented. In addition, documentation must be present that appropriate interventions for wound healing were attempted. In all cases, the care plan must identify the resident's need and demonstrate whether the wound is responding to the current treatment.

**22. What key concepts are necessary for a successful wound prevention and management program in a subacute and skilled nursing care facility?**

- Education of patient and family, focusing on early detection and intervention
- A wound care committee that aggressively manages the skin integrity of residents
- A multidisciplinary approach to prevention and management of skin integrity and wounds

**23. What is one of the most important factors for staff providing care to residents who require wound care?**

The facility must identify the educational needs of the staff. The staff must be knowledgeable in wound prevention as well as treatment modalities.

**24. What should be the goals of a facility wound care committee?**

- Ensure that a resident who enters the facility without pressure ulcer does not develop one unless the clinical condition demonstrates that it was "unavoidable."
- Ensure that a resident with pressure ulcers receives the necessary treatment to promote healing, prevent infection, and prevent new sores from developing.
- Monitor trends in wound care at the facility.
- Provide a multidisciplinary forum to plan resident care.

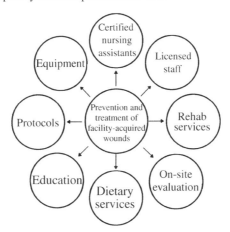

The interdisciplinary approach.

### 25. Who should be on a wound care committee?

At a minimum, the committee should include the director of nursing, infection control nurse, charge nurses, physical therapist, and dietitian. To manage and treat wounds successfully, the facility must take an interdisciplinary approach.

### 26. What role should the director of nursing play in wound care?

The director of nursing should play an active role in wound care management. Although the director's role is considered administrative, a hands-on approach is often needed for appropriate management of all skin issues in the facility.

### 27. What is a good method to identify a problem that may have a wide variety of causes?

Fishbone diagrams are useful when a team is working on a complex problem with a variety of causes. All of the causes can result in a particular problem or effect.

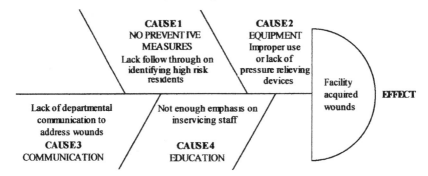

Fishbone diagram.

### 28. How does a wound care committee use a fishbone diagram?

- Draw the fishbone skeleton, and place the effect at the head.
- Brainstorm with the committee to determine four broad categories that the team believes are the major causes for the effect placed at the head of the fish.
- For each cause, ask the question, "Why?" Each reason becomes a bone on the fish.

### 29. What concept is key in approaching the issue of pressure ulcers in LTC?

The key to approaching the issue of pressure ulcers is to focus on prevention. This process starts before the resident is admitted to your facility. The facility must screen residents so that any necessary equipment and staff are in place before admission to the facility. Once the resident is admitted, interdisciplinary communication about individualized risk factors, combined with consistent implementation of risk reduction interventions and current familiarity with standards of care, decreases the resident's chance of a skin alteration.

BIBLIOGRAPHY

1. Baharestani M: Pressure ulcers in an age of managed care: A nursing perspective. Ostomy Wound Manage 45(5):18–26, 28–32, 34, 1999.
2. Castle, NG: Outcomes measurement and quality improvement in long-term care. J Healthcare Qual 21(3):21–25, 1999.
3. Fenner, SP: Developing and implementing a wound care program in long-term care. J Wound Ostomy Contin Nurs 26(5):254–260, 1999.
4. Soloway DN: Civil claims relating to pressure ulcers: A claimants' lawyer's perspective. Ostomy Wound Manage 44(2):2024, 26, 1998.
5. Turnbull GB: Update: SNF PPS and consolidated billing. Ostomy Wound Manage 45(10):12–13, 1999.
6. Xakellis GC Jr, Frantz RA, Lewis A, Harvey P: Cost-effectiveness of an intensive pressure ulcer prevention protocol in long-term care. Adv Wound Care 11(1):22–29, 1998.

# II. Ostomy

## 64. ANATOMY AND PHYSIOLOGY OF THE GASTROINTESTINAL TRACT

*Ann D. Navage, APRN, MSN, CETN, CS*

**1. What are the major parts of the gastrointestinal tract?**

The gastrointestinal (GI) tract, also known as the digestive tract, alimentary canal, or gut, may be divided into four parts:

1. The upper portion of the digestive tract consists of the mouth, esophagus, and stomach.

2. The middle portion of the digestive tract consists of the small intestine which is further divided into the duodenum, jejunum, and ileum. The small intestine is where major digestive and absorptive processes occur.

3. The lower portion of the digestive tract is made up of the large intestines, which consists of the cecum, colon, and rectum. This area's main function is storage and elimination of fecal matter.

4. An additional component of the digestive tract is the accessory structures, which include the salivary glands, liver, gallbladder, and pancreas. These structures are located outside the digestive tract; nevertheless, they contribute to the ingestion and digestion of nutrients.

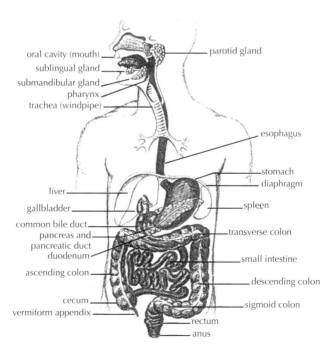

Digestive system. (From Memmler R, et al: Structure and Function of the Human Body. Philadelphia, Lippincott. 1996, with permission).

**2. What are the functions of the GI tract?**

The GI tract has six essential functions: ingestion, digestion, absorption and storage of food and nutrients, elimination of wastes, and regulation of fluid and electrolyte balance within the body.

**3. Describe the histologic composition of the digestive tract.**

The digestive tract is made up of four tissue layers:

1. **Mucosa** (the innermost layer). This layer has multiple mucus-secreting glands that lubricate and protect the inner surface of the digestive tract. If injury occurs to this layer, the mucosa has regenerative capabilities that allow the tissue to heal rapidly without the development of scar tissue.

2. **Submucosa.** This layer is made up of connective tissue, blood vessels, lymphatic tissue, nerve tissue, and structures that secrete digestive enzymes. The nerve fibers within this layer are known as Meissner's plexus.

3. **Muscularis.** The third layer consists of two layers of smooth muscle. An inner layer of circular muscle and an outer layer of longitudinal muscle facilitate movement within the GI tract. The Auerbach plexus is located between these muscle layers. The Auerbach and Meissner plexus are jointly known as the intramural plexus or enteric nervous system. The intramural plexus is primarily responsible for intestinal secretion and motility.

4. **Serosa** (the outermost layer). Also known as the adventitia, this layer forms the peritoneum. The peritoneal membrane is composed of a layer of squamous cells that rests on connective tissue. If the squamous cells are inflamed or disturbed by infection and/or surgery, adhesions (fibrous bands of scar tissue) may form and affect the normal function of the intestinal tract. The serosa lacks mucus-secreting glands. Exposure of the serosa to air results in an inflammatory response, eventual necrosis, and sloughing of the serosal layer. This phenomenon is commonly seen when a patient requires fecal diversion and a nonmatured abdominal stoma is created.

**4. What is the peritoneal cavity?**

The peritoneal cavity is the space formed between the parietal peritoneum and the visceral peritoneum. The parietal peritoneum is loosely attached to the abdominal wall, and the visceral peritoneum covers the abdominal organs. Both are made of connective tissue and are separated by a thin layer of serous fluid. This fluid prevents friction between the abdominal structures. In certain pathologic conditions, this fluid can increase in volume and causes a condition known as ascites.

**5. What is the significance of the mesentery?**

The mesentery is a double fold of peritoneum that encloses and supports the abdominal organs. It is shaped like a fan, encircling most of the small intestine and anchoring it to the posterior abdominal wall. The mesentery is vital because it contains blood vessels, lymphatics and nerve fibers that supply and innervate the intestine. The greater omentum, or fatty apron, is the part of the mesentery that extends from the greater curvature of the stomach to the transverse colon and the posterior abdominal wall. The lesser omentum extends between the stomach and the liver.

**6. What are the functions of the stomach?**

1. It is a reservoir for ingested nutrients.

2. It digests proteins by hydrochloric acid (HCl) released from the parietal cells. Proteins are broken down into pepsinogen and pepsin.

3. It secretes intrinsic factor through the parietal cells. The intrinsic factor is essential for the absorption of vitamin $B_{12}$ by the ileum.

4. It absorbs carbohydrates, alcohol and medications on a very limited basis.

5. Lastly, it protects against most ingested bacteria through acid pH.

**7. How long is the small intestine?**

The small intestine forms the middle portion of the digestive tract. In adults, the small intestine is approximately 22 feet long. This tubular organ extends from the pyloric sphincter to the beginning of the large intestine. Approximately 1 inch in diameter, it contains the four layers of tissue common to the GI tract.

**8.  What are the parts of the small intestine?**

The small intestine consists of three subdivisions:duodenum, jejunum, and ileum. The duodenum is an immobile C-shaped segment, measuring 10 inches in length and lying in the retroperitoneal cavity. Although the duodenum is the shortest of the small intestine subdivisions, it has two important features. The bile duct and the main pancreatic duct unite in the wall of the duodenum to form the hepatopancreatic ampulla or ampulla of Vater. The entry of bile and pancreatic juice is controlled by a muscular valve known as the hepatopancreatic sphincter or sphincter of Oddi.

The jejunum is the middle subdivision. It is approximately 8 feet long, $1^1/_2$ inches wide, and extends to the ileum. Although the entire small intestine is the primary organ for digestion and absorption of food substances, it is the jejunum where most of the proteins, fats, and vitamins are absorbed, along with any residual carbohydrates.

The final subdivision of the small intestine is the ileum, which is about 12 feet in length, 1 inch in diameter, and extends to the junction of the colon at the ileocecal valve. The ileocecal valve has a one way mechanism that regulates the emptying of the small intestine into the colon; it prevents reflux of intestinal contents back into the small intestine.

**9.  Is there an easy way to remember the length of each of the small intestine sections?**

An easy way to remember the overall length of the small intestine or each component is to recall the War of 1812—1 for the duodenum, 8 for the jejunum, and 12 for the ileum.

**10.  What are the major functions of the small intestine?**

1.  Completes digestion of food
2.  Absorption of nutrients
3.  Secretion of hormones that regulate the flow of bile, pancreatic juice and other intestinal secretions

**11.  What role does the ileum play in vitamin $B_{12}$ absorption?**

The terminal ileum contains the only receptor sites for the absorption of the intrinsic factor vitamin $B_{12}$ complex and bile salts. A person is placed at risk for developing pernicious anemia if this area is surgically resected. Lifelong replacement with vitamin $B_{12}$ injections is required to prevent this development. Patients may also develop fat intolerance and weight loss secondary to the inability of bile salts being reabsorbed by the ileum.

**12.  Define malabsorption syndrome.**

Malabsorption syndrome describes a group of symptoms resulting from the inability of the small intestines to absorb nutrients properly. The symptoms of malabsorption are anorexia, weight loss, anemia, diarrhea, abdominal bloating, weakness, fatigue, and vitamin deficiencies. It may occur in the following contexts: surgical removal of a portion or portions of the small intestine, interference with the production and release of bile secondary to liver disease, enzyme deficiencies due to cystic fibrosis and other genetic conditions, obstruction of the lymphatics by tumor formation, or celiac disease resulting in flattening of the microvilli in response to a substance found in grains called gluten. People with ostomies who have had surgical resection of the small intestine may have malabsorption if a large portion of the small intestine is removed.

**13.  How large is the large intestine?**

The large intestine forms the lower portion of the digestive tract. It measures approximately 5 feet in length. Its interior diameter ranges from 1 inch, where it joins the ileocecal valve, to $2^1/_2$ inches in diameter. It narrows again at the anal canal.

**14.  What are the parts of the large intestine?**

Parts of the large intestine include the cecum, colon, rectum, and anal canal. The cecum is a dilated, pouch-like structure that lies slightly lower than the ileocecal valve. The appendix is a closed-end, narrow tube that hangs from the cecum. It has no digestive function but contains lymphatic tissue to help the body resist infection. The colon consists of four parts:

1. The **ascending colon** begins with the cecum; it extends upward along the right side of the abdominal cavity to a point just below the liver. It turns to the left at the hepatic flexure, also known as the right colonic flexure.

2. The **transverse colon** extends across the abdomen from right to left. It is the longest and most mobile part of the large intestine and is held in position by the mesentery. On the body's left side, near the spleen, the colon turns downward to form the descending colon. This point, known as the splenic flexure, is often called the left colic flexure.

3. The **descending colon** extends down the left side of the abdominal cavity to the top of the pelvis. At this point, the colon forms an S-shaped curve and becomes the sigmoid colon.

4. The **sigmoid colon** is the distal end of the large intestine and terminates in the rectum. This region, which has a high incidence of bowel cancer, may necessitate colostomy.

The rectum is attached to the sacrum by the peritoneum; it extends about 5 cm below the end of the coccyx to become the anal canal.

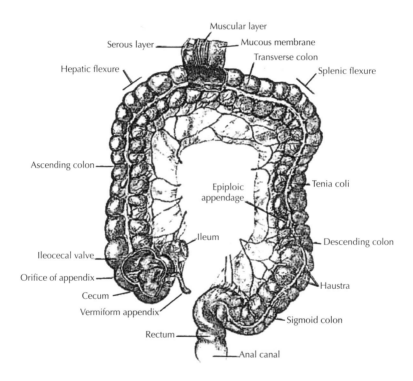

Parts of large intestine (anterior view). (From Hole J: Human Anatomy and Physiology. Dubuque; William C. Brown Publishers, 1993, with permission.)

### 15. What is the importance of the dentate line within the anal canal?

The dentate or pectinate line is the midpoint of the anal canal. It is recognized as a reference point because the tissues above and below are different in color, type, and nerve innervation.

Proximal to the dentate line, tissues of the rectum narrow to form longitudinal folds, known as the columns of Morgagni. This area is lined with columnar epithelium and has a deep purple color secondary to the internal hemorrhoidal plexus. The epithelium is innervated via autonomic nerves. This area is insensitive to tactile and painful stimuli. Distal to the dentate line, squamous epithelium lines the anal canal. The change from columnar to squamous epithelium lining of the anal canal is gradual. This area is commonly called the transition zone or cloacogenic zone. The anal mucosa is pink and very sensitive. Its innervation can differentiate between gas, liquids, and solid stool. Identification of the dentate line is important if surgical resection of this area is needed. If a patient is to have a continent ostomy, such as the ileal pouch anal anastomosis (IPAA), then the anastomosis is performed above the distal component of the dentate line to preserve anal sphincter control and allow successful continence.

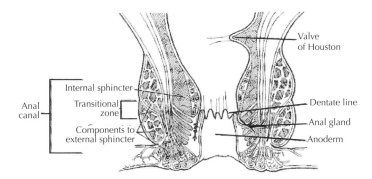

Anal canal. (From Hampton B Bryant R: Ostomies and Continent Diversions—Nursing Management. St Louis, Mosby, 1992, with permission).

### 16. What is the difference between the internal sphincter muscle and the external sphincter muscle of the anus?

These two sets of sphincter muscles allow the anus to remain closed except during defecation. The internal anal sphincter is composed of smooth (involuntary) muscle. The external anal sphincter is made up of striated (voluntary) muscle. The external anal sphincter is often affected by neurologic disorders that render the person fecally incontinent.

### 17. What are the major functions of the large intestine?

1. Absorption of water, sodium and chloride
2. Volume reduction of chyme
3. Production of vitamin K and some of the B-complex vitamins
4. Fecal matter formation
5. Fecal elimination

### 18. What is the difference between the motility of the small intestine and colon?

The principal movements within the small intestine are peristalsis and segmented contractions. Peristalsis is a propulsive activity, that results from the mucosal stretching of the circular and longitudinal muscle layers when chyme enters a segment of the small intestine. Contraction of the circular muscles occurs through Meissner's plexus and motor stimulation through Auerbach's plexus. The contraction of longitudinal muscles is due to the action of serotonin and acetylcholine. This action results in emptying of an intestinal segment.

Segmented contractions are alternating movements of the circular muscle fibers. This movement facilitates the absorption process by bringing the chyme into contact with digestive secretions and the villi. Not surprisingly, these actions are also called mixing contractions.

Within the large intestine, two processes transport ingested food. The first is a process known as haustral churning. As food passes into the ascending colon, it accumulates in the proximal haustrum, distending the ascending colon. The colon walls contract and move the food contents along from haustrum to haustrum. The second process consists of propulsive mass movements. Large segments of the colon contract as a unit to move the stool forward.

Typically, mass movements occur after a meal. Patients with ostomies frequently note stool in their pouch after eating. Abnormal irritation of the intestinal mucosa can also cause mass movements. People suffering from ulcerative colitis commonly experience this phenomenon.

**19. How does the peristaltic rush relate to diarrhea?**

Peristaltic rush is a powerful peristaltic wave. Its purpose is to relieve the intestine of an irritating substance. Extreme distention of an intestinal segment and/or chemical and mechanical irritation of bowel mucosa can cause a peristaltic rush. This rapid movement prevents the normal absorption of water, nutrients, and electrolytes. The end result is diarrhea. Patients with an ostomy who experience a peristaltic rush rapidly expel effluent in their pouch. This can cause seal failure due to the rapid force of expulsion and heaviness of the effluent.

**20. Of what significance are the normal flora found in the large intestine?**

The alkaline environment of the large intestine permits the growth of some common bacteria, such as *Escherichia coli, Clostridium perfringens, Lactobacillus* spp., and *Aerogenes* spp. These bacteria break down substances that have escaped the digestive enzymes. They also synthesize nutritional factors such as vitamin K, thiamin, riboflavin, vitamin $B_{12}$, folic acid, biotin, and nicotinic acid. Bacterial action also causes gas to form, which provides bulk and propels the feces through the remaining tract.

**21. How are nutrients absorbed?**

Absorption occurs along the entire length of the small intestine; most of it is completed by the time nutrients reach the ileum. Nutrients are absorbed through the mucosa, specifically through the villi by active transport. Within each villus, there is connective tissue containing blood capillaries, a lymphatic vessel called a lacteal, and nerve fibers. The mucosal epithelium of the small intestine has multiple mucus-secreting goblet cells to facilitate movement by lubricating nutrients and to protect the mucosa against irritation. Between the villi are intestinal crypts or crypts of Lieberkühn, which secrete approximately 2,000 ml of intestinal juices per day. This watery mixture contains mucus from the goblet cells and acts as a carrier for absorption of nutrients from chyme.

Digested nutrients such as simple sugars, amino acids, simple fatty acids, electrolytes, and water enter the capillary blood and flow to the portal vein of the liver. Most lipids are absorbed through the process of diffusion. They enter the lacteal area and are carried via lymphatic fluid to the blood.

**22. Where are nutrients absorbed?**

Absorption of all nutrients occurs within the small intestine, which is an ideal organ for this task. Length alone provides a huge surface area, and the mucosal lining has three structures that greatly enhance nutritional absorption:

- Plicae circulares or circular folds—deep folds in the mucosal and submucosal layers that mix chyme with intestinal juices.
- Villi—tiny, fingerlike projections of mucosa that are most numerous in the duodenum and proximal portion of the jejunum.
- Microvilli—tiny projections of the epithelial cells of each villus. They resemble a fine brush and increase the absorptive surface. Because of their fuzzy appearance, they are commonly called the brush border.

**23. How does the GI system receive its blood supply?**

The GI system receives approximately one-third of the body's cardiac output. The blood supply to structures within the abdominal cavity is called the splanchnic circulation. Superior and inferior mesenteric arteries and celiac arteries supply the stomach, small and large intestine, pancreas, and gallbladder. However, the duodenum is supplied with blood carried by the hepatic artery. The liver is a unique organ with a dual blood supply, receiving blood from one artery and one vein. The majority of the liver's blood flow is through the portal vein, which is rich in nutrients; the hepatic artery supplies oxygenated blood to the liver cells.

Venous drainage of the digestive system goes through the superior and inferior mesenteric veins and splenic and gastric veins to empty into the portal system. If hypovolemia occurs, the GI system suffers a devastating insult. Poor perfusion results in mucosal ischemia and eventual necrosis. Once necrosis occurs, the GI tract does not have an effective barrier against bacteria, leading to peritonitis and possible sepsis.

**24. How do the sympathetic and parasympathetic impulses affect the digestive tract?**

Branches of the sympathetic and parasympathetic divisions of the autonomic nervous system innervate the digestive tract. These nerve fibers generally innervate the muscular layer, maintain muscle tone, and regulate the strength, rate, and speed of muscle contractions. Parasympathetic impulses increase the digestive activities by stimulating GI secretions and motility, whereas sympathetic impulses inhibit various digestive actions.

**25. What two types of secretions are found within the digestive tract?**

**Mucus secretions** produced by goblet cells are found throughout the entire length of the GI tract. For this reason, people who have an ileal conduit or other urinary diversion using part of the ileum have mucous shreds in their urine. Patients need to be aware of this fact and not to confuse this normal secretion with the presence of pus. The mucus secretions protect and lubricate the walls of the digestive tract.

**Digestive secretions** are produced in the mouth, stomach, duodenum and jejunum. These secretions are often called enzymes. They break down digested nutrients for absorption.

**26. Why does lactose intolerance occur?**

Lactose intolerance occurs when there are insufficient quantities of the lactase enzyme to break down lactose (milk sugar) within the small intestine. Lactose from milk and milk products remains undigested and causes an increase in osmotic pressure. Water is drawn into the intestinal tract from body tissues. Additionally, intestinal bacteria act upon the undigested sugar and produce gas. Common symptoms are bloating, intestinal cramps, increased flatus, and diarrhea. In people with an ostomy and concomitant lactose intolerance, the consumption of lactose-containing products may cause excessive gas to build up in the pouch. This requires frequent release of the gas to avoid unnecessary tension on the pouch adhesive seal.

**27. What are the major effects of aging on the GI system?**

1. Changes in the ability to digest and absorb foods result from a decrease in the secretion of digestive enzymes and bile.

2. Atrophy of the gastric mucosa causes a decrease in hydrochloric acid secretion.

3. A decrease in bile secretion impairs absorption of fats and water-soluble vitamins such as A, D, E, and K. This leads to weight loss, altered calcium metabolism, and possible bleeding disorders secondary to inadequate vitamin K synthesis.

4. Decreases in peristalsis within the large intestine coupled with a reduction in abdominal wall muscle tone and strength cause a diminished ability to defecate and increase the incidence of constipation.

5. Ingestion difficulties due to tooth loss, gum disease, dryness of mucus membranes, and salivary gland secretions contribute to swallowing difficulties and diminished taste.

## BIBLIOGRAPHY

1. Black J, Matassarin-Jacobs E: Medical-Surgical Nursing—Clinical Management for Continuity of Care. Philadelphia, W.B. Saunders, 1997.
2. Doughty D: Urinary and Fecal Incontinence—Nursing Management. St. Louis, Mosby, 2000.
3. Guyton A, Hall J: Textbook of Medical Physiology. Philadelphia, W.B. Saunders, 1996.
4. Hampton B, Bryant R: Ostomies and Continent Diversions—Nursing Management. St. Louis, Mosby, 1992.
5. Hole J: Human Anatomy and Physiology. Dubuque, William C. Brown Publishing, 1993.
6. Marieb E: Human Anatomy and Physiology. Menlo Park CA, Benjamin Cummings Publishing, 2001.
7. Memmler R, et al: Structure and Function of the Human Body. Philadelphia, Lippincott, 1996.
8. Porth C: Pathophysiology—Concepts of Altered Health States. Philadelphia, Lippincott, 1998.
9. Thibodeau G, Patton K: Human Body in Health and Disease. St. Louis, Mosby, 1992.
10. Thompson J, et al: Mosby's Clinical Nursing. St. Louis, Mosby, 1997.

# 65. ANATOMY AND PHYSIOLOGY OF THE GENITOURINARY TRACT

*Ann D. Navage*, APRN, MSN, CETN, CS

### 1. What are the parts of the genitourinary system?

The male and female urinary systems are divided into two parts. The upper urinary tract consists of two kidneys and two ureters. The lower urinary tract consists of the bladder and the urethra. The male urinary system also includes organs of male reproduction: the prostate, scrotum, testes, epididymis, vas deferens, spermatic cord, seminal vesicles, and penis.

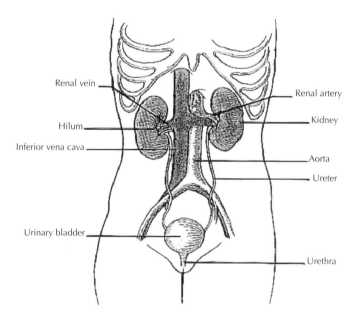

Urinary system. (From Hole J: Human Anatomy and Physiology. Dubuque; Willliam C. Brown, 1993, with permission.)

### 2. What is the major function of the genitourinary system?

The urinary system may also be called the excretory system. It functions primarily as an excretory agent to remove urine, a liquid waste containing nitrogen and salts.

### 3. What functions do the kidneys perform?

- Regulating volume and chemical composition of the blood
- Maintaining acid-base balance and balance between salts and water
- Regulating blood pressure and kidney function via renin
- Stimulating red blood cell production in bone marrow by the hormone erythropoietin
- Metabolizing vitamin D to an active form, which enables the intestinal cells to absorb calcium from the diet, keeping bones hard and strong

**4. Describe the external structure of the kidney.**

The kidneys are a pair of reddish-brown, bean-shaped organs. They lie in the retroperitoneal space against the dorsal wall of the abdominal cavity. The kidneys are positioned on both sides of the vertebral column, extending approximately from the level of the fifth thoracic vertebrae to the third lumbar vertebrae. In this location, they receive some protection from the lower part of the rib cage. The right kidney is situated slightly lower than the left kidney because of the position of the liver. Symmetrical in size and shape, the adult kidney weighs about 150 gm (5 ounces) and measures 12 cm long by 6 cm wide by 3 cm thick. Kidneys of adult females are slightly smaller than those of adult males.

The lateral surface of each kidney is convex. The medial surface is concave with a vertical cleft called the renal hilus. The hilus leads into a space within the kidney known as the renal sinus. The ureters, renal blood vessels, lymphatic tissue, and nerves enter and exit at the hilus and occupy the renal sinus.

**5. Describe the internal structures of the kidney.**

The internal anatomy of the kidney is composed of two regions:
• Renal parenchyma consisting of the renal cortex and renal medulla
• Renal pelvis

The **renal cortex** is paler in color than the rest of the kidney, granular in appearance, and composed of millions of nephrons, the basic structural and functional unit of the kidney. The **renal medulla** is a dark red-brown color and is made up of cone-shaped structures known as pyramids. The base of each pyramid lies adjacent to the cortex or periphery of the kidney, whereas the apex of each pyramid points toward the renal pelvis. Each pyramid has a striped appearance from bundles of urine-collecting tubules. The pyramids are separated from each other by extensions of cortical tissue called renal columns. Individual pyramids and surrounding renal columns form a lobe. There are approximately eight lobes per kidney.

The **renal pelvis** is a funnel-shaped tube within the renal sinus and is continuous with the ureter. The renal pelvis is divided into two or three extensions to form the major calyces which, in turn, divide into 8–14 minor calyces. These funnel-shaped extensions enclose the pyramids to collect urine and empty it into the renal pelvis.

**6. Describe the structure of a nephron.**

The nephron is the functional unit of the kidney. It is made up of the (1) the renal corpuscle, consisting of the glomerulus and glomerular capsule, commonly referred to as Bowman's capsule, and (2) the renal tubule. The renal tubule has four sections:
1. The proximal convoluted tubule
2. The loop of Henle
3. The distal convoluted tubule
4. The collecting duct, which empties into the minor calyces of the renal pelvis

**7. What is the role of the nephron?**

The major function of the nephron is to remove waste products from the blood and regulate water and electrolyte concentration within body fluids. Urine is the end product.

**8. How does the structure of the ureters contribute to their function?**

The ureters are a pair of slender tubes that convey urine from the renal pelvis of the kidneys to the bladder. They are approximately 24–30 cm (10–13 inches) long. The left ureter is slightly longer than the right because of the height of the right kidney. The ureters lie behind and below the peritoneum and follow an inverted S-shaped course. They enter the bladder at an oblique angle through the posterior bladder wall at the trigone muscle. The oblique entry of both ureters combines with pressure created by the bladder filling with urine to close the ends of the ureters and prevent backflow of urine. This point is important for the surgeon to take into account when creating a urostomy, because backflow of urine can cause hydronephrosis and damage the kidney. To help alleviate the problem with overfilling of the urostomy pouch and backflow of urine, people with urostomies are encouraged to attach the pouch to a larger bag at nighttime.

Three layers of tissue compose the ureter walls:

1. Mucosal layer (innermost layer of tissue) composed of transitional epithelial cells and continuous with the renal pelvis and bladder
2. Muscular layer, composed of two layers of smooth muscle (circular and longitudinal)
3. Outer layer, composed of fibrous connective tissue

Muscles of the ureters have the same peristaltic movement as the digestive system. The rhythmic movements of peristalsis and gravity move urine into the bladder. In patients with a urostomy, these movements propel urine into the intestinal segment that serves as a conduit to the outside of the body.

### 9. What significance does narrowing of the ureters have?

The ureters vary in diameter from 2 to 10 mm. There are three points of narrowing: (1) the ureteropelvic junction, (2) the intersection of the ureter and the iliac artery, and (3) the ureterovesical junction. These narrow segments, usually 2–4 mm wide, can be the sites of obstruction. Renal calculi or kidney stones, formed by the crystallization of calcium, magnesium or uric acid salts, can usually pass through the distendible ureter if smaller than 5 mm in diameter. Larger calculi are often the culprit of obstruction. After ostomy surgery that requires ureteral manipulation, stents are placed to prevent edema from obstructing urine flow in these narrowest of areas.

### 10. Describe the location and function of the urinary bladder.

The urinary bladder is located retroperitoneally and posterior to the symphysis pubis. It is a hollow muscular organ that acts as a temporary reservoir for urine. The size and shape of the bladder vary with its degree of fullness and with age.

### 11. How does the structure of the bladder wall contribute to its function?

The bladder wall is composed of four tissue layers: (1) mucosal, (2) submucosal, (3) muscle, and (4) serous. Transitional epithelial cells form the inner mucosal layer. The submucosal layer contains blood vessels, lymphatics, and nerves. The muscle layer is referred to as the detrusor muscle. It has three layers of involuntary smooth muscle fibers capable of great distention. Lastly, the serous layer is a fibrous connective tissue that covers the outside of the bladder, except for the superior bladder surface, which is covered by parietal peritoneum.

When the bladder is empty, its walls form into folds called rugae, similar to those of the stomach. As the bladder fills, the muscle walls expand, the rugae disappear, and the bladder becomes pear-shaped, rising in the abdominal cavity. A moderately filled bladder contains 500 ml of urine but is capable of accommodating more. The pelvic muscle floor provides the bladder primary support, and the pelvic ligaments maintain the anatomic position of the bladder.

### 12. Describe the location and function of the urethra.

The urethra extends from the urinary bladder to the external urinary meatus. The urethra is a conduit for voiding and aids in maintaining continence. The length of the urethra differs by sex. The **female urethra** is a thin-walled tube measuring 3–4 cm long and is attached to the inferior pubis by ligaments. Ligament support is essential to maintain the position of the bladder neck and urethra to prevent incontinence. The urinary meatus or orifice is anterior to the vagina and posterior to the clitoris.

The **male urethra** is approximately 20 cm long and is divided into three sections: (1) the prostatic urethra, (2) the membranous urethra, and (3) the penile or spongy urethra. The prostatic urethra extends the length of the prostate gland. The membranous urethra extends about 2 cm from the prostate gland to the beginning of the penis. This section is firmly attached and most susceptible to traumatic injury. The penile urethra is the longest section, extending 15 cm through the penis to the opening at its tip by the external urinary meatus. The male urethra also functions to deliver semen during ejaculation.

### 13. How is urine transported from the kidneys to the urinary bladder?

Urine is transported from the kidneys to the bladder via the ureters. The presence of urine in the renal pelvis of the kidney initiates peristaltic waves to force the urine through the ureters. The peristaltic waves in the ureters is directly related to the rate of urine production, which averages 1–2 ml per minute. The larger the quantity of urine produced, the more quickly it transfers to the bladder because peristaltic waves occur more frequently. Contraction of the smooth muscle fibers within the ureter walls also helps urine to flow.

### 14. Does a ureteral obstruction affect urine production?

Yes. When a ureter is obstructed, strong peristaltic waves are initiated in the proximal ureter to move the obstruction down the ureter and into the bladder. The presence of the obstruction, most commonly a renal calculus, stimulates the ureterorenal reflex. This sympathetic reflex constricts blood flow in the renal arterioles of the kidney. Urinary output by the kidney on the side of the affected ureter is reduced.

### 15. What is the normal composition of urine?

Urine is composed of 95% water and 5% dissolved solutes. The amount of the solutes is indicated by specific gravity. Specific gravity of urine can vary from 1.002 (very dilute) to 1.040 (very concentrated) compared with the specific gravity of water, which is 1.000. The dissolved solutes are nitrogenous waste products, specifically urea from the catabolic metabolism of amino acids, uric acid from the metabolism of nucleic acid, and creatinine from the metabolism of creatine. Urine pH ranges from 4.5 to 8.0. Typically, it hovers around 6, making it acidic.

Electrolytes are also found in the urine. Their concentration varies with dietary intake as well as nephron and kidney function. They are excreted to keep the blood constantly balanced. The yellow pigment known as urochrome is derived from the breakdown of hemoglobin by bilirubin or bile pigments. Urine is usually clear, and the color ranges from pale straw to amber. The greater the concentration of the urine, the deeper its color.

Abnormal constituents of urine include glucose, proteins, ketones, bile pigments, and blood cells. The presence of these substances is significant and may be an important warning of illness and helpful in diagnosis of disease.

### 16. Can urine color and odor be altered by certain foods?

Yes. Foods affect the characteristics of urine. Freshly discharged urine is mildly aromatic, but as urea metabolizes, urine takes on a distinct odor of ammonia. Some foods, such as asparagus, change the odor of urine. Other foods, such as beets, alter its color. Prescription drugs and vitamins also have the potential for altering color. People with a urostomy should be aware of this possibility, particularly if they find their urine to have an undesirable odor or sudden change in color. It is first necessary to rule out dehydration or infection as the cause.

### 17. What is a normal quantity of urinary output?

Typically, a urine output of 50–60 ml per hour is normal. Output is influenced by a number of factors, including environmental and body temperature, humidity, fluid intake, respiratory rate, and emotional stability. Output of less than 30 ml per hour, may suggest renal disease, hypovolemia, or obstruction.

### 18. What hormones influence urine volume and concentration?

Antidiuretic hormone (ADH) and aldosterone are the primary hormones that affect urine volume and concentration. The posterior lobe of the pituitary gland secretes ADH in response to stress or electrolyte or fluid imbalances. It acts on the collecting ducts of the nephron prompting reabsorption. Urine volume decreases, whereas urine solute concentration increases. Aldosterone is produced by the adrenal glands in response to stress or fluid and electrolyte imbalances. It acts on the distal tubule of the nephron, causing sodium and water reabsorption and potassium excretion.

### 19. How does the aging process affect urinary function?

The natural aging process causes a number of changes in the kidneys:
- Loss of tissue mass and decrease in size
- Loss of functioning nephrons

• Circulatory changes contributing to decreased glomerular filtration, decreased tubular reabsorption, and inability to concentrate urine

## BIBLIOGRAPHY

1. Black J, Matassarin-Jacobs E: Medical-Surgical Nursing—Clinical Management for Continuity of Care. Philadelphia, W.B. Saunders, 1997.
2. Doughty D: Urinary and Fecal Incontinence—Nursing Management. St. Louis, Mosby, 2000.
3. Guyton A, Hall J: Textbook of Medical Physiology. Philadelphia. W.B. Saunders, 1996.
4. Hampton B, Bryant R: Ostomies and Continent Diversions — Nursing Management. St. Louis, Mosby, 1992.
5. Hole J: Human Anatomy and Physiology. Dubuque, William C. Brown, 1993.
6. Marieb E: Human Anatomy and Physiology. Menlo Park, CA, Benjamin Cummings Publishing, 2001.
7. Memmler R, et al: Structure and Function of the Human Body. Philadelphia, Lippincott, 1996.
8. Porth C: Pathophysiology—Concepts of Altered Health States. Philadelphia, Lippincott, 1998.

# 66. CONDITIONS NECESSITATING AN OSTOMY

*Debra L. Dubuc*, APRN, MSN, CS, CWCN, COCN

**1. Define an ileostomy.**

An ileostomy is the surgically created bowel diversion in which the small intestine is divided at the ileum. The proximal portion of the ileum is brought through the skin surface and a stoma is created. The distal, diseased portion of the bowel is removed. Stool is expelled through the stoma and into an ostomy pouch, which needs to be worn at all times. Because this type of ostomy is relatively high in the gastrointestinal tract, the stool is liquid or soft and contains digestive enzymes that are irritating to the skin.

**2. Define colostomy.**

A colostomy is a bowel diversion in which part of the colon or large intestine is divided. The distal portion is either sutured closed or removed, depending on the reason for creating the colostomy. The proximal portion is brought to the skin surface and a stoma is created. The stool then drains from the stoma and into an ostomy pouch. Depending on where the large bowel was resected, the stool may be loose, as with an ascending colon or transverse colostomy, or formed, as with a sigmoid colostomy.

**3. Define urostomy.**

A urostomy is a surgically created urinary diversion. Various types of urostomies are discussed in detail in Chapter 67. The commonality is that all urostomies divert urine away from the bladder and empty through a stoma.

**4. Do all ostomies require that a pouch be worn to collect effluent?**

Not all ostomies require that a pouch be worn continually. Some ostomies, both bowel and urinary, are considered "continent" because they have the ability to contain the effluent. This goal is accomplished through the use of a one-way valve that is created at the time of the surgery. Such ostomies must be intubated with a catheter to drain the stool or urine. Additionally, some sigmoid colostomies, although not continent, are regulated through bowel irrigation. They may evacuate the majority of the bowel content once a day after the irrigation and require only a small dressing or stoma cap during the rest of the day. Stomal irrigation is discussed in detail in Chapter 71.

**5. What types of gastrointestinal or genitourinary problems may require ostomy surgery as part of the treatment?**

The types of problems that may include an ostomy are diseases or traumas which result in obstruction, perforation, inflammation, or neurological problems. These problems can be congenital or acquired.

**6. What types of obstructive problems necessitate a colostomy or ileostomy?**

Obstructive problems that may necessitate colostomy or ileostomy surgery include cancers or lesions that are very large or located too distally to allow for anastomosis. Such lesions may obstruct the bowel by growth from within the intestinal lumen, which limits the ability of the intestinal contents to move past the obstruction. Growths outside the intestine that put pressure on the intestine can also cause an obstruction. In this second scenario, the cancer or lesion is usually that of an adjacent organ, such as the uterus, liver, spleen, stomach, or bladder. The surgeon needs to determine whether a debulking or resection of the growth is possible without creating an ostomy or whether an ostomy is necessary. Hirschsprung's disease, a neurologic disorder, can also result in obstruction of the bowel and necessitate a colostomy or ileostomy.

**7. How does the size and location of the cancer or lesion affect the need for an ostomy?**

The size and location of the growth help to determine the best surgical procedure. If the growth involves a very low segment of the intestine or rectum, anastomosis may not be possible because there is not enough distal tissue onto which the proximal intestine can be attached. If the removal of the tumor is too near the internal rectal sphincter which would affect continence, an abdominal-perineal resection is performed and the patient will have a permanent colostomy.

If the cancer is very large or requires removal of a large portion of the colon, the patient may be left with short gut syndrome and chronic diarrhea, which can be very debilitating for the patient and are likely to cause problems with perianal skin excoriation and incontinence. For this reason, when large amounts of bowel are removed, a permanent colostomy is created. For more details about ostomy surgical procedures, refer to Chapter 67.

**8. Why do some patients with Hirschsprung's disease need a colostomy or ileostomy?**

Hirschsprung's disease is a congenital disorder affecting about 1/5000 live births with an increased prevalence in males and children with Down syndrome. Ganglionic cells are absent in the lower intestine. Most patients have an aganglionic portion of bowel involving the rectal sphincter and part of the distal bowel. About 10% of patients have an entire aganglionic bowel. This pathology results in obstruction of the intestine, gross dilation of the bowel, and toxic megacolon. The aganglionic section of the bowel is resected, but if it is too large or too low, a colostomy is necessary.

**9. What obstructive bowel problems usually do not require an ostomy as part of the treatment?**

Adhesions, large polyps, volvulus, and intussusception are usually treated with surgical modalities that do not require an ostomy.

**10. What obstructive conditions may require a urostomy?**

Obstruction from cancer or noncancerous growths is one of the leading causes of urinary diversions. Often involving the urinary bladder, obstructing growths may occur in other parts of the genitourinary tract or in adjacent organs that exert pressure on the organs of the urinary tract. Such urostomies are typically permanent. Cutaneous urostomies may be performed as a temporary measure to allow drainage of urine in obstructive conditions. Aside from tumor growth, obstruction can result from chronically dilated ureters and refluxing megaureters by impaired flow of urine.

**11. How are urinary cancers that require urostomies in children different from urinary cancers typically found in adults?**

Urinary neoplasms in children that require diversions are often rhabodomyosarcomas, which are highly malignant and have a tendency to involve local structures. If the bowel is involved, the child may also have a colostomy. Children with pelvic cancer require long-term follow-up care because radiation therapy and chemotherapy in children have late effects on growth and development. As they reach puberty, plans should be made for hormone replacement and possible restorative procedures to alleviate any sexual dysfunction.

Adults with urinary tumors may also require a urinary diversion. Bladder tumors are the most common type of urinary cancer in adults that require a urostomy, but kidney or other pelvic tumors are also possible. Bladder tumors occur more frequently in males, and the incidence increases with each decade after the age of 40. Increased bladder cancer rates have been correlated with highly industrialized urban areas and smoking. Patients with muscle-invasive bladder cancer generally have an aggressively progressing tumor. Such patients have a low 5-year survival rate, usually 40–50%, even with radical cystectomy.

**12. When does perforation of the intestine occur?**

Perforation of the intestines is another common reason for ostomy surgery. Perforation commonly occurs from trauma, ruptured diverticulitis, extensive ulcerative colitis, and fistulas. Perforation from trauma commonly includes gun shot wounds, stab wounds, and all forms of blunt trauma. Perforation from diverticulitis occurs in approximately 1–2% of cases but can carry an overall mortality rate of 20–30%. Perforation may also result from extensive ulcerative colitis. This type of perforation may result in fistula formation. Not all fistulas are managed with ostomy surgery. The creation of an ostomy is beneficial because it allows the fistula to close without the added pressure of fecal contents moving through the fistulous tract, which contributes to keeping the tract open.

### 13. Why may perforation of the intestine necessitate a colostomy or ileostomy?

When the bowel is perforated, the intestinal contents seep into the peritoneal cavity. This material contains stool, digestive enzymes, and bacteria. The bacteria cause peritonitis, resulting in the potential for abscess and fistula formation. Perforated bowel is usually inflamed and needs to be rested. If the perforation was caused by trauma, such as a knife or gunshot wound, the bowel may have sustained multiple sites of injury with extensive inflammation. The involved segment is usually removed and a temporary colostomy performed.

Ostomy surgery necessitated by intestinal perforation is often created temporarily to allow the bowel to rest. The area of damage or trauma is removed, and the proximal portion is brought to the surface to form the stoma. The distal portion is either also brought to the surface, creating a mucous fistula, or closed and left inside the abdominal cavity for future reanastomosis.

A common surgery for the creation of a temporary colostomy is Hartmann's procedure, a two-stage operation with creation of a temporary colostomy in the first stage and reversal with reanastomosis in the second stage (see Chapter 67).

### 14. Can perforation also be a cause for a urostomy?

Yes. Perforation of the bladder may require a temporary or permanent urinary diversion. Common causes of urinary perforation are typically sharp or blunt trauma.

### 15. What types of inflammatory conditions may require a colostomy or ileostomy as part of overall treatment?

- Crohn's disease
- Ulcerative colitis
- Necrotizing enterocolitis
- Ischemic bowel disease

### 16. How are Crohn's disease and ulcerative colitis different?

Although both conditions are inflammatory bowel diseases, they also have distinctive features.

*Comparison of Ulcerative Colitis and Crohn's Disease*

| ULCERATIVE COLITIS | CROHN'S DISEASE |
| --- | --- |
| Begins in rectum and progresses proximally but typically is confined to colon only | Seen in any part of the GI tract, common in terminal ileum |
| Diarrhea, often bloody and mucoid | Noncontinuous patches of pathology |
| Cramping, fever, nutritional concerns | Diarrhea, bleeding unusual |
| Ulcerations of mucosa and submucosa | Cramping, fever, nutritional concerns |
| Can cause toxic megacolon | Abscesses, fistulas, perineal ulcerations |
| Ileostomy "cures" the disease | Narrowing of intestinal lumen |
|  | Surgical resection has limited effectiveness, reserved for treating complications, with recurrence common |

Recurrence of Crohn's disease near a previously resected area occurs in as many as two-thirds of clients within 3 months of surgery. For this reason, surgical corrections are considered palliative at best. The mainstay of treatment for both ulcerative colitis and Crohn's disease focuses on controlling the inflammation with immunosuppressive agents and corticosteroids and giving antidiarrheal agents, sulfasalazine, and metronidazole, along with nutritional and emotional support.

### 17. Which other inflammatory bowel conditions are not commonly treated with ostomy surgery?

Other inflammatory bowel conditions are treated with surgical procedures other than an ostomy or nonsurgically with anti-inflammatory agents, antibiotics, and rest.
- Gastroenteritis
- Appendicitis
- Abscesses
- Anal fissures

### 18. Which inflammatory urinary conditions may be helped by urostomy surgery?
- Severe interstitial cystitis
- Urethral strictures
- Renal abscess
- Chronic pyelonephritis
- Retroperitoneal fibrosis

Patients prone to some of these disorders are even more prone to urinary tract infections after diversion surgery because of the loss of protective functions of the urethra, possible reflux of urine up the ureters, and the often chronic colonization of the urine that follows the diversion.

### 19. When may a neurologic condition necessitate ostomy surgery?

Neurogenic conditions of the bowel can cause paralytic ileus. If the ileus is chronic and results in severe problems with constipation and impaction, a colostomy may be performed. Likewise, neurogenic conditions of the bladder can cause chronic urinary retention, which can be treated with intermittent catheterization or a permanent urostomy. Some patients with impaired dexterity, such as those with high spinal cord injuries, may choose the urostomy as a more acceptable treatment option.

### 20. What neurologic conditions may be treated with ostomy surgery?

Neurologic conditions affecting the bowel that may result in a fecal diversion include Hirschsprung's disease and neurogenic bowel from spinal cord injury.

Neurologic conditions affecting the urinary system that may result in urinary diversions include neurogenic bowel from spinal cord injury, myleomeningocele, and prune-belly syndrome with hypotonic bladder.

### 21. Which congenital malformations necessitate a bowel or urinary diversion?

Some of congenital conditions may require a temporary diversion, whereas others require a permanent diversion. Congenital malformations that result in ostomy surgery are many and varied. The more common anomalies include extrophy of the bladder, posterior urethral valves, and anorectal malformation.

### 22. What determines when a temporary colostomy is reversed?

The reversal of a temporary colostomy depends on the reason that the colostomy was created in the first place. Usually, the colostomy is created to allow a diseased or inflamed section of bowel to rest and heal. Once healing has occurred, the bowel can be safely reanastomosed. Most surgeons prefer to take a conservative approach to make certain that the bowel is ready to be reanastomosed rather than reconnecting it prematurely. The time period involved depends on all of the usual factors that can delay or speed healing, including the state of the patient's overall health, the presence or absence of chronic diseases (e.g., diabetes, heart disease, malnutrition, immunologic disorders), the use of medications that may slow healing, and concurrent chemotherapy or radiation therapy. The surgeon needs to discuss the timing with the patient. Most reversal procedures occur 8–12 weeks after the temporary colostomy was created. This period may be extended indefinitely if the conditions are not conducive to a successful outcome.

**23. Are all temporary colostomies eventually reversed?**

No. Reversal may not be possible in elderly patients or patients with health concerns that make them a poor surgical risk. Additional illness after the creation of the ostomy may also make the patient a poor surgical risk, necessitating permanent status for the temporary colostomy. In other cases, the patient may opt not to have the temporary colostomy reversed. Although the reversal of the colostomy is a much less involved procedure than its original creation, some people decide that they do not wish to undergo more surgery.

**24. How is an emergent ostomy, such as occurs after a knife or gunshot wound, different from a planned ostomy, such as one created because of cancer?**

Emergent ostomy surgery has a number of negative consequences. First, the trauma did not occur under controlled conditions. The wound is contaminated by bacteria and prone to infection. The longer the period from the time of injury to the time of surgery, the more likely the wound will be contaminated.

Secondly, the amount of tissue damage caused by the trauma will be variable and may be extensive. Since the situation is a traumatic one, the patient may also have other organs damaged in addition to the intestinal injury. These injuries may be life threatening. The patient may not be in a state normally conducive to a good surgical outcome, but will need to be operated on anyway. Stabilization of all body systems will be important, with the major organs given the top priority. All of this may cause the patient to have poor healing in general.

Third, the patient will not have the benefit of having an ostomy specialist perform stoma site selection pre-operatively. The site chosen for the stoma placement will be made when the patient is in the operating room in a recumbent position. This may end up being a less than ideal because the holistic systematic assessment necessary for correct placement will not have been performed. This lack of pre-operative site selection has been correlated with increased post-operative management complications in the ostomy population.

**25. What psychological issues are involved in an emergent ostomy?**

Ostomy surgery performed as a result of trauma does not give patients time to adjust to the idea of having an ostomy. They experienced a traumatic event, went to the operating room, and awoke with a pouch on their abdomen. This makes emotional adjustment and acceptance of the ostomy more difficult. The patient who has cancer and a planned ostomy surgery may be much more in tune with the idea that the ostomy is part of a life-saving procedure in the course of removing a deadly cancer. This person is likely to be more concerned with surviving than with the loss of their normal bowel function. As the initial threat to life subsides, the cancer patient may refocus his or her concerns to living with an ostomy. For more information about emotional concerns related to ostomies, refer to Chapter 73.

**26. What is a fistula?**

Fistulas are an abnormal communication between two structures. Some fistulas are created surgically; others are a spontaneous result of injury or pathology. A fistula can be created surgically when the bowel is resected during ostomy surgery. The distal segment may be brought to the skin surface with plans for future reanastomosis. This distal segment does not expel fecal material because it is no longer attached to the food source. However, because the bowel segment retains its innervation and blood supply, it continues to act as a normal bowel with peristalsis and mucus production. Mucus may be occasionally emitted from the rectum or stoma. For this reason it is often referred to as a mucus fistula. Another type of fistula is the spontaneous, unwanted fistula that results from pathology or injury. Such fistulas can be difficult to heal and problematic to manage. Fluid and electrolytes imbalances are common. Fistulous tracts are named by identifying the anatomic sites that are abnormally connected. Examples include enterocutaneous fistulas, rectovaginal fistulas, and vesicovaginal fistulas.

Enterocutaneous fistulas, involve communication between the intestinal tract and the skin. They may drain large amounts of material that is corrosive to the skin and can result in fluid and electrolyte loss. Rectovaginal fistulas are an abnormal communication between the rectum and the vagina, and vesicovaginal fistulas allow communication between the bladder and the vagina. Patients may have more than one fistula, and multiple organs may be involved.

### 27. How are fistulas managed?

Local care centers on the management of drainage and protection of intact skin surrounding the site. Depending on the anatomic sites connecting the fistulas, cannulization with a drainage device, application of mechanical suction, or pharmacologic therapy can be used. By far, pouching is the most frequently used strategy.

### 28. Why are fistulas sometimes pouched like an ostomy?

Fistulas that drain onto the surface of the skin can be highly irritating to the skin, especially enterocutaneous fistulas, which contain enzymatic stool that is highly corrosive. To protect the skin from breakdown and to keep the patient dry and comfortable, a pouching system is often used. The pouching system may be used alone or in conjunction with suction. The skin should be prepped with a skin barrier and then the pouch applied. If the abdominal contour or fistula opening is irregular in shape, stomapaste or other adhesives help to create an effective seal. For more information about pouch application, see Chapters 68 and 69.

### BIBLIOGRAPHY

1. Colwell JC, Folkedahl B: Stoma site selection in a patient with multiple enterocutaneous fistulae. J Wound Ostomy Contin Nurs 28:113–115, 2001.
2. Davis M, Dere K, Hadley G: Options for managing an open wound with draining enterocutaneous fistula. J Wound Ostomy Contin Nurs 27:118–123, 2000.
3. Goljan EF: Pathology. Philadelphia, W.B. Saunders, 1998.
4. Hampton BG, Bryant RA: Ostomies and Continent Diversions—Nursing Management. St. Louis, Mosby, 1992.
5. Krupski T, Theodorescu D: Orthotopics neobladder following cystectomy: Indications, management and outcomes. J Wound Ostomy Contin Nurs 28:37–46, 2001.
6. McPhee SJ, Lingappa VR, Ganong WF, Lange JD (eds): Pathophysiology of Disease. New York, Lange Medical Books/McGraw-Hill, 2000.
7. Pieper B, Mikols C: Predischarge and postdischarge concerns of persons with an ostomy. J Wound Ostomy Contin Nurs 23:105-109, 1996.
8. Saibil F: Crohn's Disease and Ulcerative Colitis. New York, Firefly Books, 1997.
9. Smith DB, Johnson DE: Ostomy Care and the Cancer Patient. New York, Harcourt Brace & Jovanovich, 1986.
10. Welch JP, Cohen JL, Sardella WV, Vignati PV: Diverticular Disease—Management of the Difficult Surgical Case. Baltimore, Williams & Wilkins, 1998.

# 67.  OSTOMY SURGICAL PROCEDURES

*Janice C. Colwell, RN, MS, CWOCN*

**1.  What are the preoperative considerations for a patient undergoing a fecal or urinary diversion?**
- Stoma location and stoma creation
- Patient education related to living with a stoma
- Preoperative preparation: bowel cleansing and diet

**2.  Why is stoma location an important factor?**

A poorly located stoma can cause failure of the pouching system, resulting in leakage and peristomal skin problems. Inability to maintain a pouching system seal impedes the patient's ability to return to normal daily routines. Locating a stoma too close to the umbilicus, in an incision, or in or next to a deep abdominal crease interferes with the adhesive bond of the pouching system, causing leakage. Self-care is impeded if the stoma is not placed in an area that the patient can visualize, because problems in emptying and changing the appliance are created.

**3.  What is the ideal way to mark a patient for stoma placement?**

The ideal situation in choosing the stoma site is to assess the patient in the outpatient arena while the patient is wearing street clothes. Optimal conditions for choosing the stoma site on the abdomen include:
- Presence of 2–3 inches of flat adhesive surface
- Location in the rectus muscle
- Position in an area where the patient can visualize the stoma
- Below the belt line

To make the final site selection, the patient assumes an upright sitting position, with feet flat on the floor. The belt line is identified. It is important to differentiate between the waist and belt line, because with most men the belt line is several inches below the waist. The advantage of placing the stoma below the belt line is that the pouching system can be concealed with clothes and the weight of the pouch can be supported by underclothing.

After the belt line is identified and marked with a nonpermanent pen, the rectus muscle is identified. The rectus muscle can be visualized by asking the patient to lie down, then raise the head and shoulders off the table. The muscle can be identified by palpating the abdomen. The rectus muscle is located in a north-south orientation on each side of the umbilicus. In thin patients, the rectus muscle can often be seen. The potential for developing a peristomal hernia is lessened if the stoma is placed through the rectus muscle. The abdomen is assessed for creases and folds while the patient is in a sitting position. Ask the patient to bend forward. The chosen stoma site must allow approximately 2–3 inches of adequate adhesive surface on the abdomen, carefully avoiding deep creases and bony prominences. The preferred area for stoma siting is normally at the crest of the abdominal fold. In general, this area does not crease with weight gain or weight loss and can be visualized by the patient.

**4.  What is used to mark the stoma?**

A stoma marking disc is used to establish the best location. The plastic marking disc is held against various sites to determine whether the chosen area remains flat while the patient is bending forward and noting if the patient can see the site. The proposed stoma site is marked with a pen that will tolerate the surgical scrub. If the site is chosen more than 7 days before to surgery, the mark should be covered with a transparent dressing, which protects the mark from fading.

### 5. What important issues are related to stoma construction?

A stoma should protrude above the skin level approximately 2 cm. Such protrusion ensures that the stoma drains directly into the pouching system, which helps prevent skin problems. A stoma at skin level discharges the effluent directly on the pouching seal and can cause pouch failure. Ideally, the stoma lumen should be located straight up, directing the output directly into the pouch. These principles pertain to both fecal and urinary stomas.

### 6. What topics should be covered in planning preoperative education of the patient anticipating stoma creation?

Patients should be asked whether they would like to include a family or friend in the preoperative educational session. In this time of high stress, the support and "extra ear" that the significant other provides can be invaluable. Topics introduced in this session include the normal gastrointestinal or urinary tract functioning and surgical alterations. Description and illustration of the stoma prepare the patient for what the stoma will look like after surgery. A photograph, if appropriate, can also be used.

The patient should understand that the stoma does not have sensation when a bowel movement or urine is expelled and that a pouch is continuously worn to collect the stomal output. A stoma pouching system can be shown to the patient so that he or she can see the size and shape of a standard pouch as well as understand how it adheres to the skin and how it is emptied. Perhaps the two most frequent questions asked by patients before stoma surgery are the following:

- Will the pouch show under my clothes? Answer: It will be concealed by form-fitting underwear.
- Will I have an odor? Answer: If the pouch is correctly applied, there will be odor only when the pouch is emptied, because pouches are odor-proof.

### 7. What preoperative preparations does a patient undergo before fecal diversion?

The presurgical diet is 24–48 hours of an unlimited clear liquid diet. A bowel cleansing preparation such as GoLYTELY or Fleets Phospho-Soda is administered during the afternoon before the surgical procedure. It is also important that the patient not ingest aspirin 7–10 days before the surgery because aspirin can interfere with normal clotting.

### 8. Does the patient undergoing creation of a urostomy need a bowel prep?

Yes. The patient in whom an ileal conduit is performed will have a small bowel resection; therefore, a bowel prep is required. The patient goes on an unlimited quantity of clear liquids 24–48 hours before surgery and on the day before surgery takes Fleets Phospho-Soda. As noted previously, aspirin and aspirin-containing medications must be stopped 7–10 days prior to surgery.

### 9. How is a permanent ileostomy created?

Permanent ileostomies are less common now than a few years ago because reconstructive surgery spares the native sphincter. A permanent ileostomy may be created for treatment of Crohn's colitis, for treatment of ulcerative colitis or familial adenomatous polyposis in patients who are not candidates for a sphincter-sparing operation or, rarely, for treatment of colonic cancer. When a permanent ileostomy is created, the anus, rectum, and colon are removed (total proctocolectomy), and the end of the small intestine is brought to the skin surface and everted to create a stoma.

### 10. How is a temporary ileostomy different in its construction?

A temporary ileostomy is usually created to divert the fecal stream away from a protective anastomosis. The most common type of temporary ileostomy is a loop ileostomy. A loop of small intestine is brought to the skin, and a support bridge is temporarily secured under the loop while healing takes place. A loop ileostomy is used after the creation of an ileal pouch anal anastomosis. It may be used in the treatment of ulcerative colitis and familial adenomatous polyposis.

### 11. In what area of the colon are colostomies created?

The section of the colon used to create a colostomy depends on the purpose of the surgical intervention. The stoma is generally created proximal to the resected area or the area requiring protection. This proximal end is brought to the abdominal surface and "matured" by eversion.

Loop colostomies are most commonly created from the transverse colon, which can divert stool from the descending and sigmoid colons. Loop colostomies are created almost like a loop ileostomy. The difference, of course, is that the large intestine is brought to the surface of the abdomen. If a right-sided colonic diversion is required, a loop ileostomy is indicated.

## 12. What type of fecal stomas can be created?

An end stoma is created by dividing the bowel and suturing the proximal (also known as the functioning) end to the abdominal skin as a single opening. If the distal end of the bowel can be oversewn, the procedure is called Hartman's closure. If the distal end is brought to the skin surface and matured, the opening is called a mucus fistula (nonfunctioning proximal opening). Creation of an end stoma and a mucus fistula is called a double-barrel stoma. If the distal end of the bowel is left in its normal anatomical position, it is referred to as Hartman's pouch.

## 13. What are the options for continent fecal diversions?

The Kock continent ileostomy is made of terminal ileum and consists of an intestinal pouch serving as a reservoir for stool with an intestinal nipple valve between the pouch and the abdominal stoma. The nipple valve is surgically created using small bowel. Its function is to act like a sphincter to prevent incontinence. Patients empty the pouch periodically by intubating the stoma with a soft tube. No external pouching system is required. The patient covers the stoma with an absorbent pad. The continent ileostomy is associated with a high complication rate, related to displacement of the nipple valve, which causes involuntarily emptying of the pouch. To improve continence, the "living collar of ileum" technique wraps the ileum around the neck of the pouch. Few continent ileostomies are created because of the high rate of complications.

A continent fecal diversion, (more accurately called a restorative proctocolectomy with ileal pouch anal anastomosis) has become the treatment of choice for many patients with ulcerative colitis and familial polyposis. The ileal pouch anal anastomosis (IPAA) creates a pouch from the terminal ileum by connecting the pouch to the anus and allowing use of the sphincter muscles for continence. A temporary diverting loop ileostomy is generally created to protect the anastomosis and closed in 8–12 weeks. Once the stoma is closed, the patient can expect on average 6 stools in 24 hours. At least 50% of patients with an IPAA develop pouchitis, a mucosal inflammation of the pouch.

## 14. How is an ileal conduit type of urinary diversion created?

A segment of ileum, generally 20 cm, is resected and bowel continuity is restored. The proximal end of the ileal segment is sutured closed, and the distal end is used to create the stoma. The ureters are anastomosed to this conduit. The urine drains into and then through the piece of small intestine into an externally worn pouching system. The number of incontinent urinary diversions is decreasing because of the option for continent diversions.

## 15. What procedures create a continent urinary diversion?

A continent urinary diversion uses an internal pouch to collect urine and a stoma, which is intubated to drain the urine. The Kock pouch has been adapted from the Kock continent ileostomy procedure for use as a continent urinary diversion. Metabolic as well as nonmetabolic complications have made this procedure uncommon.

The Indiana pouch has gained popularity because of the low complication rate. It has a reservoir that is created from ileum and ascending colon, and continence is achieved by incorporating the ileocecal valve at the neck of the pouch located just under the skin. The skin level stoma is intubated periodically during the day, and a protective patch is worn over the stoma.

## 16. What are the alternatives to a urinary diversion that utilize the urinary sphincter?

The orthotopic neobladder is a newer reconstructive procedure in which a surgically constructed bladder is created from small intestine or stomach and attached to the urethra. This procedure allows the use of some of the original urinary tract, and the patient does not have a stoma. It can be offered to patients with a cancer-free trigone and urethra and a competent sphincter.

**17. After creation of a fecal diversion, what is the standard of care for abdominal assessment?**

In the immediate postoperative period, the patient has an abdominal incision, routinely closed with surgical staples. The incision should be assessed every 8 hours for signs of drainage, redness, or warmth that might indicate dehiscence or wound infection.

The stoma is assessed through the ostomy pouching system that is placed on the patient in the operating room. If a two-piece system is in place, remove the pouch to directly visualize the stoma and replace without applying pressure to the abdomen. The stoma should be a deep red and have moist, edematous tissue.

Bowel sounds, as well as flatus and stool, are absent for 24–72 hours because a paralytic ileus results from the anesthesia and bowel manipulation. The presence of bowel sounds and and the presence of flatus indicate the return of bowel function and the start of oral intake; thus bowel sounds should be assessed every 8 hours following surgery. In some cases, a nasogastric (NG) tube is used to decompress the stomach until bowel function returns. If a NG tube is needed, it is generally placed while the patient is under general anesthesia.

A closed suction drain may be placed in the abdominal space if fluid accumulation is anticipated. The drain of choice is a Jackson-Pratt (JP) drain, attached to a closed suction collection device. The drain is emptied every eight hours and remains in place until there is less than 15 cc of output in 24 hours.

A urinary catheter is routinely inserted in a patient undergoing a fecal diversion in the operating room. A distended bladder can disrupt a low anastomosis or pouch anastomosis. Thus the catheter remains in place for 1–3 days, unless impaired urinary function is anticipated.

**18. What postoperative assessment should be performed for patients who undergo urinary diversion?**

As noted above, the incision and bowel sounds should be assessed every 8 hours, and an NG tube and a JP drain may be in place. Ureteral stents (small tubes) are likely to be present in the stoma lumen. Stents are placed to protect the ureteral intestinal anastomosis and generally remain in place for 5–7 days, unless healing is delayed, or the integrity of the tissue is in question. The urine is blood-tinged for the first 24–36 hours and shows evidence of mucus threads, because the intestinal conduit sheds mucous.

Bowel function is monitored. Oral intake is started once bowel sounds and the passage of flatus are confirmed. Remember that the patient with an ileal conduit underwent a small bowel resection, which can delay the return of bowel function.

**19. Postoperative stoma assessment should include what criteria?**

- Stoma size
- Stoma mucosa: color, presence of edema, tissue turgor
- Mucocutaneous junction (place where the stoma and skin meet)
- Condition of the peristomal skin
- Presence of gas (fecal stoma) and output in pouch

**20. What postoperative complications can occur in patients undergoing urinary or fecal diversion?**

Because the gastrointestinal (GI) tract is used to create a urinary or fecal stoma, the complications that can be seen post operatively are related to GI function.

- Bowel obstruction
- High-volume stoma output
- Anastomotic leak

A bowel obstruction can result from adhesion formation or from a prolonged ileus. Treatment for a bowel obstruction can include decompression with an NG tube, decrease in the use of narcotics, bowel rest, and, as a last resort, surgical intervention.

If significant portions of the small bowel are resected or bypassed, high stoma output can result. Interventions for high stoma output include nutritional manipulation with foods that thicken the output and medications that slow transit time, allowing absorption.

An anastomotic leak can occur when the patient demonstrates an increase in abdominal pain, abdominal distention, high white blood cell count, and signs of sepsis. An anastomotic leak is generally cause for reoperation.

## 21. What are the goals in the postoperative period for a patient who has undergone stoma creation?

The primary goals in the postoperative period include:
• Pain management
• Self ostomy care
• Toleration of diet

Pain management is a critical factor in assisting the patient to achieve functional outcomes. When pain is controlled, the patient can ambulate, which speeds the return of bowel function. Respiratory complications decrease and the risk for blood clots lessens.

The patient with a new stoma must start to learn skills and procedures for self care. At the least, the patient must know how to empty the pouch at the time of discharge. It is helpful to have the patient be able to change the pouch independently.

The patient must tolerate a low residue diet and have stoma output within the normal range. Length of stay for a patient undergoing stoma creation varies, depending on the patient's overall condition and the surgical procedure. Typical length of stay in a noncomplicated patient is generally 5–7 days.

### BIBLIOGRAPHY

1. Becker JM: Indications for colectomy and choice of procedures. In Bayless TM, Hanauer SB (eds): Advanced Therapy of Inflammatory Bowel Disease. Philadelphia, Decker, Hamilton, 2001, pp 175–178.
2. Colwell JC, Gray M: An evidence based report card: What functional outcomes and complications should be taught to the patient with ulcerative colitis or familial adenomatous polyposis who undergoes an ileal pouch anal anastomosis? J Wound Ostomy Contin Nurs 28:184–189, 2001.
3. Colwell JC, Goldberg M, Carmel J: The state of the standard diversion. J Wound Ostomy Contin Nurs 28:6–17, 2001.
4. Doughty DB, Lightner DJ: Genitourinary surgical procedures. In Hampton BG, Bryant RA (eds): Ostomies and Continent Diversions. St. Louis, Mosby, 1992, pp 249–263.
5. Erwin-Toth P, Doughty D: Principles and procedures of stomal management. In Hampton BG, Bryant RA (eds): Ostomies and Continent Diversions. St. Louis, Mosby, 1992, pp 29–103.
6. Gray M, Cluff D, Johnson VY, Dixon L, Wasson D: Urinary diversions: Perspectives on nursing care. Perspectives 2:1–7, 2001.
7. McGarity WC: Gastrointestinal surgical procedures. In Hampton BG, Bryant RA (eds): Ostomies and Continent Diversions. St. Louis, Mosby, 1992, pp 349–373.
8. Wound, Ostomy and Continence Nurse's Society. Guidelines for Management: Caring for a Patient with an Ostomy. Laguna Beach, CA, Wound, Ostomy and Continence Nursing Society, 1998.

# 68. ROUTINE ASSESSMENT OF THE PATIENT WITH AN OSTOMY

*Eileen M. McCann*, RN, BSN, CWOCN

### 1. How is a stoma assessed?

Stomal assessment can be divided into two phases: the perioperative/immediate postoperative phase and the matured phase. During the immediate postoperative phase, several factors should be assessed when determining whether a stoma is healthy:

- Location
- Height
- Size
- Color
- Shape

Once a stoma has matured, it is smaller because of the resolution of postoperative edema. This point is important to remember when ordering pouching supplies, as the patient's size will change. For this reason, it is recommended that the patient recheck their size regularly and not order more supplies than needed during the initial postoperative period.

### 2. Why is stomal location important?

A poorly placed stoma causes difficulty with the patients ability to care for the ostomy and may make appliance adherence more difficult. Ideally, the stoma should not be located at the following sites:

- Within a skin fold`
- On uneven abdominal contours
- Near a bony prominence
- At the beltline

When possible, it is preferable for an ostomy specialist or someone with special training in site selection to mark the optimal location preoperatively.

### 3. How should the color of the stoma be assessed?

The color and degree of moisture of the stoma give information about the overall circulation and health of the stoma. Stomal characteristics are described below.

| APPEARANCE | SIGNIFICANCE |
|---|---|
| Red, moist | Healthy |
| Pale pink | Anemia, low hemoglobin |
| Early postoperative edema | Normal |
| Shiny, taut edema (non-postoperative) | Proximal stomal obstruction |
| Dusky dry, purple, black | Compromised circulation, ischemia |
| Dark color, history of laxative use | Melanosis coli from laxative use |

### 4. How should stoma height and shape be assessed?

Stoma height and shape are also important considerations that help determine how easy or difficult the stoma will be to maintain with a pouching system and what system is likely to work the best. An ideal stoma should look similar to a rose bud. It should protrude 2–3 cm from the abdominal wall to form a round, budded shape. The appliance can then easily form a seal around the base of the stoma. A flush stoma, (one that exits at skin level) encourages effluent to leak beneath the appliance and undermine the seal, causing skin irritation. Excessively protruding stomas are susceptible to trauma and are also emotionally upsetting to the patient.

### 5. Why is stoma size important?

In assessing the size of the stoma, proper measurement is important. A stoma measuring guide, provided by the pouching equipment manufacturer, should be used for accurate stomal measurement in inches or millimeters. This provides consistency with equipment sizes and ordering. Stomal measurement should be performed at the base of the stoma.

### 6. What are the characteristics of the ideal stoma?

Ideally, a healthy stoma should be round and beefy red. The stoma should be located on a smooth portion of the abdomen, away from belt lines, bony prominences, suture lines, and the umbilicus. The mucosa should have a moist quality, and the stoma should protrude as discussed previously. The opening should be located in the center of the stoma. If the stoma looks like the one described here, a heart-felt "thank you" to the person who selected the site and the surgeon is definitely in order.

### 7. What determines the type of effluent from the stoma?

The type of effluent from the stoma relates to the type of stoma and the section of bowel involved.

### 8. What are the typical characteristics of normal ileostomy effluent?

Ileostomy output can usually be seen by 24–48 hours postoperatively, and is initially viscous and greenish. As bowel function begins to return, the output from an ileostomy is high, often between 1000 and 1800 cc per day, because of removal of the colon being removed and the decrease in intestinal absorptive surface. Gradually the small intestine compensates and the output decreases. Normalized ileostomy output has a pasty consistency and is medium brown in color. The average amount to be expected is 500–800 ml per day.

### 9. Describe the typical characteristics of normal colostomy effluent.

Colostomy output can vary, depending on the location of the stoma within the colon. Because the main functions of the colon are to store stool and absorb water and nutrients, distal stomas (those closest to the rectum) produce thicker stool.

- Cecostomies may have projectile output because of their proximity to the ileocecal valve and have watery consistency.
- Transverse colostomies initially have watery output, which later becomes softer and pasty.
- Descending/sigmoid colostomies initially expel only light serous output and flatus. Stool output usually begins 4–5 days postoperatively. It may be pasty at first, then gradually thickens and may even have a formed stool quality. Once regulated, the patient may even return to preoperative elimination pattern.

### 10. What are the typical characteristics of normal urostomy output?

A urinary stoma can be expected to begin expelling urine immediately after surgery. Blood-tinged urine is a normal occurrence in the immediate postoperative phase. Gradually, the bleeding subsides, and clear straw-colored urine is expected from a urinary stoma. If a piece of ileum or other intestine is used in creation of the urostomy, mucus shreds are to be expected in the effluent because of the natural mucus-producing cells that line the small intestine. They should not be misinterpreted as infection or pus.

### 11. Summarize normal gastrointestinal/genitourinary stomal output.

**Gastrointestinal stomal output** is influenced by the amount of bowel resected, the location of the stoma in the bowel segment involved, medication, activity, and diet. Gradually over several months in the postoperative period, the bowel adapts and increases its absorption capacity. The volume of output decreases, and the consistency becomes thicker.

In a **urinary stoma**, urine output begins immediately after surgery is initially bloody. Gradually the urine output becomes straw-colored and clear with mucus shreds.

### 12. Besides the characteristics of the stoma, what else should be assessed?

Peristomal skin, postoperative complications, client's ability to perform self-care, and psychosocial adjustment to having an ostomy.

### 13. Describe the characteristics of healthy peristomal skin.

Normal peristomal skin should be clean, dry and intact with good turgor. There should be little or no difference between the peristomal skin and the remainder of the healthy abdominal skin.

### 14. What should peristomal skin assessment include?

1. Mucocutaneous suture line (also called the mucocutaneous junction), where the stoma is sutured to the abdominal skin. There should be no redness or erythema. Sutures may be noted and are usually self-dissolving. The edges should be well approximated around the base of the entire stoma without any separation.

2. Quality of peristomal skin: should be clean, without erythema, ulceration, rashes, blisters, denudation, or excoriation.

### 15. What kind of routine postoperative course can the patient with an ostomy expect?

Patients undergoing ostomy surgery are susceptible to the same complications as any patient facing major abdominal surgery and should be monitored for potential postoperative complications:

- Shock
- Hemorrhage
- Thrombophlebitis
- Pulmonary embolus
- Respiratory problems
- Paralytic ileus
- Wound infection
- Intra-abdominal complications
- Pain
- Psychological and emotional problems

In addition, the patient may experience stomal complications related to the particular type of ostomy surgery performed. The typical patient can look forward to successful rehabilitation and gradual return to normal daily activity. Often patients experiencing the debilitation of chronic illness preoperatively, as from ulcerative colitis or Crohn's disease, feel much better and experience a dramatic improvement in lifestyle. Patients can expect that, as their physical condition in the immediate postoperative period gradually improves, they will be progressively instructed in caring for the ostomy.

Ostomy patients need encouragement, support, and counseling to deal successfully with the alteration in body image. A multidisciplinary approach provides the most comprehensive care. The nurse provides ostomy care and instructs the patient in self-care. An enterostomal therapist or ostomy specialist can help the primary care nurse to determine an appropriate pouching system for the patient. The specialist also helps to reinforce learning of self care and provides counseling and continuity as the client gradually adjusts to the stoma and a new lifestyle.

Pain management and comfort in the initial postoperative period should be maximized for avoidance of complications. This approach provides a smooth postoperative course and facilitates the patient's ability to learn.

### 16. With shorter hospital stays, how can all of the necessary self-care be learned before the patient is discharged?

In the current health care environment, shorter hospital stays are the norm. Because of the limited time that the client is in the hospital, it is often not practical or feasible to teach every aspect of self-care management. Additionally, some issues are likely to come up only after the patient is discharged and has returned to normal routine. Home care or subacute rehabilitation often is needed to reinforce the teaching that began during hospitalization. It is important to provide close outpatient follow-up and supervision for ostomy patients during the first 6–8 weeks after surgery. During this time, the stoma routinely shrinks, requiring adjustments in stoma sizing. This also gives patients the opportunity to ask questions and obtain reassurance as they gradually adjust to an ostomy with the goal of returning to normal daily activity.

### BIBLIOGRAPHY

1. Francini A, Cola B, Stevens PJ: Atlas of Stomal Pathology. New York, Raven Press, 1983.
2. Hampton BG, Bryant RA: Ostomies and Continent Diversions—Nursing Management. St. Louis, Mosby, 1983.
3. Broadwell DC, Jackson BS: Principles of Ostomy Care. St. Louis, Mosby, 1982.
4. Hampton BG: Distinguishing among ostomy architectures and assessment findings: A primer for nurses. Progress Devel Ostomy Wound Care 4(4):3–12, 1992.

# 69. OSTOMY EQUIPMENT AND SELECTION CRITERIA

Paula Erwin-Toth, MSN, RN, ET, CWOCN, CNS

### 1. Is there much difference in ostomy equipment?

Absolutely. We are fortunate to have so many options that allow us to individualize the equipment and accessories for people with ostomies. In the early years of modern ostomy surgery, equipment was bulky and complex to assemble and manage. Variety was lacking, limiting the ability to individualize the product to the patient's needs. Skin protection was practically nonexistent and odor management, archaic. Modern ostomy equipment provides superb skin protection. Disposable equipment is lightweight and odor-proof. Accessory products range from skin barrier strips and washers to specially designed panties. The variety of sizes and features makes pouch selection both challenging and fun.

### 2. Summarize the differences in ostomy equipment.

*Pouch Options for Ostomies*

| PRODUCT | RATIONALE FOR USE | EXAMPLES |
|---|---|---|
| **Pouch system** | | |
| One-piece | Simple, minimal dexterity, personal preference | All manufacturers |
| Two-piece | Wafer and pouch may be changed at different times; can assess the stoma easier; personal preference | All manufacturers |
| **Wafer adhesive** | | |
| Gentle | Irritated, fragile skin postoperatively | ConvaTec Gentle Touch Hollister SoftFlex Barrier |
| Standard | No exceptional needs | All manufacturers |
| Extra strong | Better adherence, extended wear time | ConvaTec Durahesive and Durahesive Plus Hollister Flextend Barrier |
| Non-adhesive | Irritated skin, adhesive allergies | Cook–VPI Nonadhesive system |
| **Wafer contour** | | |
| Convex | Retracted stomas, soft abdomen | All manufacturers |
| Flat Standard | | All manufacturers |
| Low profile | Added discretion, personal preference | Coloplast Assura Ostomy System Hollister New Image Cymed-Micro Skin |
| **Wafer type** | | |
| Custom cut | Irregular shape of stoma, oval stoma | All manufacturers |
| Precut | Dexterity or visual problems, round stoma | All manufacturers |
| **Wafer flexibility** | | |
| Firm, less flexible | Soft abdomen | Most manufacturers |
| Soft, flexible | Creased or contoured abdomens | ConvaTec Flexible Wafer Hollister Contour I Cymed-Micro Skin |

*Table continued on following page*

*Pouch Options for Ostomies (Continued)*

| PRODUCT | RATIONALE FOR USE | EXAMPLES |
|---|---|---|
| **Flange** | | |
| Regular | Standard | All manufacturers |
| Floating | Tender or postoperative abdomens | Hollister CenterPoint Lock |
| | | Hollister Guardian 2-Piece |
| Locking | Added security | Coloplast Assura Ostomy System |
| | | ConvaTec AutoLock |
| | | Hollister Centerpoint Lock |
| **Pouch volume** | | |
| Large capacity | High-volume effluent | Smith & Nephew-Bongort Max-E Pouch |
| Small capacity | Pediatric, sports, intimacy | Coloplast Small Pouch |
| | | Coloplast Mini Pouch |
| | | Coloplast Pediatric Pouch |
| | | ConvaTec Mini Pouch |
| | | ConvaTec Little Ones |
| | | Hollister Mini-Pouch |
| | | Smith & Nephew-Bongort Pediatric Pouch |
| **Stoma caps** | Covers stoma when no effluent is expected | Coloplast Stoma Cap |
| | | ConvaTec One-Piece Cap |
| | | Hollister Contour 1 Cap |
| **Pouch material** | | |
| Transparent | Easy visibility of effluent and stoma | All manufacturers |
| Opaque | Added discretion | All manufacturers |
| Decorative | Individualization, fun | OPAC Ostomy Pouch Covers |
| | | Options Ostomy Support Barrier |
| Fabric-like | Less perspiration; reduces plastic irritation | Coloplast Assura System |
| | | Cymed Comfort Backing |
| | | Hollister Contour I with Comfort Wear Panel |
| | | Marlen Pouches |
| Odor filter | Increased odor control | All manufacturers |
| **Pouch closure** | | |
| Closed end | Sigmoid colostomies, small volume effluent, intimacy | All manufacturers |
| Drainable | Standard | All manufacturers |
| Spout | Urostomy | All manufacturers |

### 3. What is the difference between one-piece and two-piece ostomy systems?

In **one-piece pouch,** the skin barrier and pouch are sealed together. The backing cover is removed to expose the specially designed skin adhesive and then applied to the abdomen.

A **two-piece system** has a separate flange, also known as a wafer, with a skin barrier. The pouch secures by snapping onto the flange. The flange is applied to the abdomen first, and the pouch is then snapped on. This system gives the user the option of changing pouches between flange changes. Both systems are available in cut-to-fit or precut openings.

### 4. Explain cut-to-fit and pre-cut.

Cut-to-fit and pre-cut are the types of openings in the adhesive wafer. Both come in a variety of sizes. Ostomy patients who have a round stoma are able to get a good fit with the precut openings, which may be easier for people with limited dexterity or visual problems. If the stoma is oval or irregularly shaped, the precut type does not provide a good fit. In this instance, the wafer should be custom-cut to match the stoma (cut-to-fit).

**5. What are the other features of a two-piece system?**

Two additional features available in the two-piece system are the floating flange and the locking flange. With a floating flange, the wafer and pouch are attached so that the patients can get their fingers under the flange. The ability to have the flange "float" means that less pressure is applied directly onto the abdomen to snap the pieces together. This method of attachment is easier and more gentle for tender or postoperative abdomens. Various manufacturers have incorporated the locking flange into their appliances. The flange "locks" onto the pouch with a snap of the mechanism, ensuring extra protection from accidental dislodgment.

**6. What other features are available in ostomy wafers?**

Additional choices include the flexibility of the wafer and the strength of adhesives in the wafer. Some wafers are soft, flexible, firm, convex, and even low profile for added discretion. There are also different adhesives. Some wafers have extra-strong and long-lasting adhesion, whereas others have extra-gentle adhesives for patients who may not be able to tolerate stronger adhesion. For ostomates who react to adhesives or have irritated skin, totally nonadhesive appliance systems are available. These systems use an ostomy belt and a silicone ring to achieve control and prevent leakage (see Chapter 70).

**7. What different features are available in ostomy pouches?**

Transparent ostomy pouches allow easy visibility to help determine when to empty, whereas opaque pouches offer added discretion. The materials used to make the pouch may be the typical plastic material or have a more fabric-like quality. Some contain odor filters built into the pouch; others do not. Pouches also come in different sizes; larger pouches accommodate high-volume effluent, whereas smaller sizes can be better fitted for pediatric ostomates.

**8. How is the right product selected?**

The variety of products available for the ostomate has never been better. There is a product designed to meet essentially every need. For those who may be confused by the large selection, an ostomy specialist or enterostomal therapist can help make recommendations to individualize the product choices to the ostomate's preferences and needs.

**9. What is the difference between pouches used for a urinary stoma and a fecal stoma?**

The main difference is the manner in which the pouch is emptied. Fecal stomas, especially those with thinner, stool-like ileostomies, need a pouch with an opening in the bottom to allow the stool to drain out the bottom; hence the term *drainable*. The pouch is secured at the bottom between emptying with a closure clip or clamp. A closed end pouch is sometimes used for patients with thick, formed stool such as these with descending or sigmoid colostomies. It can also be a nice option for people with thinner stool to wear during intimacy, swimming, or traveling.

A urinary stoma, such as an ileal conduit, produces urine with mucus shreds. Urostomy pouches have a spout on the bottom that can be opened to drain the urine. The spout also comes with a connector allowing the person to attach the pouch to a leg bag or bedside drainage bag.

**10. What is convexity?**

Convexity refers to an approach which an insert is added into the pouch or flange or integrated into the wafer system to place downward pressure in the peristomal region. The bowl-shaped configuration helps to make the stoma protrude outward. Convexity is useful in people with flushed or retracted stomas to minimize leakage. It is also helpful for those with soft abdomens or peristomal creases. Convexity is available in shallow, medium, and deep convexity, with a firm or flexible base. Cut-to-fit, customized, and presized systems offer numerous options for people needing convexity to provide maximum pouching security (see question 2).

**11. Are special pouches available to manage large or irregular stomas and fistulae or draining wounds?**

Yes. Specially designed large pouches allow access to the stoma, fistula or wound bed through an access window. This window can be opened between pouch changes to examine or administer treatments. The bottom of the pouch can be attached to constant drainage, or, if the output is thicker, the drainage spout can be cut off and the pouch closure clamp applied.

**12. Describe the nonadhesive pouch system.**

Nonadhesive pouches are designed to secure to the abdomen with a ring-and-belt system. These systems accommodate large fluid volume by spreading the fluid weight across the body. The largest pouch that fits the body from hip to hip point is recommended. The system is held in place by use of a silicone O-ring and an ostomy belt. The proper belt tension is important to keep the pouch secure by placing reasonable downward force on the O-ring without excessive pressure, which may be uncomfortable for the patient. Over time, typically 3–4 weeks, the belt looses its elasticity and is no longer fully functional. For this reason it is important to change the pouch and belt when the belt becomes worn. This type of system is especially helpful in people with severe peristomal skin damage or skin conditions, such as severe psoriasis, around the stoma.

Standard pouching systems can be converted to the nonadherent configuration if the increased peristomal pressure created by the ring in the adherent system is uncomfortable or not advisable. To create this effect, an additional belt gasket is attached over a one-piece Karaya ring pouch, and a standard pectin skin barrier is affixed to the adhesive side of the pouch. This allows the clinician to treat the peristomal skin condition with the prescribed topical therapy without concern over altering adhesion. The pouch is secured to the patient's abdomen using two belts. One belt rests along the waistline, and the other rests low across the hips. The belts can be removed, the dressing changed, and the same pouch and belts reapplied.

**13. What is used to keep a drainable pouch closed?**

Each company that manufactures ostomy pouches has a clamp, closure clip, or mechanism to keep the pouch closed and secure between emptying. Not all clamps work with all pouches. It is important to select a clamp appropriate for the patient's needs. In selecting a clamp, consideration should be given to the patient's manual dexterity and visual acuity. Some patients find trying the various types of clamps to be the best way to determine their capability and personal preference. Some clamps open and close much like a barrette, another closes like a bread twist tie, and another has a Velcro closure. Some clamps are straight across, and others are curved. With so many choices, patients should use actual ostomy clamps or clips and avoid other household items to seal their pouches. Paper clips and rubber bands are not advisable because paper clips can cut the pouch and rubber bands break. A spare clamp should be readily available in case of breakage or loss (such as dropping it in the toilet.)

**14. What is recommended for people with irregular skin contours or other special needs?**

A wide variety of skin barrier strips, washers, and seal and skin sealants are available to even the peristomal skin surface by filling in creases and depressions. The more even or level the peristomal area, the more likely a secure pouch seal will be achieved. Paste and adhesive strips should be used, such as one would use to caulk defects and uneven contours. Excessive use of these adhesives can cause skin irritation and should be avoided.

*Adhesive Products for Ostomies*

| PRODUCT | RATIONALE FOR USE | EXAMPLES |
|---|---|---|
| **Adhesives** | | |
| Spray adhesive | Use on wafer for added adhesion | Hollister Medical Adhesive Spray |
| Stoma paste | Fills in cracks and irregular contours for improved seal | Coloplast Ostomy Paste ConvaTec Stomahesive Paste Hollister Premium Paste |
| Stoma adhesive strips | Moldable to fill in irregular contours for improved seal, solid form easier to use with high-volume effluent | Coloplast Ostomy Strip Paste ConvaTec Stomahesive Strip Nu-Hope Skin Barrier Caulking Strips |
| Seals, rings, Karaya | Soft and flexible, fills in contours and cracks, easier to use with high volume effluent | Bard ReliaSeal Skin Barrier Adhesive Discs Coloplast Skin Barrier Rings ConvaTec Eakin Cohesive Seals Cymed-MicroDerm Washers Hollister Soft Flex Rings Hollister Karaya Paste, Rings, Powder Marlen Mounting Ring Nu-Hope Karaya Gum Powder Perma-Type Karaya Washers Adhesive Gaskets Urocare- Tracho- Foam Adhesive Disks |
| Miscellaneous adhesives | Added adhesion | Smith & Nephew Skin-Bond Cement—can Urocare- Uro-Bond II Brush-On Silicone Adhesive |
| **Adhesive removers** | Gently removes adhesive build-up | Hollister Universal Remover Wipes, Spray Smith & Nephew Uni-solve Adhesive Remover Urocare Adhesive Remover Pads |

### 15. What is a skin sealant? When is it used?

Skin sealants are products that place a protective coating over the skin to avoid mechanical trauma and to prevent lifting of the tape collar from moisture. A variety of manufactures have skin sealant products. They are available in wipes or sprays. Some products contain alcohol; caution should be exercised in applying them on denuded skin. In this case, an alcohol-free barrier should be tried. Such products are often referred to as "nonsting". If they are not available, a light dusting of skin barrier powder can be applied before putting on the skin sealant to help avoid stinging.

### 16. How is adhesive build-up avoided?

To ease the removal of adhesives, skin solvents can be used. They are available in wipes or sprays and facilitate lifting of adhesives and adhesive residue. Caution should be taken, because excessive adhesive remover build-up can create problems with adherence of the next pouch and wafer. The adhesive remover should be thoroughly washed off the skin before attempting to apply the new pouch.

*Types of Skin Sealants*

| PRODUCT | RATIONALE FOR USE | EXAMPLES |
|---|---|---|
| **Skin protection prep** | | |
| Skin prep Standard type | Seals skin, barrier to irritation, improved surface to adhere wafer; may sting; use only on intact skin. | Bard Protective Barrier Film Coloplast Medicated Protective ConvaTec Alkare Protective Barrier Wipe Kendall Preppies Skin Barrier Wipes Smith & Nephew Skin Prep-Wipes, Swabs |
| No sting | Costs more; can be used on irritated skin without stinging | 3M Cavilon No Sting Skin Barrier, Wipes, Swab, Spray Smith & Nephew No Sting Skin Prep |
| Skin barrier wafer | Solid barrier to protect skin | Coloplast Skin Barrier ConvaTec Stomahesive Skin Wafer Hollister Skin Barrier Blankets Hollister HolliHesive Skin Barrier |
| Skin protective powder | Dries skin and protects | ConvaTec Stomahesive Powder Hollister Premium Powder |

### 17. What special equipment is needed for ostomates who irrigate?

People with descending or sigmoid colostomies may be candidates for management of ostomies with irrigation. An irrigation cone, sleeve, and bag are needed for an effective and safe procedure. This equipment is available wherever the ostomate buys ostomy supplies. Once they achieve success with this method, ostomates may elect to wear a stoma cap or small closed end pouch to collect mucus or seepage between irrigations.

### 18. What special equipment is needed for people with continent diversions?

People with continent fecal diversions require a catheter with lumen and diameter large enough to accommodate thin to pasty stool with food particles. A 28- or 30-French catheter with a bullet tip is best. The catheter has to be stiff enough to allow passage into the nipple valve but not so stiff as to risk perforation of the valve or pouch.

For people with continent urostomies a smaller catheter is used. Because continent diversions can produce a significant amount of mucus, the catheter must be large enough to allow the mucous and urine to pass easily. A 12– to 16-French straight or coude tip catheter is recommended. A water-soluble lubricant is needed to ease passage of the catheter into the stoma.

Some clinicians advise daily irrigation or flushing of the pouch with water or normal saline to remove any fecal material or excessive mucus that remains in the pouch. An irrigation syringe with a plunger can be used to accomplish this task. It is important to avoid excess pressure or overfilling of the internal pouch. Patients are advised to avoid aspiration of the contents, which may traumatize the wall of the pouch.

Because continent stomas still produce mucus, some type of stoma dressing needs to be worn. A stoma cap or continent stoma patch offers absorption, and many are waterproof. This is a good option for active people involved in exercise or water sports.

### 19. What other accessories are available for people with ostomies?

Numerous products offer both practical and fun additions to the ostomy product portfolio. Pouch covers can be useful to absorb perspiration as well as enhance coping with body image changes. They are available in a variety of materials and sizes from standard white, beige or lace, leopard, and cartoon characters. Specially designed panties, support belts, and swimwear round out the accessory selection.

### 20. Do all insurance companies pay for ostomy supplies?

The coverage for ostomy supplies usually falls under the prosthetic device or durable medical equipment clause of an insurance policy. Companies and even policies within the same company differ on coverage. Medicare Part B covers 80% of the allowable amount for ostomy supplies. The limit on the maximum allowable was increased in October 2000. The maximum number of flanges and pouches was increased from 10 to 20 per month, and the maximum number of closed-end pouches was increased from 30 to 60 per month. For people requiring more than the allowable number of supplies, a letter of medical necessity must be written and signed by the physician to petition for additional coverage.

For people on Medicare receiving skilled home nursing care, supplies are covered as part of the skilled visit. The essential ostomy supplies must be provided to the patient by the home care agency. An order placed by the patient to an outside durable medical equipment provider will not be covered by Medicare as long as the patient is receiving skilled nursing visits—even if the reason for the skilled nursing visit is not related to the ostomy or ostomy care.

### 21. Where can patients purchase their supplies?

At present, the best place to purchase ostomy equipment is through a durable medical equipment company. Some larger or specialized pharmacies may carry a limited selection of equipment or be willing to order supplies for regular customers. Mail order and discount catalogs offer a wide selection of products. Some companies bill insurance and accept Medicare assignment; others do not.

A listing of companies can be found in the *United Ostomy Association Magazine* and annual product listings in professional ostomy journals. In addition, many of the resources available for both purchasing products and obtaining information are listed in Appendix A. Products, services, and support offer a wide range of opportunities to help people with stomas lead a normal, active life.

### BIBLIOGRAPHY

1. Erwin-Toth P, Doughty D: Principles and procedures of stomal management. In Hampton B, Bryant R: Ostomies and Continent Diversions—Nursing Management. St. Louis, Mosby, 1992, pp 29–103.
2. Goldstein B, Goldstein A: Practical Dermatology. Mosby, St. Louis, 1992.
3. Hampton B: Peristomal and stomal complications. In Hampton B, Bryant R: Ostomies and Continent Diversions—Nursing Management. St. Louis, Mosby, 1992, pp 105–128.
4. Jeffers C, MacKay AT: Improving stomal management in the low vision patient. J Wound Ostomy Contin Nurs 24:302–310, 1997.
5. Lavery I, Erwin-Toth P: Stomal therapy. In MacKeighan J, Cataldo P (eds): Intestinal Stomas Principles and Management. St. Louis, Quality Medical Publishing, 1993, pp 60–84.
6. Rolstad BS, Boarini J: Principles and techniques in the use of convexity. Ostomy Wound Manage 42:24–26, 28–34, 1996.

# 70. NONADHESIVE OSTOMY SYSTEMS

*Gerald J. French*

### 1. When should a nonadhesive ostomy system be used?

A nonadhesive system can be used for any patient with an ostomy. In patients with a history of allergies to adhesive products, this system should be a first-line consideration before trying a conventional ostomy wafer. In addition, a nonadhesive system is helpful in cases of uncontrolled leakage and irritation despite best care practices. On a temporary basis, it can be used as a pouching alternative to allow the severely excoriated peristomal skin to heal.

### 2. How is the nonadhesive pouch system applied?

Put the silicone O-ring around the stoma, snap it into the flange on the pouch, and secure the pouch with a belt.

### 3. The belt and O-ring design seems to go against current trends in pouch attachment. Why return to belts?

Adhesives are not for everyone, and certainly, many pouch systems still use belts. In the VPI system (Cook Wound/Ostomy/Continence, Inc., Spencer, IN), the belt is an integral part that provides elastic support and down force to allow the O-ring to seal and support the fluid weight of the pouch.

### 4. No other pouching system has the shape and size of a VPI system. Why was it designed this way?

The VPI system consists of a silicone O-ring, a pouch, and a belt. With the VPI system, use the largest pouch that fits the body, hip point to hip point. The pouch shape has three basic functions:

1. It allows larger fluid volume, which is less likely to overflow.

2. It supports the belt design by spreading the fluid weight across the body and onto the buttons, not onto the seal.

3. It provides a more natural appearance compared with typical one-sided pouches.

### 5. Three to four weeks seems like a long time to use a pouch. What about odor?

Under normal circumstances, the daily cleaning of the pouch eliminates the odor problem.

### 6. Can the belt be too tight?

Yes. The belt buttons are positioned for proper belt tension. You need only enough tension to provide reasonable down force on the O-ring. The tension is correct when the belt is in place, and the buttons on the belt line up with the buttonholes on the pouch.

### 7. What is the right pouch size?

For day-to-day use, the best size is the pouch that reaches from hip point to hip point. A smaller pouch may be used during exercise, swimming, or other physical activity.

### 8. What can be done about perspiration?

Perspiration is more of a problem in the summer months, as with all pouch systems. Pouch covers can solve this problem, or, depending on stomal position, the pouch can be worn outside the underwear.

### 9. Do the O-rings create a problem with exposed skin?

No—the opposite occurs. The VPI system is designed for removal each day. This allows natural washing of the peristomal skin, keeping the area fresh and clean. Daily changes mean less opportunity

---

The author is Vice President of Cook Urological, Inc., and the inventor of the VPI system discussed in this chapter.

for long-term pooling of fluids on the skin. The nonadhesive aspect allows the skin to maintain epidermal integrity or to heal from earlier insults. A measuring guide is useful to order the correct size O-ring.

**10. What if the O-ring keeps popping out of the cup after the pouch has been put on?**

Check the belt position. Typically this happens with heavier patients in whom the stoma is pointed downward. The belt should be higher in the back to ensure that the belt is pulling the O-ring flat against the peristomal area.

**11. What if the O-ring seems to move left or right of the stoma?**

The usual cause is uneven belt tension. If the belt is not neutralized, it may have more tension on one side and cause the O-ring to be pulled in that direction.

**12. After a few days an indentation is created around the stoma where the O-ring lies. Is this a problem if the patient wants to return to an adhesive style pouch?**

A slight indentation forms after the VPI system has been used for a short while. It helps with positioning and sealing; however, it quickly goes away after discontinued use. It is much like the indentation on a ring finger.

**13. Can skin preps and creams be used with the VPI system?**

Yes. However, it is best to keep the management of the ostomy as uncomplicated as possible. If creams are used, they should be worked into the skin completely.

**14. What if there is a reddening around the stoma after wearing the VPI system?**

It is normal to see some reddening due to the pressure of the O-ring. There should be no blistering or peeling of skin.

**15. The VPI system seems more suited for people with trim body shapes. Can it be used on heavier people or people who are very thin?**

The VPI system will work on most anyone, but patients must pay attention to the position of the belt and O-ring. For the O-ring to work, the belt must pull the O-ring flat against the peristomal skin. The most difficult case is the very slender person, in whom the hip points protrude. In such cases, when the patient lies down, the belt can bridge the stomal area, causing leakage. Specially designed O-ring seals are available with higher profiles to assist with this problem.

**16. What about people who are physically or visually impaired?**

The application of ostomy products presents an additional challenge for physically and visually impaired people. Independence is the key issue. Because the VPI system does not rely on the accurate placement of adhesives, it can be more accommodating.

**17. What happens when the belt loses its elasticity?**

It is essential that any belt pouch system use a clean, fully functional, elastic belt. VPI pouch system are designed to be reusable for up to 3–4 weeks. When a new system is purchased, it comes with a new belt. It is suggested that the patient keep two systems and alternate them to ensure a clean, fresh belt.

### BIBLIOGRAPHY

1. Draayer E: The VPI non-adhesive ostomy system. Enterostom Thera 10(2):65–68, 1983.
2. Duffy LM, Lange PH: Evaluation of a new non-adhesive urostomy system. Urology 25:264–266, 1985.
3. Non-adhesive ostomy and incontinence products [product insert]. Cook Wound/Ostomy/Continence, Spencer, IN,1995.

# 71. ROUTINE MANAGEMENT OF THE PATIENT WITH AN OSTOMY

*Diane E. Bryant, RN, MS, CWOCN, and*
*Ilene R. Fleischer, RN, MS, CWOCN*

**1. Is it difficult to learn how to care for an ostomy?**

Time is needed to learn the care of an ostomy. Physical care is usually mastered before psychological adaptation occurs. People learn at different paces and in different ways. It is important to assess each person's learning style and adapt the care plan to best meet his or her needs. Although self-care can usually be achieved within 1–3 months, psychological adaptation may take up to 1 year.

**2. When should a person learn about ostomy care?**

Patients and their families should learn about ostomy care as soon as the decision is made to undergo the surgery. Some people know that they will eventually need the procedure and seek information before surgery. Others, they have only a few weeks to prepare. Still others undergo procedures on an emergency basis and learn about care after surgery.

**3. What should be taught before surgery?**

People facing ostomy surgery have many questions, concerns, and fears about the loss of control over bodily functions, self-care, resumption of usual lifestyle and activities, and changes in body image. During the preoperative visit, the potential location of the ostomy is chosen, and characteristics of the stoma, type of output, pouching systems, clothing, activity, diet, odor control, lifestyle, intimacy issues and support organizations are discussed. During this visit the person views an appliance and is often surprised by its low-profile appearance and the fact that it is not noticeable under clothing. This visit also provides an excellent opportunity for patients and family members to ask questions and express concerns.

**4. What should be taught after surgery?**

- How to empty the pouch
- How to change the pouch
- When pouch changes are needed
- Normal stomal care
- Normal peristomal skin care
- How to recognize and treat common complications
- When to seek professional assistance

During hospitalization, emptying and changing of the appliance are taught to the patient and family members. Patients are encouraged to practice emptying the pouch and changing the appliance while they are hospitalized. Most patients are referred to visiting nurse services for further care, teaching, and support. Many hospitals have outpatient stoma clinics where patients are seen individually for follow-up about physical and/or psychosocial care and issues. At this time the person often resumes normal activities of life, such as returning to work or school, and frequently has questions or concerns.

**5. How often is an ostomy pouch emptied?**

The ostomy pouch should be emptied when it is approximately one-third full. This practice prevents the pouch from showing under clothing and the weight of the pouch from pulling on the seal to cause leakage. The frequency of pouch emptying in a fecal diversion depends on where in the gastrointestinal (GI) tract the stoma is located. The further along the GI tract stool is passed, the more water is reabsorbed and stool becomes more formed. In patients with an ileostomy, the stool consistency usually has a thick, pasty consistency and needs to be emptied 6–8 times per day. Ostomies located in the ascending or transverse portion of the large intestine have a soft thick stool consistency and will need to be emptied three to six times per day. Ostomies located in the descending or sigmoid portion of the large intestine will have semi-formed to formed stool and will need to be emptied one to three times per day.

A urostomy is emptied 4–6 times per day. At bedtime, the person is encouraged to connect the pouch to a continuous drainage system to prevent it from becoming too full during sleep and waking during the night to empty it.

**6. What is the best position for emptying an ostomy pouch?**

Whatever position people select to empty the pouch, whether it is standing or sitting, they should be comfortable. Some people like to sit on the toilet and empty the pouch between their legs, whereas others prefer to stand and face the toilet while emptying and others sit on a chair facing the toilet when they are in their own home. Toilet paper placed in the bowl helps prevent splashing.

**7. Should the pouch always be emptied from the drainable end?**

Not necessarily. One option for patients who wear a two-piece appliance is to snap the pouch off the wafer to empty it. Often a tab on the pouch facilitates this maneuver. This technique can also be used to release gas for patients with fecal diversions.

**8. How is a fecal ostomy pouch emptied?**

Lift the bottom of the pouch slightly to avoid accidental spilling while removing the clip. The end of the pouch may be cuffed to help keep the tail end clean. After emptying the pouch, wipe the cuff with toilet paper, damp tissue, or paper towel. The ultimate goal is to keep the end of the pouch clean. For most clamps, folding the pouch over the clamp once promotes a tight closure. It is not necessary to rinse the pouch after emptying; however, if the stool is very thick, a small amount of tepid water added into the pouch before emptying helps the stool flow out more easily. Some ostomates spray the inside of the pouch near the top portion of the pouch lightly with a vegetable oil cooking spray. This allows the stool to be emptied more completely and makes cleaning a bit easier.

**9. How is an ostomy pouch rinsed?**

Use warm water and introduce it from the drainable end. A paper cup or irrigating syringe can be used. If the pouch is rinsed, avoid water near the stoma because it may loosen the seal. Hot water should not be used because it destroys the odor-proofing of the pouch.

**10. How is a urostomy pouch emptied?**

Urinary pouches have a spout at the bottom that is opened to release the flow of urine. To ensure that the end of the pouch is completely dry, patients may wipe the spout with toilet paper. Urinary pouches are designed with antireflux valves inside the pouch to prevent the backflow of urine.

**11. How often is the appliance changed?**

The frequency of changing the appliance depends on the type of stoma, the effluent, and the patient's body contours. Patients are strongly encouraged to have a set time to change the appliance and not to wait until the appliance leaks. The maximum wearing time for most appliances is 1 week. However, most people change the appliance twice weekly. Patients should be taught to change the appliance if they notice any undermining or leakage of effluent under the wafer. Other signs of leakage include burning, pain, itching, or odor.

**12. What determines the amount of wear time for an ostomy wafer?**

When evaluating for wear time, the patient must assess the back of the wafer for the melting down of wafer material around the stoma. Most wafers are made of a pectin-based material. With time, the effluent wears away at the seal around the stoma. Wafers should protect the peristomal skin and maintain an effective seal so that the effluent does not leak under the wafer.

If the wafer around the stoma is intact, the wear time may be extended by 1 day. It is important to extend the wearing time only by 1 day and to evaluate it a few times before extending it another day.

**13. What supplies should be gathered when preparing to change an ostomy appliance?**
- Skin barrier wafer
- Pouch                           • Pen or pencil
- Skin sealant                    • Template (pattern) or measuring guide
- Skin barrier paste              • Washcloth and warm water
- Clamp                           • Rolled gauze wick or tampon (for urostomy)
- Scissors                        • Clean gloves, if desired

If the patient is doing the procedure, gloves do not need to be worn. Additional products may be needed to achieve an effective seal or extend the wear time of the appliance.

**14. Once the supplies are gathered, what is the first step to changing an ostomy appliance?**
The first step is to prepare a new appliance before removal of the existing appliance. Most skin barriers must be cut to fit $^1/_8$ to $^1/_{16}$ inch larger than the shape and size of the stoma. A template can be easily made using a measuring guide. Measure the length and width of the stoma. Mark the measurements on an index card, piece of paper, or plastic from the appliance package, and cut the opening in the card. Place the cut opening against the stoma to check for a correct fit, and make any necessary adjustments. Date and label the template top, left and right on the face-up side of the card. This card can be used for future appliance changes.

Revisions may be needed in the template because a newly created stoma changes in shape and size for the first 1–2 months or with a weight gain or loss of approximately 10 pounds. Using the template, trace the opening on the paper side of the wafer and mark the top of the wafer. Cut the wafer outside the traced line.

**15. When the new pouch is prepared, how is the old appliance removed?**
Wearing gloves, remove the clamp or open the spout and empty the contents in the appropriate receptacle. Remove the old appliance by gently peeling back the wafer and pushing down the skin. Using a warm face cloth may add comfort to the procedure. Wash the skin with warm water. Avoid soap, if possible, as it may leave a residue that interferes with wafer adhesion. The peristomal skin should be dried thoroughly. If the patient has a urostomy, use a tampon or other wick to keep the skin dry during the pouch change. During this time the stoma and peristomal skin should be inspected. Skin changes should be noted, and adaptations needed in the pouching system may be made at this time.

**16. Can baby wipes or other prepared cleansing cloths be used to clean around the stoma?**
Most of these products contain oils and lotions that interfere with the adhesion of the appliance. For this reason, it is recommended that the wipes or prepared cloths are not used. Many also contain fragrances that may irritate the skin.

**17. Once the skin is clean, what are the next steps?**
Apply one coat of the skin protective barrier wipe to the area where the tape portion of the wafer comes in contact with the skin and let dry. Peel off the backing of the adhesive wafer. If using paste, apply a bead around the cut opening of the wafer. Paste is used to achieve a more effective seal around the stoma, especially with flush or retracted stomas. Some people prefer to place the paste directly onto the skin to ensure that it ends up in an exact place. With this method, there is a chance that effluent may flow onto the paste before the appliance is placed; if used directly around the stoma, it may be difficult to center the appliance because the mucocutaneous junction cannot be well visualized. Some manufacturers recommend waiting approximately 1 minute for the paste to set. Apply the clamp to the bottom of a drainable pouch, or close the spout of a urinary pouch.

Center the wafer around the stoma, and press down gently on the wafer around the stoma to ensure a good seal. If using a two-piece appliance, snap on the pouch at this time. To ensure that the pouch is securely attached to the wafer, gently pull on the pouch. If using a belt, attach it at this time. Pouch deodorants may be put in the pouch if desired. It is important to follow the manufacturer's guidelines for use on selected products. If a wound, ostomy, continence (WOC) nurse specialist is available, incorporate his or her recommendations into the pouching procedure and plan of care.

**18. What care does the stoma require?**

The stoma requires little care. It normally produces small amounts of mucus that can be gently wiped off with a tissue or cleansed with water. Showering does not harm the stoma and the stoma's gentle outward peristaltic contractions prevent water from flowing inside the lumen. It is best to avoid the direct stream of water onto the stoma because a strong pressure may cause slight bleeding. Lying on the stomach, clothing, hugging and intimacy, and other normal activities of daily living should not harm the stoma.

**19. Why may the stoma bleed if washed?**

It is not uncommon to see a little bit of bleeding during an appliance change if a washcloth or tissue rubs the stoma, which has a rich blood supply. This is similar to bleeding from gums when some people brush their teeth. The peristomal skin must be cleansed and protected from the effluent, not the stoma.

**20. Does the stoma hurt?**

The red or pink color of the stoma often makes people think that it will be painful to touch. However, the stoma has no nerve endings and is not painful. For this reason, it is important to inspect it and ensure that no lacerations, ulcers, or other irritations are present. Teach the patient this important concept.

**21. Do all stomas look alike?**

Stomas vary in size, shape, and location. Contributing factors include individual anatomy and what part of the intestine is used to create the stoma surgically. Stomas from the large intestines are often larger than stomas from the small intestines. All stomas are swollen after surgery and usually reach their permanent size approximately 2 months after the operation.

**22. Should the stoma protrude?**

Ideally, a stoma should protrude 2–3 cm, to allow the effluent to flow out of the lumen and into the appliance, avoiding contact where the adhesive of the appliance meets the skin. This helps protect the peristomal skin from the drainage.

**23. What may cause a stoma to become retracted?**

Retraction of the stoma can be caused by a variety of factors. Most commonly it is due to a thickened abdominal wall, insufficient mobilization of the mesentery and bowel, or excessive scar formation, all of which can cause the stoma to be flush with the abdomen or retracted rather than protruding. In this case, the effluent more readily undermines the seal of the appliance, necessitating more frequent appliance changes or additional accessories to prevent irritant dermatitis.

Conversely, a stoma may be excessively long, and extra care may be required to avoid trauma to the stoma when applying the appliance. A prolapsed stoma is excessively long and edematous and should be evaluated by a health care provider.

**24. Can the appliance irritate the stoma?**

The opening in most appliances should leave *no more than* $^1/_{16} - {}^1/_8$-inch of peristomal skin exposed. This allows for maximum skin protection without irritating the stoma. If the stoma is not round, a customized template should be made that matches the size and shape of the stoma. The template can be used to ensure that the correct size opening is made in the appliance to avoid peristomal skin irritation.

**25. What type of care does the peristomal skin require?**

The peristomal skin should appear healthy, intact, and without erythema or rashes. Its appearance should be no different from that of skin beyond the appliance. Cleansing is done at the time of the appliance change. Soaps are generally avoided because many have oils, fragrances, and chemicals that may be harmful to the skin. If soap is used, it should be mild and completely cleansed with water before a new appliance is applied. Many people prefer to do this procedure while showering. Some manufacturers recommend the use of an adhesive remover on the peristomal skin when the appliance is changed. This, too, must be thoroughly rinsed off the skin before applying a new appliance.

**26. What causes peristomal skin irritation?**

Effluent undermining the seal of an appliance is a common cause of irritation. The effluent causes the skin to become erythematous and denuded (irritant dermatitis). Rather than just treating the skin with barrier powders, skin sealant, pastes, or gels, it is essential to identify and correct the cause of the problem. Common causes include incorrect appliance size, wrong template size, not changing the appliance frequently enough, or not using convexity to provide a more effective seal. For more information, see Chapter 72.

**27. Is it possible to have an allergic reaction to ostomy products?**

A sensitivity reaction can certainly occur. It usually manifests as erythema or an erythematous rash matching the size and shape of the product to which the person is allergic. It is not uncommon for the person also to complain of pruritus. An example is a sensitivity reaction to the outer tape of the appliance. In this case, the skin under the barrier part is healthy and intact, whereas the skin beyond this point and under the tape is irritated.

**28. How can one determine whether if the peristomal skin rash has a fungal etiology?**

Candidiasis may develop under an appliance, especially with leakage of effluent, which keeps the area warm and moist. People who are undergoing treatments with immunosuppressive medications, corticosteroids, or prolonged antibiotics may also be more susceptible to developing candidiasis. Peristomal skin presents as a maculopapular rash with satellite lesions and will not heal until an antifungal powder is used to treat the affected sites. Satellite lesions can be identified as red papules on the periphery of the confluent rashy area. Creams must be avoided because the appliance will not effectively seal because of their oily nature.

**29. Why do most people use skin sealant on the peristomal skin?**

Skin sealant places a breathable, protective film on the epidermis. It helps prevent mechanical irritation and skin stripping, which may occur when tapes are taken off.

**30. Is it necessary to shave the peristomal skin?**

It is strongly recommended that the peristomal skin be shaved with an electric razor or clipped with scissors to prevent folliculitis and discomfort when the appliance is removed.

**31. What should be done to treat the peristomal skin if it does not appear healthy?**

The cause of the peristomal skin irritation must be identified to correct the problem and treat the skin appropriately. Evaluation by a nurse who specializes in ostomy care is often necessary. Many hospitals have stoma clinics where this problem can be assessed and treated. Increasingly, home care agencies also have ostomy specialists to help with such problems. If a specialist is not available, the United Ostomy Association has a listing of local ostomy chapters throughout the United States. Local chapters may have a directory of local stoma clinics or may be able to recommend ostomy nurse specialists who can see patients on an outpatient basis.

**32. What should the patient be taught about ostomy care during travel?**

There are no limitations in travel, but before beginning the patient should know how to manage the ostomy for traveling. The pouch should be emptied just as one would empty the bladder. Depending on the length of the trip, short stops may be needed because the pouch should be emptied when it is approximately one-third full. Seat belts are important to wear and should not harm the stoma. If an appliance fits well and is changed on a predictable schedule, various movements and activities should not loosen the seal. Extremes of heat and cold, as occur in the trunk of a car, should be avoided when ostomy supplies are stored.

**33. What guidelines should be followed for packing supplies?**

It is best to pack extra supplies for any unexpected delays or problems that may arise during travel. Although supplies are available in most places, it is helpful to find out where appliances are available if an extended trip is planned. This information may be obtained from a local supplier, an ostomy nurse specialist, or the United Ostomy Association.

For air travel, appliances should be packed with carry-on luggage, just as medicine would be. In the event of lost luggage, the patient still has the necessary supplies for proper care of the ostomy.

For foreign travel, a note from one's physician should be readily available, stating that ostomy supplies are medically necessary. This should help prevent problems while going through customs.

If a colostomy is being irrigated, the safety rule is that the water must be safe to drink. When in doubt, the water can be boiled and allowed to cool.

**34. Should ostomy supplies be kept at work or school?**

Yes. It is recommended that an extra pouch change kit be available whenever the person leaves home. It should include a precut appliance and supplies for any unexpected pouch change. Supplies may be placed in a small bag, pencil case, cosmetic case, or any container with which the person is comfortable. This may be kept in a drawer at work, a locker at school, a pocketbook, a briefcase, or anywhere that is accessible and convenient. If the supplies are not used, the person has the comfort of knowing that they are available. If the supplies are not used for a long period, they should be checked to ensure the materials have not suffered from temperature variations or undergone other changes that may impair their usefulness.

**35. Can work continue after ostomy surgery?**

An ostomy should not affect occupation. It is normal to need some time off during the postoperative recuperative period. The patient and surgeon determine this period. The decision to tell fellow employees about the surgery is a personal one; there is no right or wrong answer. If the job involves heavy lifting, good body mechanics must be stressed and the use of a supportive device may be considered. If the person is employed in a rough contact sport, padding for the stoma may be recommended. Returning to work often contributes to positive feelings and aids adjustment as life begins to return to normal.

**36. Can children participate in activities after ostomy surgery?**

It is recommended that the school staff be informed of a child's surgery, as they would be informed about medications, allergies, asthma, or other health conditions. If the child is not old enough to keep an extra kit of supplies, an extra set-up can be kept with the school nurse or a designated teacher. Education can be provided to the staff as needed. Limitations are rare, and the child should be encouraged to resume usual activities both in and out of school. The rare times when extra padding may be required over the stoma to protect it are when the child is older and involved in rough contact sports, such as hockey or football. It is up to the parents and child to decide whether the presence of the ostomy is shared with friends or classmates.

**37. Should friends, family, and other significant people be told of the ostomy surgery?**

This decision varies from person to person. Often explaining the surgery to a spouse, loved ones, and children can help dispel incorrect information and fears, as well as help the patient cope with feelings as he or she adjusts. Most people find it helpful to talk with people to whom they are close and can trust. It is normal to initially have some feelings of insecurity. With time, this changes. For most people, the adjustment period takes from 6 months to 1 year.

**38. What type of counseling and information should be provided about social relationships?**

The ostomy should not affect social relationships. A change in body image has occurred, and time is needed to adjust. It is not uncommon to have initial feelings of anger, depression, loss of control, and decreased self-esteem. It is important to reassure patients that these feelings are normal and will subside as the ostomy is integrated into their self-concept.

Confidence and security come with time as patients gain independence and skill with physical care, as well as psychological comfort. A positive attitude and taking pride in progress contribute to full and complete recovery and adjustment. The ostomy should not change who one is or the relationships one has—it changes only the way elimination occurs. All types of relationships are still possible, whether with family, friends, dating, or marriage. People told this information may need time to adjust, just like the person who underwent ostomy surgery. It should certainly not affect a relationship negatively.

### 39. How does ostomy surgery affect sexuality?

Communication is a key component of sexual adaptation after ostomy surgery. In the initial postoperative period, patients may ask their partner not to be intimate because of abdominal discomfort from the surgical procedure. Later, if the patient has not informed his or her partner of progress, the physical distance may be interpreted as rejection. In reality, the partner is sensitive to the thought that the loved one still has pain. Sharing information related to progress and feelings is essential and contributes to resumption of emotional closeness and affection after ostomy surgery.

### 40. Can the pouch be concealed?

There are a variety of ways to alter the appearance of the pouch. Most important is finding the option that works best for each person and his or her partner. Shorter, opaque pouches are used successfully by many people for intimate times. Pouch covers, available in different colors, patterns, prints, and materials, are available in many sizes. Specialty undergarments are a choice for some people. For more information, see Chapter 69.

### 41. When can sexual activity be resumed?

Patients should check with their physician to find out how soon after surgery sex can be resumed. If possible, it is a good idea to empty the pouch before beginning sexual activity, as most people empty their bladder. When the appliance has a good seal, it remains in place during sexual activity. Experimenting with different positions may be helpful to find what works best. Hugging and other forms of physical contact do not harm the stoma or the appliance. The United Ostomy Association and the American Cancer Society have pamphlets and books about sex after ostomy surgery.

### 42. What about pregnancy with an ostomy?

An ostomy does not preclude pregnancy. However, the medical reason for the ostomy surgery may impact the ability to conceive or maintain a pregnancy. In cases of extensive malignancy, the female reproductive organs may be removed. Certain medications, such as some chemotherapy drugs, may make pregnancy contraindicated. During a normal pregnancy with an ostomy, the most common change is enlargement of the stoma as the woman's abdomen grows and the need to alter the appliance fit to the appropriate size or to use an appliance with more flexibility. Extra appliances that are ready for use should be packed with other items that will go to the hospital once labor begins. If possible, in the early stages of labor, a new appliance can be applied to help ensure a good seal during delivery.

### 43. What about erectile dysfunction?

Men may have erectile dysfunction after some extensive surgeries for bladder or rectal cancer. Most surgeons use a nerve-sparing technique whenever possible to try to prevent this problem. Before concluding that erectile dysfunction is present, much time is needed, often up to 6 months or more, because both physical and psychological comfort play a role in achieving and maintaining an erection. Some men can still experience an orgasm with or without ejaculation, even if they cannot maintain an erection. Variations to the traditional penile-vaginal penetration may be fulfilling ways to enjoy sex. When impotence is a problem, medical or surgical treatments are available and should be discussed with the health care provider.

### 44. Should people with ostomies follow a special diet?

Most people with ostomies do not follow a special diet and enjoy the foods that they did before surgery. Teaching about diet focuses on the health history with consideration of the type of stoma. For people with fecal diversions, food types are added slowly into the diet after surgery, and information is given about odor- and gas-producing foods. Foods that cause odor and gas include asparagus, cabbage, fish, garlic, onion, beans, spicy foods, string beans, and cucumbers. If the person enjoys spicy foods, they do not need to be eliminated from the diet, but stool output may have an odor. People with ileostomies need to be careful to avoid food blockages and dehydration. Teaching and counseling stress eating a well-balanced diet with adequate fluid intake for most patients.

### 45. What is a food blockage?

Only people with ileostomies are at risk for developing a food blockage. Ileostomies are created at the end of the small intestine and are approximately 1 inch in width. Scar tissue may develop at the fascia layer, causing the lumen to be smaller. Foods that are high in fiber or not digested completely may accumulate and not pass through the lumen, thus causing a food blockage. Foods associated with blockage include apple peel, celery, coconut, Chinese food, corn, popcorn, seeds, meats in casings, wild rice, grapes, raisins and fresh pineapple. People are taught to prevent food blockages by chewing foods thoroughly, avoiding large quantities of high-fiber foods, and having plenty of fluid intake.

### 46. What are the signs and symptoms of food blockage?

Signs and symptoms of food blockage include cramping abdominal pain, watery or no stool output, stomal swelling and abdominal distention. Home measures to treat the blockage include a warm bath to relax the abdominal muscles, drinking warm fluids, avoiding solid foods until the blockage resolves, and massaging the peristomal area. Assuming different positions such as knee to chest to dislodge the obstruction may also be helpful. If the blockage does not resolve in 24 hours, the patient should contact a health care provider and be evaluated.

Further treatment that may be done by a health care professional include an ileostomy lavage, which is an instillation of saline into the ileostomy to dislodge the food blockage. This is done by using a 14- or 16-French catheter and instilling approximately 50 ml saline into the ileostomy until the blockage is resolved. It is important to note that lack of stool output or abdominal cramping may be signs and symptoms of a different problem.

### 47. Is dehydration a problem with people who have an ileostomy?

Dehydration and electrolyte imbalance may occur because stool is diverted before to passing through the colon, where fluid and electrolytes are absorbed. The average ileostomy output ranges from approximately 500 ml to 750 ml in a 24-hour period. Patients are taught to drink 10–12, 8–ounce glasses of fluid per day and are encouraged to drink fluids that contain electrolytes. The greatest risk for developing fluid and electrolyte imbalance occurs during the postoperative phase because the body is trying to adapt to the ileostomy.

Conditions such as vomiting and diarrhea also may lead to dehydration in people who have had an ileostomy for a long period. Symptoms of dehydration include increased thirst, loss of appetite, lethargy, decreased urine output, sunken eyes, muscle cramps, feeling faint, abdominal cramps, dry mouth, and sometimes confusion. Fluid replacement is the treatment for dehydration. Patients should be taught to recognize the signs of dehydration and to contact their health care provider promptly for treatment.

### 48. Are medications absorbed with an ileostomy?

Many medications are enteric-coated or time-released and may not be completely absorbed by people with an ileostomy. People are taught to inform healthcare providers that they have an ileostomy and may need an alternative such as a liquid form of the medication. If there is a question whether the medication is being absorbed, it may be helpful to do a simple test. Place the tablet or capsule in a glass of water and time the rate of dissolution. If the medication has dissolved or has started to dissolve in 30 minutes, it usually will be absorbed. Never crush any medication unless instructed to do so by a pharmacist.

There is no need for people with an ileostomy to take a laxative. Laxatives may cause fluid and electrolyte imbalance. If people with ileostomies are having a procedure that normally requires a bowel preparation, they limit oral intake to clear liquids for 1–2 days.

**49. What is colostomy irrigation?**

This procedure is performed by the patient with a sigmoid or descending colostomy to regulate the elimination of stool. The goal is to prevent the elimination of stool between irrigations. Ideally, the patient performs the irrigation with water daily or every other day. Between irrigations, the patient is able to wear a small, closed-end pouch or cap. There is an adjustment period when the patient is learning the procedure and the colon is trained only to eliminate stool when water is instilled. Many people find this an ideal procedure with a good fit into their lifestyle, while others are not interested. Colostomy irrigations are optional. People may discontinue them at anytime.

**50. Who is a candidate for colostomy irrigation?**

People with descending or sigmoid colostomies are candidates and have the option of performing colostomy irrigations, because stool output from a sigmoid or descending colostomy occurs 1–3 times per day and is formed. The nurse must also assess the bowel function, preference, motivation, and ability to learn the procedure. People with a history of diarrhea or irregular elimination patterns are not usually good candidates. Contraindications to colostomy irrigations include stoma prolapse or parastomal hernia, chemotherapy or radiation, and temporary colostomies.

**51. How is the irrigation performed?**

Lifestyle issues and personal preferences determine what time of day the person chooses to perform the irrigation. The best results are achieved if the irrigation is performed at the same time each day. Colostomy irrigation kits, available from manufacturers, contain a cone tip catheter, irrigating bag, and irrigation sleeve. Most people sit on the toilet and, if wearing a two-piece appliance, snap off the pouch and snap on the irrigation sleeve. The bottom of the sleeve is placed in the toilet.

Initially, the colostomy is irrigated with approximately 500 ml of lukewarm tap water daily; the fluid is gradually increased to 1000 ml. The water should run in over a period of approximately 10 minutes. Patients are taught to stop the irrigation if they feel discomfort or abdominal cramping. Initial stool output occurs within the first 10–15 minutes, but the patient is taught to wait 30–45 minutes for the results to be completed. The patient is able to get up and move around after the initial returns. When irrigation is completed, the sleeve is removed and the closed-end pouch or stoma cap is placed back on.

**52. What is urinary crystal formation? How is it treated?**

Crystal formation, or alkaline encrustation, is sometimes seen with urostomies. The usual cause is alkaline urine that bathes the stoma or peristomal skin when the appliance does not fit correctly and is not protecting the skin. The crystals appear as white, gritty deposits. Prevention can be achieved by providing an effective seal with the appliance to prevent urine from contacting the peristomal skin. The average pH of urine is 6.0. Acidification of the urine with vitamin C may be prescribed to treat alkaline urine. The peristomal skin and stoma can also be treated with $^1/_4$ to $^1/_2$ strength white vinegar soaks with each appliance change. The vinegar helps dissolve the gritty crystals. During the initial treatment period, the soaks should be done with each appliance change or as recommended by an ostomy nurse specialist. The stoma may temporarily blanch from this treatment but will not be harmed.

**53. Why is mucus present in the urostomy pouch?**

Ileal conduits are common types of urinary diversions. These procedures create a new passageway for urine to flow into an external collection pouch. A piece of the intestines is used to create this passageway. The intestines normally secrete mucus; therefore, mucus will be present in the urostomy pouch. Drinking 2000 ml–2500 ml of fluid per day can thin excessive amounts of mucus. Agents that can be instilled into the pouch to help disperse the mucus are also available at some medical supply stores.

**54. What is a nighttime drainage system?**

A night drainage system is a large collection bag that allows more output to be collected. A smaller pouch is likely to become overfilled during the course of the night. When the pouch is full, the urine cannot drain properly. Usually a full pouch causes leakage. With the antireflux pouches and the stoma's outward contractions, it is unlikely that the pouch will become so full that it will not leak and that urine will flow retrograde into the kidney.

Nighttime collection units are typically similar to a catheter drainage bag. A special adapter is placed onto the end of the urostomy pouch spout and connects to the drainage bag tubing. The only alternative to using a nighttime drainage system is to set an alarm and get up during the night to empty the urostomy pouch. Because this alternative is arduous, most urostomy patients elect to use a nighttime system.

### 55. What recommendations help prevent a urinary tract infection (UTI) with a urostomy?

Symptoms of UTI include fever, cloudy or foul-smelling urine, fatigue, nausea and vomiting, and flank pain. To help decrease the incidence of UTI, people with a urinary diversion should drink 2000–2500 ml of fluid per day. Sufficient hydration ensures an adequate flushing of the urinary system, dilutes bacteria, and promotes acidic pH of the urine to help prevent bacterial growth. Hands should be washed before and after caring for a urostomy. The use of a pouch with an antireflux valve and emptying the pouch when it is approximately one-third full help prevent urine from bathing the area around the stoma and contributing to bacterial overgrowth.

### 56. How is stasis in a urostomy detected?

Radiologic exams, such as intravenous pylegrams (IVPs) or loopograms, identify whether urinary stasis is present. Urinary stasis can contribute to UTIs and occur if the conduit is excessively long, if there is inaccurate angulation of the conduit or ureters, or if the uretero-conduit anastomosis is not optimal. Accurate identification of UTI is best obtained via a catheterized sterile specimen from the conduit. The specimen should not be taken from the bottom of a urostomy pouch, where contaminants are present.

### 57. What is a continent diversion?

A continent diversion is a surgical alternative to ostomy surgery. It is not appropriate for everyone. It creates an internal reservoir for storage of urine or stool when the bladder or rectum must be removed. There are various types of continent diversions, some with a catheterizable stoma and some without. In those without a catheterizable stoma, urine or stool is released via the meatus or anus, respectively.

### 58. How often is the stoma catheterized to drain the urine or stool in a continent diversion?

During the postoperative period, numerous drains and tubes are often present. Continence is not established until they are removed, usually a few weeks after surgery. In this initial period, catheterizations are more frequent to prevent overdistention of the new reservoir. Depending on the type of continent diversion and whether it is urinary or fecal, the frequency of catheterizations may be every 2–3 hours. Each week it is recommended that the schedule be increased by 1 hour if there have been no problems with leakage or discomfort. This interval is advanced until catheterizations are done approximately every 6 hours. Once this has been successful, people often begin to vary the schedule slightly based on activities and eating and drinking routines. Most people feel some distention or slight cramping to indicate that the reservoir is full and needs to be emptied. A common catheterization schedule may be on rising in the morning, after lunch, after dinner, and before bedtime. Catheterization is also known as intubation in this setting.

*Sample Catheterization Schedule*

|  | DAYTIME | OVERNIGHT |
| --- | --- | --- |
| Week 1 | Every 2–3 hrs | Every 3–4 hrs |
| Week 2 | Every 3–4 hrs | Every 4–5 hrs |
| Week 3 | Every 4–5 hrs | Every 5–6 hrs |
| Week 4 | Every 5–6 hrs | Every 6–8 hrs |
| Week 5 | Every 6 hrs | Every 7–8 hrs |
| Week 6 | Approximately 4 times per day | Possibly no need to catheterize |

## 59. What is the role of the ostomy nurse specialist?

The ostomy nurse specialist is a registered nurse who has attended and completed a wound, ostomy, and continence accredited professional education program. In addition, many are certified in ostomy care. Ostomy nurse specialists may also hold additional advanced nursing degrees. In their role as ostomy nurse specialists, many provide direct care, education, support, and counseling to assist patients and those close to them with management, rehabilitation, and adaptation to the ostomy. This is an ongoing process that often begins before surgery and may continue throughout the persons lifespan. The ostomy nurse specialist is a resource for many health care providers who care for patients with ostomies.

### BIBLIOGRAPHY

1. Bradley M, Pupiales M: Essentials of ostomy care. Am J Nurs 97(7):38–46, 1997.
2. Bryant D, Fleischer I: Changing an ostomy appliance. Nursing 2000 11:51–53, 2000.
3. Choudhury MS: The Indiana pouch: A continent urinary reservoir. Progressions 1(3):12–15, 1989.
4. Colwell JC, Goldberg M, Carmel J: The state of the standard diversion. J Wound Ostomy Contin Nurs 28(1):6–17, 2001.
5. Fleischer I, Wise P: Continent Urostomy: A Guide. Atlanta, American Cancer Society, 1994.
6. Golis AM: Sexual issues for the person with an ostomy. J Wound Ostomy Contin Nurs 23(1):33–37, 1996.
7. Hampton BG, Bryant RA (eds): Ostomies and Continent Diversions: Nursing Management. St. Louis, Mosby Year Book, 1992.
8. Hill MJ: Skin Disorders. Mosby's Clinical Nursing Series. St. Louis, Mosby, 1994.
9. Turnbull GB, Erwin-Toth P: Ostomy care: Foundation for teaching and practice. Ostomy Wound Manage 45(1A Suppl):23S–32S, 1999.
10. Williams O, Vereb MJ, Libertino JA: Noncontinent urinary diversion. Urol Clin North Am 24(4):735–744, 1997.
11. Wound, Ostomy and Continence Nurses Society. Guidelines for Management: Caring for a Patient with a Continent Diversion. Laguna Beach, CA, Wound, Ostomy and Continence Nurses Society, 1996.
12. Wound, Ostomy and Continence Nurses Society. Guidelines for Management: Caring for a Patient with an Ostomy. Laguna Beach, CA, Wound, Ostomy and Continence Nurses Society, 1998.

# 72. COMMON OSTOMY PROBLEMS

*Eileen M. McCann*, RN, BSN, CWOCN

**1. What common problems are related to stomas? How do you troubleshoot them?**

Common problems related to stomas can be divided into two categories: those related to the stoma, such as prolapse, retraction, and stenosis, and those related to the peristomal skin, such as excoriation, candidiasis, and irritation. In solving stoma-related problems, treating the problem itself is often not enough. You must play detective and attempt to find and eliminate the cause. Determining and treating the cause will prevent recurrence of the problem as well as a cycle of leakage and skin breakdown.

**2. What is a retracted stoma? Why is it a problem?**

A retracted stoma is a stoma that has "caved in" below the skin layer. Causes include insufficient length of the stoma, excessive tension on the mesentery, and inadequate fixation of the bowel to the parietal peritoneum. Retraction is common in people with a thick abdominal wall and can occur with any type of stoma. Retraction can cause serious stoma management problems because the effluent stagnates near the opening and forces leakage under the appliance. It becomes difficult to maintain an adequate seal. In severe cases of retraction, surgical revision of the stoma may be indicated.

**3. What nonsurgical approach can be used to manage a retracted stoma?**

A retracted stoma can often be managed by using a firm convex appliance and wearing an ostomy belt. Convexity helps to increase the protrusion of the stoma by adding pressure to the surrounding tissue. Stoma paste is also indicated to help fill in uneven creases and abdominal contours. Appliance belts provide additional support by holding the appliance securely against the outer wall of the patient's abdomen.

**4. What causes a stoma to prolapse?**

Prolapse is the excessive protrusion of the stomal loop out of the abdominal wall in a telescoping fashion. A prolapsed stoma can result when the stoma is not adequately supported as it is brought through rectus muscle, when the stoma is placed through an oversized opening in the abdominal wall, or when insufficient sutures hold it in place. Prolapse occurs more commonly in loop colostomies and in children.

**5. How is stomal prolapse managed?**

A prolapsed stoma can be frightening and emotionally upsetting for the patient. It can often be managed conservatively, as long as no ischemia or obstruction is noted. Having the patient lie down and application of gentle pressure while the patient lies down returns the bowel to its place, effectively reducing the prolapse.

Cold compresses may be useful in reducing associated edema. Support over the stoma with an abdominal binder or belt helps hold the reduced prolapse in place. The prolapsed large stoma must be protected from trauma, which can be caused by ill-fitting equipment. A two-piece appliance must be used with caution to prevent pinching. Openings should be evaluated carefully to ensure no rubbing or trauma harms the stomal mucosa. A progressively prolapsing stoma or a prolapse with concurrent ischemia and abdominal pain may be indicative of incarceration and usually requires immediate surgical intervention.

**6. What is mucocutaneous separation? How is it treated?**

Mucocutaneous separation is an early postoperative complication consisting of a superficial detachment or separation of the suture line that secures the base of the stoma where it meets the abdominal surface. The separation can be total or partial. It is often seen in patients who are at risk for poor healing, such as those who are malnourished, receiving steroid therapy or diabetic. The separation can lead to total retraction as well as infection. Symptoms often include pain, burning, and discomfort, accompanied by purulent drainage. Surgical intervention may be necessary if peritoneal contamination is a potential problem.

In most cases, treatment consists of gentle cleansing of the defect with normal saline and application of a "filler" to the wound bed. Fillers can be in the form of powder, paste, or an absorptive dressing to absorb drainage and keep the wound bed moist. A secondary covering to create a pouching surface is then placed over the filled wound. Adhesive strips, transparent dressing, or tape can be used. If frequent wound cleansing or dressing changes are necessary, a two-piece appliance or a wound pouch with a front access port can be used to allow access to the wound without constant appliance changes. The outcome is usually favorable, and the separation typically heals well with moist wound-healing techniques.

### 7.  What is stenosis of the stoma?

Stenosis of the stoma occurs when the stomal lumen becomes narrow and rigid. It is caused by several contributing factors: insufficient skin excision to bring the stoma through, alkaline urine in a urinary stoma, radiation tissue damage, or stomal necrosis and mucocutaneous separation. One short-term management option is stoma dilatation. Stool softeners or irrigations are often indicated to ease stool passage. Urinary stents help to maintain the patency of urinary stomas. Severe stenosis leading to frequent episodes of obstruction may require surgical revision of the stoma.

### 8.  Is stomal necrosis a problem?

Stomal necrosis is usually an early postoperative complication. A necrotic stoma may appear dark red, purple, or bluish. Brown or black discoloration may also be present. The stoma looks unusually dry due to poor tissue hydration. Necrosis may involve only the exteriorized portion, of the stoma (terminal or partial ischemia). It may also involve the entire stomal loop. Exterior necrosis usually results from excessive tension on the stoma or mesentery. Obesity, abdominal distention, or edema of the abdominal wall may also contribute to stomal tension and necrosis. In this case, immediate reoperation is required to resect the necrotic portion and construct a new stoma as a precaution against perforation and peritonitis.

Partial ischemia may result from compression on the bowel by an excessively narrow opening or insufficient mobilization. It often does not require further surgery and usually is managed conservatively with careful monitoring, the use of a soft appliance with gentle cleansing, and odor management. The necrosis gradually sloughs off to reveal a healthy, intact stoma.

### 9.  What is considered a high volume of effluent? How is it managed?

Normal output is measured in terms of frequency, volume, and consistency. A urinary stoma drains urine immediately after surgery and is almost constant. Patients with an ileostomy have higher output during the first few weeks postoperatively. The consistency will be mostly liquid and may be up to 2 quarts per day.

Gradually, as the body adapts, the consistency, thickness and volume decrease to approximately 1 quart per day. In addition to causing a fluid and electrolyte imbalance, high-volume effluent can cause skin damage if allowed to pool on the skin. Maceration and peristomal skin breakdown result.

The pouch opening should be sized appropriately to eliminate peristomal skin exposure. Skin barriers that are more durable and resistant to meltdown should be used. An ostomy belt provides extra support for higher-volume output, which adds weight and can weaken the barrier. Pouches made specifically for larger output have greater capacity. They can even be connected to bedside drainage. Urinary pouches should also be connected to bedside drainage during sleep to avoid overexpansion, leakage, and potential retrograde urine flow. Patients who choose not to use a larger-capacity pouch or connect to bedside drainage should be taught to empty the pouch more frequently, whenever it is one-third full, even during the night. If the output is very watery, packets can be placed in the pouch to absorb the fluid and change it to a more gel-like consistency.

**10. What is the significance of lack of effluent from the stoma?**

The onset of stoma function varies, along with the amount and consistency of output. A urinary stoma begins expelling urine immediately. Lack of output in a urinary stoma can be indicative of obstruction, infection, or dehydration.

Gastrointestinal stomal output depends on the location of the stoma in the intestinal tract. Proximal intestinal stomas (jejunostomy or ileostomy) usually begin to function within 48–72 hours postoperatively. Distal stomas begin to function 72–96 hours postoperatively. Distal stomas produce stool of thicker consistency and lower volume than proximal stomas. Bowel function may return to individual, normal, preoperative patterns. Lack of output from an intestinal stoma, accompanied by abdominal distention, high-pitched hyperactive or hypoactive bowel sounds, pain, nausea, and vomiting is a cause for concern. Patients should be assessed for possible obstruction or an improperly functioning stoma.

**11. Is it normal for the stoma to bleed?**

The stomal mucosa contains many small vessels close to the surface of the mucosa. Superficial bleeding from even minimal trauma, such as friction during cleaning or an appliance change, can be expected and should stop spontaneously. Occasionally, superficial bleeding may not spontaneously resolve and requires interventions such as sutures, cautery, or direct pressure.

Hemorrhage or profuse bleeding from the stoma site may be indicative of more serious conditions, such as portal hypertension, trauma, recurrent disease, medication side effects, or a consequence of a treatment regimen. The bleeding should be assessed for severity and cause, along with previous measures to reduce and control the source. Gentle appliance changes and stoma care are required if portal hypertension or trauma is suspected. Medication use needs to be evaluated, including drug–drug and drug–nutrient interactions, as a contributing cause. At one time patients were encouraged to place aspirin tablets in the pouch for odor control. This practice was found to cause bleeding and stomal ulcerations and is no longer advised but is occasionally still seen in the clinical setting.

**12. What should patients do if they experience problems with irrigation?**

Irrigation is a method to establish regular bowel elimination through instillation of warm water into the bowel, thus stimulating evacuation. It is *not* a requirement to maintain normal bowel function, and is not appropriate for everyone.

Irrigation has both advantages and disadvantages. The physician, ostomy specialist, and patient should decide collaboratively if irrigation is appropriate. Before beginning a routine of irrigation, normal bowel function needs to have returned postoperatively. Patients with stomal prolapse and hernias should not irrigate because results are poor and perforation is a risk. Children, young adults, and patients with a transverse colostomy are likely to become dependent on irrigation, producing the same effects as laxative dependency. Pelvic or abdominal radiation precludes irrigation because of risk for perforation due to tissue fragility and friability. Elderly patients and patients with a poor prognosis may choose not to irrigate because the procedure can be tiring and time-consuming.

Vasovagal reactions are another problem with irrigations. Sometimes they can be avoided by placing the patient in a supine position during irrigation rather than seated on a toilet or standing. The first irrigation can be done in bed.

It is also important to give the anastomosis time to heal before beginning irrigation. Irrigations need to be performed on a regular basis for optimal results. Cramping pain may occur. Slowing the fluid instillation, encouraging the patient to take deep breaths, and using lukewarm water help relieve cramping.

**13. What if little or no irrigant is returned?**

If there is little or no return after irrigation, the patient may be dehydrated and absorbing the fluid. Increasing oral intake will help. When the irrigation fluid is difficult to instill, reposition the direction of the cone tip, and check for hard stool returns. A patient with a colostomy can still experience constipation and stomal impaction.

### 14. What peristomal skin problems can be expected in ostomy patients?

Peristomal skin management can often be a challenge. A number of peristomal skin irritations may be encountered for various reasons. Along with treating the condition, the clinician must be adept at using detective skills to determine the cause of the skin irritation. Eliminate the cause, eliminate the problem. This approach often requires creativity, using different types of appliance and pouching techniques to assess leakage problems.

### 15. What is candidiasis?

Candidiasis is a skin infection caused by yeast-like fungi. This fungus, *Candida albicans*, is part of the normal body flora in several areas. Candidal organisms love areas that are moist, warm, and dark. Patients who are immunosuppressed, diabetic, or receiving antibiotics are particularly susceptible to fungal overgrowth. A poorly fitting appliance or moisture build-up after bathing can set the stage for a candidal infection to proliferate.

### 16. What are the symptoms of candidiasis? How is it treated?

Patients with a candidal infection have lesions that appear red and splotchy. Typically satellite lesions are seen in the surrounding area. Patients complain of burning and itching. Treatment involves use of antifungal powder and skin sealants to keep the skin dry and treat the infection. Drying after a shower with a hair dryer is often effective in preventing moisture problems. The appliance and stoma must also be examined for the proper fit, and the patient should be questioned about daily routines. A poorly fitting appliance can allow moisture to seep beneath the appliance and encourage fungal growth.

Pouch covers are another solution for the patient with perspiration problems and moisture build-up. Antiperspirant can be applied to the abdominal skin that touches the pouch to help control moisture. It is advisable to change the appliance more frequently during a fungal infection so that the skin may be treated more often.

### 17. What is excoriation?

The technical definition of excoriation is a linear abrasion of the epidermis. Excoriation is also called denudation or erosion. This superficial skin irritation can result from slight seepage of stomal output under the appliance, prolonged wearing time of an appliance during which meltdown occurs, or skin stripping or trauma due to an ill-fitting appliance. Mechanical problems such as pressure, friction, and slipping may also contribute to excoriation of the peristomal skin.

### 18. How is excoriation treated?

The first step is to eliminate the cause. Appliance fit and pouching regimen need to be checked. Pressure from a belt can cause erosion, as can changing the appliance too frequently. "Less is more" is often a good policy.

Skin can become excoriated by use of too many accessory products, such as film barrier, preps, powders, pastes, belts, and tapes. Removal and application technique can also cause excoriation. If the skin is not broken, application of stoma or karaya powder, sealed onto the skin with nonstinging liquid skin barrier spray or wipe, along with repouching with the correct size opening, effectively treats the skin. Karaya powder works well but causes stinging of the skin if it is severely broken and in such cases should be avoided.

### 19. Is dermatitis of the peristomal skin a concern?

Yes. Dermatitis can cause ongoing skin irritation. There are two types of peristomal dermatitis: allergic and irritant.

### 20. What is allergic dermatitis?

A patient can develop an allergic response from exposure to any component of the pouching system—barriers, skin prep, pouches, or flanges. Once the patient develops an allergy or sensitivity to a product, it may remain forever. The skin becomes red, itchy, scaly and inflamed. Blisters and pain can also result.

Patients with known allergies should be patch-tested with products prior to their use whenever possible. The skin on the other side of the abdomen should be used for comparison. Whenever the area of skin irritation mirrors the appliance or part of the appliance in use, such as the tape border, allergic dermatitis should be suspected.

### 21. How is allergic dermatitis treated?

Treatment consists of identifying and removing the offending agent. Corticosteroid agents may be necessary in severe cases. Accessory products in use may also contain potential allergens. They should be eliminated while the skin is healing. If needed for an effective seal, the accessory products should be re-introduced one at a time to determine which product is the causative factor. Containing the effluent is also important so that the irritation does not worsen.

### 22. What is irritant dermatitis?

Irritant dermatitis results when inflammation of the peristomal skin develops in response to prolonged exposure to toxic substances, such as urinary or fecal drainage, pH variations, digestive enzymes in ileostomy output, and through use of accessory products, (e.g., solvents, glues, deodorants). Irritant dermatitis is inflamed, moist, and painful. Severe irritant dermatitis can take months to heal because the skin is fragile, similar to skin healing from a burn.

### 23. How is irritant dermatitis treated?

The inflammation can be treated with steroid creams, but caution should be used because they can cause thinning and further weakening of the skin. The skin may be dried by means of applying a skin barrier powder. The pouching system as well as the patient's application and removal technique should be reviewed. It is often helpful to eliminate as many accessory products as possible and to stick to the basics to avoid irritation.

### 24. What is folliculitis? How is it managed?

Folliculitis is the inflammation of a hair follicle. The lesions may appear inflamed, and erythematous and contain pus. Trauma to the hair follicle is caused through frequent shaving or careless pouch removal. Coagulase-positive staphylococci are often the offending organism. Folliculitis tends to be superficial but can extend into the hair follicle itself. The ensuing rash may resemble Candidiasis; therefore cultures may be indicated to distinguish the two before treatment is begun.

### 25. What is caput medusae?

Caput medusae is a peristomal skin condition caused by dilation of the cutaneous peristomal veins, which are really peristomal varices. The name refers to the resemblance of the dilated vessels to the head of the snake-haired Medusa. The skin has a bluish purple hue and is thin and fragile. Ostomates with concomitant liver disease are at risk for the development of these varices. They are also at risk for bleeding from the stoma and peristomal skin. Minor bleeding may stop spontaneously, but occasionally cautery is indicated, along with direct pressure. Severe bleeding may require suturing or surgical intervention. Patients are also at risk for massive gastrointestinal bleeding. Interventions include less frequent pouch changes, gentle stoma care, and flexible appliances without belts or tension to avoid trauma to the stoma.

### 26. What does a peristomal hernia look like?

Hernias appear as a bulge around the stoma. The bulge is a loop of bowel that has protruded through a fascial defect. Causes of a peristomal hernia include placement outside the rectus muscle, an excessively large fascial defect, placement of the stoma in the midline incision, and wound infection. Excessive weight is a predisposing factor. The patient is often asymptomatic.

### 27. What interventions should be initiated in patients with a peristomal hernia?

Support belts may help provide support to the abdominal wall. A change in pouching equipment may also be indicated. Flexible pouching systems tend to work best because of their ability to stay in place over the abdominal contours. Irrigation returns may be difficult and minimal. Irrigation should be discouraged, but if a patient insists it can be done. A cone-tipped irrigation set-up should be used to avoid perforation. Surgery is a treatment option, if desired.

### 28. What is peristomal hyperplasia?

Hyperplasia is the response of peristomal skin to chronic exposure and irritation by effluent. It presents with silver, wart-like, raised nodules and papules. They may be 2–10 cm in height and are often painful. They also bleed easily.

### 29. How is peristomal hyperplasia treated?

Treatment of peristomal hyperplasia consists of correcting the underlying problem—the chronic exposure of effluent on the skin. Pouching equipment must be evaluated. Often the stomal opening is too large. The pouch should be sized correctly, allowing minimal exposure of the peristomal skin to the effluent.

### 30. What are common causes of mechanical trauma to the peristomal skin?

Common causes of mechanical peristomal skin trauma include abrasive cleaning and removal techniques. Traumatic tape removal can result in stripping of the epidermis. Friction can result from equipment that is improperly fitted or changed too often. The peristomal skin becomes reddened and excoriated and may develop bloody, oozing areas.

### 31. What can be done about mechanical trauma?

In patients with evidence of mechanical trauma, stoma care techniques should be evaluated. The nurse must also evaluate the fit of faceplates, belts and pouches. Excessive weight gain or loss, hernias, and prolapse can also cause mechanical trauma. Barrier powders can be used to treat denuded areas, along with a non-stinging skin sealant to create an effective surface for adherence.

### 32. What is a continent ostomy?

Continent ostomies have become possible in recent years, thanks to advanced surgical techniques and evolving technology. As discussed in earlier chapters, continent ostomies include the following: Kock urinary pouch, Indiana urinary pouch, orthotopic neobladder, ileo-anal reservoir procedure, and Kock continent ileostomy. Continent ostomy diversions refer to the construction of an internal reservoir to contain body waste, giving the patient a measure of control or continence. Several different types of continent diversions, with and without stomas are available. This type of surgery is not without complications (see questions 33–35).

### 33. What is pouchitis? How is it treated?

Pouchitis is a long-term complication for patients who have had ileo-anal reservoir surgery. Incomplete emptying of the reservoir over a prolonged period can lead to bacterial overgrowth and infection. Symptoms include sudden increase of bowel movements and watery stool, accompanied occasionally by crampy lower abdominal pain. Stool is sometimes bloody. Metronidazole, the drug of choice, controls the bacterial overgrowth. Further treatment includes increasing fluid intake and prompt emptying of a full reservoir. The site of the ileo-anal anastomosis is also checked. Stenosis in this area can contribute to incomplete reservoir emptying.

### 34. What intubation problems are associated with a continent ostomy?

Intubating a stoma can be intimidating and frightening to both patients and clinicians.

Anxiety can lead to intubation difficulties. The first step is to teach the patient to relax. Taking slow deep breaths will help. The catheter can be advanced while the patient is exhaling. It is important to use a well-lubricated catheter. A pouch that is too full can place pressure on the nipple valves, making intubation more difficult. Changing positions will help, along with instilling a small amount of air with a syringe into the catheter. This approach relaxes the pouch valve. Intubation takes practice and patience.

Patients must be compliant with an intubation schedule, which is adjusted according to individual needs. The pouch must be sufficiently emptied to prevent pouchitis. The pouch must be emptied promptly when full to avoid incontinence. With time and experience, patients learn to recognize what a full pouch feels like. Their confidence increases, and they become better able to modify their routine in accordance with their own food and fluid intake habits.

### 35. When is a "continent" ostomy, incontinent?

Continence in ileo-anal pouch procedures is usually complete or nearly complete in approximately 80-90% of patients. Most of the incontinent population report mild incontinence or staining and are able to manage with the use of an absorbent pad.

### 36. What interventions reduce incontinence episodes?

Approximately half of the patients with a continent ostomy who have incontinence issues take medications, including antidiarrheal agents, such as loperamide and diphenoxylate, or bulk-forming laxatives, such as methylcellulose and psyllium, to modify bowel function. Dietary assessment is also important. Stool characteristic is an important assessment, because it can easily be modified. Treatment for incontinence depends on the type and amount of incontinence. Antidiarrheal medications and limiting of food intake near bedtime are helpful.

The ileo-anal anastomosis may be responsible for incontinence if a stricture is present. Treatment may require dilation and reservoir irrigation. Patients with seepage must perform meticulous perianal skin care. The seepage contains digestive enzymes that can cause denudation and irritation just as severe as leakage of effluent around a conventional ileostomy stoma.

### 37. What about equipment issues for a continent stoma?

Catheters and irrigation equipment should be carried with the patient at all times. Small-lumen catheters made of various materials are manufactured specifically for continent stomas. Water-soluble lubricant is also needed. Depending on the patient's continence status, the stoma may require only a small bandage covering. In some cases, stoma caps, which are small coverings to fit over the stoma in one or two pieces, may be worn. They are recommended for patients with seepage or mucous discharge between catheterizations. Catheters should be washed after use with warm water and soap. They should be rinsed well with running water through the inside of the catheter. The catheter should be hung to drip dry over a clean surface. Catheters can then be stored in a clean, dry, plastic bag. They should be replaced regularly, at least once per month, or discarded sooner if they show cracks, softened areas, or discolorations. Patients should also wear a medic alert bracelet and carry a card with catheterizing instructions. Skin sealant and barrier creams are necessary equipment for patients with ileoanal pouch diversions to provide perianal skin protection.

### BIBLIOGRAPHY

1. Francini A, Cola B, Stevens PJ: Atlas of Stomal Pathology. New York, Raven Press, 1983.
2. Hampton BG, Bryant RA: Ostomies and Continent Diversions—Nursing Management. St. Louis, Mosby, 1983.
3. Broadwell D, Jackson B: Principles of Ostomy Care. St. Louis, Mosby, 1982.
4. Mueller V: Quality of life with an ostomy: Building a model for assessment and care. Progr Develop Ostomy Wound Care 5(1):3–13, 1993.
5. Doblin-Brown K, Davidson M: Nursing care of the patient with an ileo-anal reservoir: A progressive teaching approach. Progr Develop Ostomy Wound Care 2(3):3–10, 1990.
6. Hampton B: Distinguishing among ostomy architectures and assessment findings: A primer for nurses. Progr Develop Ostomy Wound Care 4(4):3–12, 1992.

# 73. PSYCHOSOCIAL ISSUES: A DEVELOPMENTAL APPROACH

*Paula Erwin-Toth*, RN, MSN, ET, CWOCN, CNS

**1. What common psychosocial challenges are faced by children with an ostomy?**

The psychosocial implications of childhood ostomy surgery are widely varied. The underlying condition requiring an ostomy significantly affects the challenges that the child faces. Children have unique physical, psychological, social, and economic considerations that need to be addressed within the context of living and growing up with an ostomy. Counseling and support of families, friends, and caregivers are critical to the child's successful adjustment. Most clinicians advise that children with any physical challenge be raised like "normal" children. They *are* normal; they just happen to have an ostomy.

**2. What age-specific recommendations are helpful?**

It is important to treat children as unique individuals. Developmental and cognitive developmental theories can assist the clinician in identifying common challenges that face ostomates across the life span. These theories only offer a guide, not a template for practice.

**3. What approach is best with infants?**

Infants are developing a sense of trust vs. mistrust. They learn about the world through sensory input. Feeling loved and accepted begins at birth—some argue before birth.

Early interventions to promote bonding among the infant, parents, siblings, and other family members help to promote a sense of trust in the child. The world is a colorful, noisy place filled with new sights, smells, and sensations for the infant to experience. Ensuring that caregivers maintain a pleasant demeanor while interacting with the infant can enhance the child's sense of security. Accepting and warm facial expressions during ostomy care can convey a sense of acceptance of the stoma.

**4. Are interventions different for toddlers?**

Yes. As children develop, they gain a sense of mastery over themselves and their environment. They learn about the world through sensory input and the beginning of concept formation. To promote a sense of autonomy, the toddler should be included in care and instruction. At this age, a limited attention span necessitates short, focused, and positive attention to the ostomy.

Toddlers begin to be aware they are not quite like everyone else anatomically and need assurance that the ostomy is perfectly normal for them. Short, basic information and positive reinforcement are important at this stage.

**5. What challenges face preschoolers?**

Preschool children are developing a sense of initiative. They are still in the concept formation stage of cognitive development. Positive reinforcement and basic information are helpful during this phase of development. Active involvement and encouragement during pouch changing can assist children as they become more involved and aware of the ostomy. Children should be encouraged to play and participate in activities with peers. Let them know that the ostomy is normal for them but just as some things are kept private, they may want to keep the ostomy private as well. Be careful to avoid having the child feel that the ostomy is something shameful. Bathroom habits do not need to be explained. If the child attends preschool, the teacher needs to be aware of the ostomy and plans should be made to assist the child to empty the pouch until the technique is mastered. Extra equipment should be made available, and a responsible adult should be knowledgeable of how to change the pouch.

**6. Do school-aged children require some special attention?**

Apply and build on the techniques used for the preschool child. School-aged children are establishing a sense of industry and are advancing in the ability to form concepts. Once children enter school, they should be able to empty the pouch independently but may need some assistance if a complete pouch change is needed. Some clinicians recommend the use of a closed-end pouch in lieu of a drainable fecal pouch to ease management at school. Urinary pouches may be easily emptied via the spout. Children should be encouraged to participate in peer activities. Treating children as normal is especially critical during this phase of development. They may need some accommodations, such as more frequent bathroom privileges, but these needs should be planned in advance without placing undue attention on differences from peers. Body image, especially in a body conscious society, needs to be addressed honestly and in a matter-of-fact manner.

Emphasizing the child's attributes as a person and reinforcing that the ostomy restores or improves health can assist the child through these growing years.

**7. What advice may be given to teenagers with an ostomy?**

Adolescence is an especially challenging time to undergo ostomy surgery and poses special readjustment requirements for the child with an existing stoma. Teenagers are attempting to form an identity. Cognitively they begin to enter the abstract phase of development. An altered manner of elimination and threats to body image make teenagers especially vulnerable to coping with difficulties. Individual, family, and peer support and advocacy can enhance their ability to cope. Accentuate the positive aspect of the ostomy (for instance, the surgery resulting in the ostomy may significantly improve the way they feel). Encouraging them to participate in peer activities, and discussing body image and dating concerns with a trusted adult or another teenager with an ostomy can help teenagers with a stoma through these challenging times. A summer event or camp offered by support organizations, such as the Youth Rally offered annually by the United Ostomy Association and the Crohn's and Colitis Foundation, can be a valuable resource to help teenagers cope with an ostomy or inflammatory bowel disease.

**8. Are the needs of children with profound physical or developmental challenges different from those of other children?**

The critical point to remember is that the child is a child first. The ostomy and other physical or developmental challenges should be taken within the context of the individual. Encouraging the positive and building on accomplishments within the context of the child's uniqueness are essential.

**9. How can parents be supported to help themselves and their child cope with an ostomy?**

Assisting parents to cope with their own emotions is the first step to helping them effectively support their children. Raising a child with special needs, like an ostomy, can pose a strain on the family structure. Successful parenting entails meeting the child's needs within the context of the family. The child's ostomy should not become the focus of the family, but a part of the family's normal routine. Siblings can assist the child in gaining the acceptance and support of other children. Parents need to be active advocates to help their child lead as normal a life as peers without an ostomy.

**10. What are the psychosocial implications of ostomy surgery in adults?**

As with children, the psychosocial challenges facing adults are as varied as the patients themselves. Past coping abilities, diagnosis and prognosis, support systems, and developmental, cognitive, cultural and socioeconomic factors play a role in how an adult copes with an ostomy.

**11. How can psychosocial support be provided to a young adult with a new ostomy?**

Young adults with an ostomy are establishing a career path, intimacy with a partner, and independence from their family of origin. Threats to health and body image at this stage can pose challenges to the accomplishment of these goals.

Assisting the young adult to build on past effective coping skills and develop new ones requires individualized attention from the clinician. Frequent concerns of young adults include the ability to return to work or college, dating, marriage, reproduction, sports, and social activities. Peer visitors can provide valuable networking opportunities for the young adult with an ostomy. Expressing fears and concerns in an unhurried and supportive atmosphere can aid the clinician in determining appropriate interventions.

**12. What special psychosocial challenges are faced by people in their middle years with a stoma?**

This generation is typically called to "sandwich" generation. People in their middle years may be in the process of launching their teenager and young adult offspring and caring for aging parents. They tend to be at the peak of their careers and financial earning power. Mid-life is also a time of reflection on past accomplishments and goals yet to be achieved. An ostomy at this stage of life can cause emotional and financial upheavals. Many people in mid-life experience age-related body image challenges. An ostomy at this stage of life can deepen such concerns. Encouraging patients to focus on their own needs is a first step toward successful adjustment to living with an ostomy.

**13. What common psychosocial concerns are faced by older persons undergoing ostomy surgery?**

Maintaining independence and ego integrity are key concerns of older people undergoing ostomy surgery. Fears tend to revolve around inability to care for oneself, the ability to learn new tasks, and whether the ostomy will limit social activities. An individualized plan to address particular challenges can ameliorate the impact of many concerns and deficits. Body image issues continue to be of importance throughout the life span. Assisting the older person to view the ostomy as a lifesaving or life-improving procedure rather than evidence of a disorder or disease can support efforts to integrate the ostomy into a positive body image.

Accommodations for people with an existing stoma may need to be made as they age. Changes in visual acuity and manual dexterity may require modification of the pouching system to help the older person maintain independence in self-care. People are living longer, healthier lives. Dating and sexuality are areas that need to be addressed with older adults.

**14. What tips can be offered to the partners of people with stomas?**

Partners and potential partners of persons with stomas need information to enable them to understand and support their partner. A supportive, loving relationship is not negatively affected by an ostomy. However, in a relationship that is not well established or in which problems already exist, an ostomy may be perceived as a problem or serve as an excuse to end an unstable union.

**15. Are some concerns more prevalent than others?**

Many partners worry about what to say or not to say; what to do or not to do. This is a fairly typical feeling in any relationship but is especially difficult when coping with an ostomy. The most important consideration is how well the person with the stoma has accepted the ostomy. People with ostomies cannot rely on the support of another to come to terms with something so intimate to themselves. A partner can offer loving support and reinforcement that can help the person cope with the stoma, but ultimately adjustment comes from within. Reassure the couple that an ostomy will not interfere with normal sexual activity.

**16. Does sexual orientation influence advice given to partners?**

It is important to offer open discussion and support according to the sexual orientation of the client. Appropriate referrals to gay/lesbian ostomy support groups through the United Ostomy Association can be especially helpful.

**17. What practical tips can be offered to help ease the return to intimacy?**

Numerous aids can enhance the romance for people with ostomies and their partners. Commercially available pouch covers, lingerie, and small mini-pouches are designed to enhance intimacy. The most important activity is focusing on the loving relationship with a sense of love, joy and adventure as sexual activity is resumed.

**18. What common cultural influences may affect how a person copes with an ostomy?**

As with life span issues, no generalizations can be made about culture and coping with an ostomy. Some general influences can be related to gender, age, personality, and culture. A cultural assessment is an integral part of the assessment process. Self-care may be the common expectation in Western cultures but may not be standard in others. Sharing of feelings and referrals for support may or may not be acceptable based on cultural values. It is beyond the scope of this chapter to examine all of the cultures and potential influence on coping with an ostomy. Texts and articles about transcultural nursing can offer the clinician helpful support.

**19. How can social issues influence a person's ability to cope with an ostomy?**

Social and economic factors can have a significant impact on a person's ability to cope with and manage a stoma. The ability to purchase appropriate supplies and have access to professional and family/caregiver support varies greatly. Ensuring that the person with an ostomy is aware of services and support is an integral part of care. Some people are unaware of insurance and Medicare coverage of ostomy supplies. Additionally, they may be eligible for equipment through other state- and industry-sponsored programs.

**20. What role can support groups play in the psychosocial adjustment of people with ostomies?**

Referral to a support group before and after surgery can offer a tremendous resource for people with ostomies and their significant others. A well-adjusted ostomy visitor of the same gender, age, and diagnosis can offer a tremendous psychological boost. Support groups should be offered at regular intervals in both the short-term and long-term rehabilitation process. Disease-specific, family, and caregiver support groups can offer additional resources for the patient, family, and clinician.

## BIBLIOGRAPHY

1. Erwin-Toth P, Doughty D: Principles and procedures of stomal management. In Hampton B, Bryant R: Ostomies and Continent Diversions—Nursing Management. St. Louis, Mosby, 1992, pp 29–103.
2. Erwin-Toth P: The effect of ostomy surgery between the ages of 6 and 12 on psychosocial development in childhood, adolescence and young adulthood. J Wound Ostomy Contin Nurs 26(2):77–85, 1999.
3. Golis AM: Sexual issues for the person with an ostomy. J Wound Ostomy Contin Nurs 23(1):33–37, 1996.
4. Hampton B, Bryant R: Ostomies and Continent Diversions—Nursing Management. St. Louis, Mosby, 1992.
5. Jenks JM, Morin KH: The influence of ostomy surgery on body image in patients with cancer. Appl Nurs Res 10(4):174–80, 1997.
6. Lavery I, Erwin-Toth P: Stoma therapy. In MacKeighan J, Cataldo P (eds): Intestinal Stomas Principles and Management. St. Louis, Quality Medical Publishing, 1993, pp 60–84.
7. Manworren RC: Developmental effects on the adolescent with a temporary ileostomy. J Wound Ostomy Contin Nurs 23(4):210–217, 1996.
8. VanHorn C, Barrett P: Pregnancy, delivery and postpartum experiences of fifty-four women with ostomies. J Wound Ostomy Contin Nurs 24(3):302–310, 1997.
9. Zoucha R, Zamarripa C: The significance of culture in the care of the client with an ostomy. J Wound Ostomy Contin Nurs 24(5):270–276, 1997.

# III. Continence

## 74. PHYSIOLOGY OF VOIDING

*Sharon A. Aronovitch, PhD, RN, CETN*

### 1. What three muscles are involved in urination? How do they differ?

Voiding, also known as micturition, involves the coordination of activity among three bladder muscles: the detrusor and the internal and external sphincter muscles. The detrusor muscle is smooth muscle. The internal sphincter is composed of circular smooth muscle. The external sphincter is circular striated muscle.

### 2. What are the roles of the bladder muscles in voiding? How does voiding occur?

Both the detrusor and internal sphincter are smooth muscles and are not under voluntary control. The detrusor muscle is located within the body of the bladder. This muscle relaxes to allow urine into the bladder from the ureters. At a predetermined capacity, usually 600 cc, the detrusor muscle contracts to push out the urine. The internal sphincter is a continuation of the detrusor muscle onto the neck of the bladder. As urine fills the body of the relaxed bladder, the internal sphincter contracts (closes off the bladder neck) to prevent leaking of urine (fill phase). It relaxes to allow urine to flow out when the bladder contracts. The external sphincter is under voluntary control. During the empty phase, the sphincter remains contracted to prevent urine leakage until the person consciously relaxes it, thereby allowing voiding of urine.

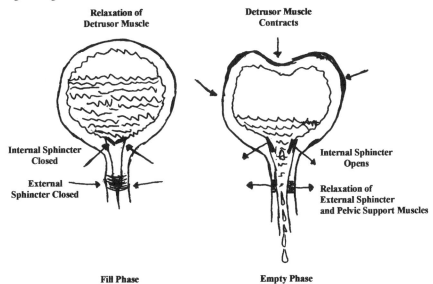

Muscles of the bladder.

### 3. Why is the detrusor muscle important to the voiding process?

The importance of the detrusor muscle is twofold. First, it acts as an expanding balloon to allow urine into the bladder; secondly, it contracts once the bladder is full to expel the urine. Within the cerebral cortex is a detrusor motor area that modulates bladder emptying, thereby permitting social continence.

### 4. How are the bladder muscles innervated?

The bladder muscles are innervated via both the sympathetic and parasympathetic divisions of the autonomic nervous system. The detrusor muscle is the only bladder muscle that is innervated by both sympathetic and parasympathetic systems. The acetylcholine receptors (parasympathetic system) stimulate the detrusor muscle to contract and expel urine. The beta-adrenergic receptors (sympathetic system) stimulate the bladder muscle to relax, thereby allowing the detrusor muscle to expand and the bladder to fill with urine. Contractions of the internal sphincter are regulated by the alpha-adrenergic receptors (sympathetic system) to maintain continence. The external sphincter is regulated by the acetylcholine receptors (neurotransmitter at cholinergic synapses of parasympathetic and sympathetic system) but is also under the voluntary control of the cerebral cortex, which controls its relaxation or contraction.

### 5. What is the micturition reflex?

This complex reflex is composed of the brainstem, spinal cord, bladder and urethral nerve structure that permits voiding. All components of the voiding system need to be intact for micturition to occur. As sensory receptors located in the bladder and urethra become stretched by the filling of the bladder with urine, signals are sent via the pelvic nerves to the introspective nerves in the sacral spinal cord (segments 2, 3, 4) and then to the brainstem that the bladder needs to empty. The parasympathetic nervous system (extrovert nerves) respond to the bladder via the same nerve track, and micturition occurs. However, micturition can be inhibited by the cerebral cortex by contraction of the external sphincter.

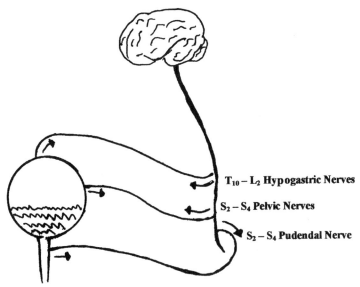

$T_{10} - L_2$ **Hypogastric Nerves**

$S_2 - S_4$ **Pelvic Nerves**

$S_2 - S_4$ **Pudendal Nerve**

Micturition reflex.

### 6. When does a child become continent?

A child obtains continence only when conscious neurologic awareness occurs, typically at the age of 1–2 years. Until this age, a child becomes aware that a voiding episode has occurred immediately after urination. Full mastery of the skills required for continence begins at age 5. Continence is achieved when the child is able to identify, contract, and relax the pelvic floor muscles to control voiding.

**7. Is it normal for a child of 5 years age to wet the bed?**

Nocturnal enuresis (bedwetting) is normal in children until the age of 3 years. Up to 15% of children continue to experience episodes of urinary incontinence until age 5 years. The majority of these children are male. Less than 1% of older children still have episodes of nighttime incontinence at 12 years of age. A recent study from Scandinavia reported evidence of a genetic predisposition toward nocturnal enuresis.

**8. Does normal aging lead to incontinence?**

The aging process does not cause urinary incontinence. However, there is an increase in nocturia because elderly people void smaller amounts of urine during the day. The aging process also results in changes in the central nervous system, bladder, and adjacent organs.

**9. Why are voiding problems present with benign prostatic hypertrophy (BPH)?**

BPH, an enlargement of the glandular components of the prostate, causes bladder outlet obstruction because the gland encroaches on the lumen of prostatic urethra and increases smooth muscle tone in the bladder neck and prostatic urethra. In mild cases of BPH, the detrusor muscle is able to compensate for the increased outlet resistance by increasing the intensity of the contractions. Severe cases of BPH result in obstruction of the outlet and, over time, decompensation of the detrusor muscle and a change in the urinary stream. The changes in the urinary stream include a decrease in flow of urine, intermittence of flow, frequency of urination, and incomplete bladder emptying. In elderly men, BPH is thought to preserve continence.

**10. How often should a person void?**

On average, most people void every 3 or 4 hours during the day with one void at night. It is normal for the elderly to get up twice during the night to urinate.

**11. What is considered an abnormal voiding pattern?**

Any interval of 2 hours or less between voids or more than 8 voids per day is considered aberrant.

BIBLIOGRAPHY

1. Continence Facts: http://www.rpromise.com/tena/facts.html
2. Gray M: Physiology of voiding. In Doughty DB (ed): Urinary and Fecal Incontinence: Nursing Management, St. Louis, Mosby, 2000, pp 1–24.
3. Wiener JS: Incontinence: Is it inherited? Qual Care Newslett 18(3):1, 2000.

# 75. PHYSIOLOGY OF DEFECATION

*Catherine T. Milne, APRN, MSN, CWOCN, CS, ANP,*
*and Lisa Q. Corbett, APRN, MSN, CWOCN, CS*

### 1. What are the physiologic components of defecation?

Intestinal contents, motility, and distensibility, coupled with an intact sensory pathway and sphincter control, are essential to the normal defecation process.

### 2. What are the anatomic components of defecation?

The rectum is 3–4 cm in length and lies slightly anteroposteriorally low in the pelvic floor. This position assists in acting as a barrier to fecal seepage. Attached to the symphysis pubis at one end, the puborectalis muscles wraps around the anorectal junction, causing a right-angle flexure at the posterior end. This, too, acts as a physical barrier to fecal flow in its state of normal tonic contraction.

### 3. What are the roles of the internal and external anal sphincters, anal canal, and rectal sensation in defecation?

The **internal sphincter** is composed of circular smooth muscle. Receiving input from the sacral nerves, it is under involuntary control. It remains closed, giving resting tone to the area, until nervous innervation relaxes the sphincter.

The **external sphincter**, consisting of striated muscle, lies below the internal sphincter. Although its normally contracted state adds little to resting tone, its purpose is to augment tone in periods of rectal distention or increased intra-abdominal pressure. The external sphincter helps maintain social continence because of voluntary control from the cerebral cortex.

The **anal canal** can distinguish among flatus, liquid, and solid stool. This process is called *anal sampling*. **Rectal sensation** allows selective, conscious passage of some material and not others.

### 4. How does defecation occur?

Stool enters the rectum, causing it to enlarge. The distended anal canal sends signals along the sacral nerves to the spinal cord. The internal sphincter relaxes reflexively. The contents descend a bit so that anal sampling can occur. During this process, the external sphincter increases its tone and pulls on the puborectalis and the levator ani muscles to further angulate the rectum to prevent fecal seepage. Once the cerebral cortex signals the pudendal nerve to relax, sitting or squatting straightens the anorectal angle to facilitate passage of stool. Bearing down during this time relaxes the puborectalis muscles to straighten this angle even more. The pelvic floor descends at this time, and the anal canal contracts simultaneously, with full relaxation of the internal and external sphincter, to expel stool.

### 5. What other factors influence the defecation process?

The social setting, availability of a bathroom, and intact cognition and functional mobility also affect the defecation process. The rectum can stretch and hold stool for quite some time until a conscious decision is made to defecate at an appropriate, socially acceptable time and place.

### 6. How often should normal defecation occur?

Stool frequency is highly individualized. A range of one or two bowel movements per day to one stool every 3 or 4 days is considered normal.

### 7. Can stool be defined by its characteristics?

Many patients report having "diarrhea" as a method to bring up the subject of fecal incontinence. The classic definition of diarrhea is more than two bowel movements per day or liquid stool. Stool can be described based on its consistency.

Type 1: separate, small hard lumps that are difficult to expel
Type 2: hard, sausage-shaped lumps, formed together and difficult to expel
Type 3: sausage-like but with cracks on the surface; may be somewhat difficult to expel
Type 4: smooth, soft, formed, easy to expel
Type 5: soft, formed pieces that are easy to expel
Type 6: mushy, puffy pieces with ragged edges
Type 7: liquid with no formed pieces

## 8. When is defecation abnormal?

Certainly defecation is abnormal when performed in a socially unacceptable place or time. A change in the consistency or frequency from the patient's usual habits is also considered aberrant. Abnormality, however, does not necessarily indicate disease. A change in routine or usual foods may be enough to change defecation patterns temporarily. Clinical suspicion for malignancy is high with an unexplained change in bowel habits in any patient who is older than 40 or at high risk, such as patients with familial polyposis.

## 9. Can you have two bowel movements a day and still be constipated?

Patients often define constipation as stool infrequency. However, stool that is hard and difficult to pass, regardless of frequency, is true constipation. If the patient spends an inordinate amount of time on the toilet and strains to defecate two times per day, constipation is present.

## 10. Why do elderly people become constipated?

As a normal consequence of aging, colonic transport time slows somewhat. This reduces the frequency of bowel movements. More often, constipation in this population results from reduced exercise, limited fluid intake, and poor dietary habits and as an undesirable side effect of medications used to treat other comorbidities.

## 11. When does social continence occur?

Youngsters can develop the cognitive pathways to become socially continent between the ages of 2 and 4 years. Most children reach this milestone by the age of $3\frac{1}{2}$ years.

### BIBLIOGRAPHY

1. Bliss, D, Larson, S, Burr, J, Savik, K. Reliability of a stool consistency classification system. J Wound Ostomy Contin Nurs 28(6):305–313, 2001.
2. Doughty D: A physiological approach to bowel training. J Wound Ostomy Contin 23(5):46–56, 1996.
3. Jensen L: Assessing and treating patients with complex fecal incontinence. Ostomy Wound Manage 46(12): 56–60, 2000.
4. Norton C, Chelvanayagam S: A nursing assessment tool for adults with fecal incontinence. J Wound Ostomy Contin Nurs 27(5):279–291, 2000.

# 76. CLASSIFICATION OF URINARY INCONTINENCE

*Nancy Tomaselli, RN, MSN, CS, CRNP, CWOCN, CLNC*

### 1. What is a urinary incontinence?

Of the several types of urinary incontinence, all are associated with the inability to restrain or control urinary voiding, leading to the involuntary loss of urine. The term *incontinence* can be used to describe a symptom (the patient's report of involuntary loss of urine), a sign (observed leakage of urine), or a condition (pathology as demonstrated by clinical or urodynamic studies).[3]

### 2. How common is urinary incontinence?

Millions of people are affected by urinary incontinence. As the population ages, the overall incidence is expected to rise. Urinary incontinence is more prevalent in women by a margin of 3:1; over half of all women experience urinary incontinence at some time during their life.

### 3. Describe the social impact of incontinence.

Incontinence is the leading cause of institutionalization in the elderly. In attempt to hide the problem, people who are incontinent withdraw from social activities and intimate relationships, adding to depression and medical concerns.

### 4. How is incontinence classified?

The International Continence Society (ICS) has developed a physiologically based classification system for types of incontinence that is widely used by clinicians.[1] This system was used by the Agency for Healthcare Research and Quality to develop clinical practice guidelines for urinary incontinence (AHCPR, 1996). The Urodynamic Society and the American Urologic Association also advocate the use of this classification system.

### 5. What are the components of the ICS classification system?

The ICS classification system is based on two functions of the lower urinary tract: urinary storage and urinary elimination. Incontinence is considered a problem with storage or a problem with elimination. Problems are further categorized by the cause of bladder or sphincter dysfunction. Types of incontinence are defined within the framework of a storage problem or emptying problem and the area of dysfunction. For example, urge incontinence is a storage problem caused by bladder dysfunction. Much like a car, which needs both an engine (mechanical) and a battery (electrical) to run properly, the causes of incontinence can be simply a mechanical (filling or emptying) or an electrical (neurologic) malfunction. On occasion, both mechanical and electrical systems become dysfunctional.

*ICS Classification System*

| PROBLEM | ETIOLOGY | RESULT |
|---|---|---|
| Problems with storage | Bladder dysfunction | Urge incontinence |
| | Sphincter dysfunction | Stress incontinence |
| | Other | Mixed and functional incontinence |
| Problems with elimination | Bladder dysfunction | Overflow incontinence |
| | Sphincter dysfunction | Overflow incontinence |
| Mixed problems with storage and emptying | Bladder and sphincter dysfunction | Reflex incontinence |

Adapted from Doughty DB, Waldrop J: Introductory concepts. In Doughty DB (ed): Urinary and Fecal Incontinence: Nursing Management, 2nd ed. St. Louis, Mosby, 2000, pp 29–45.

**6. What diagnostic tools are used to determine the type of incontinence?**

Urodynamic tests are performed to determine the anatomic and functional status of the urinary bladder and urethra. They measure bladder filling, detrusor function, and function of the urinary sphincters and accessory muscles involved in voiding. Testing modalities are further described in Chapter 77.

**7. Name the types of urinary incontinence.**

*Types of Urinary Incontinence*

| TYPE | PATHOPHYSIOLOGY |
| --- | --- |
| Stress | Involuntary loss of urine from the urethra as intra-abdominal pressure increases above urethral resistance during physical exertion, such as coughing, laughing, sneezing, lifting, bending or changing positions. |
| Type I | Stress incontinence caused by urethral hypermobility. There is loss of the posterior urethrovesical angle during stress maneuver but maintenance of the anterior support (see figure below). |
| Type II | Stress incontinence caused by urethral hypermobility. There is loss of both the posterior urethrovesical angle and anterior support (see figure on following page). |
| Type III | Stress incontinence caused by intrinsic sphincter deficiency (see figure on following page). |
| Urge | Involuntary loss of urine from overdistention of the bladder due to urinary retention. |
| Mixed | Combination of urge and stress incontinence. |
| Overflow | Involuntary loss of urine from overdistention of the bladder due to urinary retention. |
| Transient | Temporary episodes of urinary incontinence that are reversible once the cause is identified and treated. |
| Functional | Inability for a normally continent person to get to the toilet. |
| Reflex | Loss of urine without any warning or sensory awareness. |

Adapted from Wound, Ostomy and Continence Nurses Society: Standards of Care: Patients with Urinary Incontinence. Laguna Beach, CA, WOCN Society, 1992; and Doughty DB, Waldrop J: Introductory concepts. In Doughty DB (ed): Urinary and Fecal Incontinence: Nursing Management, 2nd ed. St. Louis, Mosby, 2000, pp 29–45.

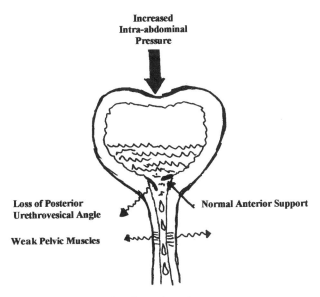

Type I stress incontinence.

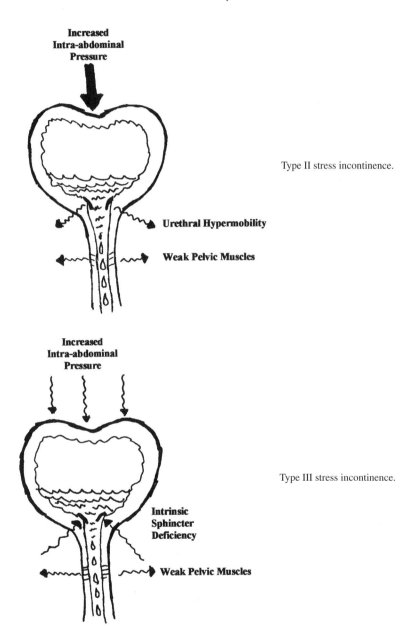

Type II stress incontinence.

Type III stress incontinence.

### 8. What are the urodynamic findings for stress incontinence?

There is a loss of urine with increase in abdominal pressure without detrusor contraction or an overdistended bladder. The pelvic floor muscles are weak.

### 9. How does hypermobility of the bladder neck contribute to type I and type II stress incontinence?

High intra-abdominal pressure, produced by seemingly normal activities such as laughing, place a downward pressure on the bladder and urethra. As the pressure descends deep into the pelvic floor, the normal urethral resistance is no longer present and leakage results. Weak pelvic floor muscles contribute greatly to type I stress incontinence.

## 10. How does intrinsic sphincter deficiency (ISD) contribute to type III stress incontinence?

The urethral sphincter cannot contract to create sufficient resistance in response to the storage of urine in the bladder. The cause may be congenital sphincter weakness (myelomeningocele or epispadias), prostatectomy, trauma, radiation therapy, sacral cord lesions, urologic procedures affecting sphincter function, atrophic vaginitis, or urethritis. ISD is characterized by leakage under minimal increases in intra-abdominal pressure, such as walking or getting up from a chair.

## 11. List factors contributing to weak pelvic floor muscles.
- Multiple pregnancies
- Difficult deliveries
- Previous gynecologic procedures
- Obesity

## 12. Define urge incontinence.

Urge incontinence is the involuntary loss of urine from an abrupt and strong desire to void. It is sometimes called "key in the lock" syndrome because when the person hears the sound of a key in a doorlock when he or she arrives home, there is a severe, sudden urgency to urinate.

## 13. Describe urgency.

Urgency results from bladder hypersensitivity with no demonstrable detrusor instability. This abnormal sensitivity to bladder filling causes the patient to feel uncomfortable with only a moderately full bladder. The brain signals the urge to void frequently and small voided volumes are expelled. Detrusor contractions are normal. Sensory urgency can result from decreased bladder compliance due to a non-neurogenic etiology such as chemical or radiation cystitis. Loss of bladder wall elasticity and lack of bladder accommodation cause a steep rise in the intravesical pressure during bladder filling without detrusor contraction. In patients with a compromised urethral sphincter mechanism, this abnormal increase may overcome the urethral pressure and produce urinary incontinence. A major concern with poor detrusor compliance is the development of vesicoureteral reflux and hydronephrosis.

## 14. What factors contribute to bladder irritability and the sensation of urgency?
- Acute urinary tract infection
- Dietary irritants such as caffeine, artificial sweeteners, or alcohol
- Medications such as diuretics
- Inadequate fluid intake
- Habitual frequent voiding
- Fecal constipation and impaction
- Benign prostatic hypertrophy
- Atrophic vaginitis
- Pelvic tumors
- Bladder prolapse
- Medical conditions resulting in increased urine production such as diabetes insipidus
- Factors of idiopathic origin, seen predominantly in children and the elderly, with uncertain neurologic or other coexisting factors

## 15. What are the urodynamic findings for urge incontinence?

Detrusor instability, detrusor hyperreflexia, detrusor overactivity, and detrusor sphincter dyssynergia can be found on urodynamic studies. Detrusor instability is a result of involuntary detrusor contractions in the absence of associated neurological disorders. The bladder contracts and empties when it should be relaxed and storing (see figure on following page).

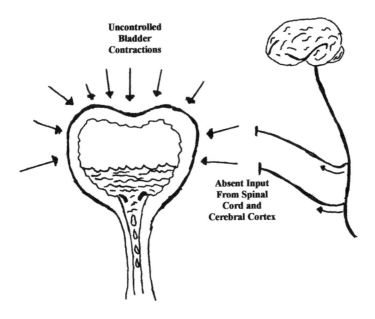

Detrusor instability.

Detrusor hyperreflexia is caused by involuntary detrusor contractions associated with a neurologic disorder such as a stroke. It is often accompanied by detrusor sphincter dyssynergia in patients with suprasacral spinal cord lesions and multiple sclerosis. Detrusor overactivity is caused by involuntary detrusor contractions. Its specific cause is unclear. Detrusor sphincter dyssynergia is the inappropriate contraction of the external sphincter simultaneously with an involuntary contraction of the detrusor muscle (see figure below). This is a common feature of neurologic voiding disorders.

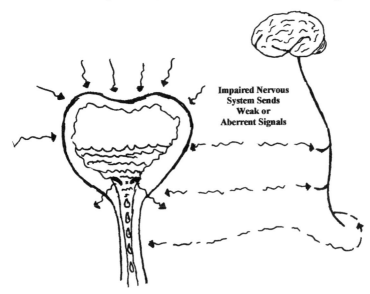

Detrusor hyperreflexia with detrusor sphincter dyssynergia.

**16. What happens in detrusor hyperactivity with impaired bladder contractility (DHIC)?**

Involuntary detrusor contractions in which the patient is either unable to empty the bladder completely or can empty their bladder completely only with straining due to poor contractility of the detrusor. Patients with DHIC may have symptoms of urge incontinence and an elevated postvoid residual (PVR) volume; they may also exhibit obstruction, stress, or overflow incontinence. Therefore, it must be distinguished from other types of incontinence to avoid inappropriate diagnosis and treatment.

**17. What factors reduce the ability to inhibit bladder contractions?**

- Cerebrovascular accident
- Dementia
- Parkinson's disease
- Diabetes mellitus
- Brain injury/tumor

**18. What is mixed incontinence?**

The combination of urge and stress incontinence. Patients have symptoms of both entities: leakage with high intra-abdominal pressures and urinary frequency with urgency.

**19. Define overflow incontinence.**

Overflow incontinence is the involuntary loss of urine from overdistention of the bladder resulting from urinary retention. There is continuous or intermittent leakage of small amounts of urine. It can present as frequent or constant dribbling or with symptoms of urge or stress incontinence.

**20. Describe the pathophysiology of overflow incontinence.**

Overflow incontinence is caused by an outflow obstruction or reduced bladder contractility. It is a failure to empty adequately. In the "overfull" bladder, intrabladder pressure eventually overcomes urethral resistance, resulting in urine release. Pressures quickly fall after small amounts are released, and full emptying cannot be achieved.

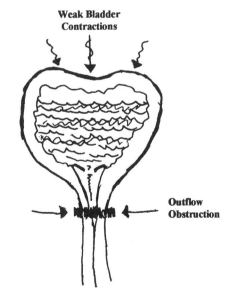

Overflow incontinence.

**21. List factors causing outflow obstruction.**

- Prostatic hypertrophy
- Detrusor external sphincter dyssynergia
- Mechanical obstruction of the urethra (e.g., urethral stricture)
- Anti-incontinence procedures or pelvic organ prolapse in women

**22. List factors causing reduced bladder contractility (also known as acontractile detrusor, detrusor areflexia, or detrusor underactivity).**

- Sacral cord lesions or injuries
- Neurologic conditions (e.g., diabetic neuropathy)
- Multiple sclerosis
- Low back syndrome
- Pelvic trauma resulting in denervation
- Abdominal perineal resection
- Hip surgery
- Drugs
- Idiopathic causes

**23. What is transient incontinence?**

Transient incontinence is defined as temporary episodes of urinary incontinence that are reversible once the cause is identified and treated. All reversible factors should be addressed before assessing for other types of incontinence. Using the mnemonic **DIAPPERS**, described by Resnick in 1996, a clinician can easily remember the common reversible causes of transient incontinence.

**D** = **D**elirium
**I** = **I**nfection or inflammation
**A** = **A**trophic vaginitis and urethritis
**P** = **P**harmaceuticals
**P** = **P**sychologic conditions
**E** = Conditions resulting in **E**xcessive urine production
**R** = **R**estricted mobility
**S** = **S**tool impaction

**24. Describe other conditions that contribute to transient incontinence not covered by the DIAPPERS mnemonic.**

Pregnancy, vaginal delivery, episiotomy, and prostatectomy.

**25. List medications that commonly cause transient incontinence.**

- Diuretics
- Caffeine
- Anticholinergics
- Psychotropics
- Narcotic analgesics
- Alpha-adrenergic blockers
- Alpha-adrenergic agonists
- Beta-adrenergic agonists
- Calcium channel blockers
- Alcohol

**26. Define functional incontinence.**

Functional incontinence is the inability for a normally continent person to get to the toilet. There is loss of bladder control due to a functional deficit rather than an organic dysfunction. Normal physiology and structure of the urinary tract are usually intact. This diagnosis is usually one of exclusion because some immobile and cognitively impaired patients have other types of urinary incontinence.

**27. Does functional incontinence overlap with transient incontinence?**

Certainly some of the functional deficits that contribute to transient incontinence occur in functional incontinence. However, in functional incontinence, the deficit caused by restricted mobility is temporary.

**28. List causes of functional incontinence.**

- Cognitive impairments: altered mental status, dementia
- Mobility/dexterity impairments: arthritis, visual impairment, compromised pulmonary function, hip fracture, pain
- Psychological impairments: depression, withdrawal, lack of motivation
- Environmental barriers: distance to bathroom, side rails, restraints, lighting, clothing that is difficult to remove
- Dependence on caregiver for toileting
- Lack of caregiver responsiveness to voiding needs

**29. What specific metabolic conditions cause an increase in the production of urine?**
- Metabolic disorders such as hyperglycemia, hypercalcemia, and diabetes insipidus
- Excessive fluid intake
- Volume overload

**30. What factors restrict mobility?**
- Impaired ability or willingness to get to the toilet
- Delirium
- Chronic illness
- Injury
- Deconditioning
- Physical or chemical restraints

**31. Discuss reflex incontinence.**

Reflex incontinence is the loss of urine without warning or sensory awareness. The patient is unaware of bladder filling and can neither delay nor voluntarily initiate voiding. There is postmicturitional or constant dribbling. Detrusor hyperreflexia in the form of uncontrolled, overactive bladder contractions caused by a centrally located neurologic lesion and an involuntary urethral relaxation in the absence of the sensation associated with the desire to micturate are the pathophysiologic causes.

**32. What conditions are associated with reflex incontinence?**
- Spinal cord injury above the level of the sacral micturition center (S2–S4)
- Neurologic lesion involving suprasacral spinal cord, such as multiple sclerosis, transverse myelitis, or spina bifida

**33. Is there any good news?**

Incontinence is a highly treatable condition. A thorough and accurate assessment of the type of incontinence, designed to identify reversible factors or established incontinence, is essential for the development of an effective treatment plan.

### BIBLIOGRAPHY

1. Abrams P, Blaivas JG, Stanton SL, Anderson JT: The standardization of terminology of lower urinary tract function. Scand J Urol Nephrol 114(Suppl):5–19, 1988.
2. Agency for Health Care Policy and Research, Public Health Service, U.S. Department of Health and Human Services: Urinary Incontinence Guidelines Panel: Urinary Incontinence in Adults: Clinical Practice Guideline Update. AHCPR Pub. No. 96-0686, Rockville, MD, 1996.
3. Blavis J, Appell R, Fantl JA, et al: Definition and classification of urinary incontinence: Recommendations of the urodynamic society. Neurourol Urodyn 16:149–151, 1997.
4. Doughty DB, Waldrop J: Introductory concepts. In Doughty DB (ed): Urinary and Fecal Incontinence: Nursing Management, 2nd ed. St. Louis, Mosby, 2000, pp 29–45.
5. Resnick N: Geriatric incontinence. Urol Clin North Am 23(1):55–71, 1996.
6. Wound, Ostomy and Continence Nurses Society: Standards of Care: Patients with Urinary Incontinence. Laguna Beach, CA, WOCN Society, 1992.

# 77. ASSESSMENT OF URINARY CONTINENCE

*Lisa M. Oliveira*, APRN, MSN

### 1. How common is urinary incontinence?

Urinary incontinence affects 15 million Americans; 85% are female. At least 26.3 billion/year is spent on continence care. It is estimated that urinary incontinence affects 15–30% of people over age 65 who live in the community. The problem affects 50% or more of nursing home residents.

### 2. How does a clinician determine what type of urinary incontinence a patient has?

Determining the type of urinary incontinence (UI) depends on a good history and physical exam. Although UI is a symptom and not a disease, it is still important to determine its cause is. A basic evaluation must include a medical, neurologic, and genitourinary history. The examiner must keep in mind the transient causes for UI discussed in Chapter 76 under functional incontinence. A careful review of medication history is essential.

### 3. What specific questions can be asked during the historical assessment?

1. *Do you leak urine or have damp underwear or occasional wetness?* Many people do not understand the word "incontinence" or associate incontinence with total loss of urine control.

2. *How do you cope and manage urine leakage?* People suffering from incontinence withdraw socially to avoid potentially embarrassing moments. Others plan activities so that a bathroom is nearby at all times. The use of pads, diapers, or other self-made methods to control urine may be disclosed. The answers to this question may be the first hint as to whether the patient has stress or urge incontinence.

3. *Where in your house or apartment is the toilet? Do you ever use a commode or urinal? Do you have a problem getting to the toilet or any problems getting your clothes on or off at the time of urination?* These questions assess the environment as well as the mobility and dexterity skills necessary for continence. Perhaps the toilet is upstairs, and severe arthritis prevents the person from reaching the toilet. Positive responses may point toward a functional cause of incontinence.

4. *Have you had any of the following: multiple pregnancies, difficult deliveries, genitourinary surgery, neurosurgery, back operations, diabetes, neurologic disease, urinary tract infections, leakage of stool, or radiation therapy for cancer in the pelvic region?* Positive response to any of the above requires further probing. Medical history often helps the clinician identify the type of incontinence. For example, a patient with recurrent urinary tract infections may have transient incontinence. Another may have experienced pudendal nerve damage during a difficult delivery.

5. *What medications (prescription and over-the-counter) do you take? What natural, homeopathic or herbal preparations do you take?* Many medications, including nonprescription and "natural" products, can cause or contribute to incontinence.

6. *How many cups of fluid do you drink every day? What types of liquid?* Insufficient fluid intake prevents adequate dilution of bladder irritants and causes urge incontinence. Certain liquids, such as caffeine, diet carbonated beverages, and alcohol, directly irritate the bladder.

7. *How often do you have a bowel movement? Is the movement hard or soft? Do you find yourself straining to have a bowel movement?* Constipation is a frequently overlooked factor in urge or overflow incontinence.

8. *Does your urine burn or smell? Do you ever see blood in your urine?* A positive response may be related to a urinary tract infection. Hematuria can also be present in bladder cancer.

9. *When did the symptoms start? How often are you wet? When there is leakage, is it a few drops, enough to dampen your clothes or saturate them? How many pads do you use? When do you use them? Are you free from leakage when you sleep? Does a certain activity, such as sneezing or exercise, cause leakage?* These general questions specific to voiding patterns help focus the clinician to begin a differential diagnosis between the various types of incontinence.

10. *How often do you urinate during the day? At night? Are there any problems with having your stream start or stop? Does the urine dribble out or come out as a forceful stream? Do you have to strain to urinate? Do you feel as though your bladder is not empty after you finish urinating?* Positive responses may indicate overflow incontinence or incomplete emptying.

11. *Do you find yourself rushing to urinate? Is there no time between "feeling the urge to go" and voiding? Do you always make it to the toilet on time?* Urge incontinence may present with these symptoms.

Take the time to get a good history. The end result will save the clinician time later, identifies patient knowledge deficits, and may save the patient from undergoing time-consuming and expensive clinical procedures.

**4. What are the components of the physical assessment of an incontinent patient? How do abnormal findings correlate with a specific diagnosis?**
- A physical exam includes a general exam with a focused abdominal and genitourinary exam.
- Clinical suspicions of depression, confusion, and dementia can be easily confirmed using valid clinical tools, such as a Mini-Mental Status exam or depression scale. Noncognitively intact or depressed patients may have functional incontinence.
- Neurologic evaluation of cranial and peripheral motor and sensory nerves, intact reflexes, two-point discrimination, presence of tremors, and motor strength is essential.
- Assess dexterity, range of motion, and gait for any abnormalities. Deficits in this area point to functional incontinence.
- Look for the presence of edema in extremities. Edema may subside during the night in a supine position. This increases urine output and contributes to nocturia.

**5. What should a focused abdominal examination include?**
A general abdominal exam includes inspection, palpation, and auscultation to evaluate for organomegaly, masses, suprapubic tenderness, peritoneal irritation, bladder fullness, or fluid collections. Diastasis recti (separation of the rectus muscles in the abdominal wall) can be determined by having the supine patient attempt to place the chin on the chest. This maneuver tightens the rectus muscles. The examiner palpates the rectus muscles for soft, separated areas.

**6. Describe the abnormal findings of a rectal exam.**
Abnormal visual and digital rectal exam findings include internal or external hemorrhoids, rectal masses, fecal impaction, enlarged prostate, boggy or hard prostate, rectal prolapse, anal fissures, poor rectal tone, or absence of an anal wink.

**7. How do you test for an anal wink?**
Lightly touch the anus with a wisp of cotton. Intact anal innervation is demonstrated when the anus contracts slightly (winks) at this external stimulus.

**8. How can hemorrhoids, anal fissure, or rectal prolapse be visualized more clearly?**
Have the patient bear down slightly. The increases in abdominal pressure put pressure on the anus, causing it to bulge outward somewhat. At this time, a fissure, hemorrhoid, or overt prolapse can be seen.

**9. How is rectal tone tested?**
Once a lubricated, gloved finger is inserted in the rectum, the patient is asked to tighten the muscles around the examiner's fingers. Lax tone indicates a neurologic deficit. Extreme tone may result from a spastic disorder, pain from a lesion or fissure, or examination anxiety.

**10. Describe the genital exam for men.**
In addition to the prostate exam, the genital exam for men determines testicular tenderness or any abnormalities of the foreskin.

**11. What is the purpose of the genital exam in women?**

A genital exam for women determines the condition of perineal skin, looks for signs of atrophic vaginitis/urethritis, assesses for pelvic prolapse (cystocele, rectocele or enterocele), and determines perivaginal muscle tone.

**12. How is the pelvic muscle floor evaluated in women?**

Strength assessment of the pelvic muscles is essential, because loss of tone or strength contribute to both stress and urge incontinence. By inserting the index and middle finger into the vagina and asking the patient to contract the muscles as tight and as long as possible around them, the clinician can determine muscle strength and endurance. Patients with both strength and endurance actually lift the clinician's fingers in the vagina.

**13. What is atrophic vaginitis/urethritis?**

The lack of estrogen in postmenopausal women produces atrophy of the urethral and vaginal mucosa. Atrophy causes a decrease in mucus production and tissue thinning, which weakens the ability of the urethra to maintain closure. Because blood supply and urethral tone are also affected, the urethra is rigid. These factors contribute to increased susceptibility to urinary tract infections.

The vaginal wall in the waning and eventual absence of estrogen also loses tone. The natural ripples (rugae) in the vaginal wall flatten. Vaginal tissues become dry and pale. Occasionally there may be irritation with red, petechial areas with or without erosions.

**14. What symptoms are associated with atrophic vaginitis/urethritis?**

Not all women notice symptoms. Urinary urgency, itching, dysuria, and painful sexual intercourse are the most frequently reported.

**15. What is the difference between a cystocele, rectocele, and cystourethrocele?**

A **cystocele** is the loss of pelvic tone, allowing the bladder to bulge into the anterior wall of the vagina. This bulge can be felt during distal vaginal exam when the patient performs the Valsalva maneuver. Severe protrusion can be seen on visual examination.

A **rectocele** is the loss of pelvic tone allowing the rectum to bulge into the posterior wall of the vagina. This, too, can be felt by vaginal exam or, if severe, seen visually.

A **cystourethrocele** is the bulging of both the bladder and urethra into the anterior vaginal wall.

**16. How is uterine prolapse assessed?**

By digital exam and visual inspection, the clinician can determine the severity of the prolapsed uterus. In a first-degree prolapse, the uterus and cervix descend into the vaginal canal but remain within. In a second-degree prolapse, the cervix is at the introitus. The most severe, a third-degree prolapse, occurs when the cervix and vaginal canal descend outside the vaginal opening.

**17. What procedures should be performed at the initial evaluation of all patients with incontinence?**

A cough stress test, postvoid residual urine and dipstick urinalysis.

**18. What information does a dipstick urinalysis provide?**

Dipstick urinalysis tests for the presence of infection, hematuria, proteinuria, glycosuria, pyuria, or bacteria. The presence of nitrates, the hallmark of bacterial infection, compels the clinician to send a clean-catch urine specimen or a specimen obtained via catheterization for culture and sensitivity. Any urinary infection must be treated before therapy is started. Other abnormalities, such as glucose or protein, must be investigated, and associated underlying conditions must be treated.

**19. What blood test may be helpful in determining a cause for urinary retention?**

Vitamin $B_{12}$ levels. A deficiency can cause urinary retention.

**20. What is a cough stress test? How is it performed?**

A cough stress test detects stress incontinence. The patient must have a full bladder for the test to be accurate. In the lithotomy position, the patient is asked to cough vigorously or perform a Valsalva maneuver. The clinician observes for urine leakage during the cough. The procedure is repeated in the standing position. If leakage is delayed after the cough, an inappropriate (timing or strength) bladder contraction is the cause of urinary leakage.

**21. Give another name for the cough stress test.**

Provocative stress test.

**22. Define postvoid residual (PVR).**

PVR should be done immediately after a patient voids voluntarily. This measurement can be taken by catheterizing the patient or performing a pelvic ultrasound or "bladder scan" to determine the volume of urine left in the bladder. A PVR of 150 cc or more is considered abnormal. Neurogenic causes or outflow obstructions are the most common etiologies of an excessive PVR.

**23. When is a voiding diary used?**

A voiding diary is an important tool to determine the type and severity of incontinence. Kept by the patient, it measures how often the patient urinates, how many leakage episodes occur, how often the patient gets a urinary urge, what type of fluids the patient drinks, and how much fluid is taken in. It is important for patients to see on paper what their voiding habits are. The diary can be used to compare incontinence episodes after treatment as a way to measure outcomes. Patients are asked to keep at least a 3-day diary, although many clinicians prefer to evaluate a 7-day diary.

**24. What additional tests can be performed?**

In conjunction with a good history and physical exam, urodynamic studies (UDS) can provide up to 90% of the information necessary to develop and implement an incontinence treatment plan.

**25. Describe the differences between simple and complex UDS.**

Simple UDS, also known as bedside UDS, is performed without machines. Complex UDS is a high-tech approach, using electronic machinery to record and graphically display or print test results. Complex UDS is more expensive to perform.

**26. What are complex urodynamics?**

Urodynamics consists of several bladder function tests. They are not routinely performed on every patient but are used to help determine a diagnosis when the patient has a variety of symptoms or has not responded to one or more treatment options. The tests include electronic uroflometry, multichannel cystometry, and electromyographic measurements of pelvic floor and sphincter activity. A stress cystogram is usually done using a radiographic dye to measure bladder descensus.

**27. Who is best suited for bedside UDS?**

Patients with stress or urge incontinence who have not had genitourinary surgery to correct incontinence are the best candidates for bedside UDS.

**28. So UDS is a simple test?**

In reality, UDS is a series of tests, including evaluation of the voiding diary and functional capacity, uroflometry, PVR measurement, bedside cystometry, provocative stress test, pad tests, and Q-tip testing. The voiding diary is discussed in greater detail in Chapter 79.

**29. Why is functional capacity important?**

Functional capacity is measured periodically during a bladder retraining program. Knowing the average voided volume at the start helps to gauge progress.

### 30. What is uroflometry?

Uroflometry is the measurement of voiding speed and volume to determine a flow rate. The result is called a $Q_{AVE}$. This test can be performed with an electronic printout or manually. Uroflometry can be used to assess the flow of urine if bladder outlet obstruction or deficient detrusor contraction strength is suspected.

### 31. What is the mathematical formula to determine $Q_{AVE}$?

Voided urine volume, divided by voiding time, equals average ml per second or $Q_{AVE}$.

### 32. What is normal $Q_{AVE}$?

Males under the age of 50 have an average $Q_{AVE}$ of 10.5 ml per second. An elderly male has a $Q_{AVE}$ of 5.5 ml per second. Female $Q_{AVE}$ is not age-dependent. It ranges between 20 and 36 ml per second.

### 33. How does an electronic uroflometer work?

The patient should have a full bladder and void in his or her normal position. The uroflometer is positioned to catch the stream. Shaped like a urimeter, it electronically measures the force and volume of the urine steam as the void passes through it. A printout graphically depicts the entire void.

### 34. How is uroflometry performed manually?

The clinician uses a stopwatch to measure voiding time. While allowing patient privacy, the clinician listens to the force of the urinary stream during the entire micturation process. Evidence of straining is observed as an additive to voided volume and $Q_{AVE}$. Urinary stream should be continuous until nearly the end, at which point there may be short urine spurts.

### 35. What are the limitations to uroflometry?

An overdistended bladder causes falsely low flow rates because detrusor contractility is limited. An underfilled bladder produces falsely high flow rates. Poor flows or interrupted streams do not specify which problem is causing poor emptying; however, normal results rule out a number of disorders.

### 36. How many flow measurements are taken?

Because many patients are nervous urinating in front of another person, it may take several attempts to arrive at a valid and reliable $Q_{AVE}$.

### 37. It is hard enough to listen for the quality of a urinary stream in men. Do you have any tips to determine the amount of force in a woman's urinary stream?

Putting a layer of tinfoil in the measuring device amplifies the sound of the force of urine stream and allows the clinician to hear the urine stream quality. Remind the patient that urination will be louder than normal if you choose to use this technique.

### 38. Describe bedside cystometry (CMG).

Bedside CMG evaluates filling, capacity, and the presence of detrusor instability using the patient's reported sensations of bladder fullness.

### 39. When is CMG performed?

CMG is usually performed as a component of the initial evaluation or after failure of empirical treatment in patients with clear symptoms of stress or urge incontinence. Detrusor instability can also be evaluated.

### 40. What is the difference between multichannel CMG and bedside CMG?

Multichannel CMG electronically records results on graph paper sent from transducers connected to rectal catheters, electromyography, and surface electrodes. Patients who have had failed incontinence surgery, prostatectomy, or PVR over 150 cc or who have been unresponsive to behavioral and medical therapies should have a multichannel CMG rather than bedside CMG.

**41. How is a bedside CMG done?**

The patient empties the bladder. PVR is performed, using a 12- or 14-French red rubber catheter. A 60-cc piston syringe is attached to the catheter. While holding the syringe about 6 inches above the symphysis pubis, the clinician fills the barrel with saline or water by 50-cc increments until the patient reports the first sensation of bladder filling. Fluid instillation continues until the patient reports both the first desire to void and then a strong voiding urge.

**42. When should normal sensations of filling and voiding urge occur?**
- First sensation of bladder filling: 90–150 cc
- First urge to void: 200–300 cc
- Strong urge to void: 300–600 cc

**43. What do delayed or absent sensations during the bedside CMG indicate?**

Delayed bladder filling sensation is indicative of neuropathy or chronic overdistention of the bladder. Absent sensation is seen in spinal cord abnormalities.

**44. Sometimes bladder capacity is smaller in a bedside CMG than voiding diaries. Why?**

Any detrusor instability ("overactive bladder") is easily discerned because of a more rapid filling in the bedside CMG.

**45. Bladder filling is fast at the beginning of the CMG but slows down later in the test. Is this finding normal?**

It is normal for the bladder to fill rapidly at first but more slowly as bladder capacity is reached. The resistance against filling as the muscle is stretched is a normal physiologic response to prevent overfilling and bladder rupture. This respond is termed *compliance*.

**46. What if bladder filling during the CMG is slow throughout the exam?**

Sluggish filling is usually related to decreased bladder compliance. When it is observed, a multisystem complex urodynamic testing is advised.

**47. Decreased compliance puts the patient at risk for what three problems?**

Urinary tract infection, urinary reflux, and upper urinary tract dilation.

**48. During the filling phase of the CMG, the fluid in the syringe barrel fluctuates up and down or sometimes rises and overflows the syringe. What does this finding indicate?**

Detrusor instability. Uninhibited bladder contractions force fluid out the catheter and up the barrel of the syringe. If a clinician strongly suspects detrusor instability by history but is unable to elicit a positive response, usually due to patient anxiety, the CMG is repeated in a standing position.

**49. What is a pad test?**

A pad test can be done to determine the amount of urinary leakage and can be used to measure the outcome of a certain treatment. The pads are weighed after use to determine the amount of urinary leakage. This test is done more commonly in research than in daily clinical practice.

**50. What is the Q-tip test?**

The Q-tip test can be used to determine the loss of support of the bladder neck. After the Q-tip is coated with K-Y jelly mixed with lidocaine, the clinician inserts it into the urethra up to the urethral vesicle junction and asks the patient to bear down. The Q-tip should not rise more than 30°. A rise > 30° is considered a positive test for urethral hypermobility.

**51. Why is the Q-tip test inappropriate for male patients?**

Urethral hypermobility does not occur in men.

**52. What controversies are associated with Q-tip testing?**

The Q-tip test alone does not establish the cause of stress incontinence. Many women have ure-thral hypermobility but are continent. Some clinicians think that the Q-tip test represents anterior pelvic muscle relaxation rather than sphincter incompetence due to hypermobility. Additionally, up to 30% of elderly women have a false-negative response.

**53. Are men affected by incontinence?**

Men also suffer from incontinence, albeit less often than women. There is one exception, how-ever. The majority of postoperative prostatectomy patients experience incontinence for 1–3 months after surgery. Although continence improves over time in this population, some men report inconti-nent episodes 1 year after the procedure.

BIBLIOGRAPHY

1. Agency for Health Care Policy and Research: Urinary incontinence in adults: Acute and chronic management. Rockville MD, U.S. Department of Health and Social Services, AHCPR Publication No. 96-0682, 1996.
2. Chai T, Steers W: Neurophysiology of micturation and continence. Urol Clin North Am 23:221–236, 1996.
3. Shinopulos N: Beside urodynamic studies: Simple testing for urinary incontinence. Nurse Pract 25(6):19–37, 2000.
4. Hoffman E: Overactive bladder: Diagnosis of a hidden disorder. Patient Care Nurse Pract Spring Suppl:15–21, 2001.
5. Newman D: Continence for Women: Research-based Practice. Washington, DC, Association of Women's Health Obstetric and Neonatal Nurses, 2000.

# 78. ASSESSMENT AND DIAGNOSIS OF FECAL INCONTINENCE

*Catherine T. Milne, APRN, MSN, CWOCN, CS, ANP, and Lisa Q. Corbett, APRN, MSN, CWOCN, CS*

**1. What is fecal incontinence?**

Fecal incontinence is the inability to voluntarily maintain gas and/or stool in liquid or solid form in the rectum. It can take place as stool seepage or large bowel movements. In the case of flatus, the passage of gas is uncontrolled.

**2. Is fecal incontinence common?**

Two percent of the general population is fecally incontinent. This rate rises to greater than 7% in healthy independent people over the age of 65. Fecal incontinence affects well over one-third of elderly patients in skilled nursing facilities. Of course, most toddlers and all infants are fecally incontinent, although society does not view this age group as having aberrant behavior.

**3. How does fecal incontinence affect quality of life?**

Fecal incontinence isolates people from family, friends, social activities, and essential daily activities such as food shopping or banking. Like those with urinary incontinence, people with fecal incontinence often plan their day around their bowel movements. Attempts to keep the incontinent episodes secret often entail elaborate excuses, the use of costly pads or diapers, and extensive use of odor eliminators, powders, or perfumes. Fecal incontinence is the second most common reason for admission to a skilled nursing home.

Most patients will not confess their problems to their health care provider for fear that they will be placed in a skilled nursing facility and forced to give up what little independence they have left. Others believe fecal incontinence is a normal part of aging or think that no cure is available. Many are embarrassed or ashamed.

**4. What causes fecal incontinence?**

The many causes of fecal incontinence can be categorized into the following areas:
- Impaired sphincter muscles
- Impaired or absent nervous system innervation
- Anal pathology
- Rectal pathology

**5. What is the most common cause of fecal incontinence?**

Childbirth via a vaginal delivery is one of the most common causes of fecal incontinence. During delivery, especially with forceps use or episiotomy, damage to the anal sphincter muscle can result. These injuries can cause partial or full tears. Up to 35% of patients experience some anal sphincter dysfunction. Most childbearing women do not show symptoms at the time of delivery, but as they age, the development of pelvic floor weakness can no longer compensate for the injury to the anal sphincter.

**6. How else can sphincter muscles suffer damage?**

Surgical procedures, such as a hemorrhoidectomy, can damage the internal or external sphincter. Rectal prolapse, physical trauma, or other anal surgical procedures interfere with intact sphincter musculature.

**7. What pathologies are involved with impaired or absent nervous innervation?**

Injury to the pudendal nerve during childbirth can disrupt nervous innervation pathways to and from the spinal cord. Cord injuries, tumors, and central nervous system diseases such as dementia or multiple sclerosis additionally affect these tracts. Pathology results from impaired nervous innervation to the sphincter, pelvic floor muscles, or rectal areas that activate sphincter contractions necessary for continence. Severe and protracted straining to produce stool can also physically damage the nerves.

### 8. Why is diabetes mellitus a risk factor for fecal incontinence?

Diabetes, in addition to alcohol and heavy metal toxicity neuropathies, has been shown to disrupt the nervous innervation to the pelvic floor. Up to 5% of all diabetic patients experience fecal incontinence. Neuropathy also impairs rectal sensation, distention, and anal sampling.

### 9. Why is fecal incontinence of sudden onset a concern?

Sudden onset of fecal incontinence may be a grave sign of cauda equina syndrome. A rapidly developing tumor on the spinal cord presents with low back pain, lower extremity weakness, and sudden onset of fecal or urinary incontinence. Emergent evaluation is required.

### 10. What anal pathologies cause incontinence?

Congenital abnormalities, anal carcinoma, protruding internal hemorrhoids, perianal infections, fistula in ano, and Crohn's disease can affect anal sphincter control, rendering the patient incontinent.

### 11. What rectal pathologies cause incontinence?

Rectal cancer, ischemia, proctitis, inflammatory bowel disease, or infection cause fecal incontinence by affecting distensibility and normal rectal sensation.

### 12. How does diarrhea or constipation cause incontinence?

**Diarrhea** shortens anal sampling time. In turn, there is dramatically less time for the cerebral cortex to make the decision as to "hold" or "let go." Impaired rectal sensations as a result of rapid stool influx and distention may contribute to a judgment error in the cerebral cortex.

**Constipation**, if severe enough, leads to impaction. The overflow stool, usually liquid, seeps around the stool bolus stuck in the rectum. Distention signals sent to the spinal cord have not been interrupted because of the impaction and eventually are ignored. Any liquid spilling around the hard stool does not set off additional distention or anal sampling signals to the brain. The external sphincter, then, does not increase tone and fecal incontinence occurs.

### 13. Does the rectum ever become nondistensible?

Patients who have received radiation to the pelvic floor develop a "stiff" or a noncompliant rectum. Radiation causes scar tissue to form. Scar is nonelastic. Surgical procedures in the rectal area can also result in a nondistensible rectal vault.

### 14. Are there different types of fecal incontinence?

Some authors classify fecal incontinence into minor or major categories, whereas others organize the disorder into cases with or without an intact sphincter mechanism. Still others describe fecal soiling as either passive or urge incontinence.

### 15. Describe the difference between major and minor incontinence.

**Minor fecal incontinence** occurs after a bowel movement with slight soiling on the underwear. Small seepage of stool can also occur with coughing, heavy lifting or other straining movements. The likely cause is related to a local anal problem that prevents the external sphincter from forming a strong, taut seal, such as hemorrhoids. An incompetent internal anal sphincter is another cause of minor fecal incontinence.

**Major fecal incontinence** is the complete loss of stool. It is indicative of sphincter failure or incompetent nervous innervation.

### 16. What is the difference between passive and urge fecal incontinence?

In urge incontinence, there is little time between anal sampling and expulsion of feces. The inability to contract the external sphincter in response to a distended rectum starts the urge response. Diarrhea often causes urgency because of its associated high colonic peristaltic pressures. These waves overpower the normally contracted external sphincter and reduce the angularity of the anorectal junction, leading to urge sensations and possible incontinence. Passive fecal incontinence is another term for minor fecal incontinence.

### 17. How is the diagnosis of fecal incontinence made?

The diagnosis of fecal incontinence is based on the history, physical examination, and diagnostic tests that measure anal and rectal function.

### 18. Describe the essential components of the patient history?

Asking the right questions to elicit subtle clues about symptoms assists in determining the cause of fecal incontinence and guides treatment options. The following questions are helpful:

1. *What is the most problematic issue with your bowels? Do you leak stool into your clothing? How often? Do you wear a pad or diaper to contain the stool?* Such questions determine coping status and strategies and obtain information about the patient's quality of life. Description of most prominent symptoms allows the clinician to focus on what is important to the patient. It is important to discern whether pad or diaper use is related to concurrent urinary incontinence, actual fecal incontinence, or fear of soiling.

2. *When did the problems start?* Onset of symptoms may be related to an incident that affects sphincter function, such as childbirth or an anal surgical procedure. Casual relationships as seen in medication or dietary changes may also affect fecal continence.

3. *How often do you have a bowel movement? Has this pattern changed?* These questions determine whether bowels move in a distinct pattern or are variable. Pattern changes may reflect a more serious pathology, such as carcinoma. Patients with a long-standing history of a variable bowel pattern, but no nocturnal movements, may have irritable bowel syndrome (IBS).

4. *Describe the normal consistency of your stool. Does its consistency vary?* Variable stool consistency is another classic sign of IBS. Liquid stool increases the possibility of fecal urge incontinence and fecal passive incontinence from postmovement soiling. Hard pellet-like stools point to slow colonic transport time that can result from medication, inadequate fluid intake, or aberrant or absent nervous innervation.

5. *Once you are aware that your bowels need to move, is the urge strong and sudden? Can you overcome the urge?* A poorly functioning external sphincter has been shown to contribute to fecal urge incontinence. Damage to the external sphincter may occur during obstetrical or surgical procedures or as a result of a traumatic injury. Additionally, a patient may inadvertently retrain the bowels to respond to any rectal sensation as "urgent" for fear of soilage.

6. *Are you aware of fecal soiling when it occurs or do you find fecal stains or movements in your undergarments? Does the leakage occur just after moving your bowels on the toilet, is it associated with any activity, or is it continuous?* A positive response to these questions indicates symptoms of passive or minor incontinence. Impaired internal anal sphincter, idiopathic smooth muscle degeneration, or rectal prolapse may be the cause.

7. *Can you discern the difference between gas and stool? Are there any times when you cannot control when you pass gas?* Damage to sensory nerves in the anal canal prevents normal anal sampling from occurring. High intra-abdominal pressures during lifting, straining, or hearty laughing in conjunction with weak pelvic floor muscles additionally contribute to this socially embarrassing phenomenon.

8. *Describe any pain you have with your bowel movements.* Pain while passing stool may indicate hemorrhoids or an anal fissure. Pain that is relieved with the passage of stool is associated with inflammatory bowel diseases and IBS. Patients often describe the latter discomfort as a bloating, colicky, or crampy feeling.

9. *Is there any blood or mucus in your bowel movements?* Although there are many reasons for blood or mucus to be passed, including hemorrhoids, anal fissures, rectal prolapse, IBS, and inflammatory bowel disease, the clinician must first rule out the presence of malignancy. The first presenting symptom in over 25% of colorectal cancer cases is fecal incontinence. Referral to an appropriate physician for evaluation is imperative.

10. *Do you need to strain to pass your stool? Do you feel the need to push the skin near your rectum to help pass stool? Do you need to insert anything into your rectum to get the stool out? Do you feel as if your bowels are never emptied completely?* Constipation frequently causes staining and evacuation difficulties. The presence of a rectocele and weak pelvic floor muscles contribute to constipation.

11. *What medications are you taking? Name the nonprescription medications, herbs, and vitamins that you are taking.* Prescription and nonprescription medications can easily influence stool consistency or frequency. Analgesics, anticholinergics, antidepressants, calcium channel blockers, calcium-containing vitamins, and antiosteoporotic agents are constipating. Laxatives, NSAIDs, and antibiotics tend to have an opposite effect.

12. *Tell me about your medical and surgical history.* Diabetes mellitus, thyroid disorders, neurologic disease, spinal cord or sacral trauma, obstetric history, and unwanted anal intercourse can contribute to impaired nervous innervation or incompetent internal or external sphincter control.

13. *Do you have any problems getting to the toilet?* Fecal incontinence in patients with mobility problems may be related strictly to toilet access rather than a pathologic disorder. The lack of an available caregiver, fear of falling, inability to get into a narrowed door bathroom, or difficulty in transferring to the commode or toilet are frequent reasons of incontinence in this population.

14. *Review your normal daily diet and fluid intake. Do you smoke?* Low fluid intake can lead to hard stools. High-fiber intake can soften stools excessively. Caffeine in coffee, tea, and cola drinks has been shown to increase colonic peristalsis while paradoxically decreasing upper GI tract motility. Some patients are able to identify certain foods that slow or speed stool transit time.

15. *Do you have any soreness or itching around your rectum?* Skin irritation is common in patients with passive fecal incontinence. Both diarrhea and mucus cause excoriation. If a positive response to the question is elicited, teaching the patient perineal hygiene techniques with emphasis of skin care is imperative (see Chapter 82).

16. *Do you leak urine in addition to stool?* Double incontinence, the simultaneous presence of urinary and fecal incontinence is significant for severe pelvic muscle floor dysfunction. In many of these instances, biofeedback and pelvic muscle floor exercises dramatically reduce severity.

**19. What are the components of the physical assessment of patients with suspected fecal incontinence?**

- **General assessment that includes evaluation of cognitive status and mobility.** Intact cognition is necessary to sense rectal fullness. Ability to maneuver oneself to the toilet or commode in a reasonable time frame is also essential.
- **Abdominal exam.** Observation, auscultation, and palpation should reveal normal contours, normal bowel sounds, the absence of bruits, and no masses. In patients with severe constipation, a mass of feces can sometimes be palpated.
- **Visual inspection of the perineum.** The skin should be free of rashes or excoriation. Congenital abnormalities, such as a pilonidal cyst, and scars from surgical procedures should be noted because they lead the clinician closer to a diagnosis. In women, a vaginal exam is performed to observe for the presence of a rectocele.
- **Visual inspection of the anus.** The presence of soiling on the anus may indicate leakage and an incompetent sphincter. Hemorrhoids and skin tags, if seen, suggest physical causes for passive incontinence.
- **Cotton ball test.** Wiping the anus with a damp cotton ball reveals fecal soiling that was not visualized. Stool that is insufficiently removed from the anus can cause itching or excoriation. Passive incontinence from sphincter damage is often the cause.
- **Valsalva maneuver.** Performed in the supine, sitting, and standing positions, the Valsalva maneuver allows visualization of rectal prolapse. During the maneuver, the pelvic floor muscles are observed. If downward movement of the pelvic floor is 2 cm or greater, the pelvic floor is weak and unable to support the normal defecation process. Uncoordinated pelvic floor muscle function may indicate a neurologic disorder. If the anus moves anteriorly during this process, sphincter muscle damage is likely. A cystocele or rectocele may also be visualized.

- **Anal wink.** The anal wink, performed by gently stoking the anus with a cotton ball and observing a normal puckering or quivering motion in response, assesses for intact nervous innervation. Absence of the anal wink indicates a neurologic problem affecting continence.
- **Digital rectal exam.** Resting and active sphincter tone, the presence of fecal impaction, and the presence of rectal masses aid the clinician in determining cause or contributing factors to fecal incontinence.

## 20. During the digital rectal exam, what does low resting tone indicate?

When the lubricated, gloved index finger is gently inserted into the rectum without resistance and minimal "squeeze" is felt around the finger, low rectal tone is present. This finding correlates with passive fecal incontinence related to sphincter abnormalities.

## 21. How is active sphincter tone tested?

After resting tone is evaluated, ask the patient to squeeze as hard a possible around your finger. While noting the strength, you should also evaluate the length of time of the contraction. Ability to hold a voluntary contraction evaluates pelvic muscle and sphincter endurance. Poor strength or reduced endurance correlate highly with urge incontinence. Contraction symmetry of the around the finger, if absent, indicates impaired sphincter musculature.

## 22. Is the digital rectal exam a reliable way to determine how much stool is in the rectum?

No. Especially if the stool is soft, there is no reliable way to determine stool volume in the rectum. An abdominal x-ray is recommended if physical exam suggests impaction or a large amount of stool.

## 23. Describe the diagnostic tests used in determining fecal incontinence.

Anorectal physiology tests include anorectal manometry, electromyographic (EMG) testing, defecography, and endoanal ultrasound. These tests help to determine diagnosis but also assist in the selection of the best course of treatment.

## 24. What is anorectal manometry? How is performed?

Used to evaluate sphincter pressure, length of the anal canal, and anorectal sensation, anorectal manometry uses highly specialized equipment. A small catheter, connected to a transducer that can measure pressures, is inserted. Pressures at rest are measured in 1-cm intervals in all four quadrants of the anal canal. The pressures are taken at rest and during repeated Valsalva maneuvers and voluntary muscle tightening. Resting internal sphincter tone is assessed with normal readings between 40 and 80 mmHg. External sphincter tone, evaluated during squeeze motions, should have readings 40–80 mmHg greater than resting pressures.

Length of the anal canal is determined when resting pressures decrease as the catheter is progressed upward. Men tend to have a longer anal canal as well as higher resting pressures.

Anorectal sensation is evaluated by placing a balloon-tipped catheter into the rectum. Saline is infused into the balloon, and the patient is instructed to report when rectal sensation is first felt and when the urge to defecate is present. Rectal sensation commonly occurs when infusion has reached 40–80 cc, whereas defecation urge is normally present between 120 and 150 cc.

## 25. What do abnormal anorectal manometry results indicate?

Abnormal anorectal manometry can demonstrate low resting and squeeze pressures as well as a short anal canal. Treatment options for patients with overall low pressures include biofeedback. Patients with pressure deficits in specific areas of the anal canal can be referred to a colorectal surgeon to evaluate the response to surgical repair.

## 26. What is anal EMG? How is it performed?

Anal EMG (also called pudendal nerve terminal motor latency study) is used to assess neuropathy of the pelvic muscle floor. A gloved electrode is inserted into the anal canal and connected to a machine that sends electrical impulses to the area to stimulate muscle contraction. The time from stimulation to muscle contraction (called the latency time) is recorded. Normal latency times should be between 1.8 and 2.2 milliseconds.

### 27. What do abnormal anal EMG readings indicate?

Abnormal latency times indicate neuropathy of the pudendal nerve. Patients with this disorder may benefit from a post-anal repair surgical procedure as the anal canal is elongated and narrowed through surgical manipulation to improve function.

### 28. What is a defecating proctography? How is it performed?

A barium paste is inserted into the rectum. The process of defecation is subsequently captured radiologically. This procedure is reserved for patients with suspected rectal prolapse that cannot be externally visualized. Sphincter muscles are unable to close in the presence of a prolapse.

### 29. How is an endoanal ultrasound performed?

An ultrasound probe is inserted into the anal canal, anal structures are identified. Detailed ultrasound images are taken of the sphincters to identify any anatomic thinning or disruption in structures.

### 30. How do the results of the endoanal ultrasound guide treatment?

Thinning of the sphincter mechanism responds best to treatment with biofeedback. Anatomic disruptions of either the internal or external sphincter require surgical repair.

### BIBLIOGRAPHY

1. Jensen, L: Fecal incontinence: Evaluation and treatment. J Wound Ostomy Contin Nurs 24(5):277–282, 1997
2. Jensen L: Assessing and treating patients with complex fecal incontinence. Ostomy Wound Manage 46(12):56–60, 2000.
3. Jensen L: Assessment and management: Patients with bowel dysfunction and fecal incontinence. In Doughty DB (ed): Urinary and Fecal Incontinence: Nursing Management, 2nd ed. St. Louis, Mosby, 2000.
4. Norton C, Chelvanayagam S: A nursing assessment tool for adults with fecal incontinence. J Wound Ostomy Contin Nurs 27(5):279–291, 2000.

# 79. BEHAVIORAL METHODS TO ACHIEVE CONTINENCE

*Michelle B. Mayer, PT, OCS, ATC, and Julie M. Peinhardt, MS, PT*

### 1. Describe the importance of using behavioral methods to improve continence.

Behavioral methods demonstrate superior outcomes compared with pharmacologic therapy in improving continence. More people are continent or have fewer incontinent episodes with behavioral techniques.

### 2. List the six simple steps for bladder health.

1. Drink water.
2. Avoid caffeine.
3. Maintain bowel regularity.
4. Keep a bladder schedule.
5. Perform a pelvic floor exercise program.
6. Maintain urge control.

### 3. Are these steps behavioral methods?

Yes. However, it is important to educate the patient about the anatomy and function of the bladder as well as the pelvic floor musculature. Some of the behavioral methods appear contradictory to maintaining incontinence unless bladder physiology and pelvic anatomy are understood.

### 4. Why is drinking water so important as part of bladder treatment?

It is important to drink water on a regular basis because it maintains a decreased concentration of urine. Increased urine concentration can increase urgency and frequency by irritating the bladder. It also helps to decrease the risk of urinary tract infections.

### 5. What substances are considered bladder irritants?

- Caffeine
- Alcohol
- Tobacco
- Spicy foods
- Tomato-based products
- Citrus juices
- Artificial sweeteners
- Sugar/honey

### 6. What happens to someone who ingests irritants?

Irritants can contribute to increased urge incontinence and frequency of voiding.

### 7. What is the rule of thumb for fluid intake?

The rule of thumb for fluid intake is one-half of body weight in ounces of fluid per day. For example, a patient who weighs 100 pounds should drink 50 ounces of fluid per day. One-half to two-thirds of this fluid should be water.

### 8. Why should patients prevent constipation?

Increased pressure from an overfilled rectum pushes into the bladder, causing increased urgency, frequency, and incomplete bladder emptying, all of which contribute to incontinence.

### 9. What is the best way to prevent constipation?

Dietary manipulation works best. First obtain a history of bowel habits from the patient. If there is a long-standing history of laxative use for bowel stimulation, dietary interventions are not likely to be successful. The following foods are helpful:

- Bran
- High-fiber foods, such as oatmeal and dark green leafy vegetables
- Prunes
- Dried apricots (3 per day are better than prunes)
- Adequate fluid intake, preferably water

If the patient is reasonably compliant with these measures and still has constipation, an in-depth examination by the health care provider is recommended. Many medications, especially calcium channel blockers, are constipating. There is always a possibility of a polyp or tumor in the colon. Collaboration with the patient and attending physician can usually reach a solution to this problem.

**10. What about stool softeners and bulky agents?**

Pharmacologic therapy for constipation is a potential intervention. Many of these agents require the patient to drink lots of fluid. Most incontinent patients are reluctant to do so, because they believe that it will increase frequency and urge sensations. Inadequate fluid intake results, and constipation is worsened. Additionally, patients should avoid pharmacologic therapy unless absolutely needed to minimize drug-drug and drug-food interactions and side effects.

**11. My patient drinks coffee because it makes her have a bowel movement and prevents constipation. What do I do?**

Education is key in this situation. One reason that coffee stimulates the bowels is that it is a hot liquid. The temperature helps initiate the gastrocolic reflex, which, in turn, begins the peristaltic process. Another hot liquid, even something as simple as hot water, can do the trick. Remind the patient about the high bladder irritation effect of coffee (even the decaffeinated kind).

**12. Bladder diaries include what type of information?**

| | |
|---|---|
| • Time of voids | • Activity during leaks |
| • Amounts of voids | • Number and type of pads used per day |
| • Times and size of leaks | • Amount and type of fluid intake |

*Sample Bladder Diary*

| TIME | TYPE OF FLUID AND AMOUNT | VOID AMOUNT (SM, MED, LG) | LEAKAGE ACCIDENT (SM, MED, LG) | URGE PRESENT? | ACTIVITY DURING LEAKAGE EPISODE | NO. OF PADS USED | TYPE OF PAD |
|---|---|---|---|---|---|---|---|
| 8:00 PM | 8 oz coffee | Medium | No | Yes | Walking | — | — |
| 10:30 AM | 12 oz diet soda | Large | Yes (Medium) | No | Sneezed | 1 | Maxi |
| 2:00 AM | — | Small | Yes (Small) | Yes | Sleeping | 1 | Mini |

**13. Why is a bladder diary helpful?**

- The patient becomes more aware of environmental issues that affect continence, such as coughing or consuming bladder irritants.
- The patient can use the diary to measure success of behavioral methods.
- The clinician can use the data to assist in the assessment and diagnosis of the type of incontinence that the patient is experiencing.
- The clinician uses the bladder diary as a tool to identify modifiable behaviors.
- The bladder diary serves as a teaching tool for the clinician to use with the patient.
- The diary can help the clinician identify and modify nonbehavioral treatment options.

**14. How often should a patient complete a bladder diary?**

It is usually left to the clinician's discretion. Some clinicians have the patient do a 3-day diary initially and repeat it just before each appointment for comparison. Others have the patient record a 7-day diary. Much depends on the patient's willingness and motivation.

**15. What is the normal number of voids during the night (nocturia)?**
- 0–1 per night under the age of 65
- 1–2 per night over the age of 65

**16. What is urge control?**
Urges are signals that people feel as the bladder stretches to fill with urine. Urges are felt even if the bladder is not completely filled. Urges are reminders, not commands. Urge control is a behavioral method used as part of a bladder retraining program.

**17. What is bladder training/retraining?**
It is a program of mandatory, scheduled voiding with progressive increases or decreases in small intervals between voiding. This program helps patients to develop appropriate voiding schedules.

**18. Why should a patient perform bladder training or retraining?**
It is important to perform bladder training to help establish bladder homeostasis and reeducate the brain to bladder signals. Continence is a learned behavior. It also helps the patient to avoid straining to completely empty the bladder and prevents "just-in-case" voids.

**19. What content is taught to the patient who uses bladder retraining as a behavioral method to achieve incontinence?**
In bladder retraining the patient is instructed to keep to a strict schedule of voiding. Its goal is to learn continence by having the patient voluntarily suppress urge feelings. This strategy eventually increases bladder capacity, much as exercises increase the biceps muscle. Teach the patient the following:
- Void at predetermined times, even if there is no urge to urinate.
- Start with 1-hour intervals. Gradually increase the interval between voiding times over 2–3 weeks until an interval of 3 hours between urination is reached.
- If a voiding urge is felt before predetermined voiding time, the patient is encouraged not to give into the urge. The brain must show the bladder who is in charge. Stopping any current activity and performing a mental distraction exercise, such as backward counting from 100 by 7 while simultaneously performing Kegel exercises, suppresses the urge. Normal activity can then be resumed.

**20. How is habit training different from bladder training?**
Habit training is used to improve urges resulting from an over distended bladder. Many people—women in particular—are so busy they do not take the time to urinate every 3 or 4 hours. The bladder becomes severely overdistended, and the sudden urge cannot be controlled. Leakage results. When teaching habit training, set up a strict schedule of voiding every 3 hours. Instruct the patient to bend forward while sitting on the toilet to assist the bladder in complete emptying.

**21. How is prompted voiding different from habit training or bladder retraining?**
Prompted voiding is indicated in patients with mild-to-moderate dementia. It is commonly implemented in skilled nursing facilities but can be done in a home or assisted living setting. Parents who are "potty training" a child are familiar with this behavioral method. It is caregiver-intensive. The patient is a passive recipient of prompted voiding.

When initiating prompted voiding, the caregiver checks the patient for wetness on an hourly basis. The patient is asked if there is a need to urinate at this time. If so, the patient is toileted. If the patient is dry or voids at the time of caregiving assessment, the patient is given praise and positive feedback or a reward. If the patient is wet, no positive or negative response is given. The patient is given perineal hygiene, and a wetness check is done at the next previously scheduled time.

**22. What is the objective of pelvic floor muscle exercise (PFME)?**
The pelvic muscle floor provides the "sling" that keeps the bladder in the correct anatomic position so that filling and emptying can occur in a normal fashion. A well-functioning pelvic floor improves urethral sphincter function, reduces detrusor contractions, and enhances sexual satisfaction.

**23. When is PFME helpful?**

PFME is useful in treating stress and urge incontinence. The literature supports that initiating PFME in high-risk populations can delay onset, reduce severity, and in some cases prevent incontinence.

**24. List characteristics of people at high risk for incontinence.**
- Postprostatectomy
- Multiparous
- Postmenopausal
- Obesity
- Chronic neurologic disease
- Increased age
- Chronic strain with bowel movements
- History of heavy lifting
- Cigarette smoking
- Participation in high-impact physical activities

**25. What is the best way to initiate PFME?**

As for all muscles, strength and endurance training is necessary. The three most common ways to train the pelvic floor are Kegel exercises, biofeedback, and electrical stimulation. Success rates of the different methods vary among patient populations and patient motivation.

**26. What is the most common patient expectation about PFME?**

Most patients think that PFME provides results in a few days or sessions. Like all exercise, it may take up to 6 weeks to see any benefit. Inform the patient before starting therapy to improve compliance with the prescribed program. Faithful exercisers see maximum benefits between 12 and 16 weeks.

**27. Describe the physiology behind PFME.**

PFME involves intense repetitive contractions of slow-twitch (type I) and fast-twitch (type II) muscle fibers. Type I fibers are associated with endurance. Type II fibers are strength-oriented. The contractions of type I are slower to start and less intense but last longer than those initiated by type II fibers. The objective of PFME is to improve both endurance and force of muscle contraction.

**28. Why is it important for a patient to develop good technique with Kegel exercises?**

Proper training in the Kegel technique helps to maintain urine and fecal continence even with increases in abdominal pressure (e.g., coughing, sneezing). It also inhibits urge incontinence.

**29. How are Kegel exercises performed?**

Kegel exercises consist of "quick flicks" that improve type II fibers and long, sustained tonic contractions to work type I fibers. Instruction should take place after the patient can correctly identify the pelvic floor muscles by imagining the attempt to prevent urination by "pulling up" on the pelvic muscles. The abdominal muscles should not simultaneously tighten. Once the patient masters this technique, the real exercise can begin as follows:
1. Empty the bladder.
2. Contract the pelvic floor muscles and hold 3–5 seconds.
3. Relax for 10 seconds.
4. Repeat.
5. Partially contract the pelvic floor muscles. Hold for 2 seconds. Contract the muscle some more. Hold for 2 seconds. Continue until the muscle is fully contracted and hold for 10 seconds. Repeat. It is helpful to tell the patient to imagine this exercise as an elevator that makes frequent stops as it goes up a skyscraper. Rest periods of double the total contraction time of the previous exercise should be taken between each activity.
6. Do not hold your breath during these exercises.

**30. How often should Kegel exercises be performed?**

Kegel exercises should be performed in three different positions—lying, sitting, and standing—at least 10 and preferably 20 times daily for functional carryover.

**31. What is biofeedback?**

Biofeedback is a learning technique that uses specialized equipment to assist the patient in gaining control of natural body functions. It also enables the patient to see or hear how the musculature is responding. Becoming aware of these responses is the first step in learning to control them.

**32. What are the goals of biofeedback?**
- Increase the patient's awareness, recruitment, and proprioception of pelvic floor musculature.
- Learn control of pelvic floor muscles: phasic (quick) and tonic (endurance) contractions, coordination/quality of contractions, and/or relaxation.
- Progress the patient to a level where pelvic floor contractions are carried over into activities of daily living.

**33. What are the benefits of biofeedback?**
- Noninvasive, painless, and easy to use
- Ease of ability to test in functional positions
- Offers patients an alternative to perceive muscular activity
- Offers patients a motivational tool
- Provides baseline objective data

**34. How does biofeedback work?**

Biofeedback uses either internal vaginal/rectal or external adhesive sensors that record muscle action potentials from the skin surface. The patient is asked to contract the pelvic floor muscles. The sensor measures quality and length of the contraction. It is beneficial in patients who are unable to locate and exercise the pelvic muscle floor. The machine then provides visual and/or audio feedback regarding success.

**35. What components of pelvic floor function does biofeedback test?**
- Resting baseline
- Quick/phasic contractions (i.e., 2 seconds)
- Endurance/tonic contractions (i.e., 10 seconds and 60 seconds)
- Quality of the contraction in terms of initiation, holding, relaxation, and isolation of the pelvic floor muscles and the ability to avoid Valsalva.

**36. What is surface electromyography (EMG)? Does it represent muscle strength?**

Surface EMG monitors events that lead to the generation of musculature tension and assesses motor recruitment and firing rate of motor units. There is no direct correlation to muscle strength. However, it does provide information about the quality of the contraction and endurance of the musculature.

**37. Who is the ideal candidate for biofeedback?**

The ideal candidate for biofeedback is highly motivated, has good muscle innervation, and is cognitively intact. This patient may also have decreased body awareness, lack of coordination, muscle weakness, hypertonic muscles, and/or decreased sensory awareness.

**38. What are the contraindications for biofeedback?**

| | |
|---|---|
| • Menstruation | • After surgery prior to 6 weeks |
| • Vaginal infection/urinary tract infection | • Atrophic vaginitis |
| • Hemorrhoids | • Vaginal/rectal pain |
| • Pregnancy | • After radiation treatment |
| • Postpartum prior to 6 weeks | • Active herpes or venereal disease |

**39. Can biofeedback help a hypertonic muscle?**

Yes. Biofeedback can be used for "downtraining" the muscle. The patient can learn to decrease the resting tone of the pelvic floor musculature.

**40. What is the most important consideration before starting biofeedback?**

The patient must be able to perform Kegel/pelvic floor contractions properly. Technique is everything. Otherwise, bad habits can be reinforced.

**41. What is electrical stimulation? What is its role in treating incontinence?**

Electrical stimulation is used for pelvic floor muscular reeducation related to stress incontinence and inhibition of an unstable detrusor muscle as seen in urge incontinence. It inhibits involuntary detrusor contractions and decreases the intensity of urge to void.

**42. What are the five indications for electrical stimulation?**
1. Muscle testing grade of 0–2/5
2. Lack of progress with Kegel strengthening program
3. Documented detrusor instability
4. Normal sensation and reflexes
5. Decreased proprioception

**43. How does electrical stimulation work?**

Electrodes are placed on the external skin over the pelvic floor muscles (an indwelling rectal/vaginal sensor also can be used). Small electrical currents are sent from a machine to cause passive contraction of these muscles. In addition to improving type I and type II fiber function, electrical stimulation assists the patient in identifying the correct muscles involved.

**44. Does it hurt?**

No. The clinician slowly increases the intensity of the electrical current until a tingling sensation is felt. Then intensity is turned down to one notch below that point. This technique maximizes muscle contraction without causing discomfort or fatigue.

**45. What are the contraindications for electrical stimulation?**

There are multiple contraindications for electrical stimulation: pacemaker, metal implants (including intrauterine devices), vaginal and urinary infection, anticoagulation therapy, arrhythmia, atrophic vaginitis, pediatric patients, active genital herpes, active menstruation, history of urinary retention, lack of consent, cognitive impairment, and absent or diminished sensation.

### BIBLIOGRAPHY

1. Agency for Health Care Policy and Research: Urinary Incontinence in Adults: Acute and Chronic Management, Clinical Practice Guideline, No. 2, 1996 Update. Rockville, MD, AHCPR Publication No. 96-0682, 1996.
2. McCallig-Bates P: Helping women manage urinary incontinence. Adv Wound Care 13(6):285–289, 2000.
3. McDowell BJ, Burgio KL, Dombrowski M, et al: An interdisciplinary approach to the assessment and behavioral treatment of urinary incontinence in geriatric patients. J Am Geriatr Soc 40(4):370–374, 1992.
4. Newman D: The Urinary Incontinence Sourcebook, 2nd ed. Los Angeles, Lowell House, 1999.
5. Newman DK: Continence for Women: Research-Based Practice. Washington, DC, Association of Women's Health, Obstetric and Neonatal Nurses, 2000.

# 80. NONBEHAVIORAL TREATMENTS FOR URINARY CONTINENCE

*Lisa M. Oliveira, MSN, APRN*

### 1. How is urinary incontinence best treated?

Depending on type, severity, and other assessment findings, there are many options for treatment. The patient's lifestyle and treatment preferences are key to success. Treatment options include referral to a specialist, behavioral therapies, and nonbehavioral therapies.

### 2. When should a patient be referred to a specialist?

- Recurrent urinary tract infections
- Gross or microscopic hematuria without evidence of infection
- Urinary retention with a postvoid residual more than 150 cc
- Severe pelvic organ prolapse
- Symptomatic pelvic organ prolapse
- Patient desires surgical intervention to correct incontinence
- Neurologic conditions or deficits
- Uncertain diagnosis

### 3. Should one start with behavioral methods?

All nonbehavioral methods have improved outcomes when behavioral methods are used first (see Chapter 79).

### 4. What nonbehavioral methods treat stress incontinence?

- Vaginal cones
- Intraurethral plugs
- Penile clamps
- Pessary
- Periurethral collagen
- Pharmacologic therapy
- Surgical interventions

### 5. Discuss the use of vaginal cones.

Vaginal cones are tampon-shaped weights. Available as a set, they are weighted from 20 to 100 gm each. The woman inserts the lightest vaginal cone and attempts to retain it for 15 minutes twice a day. Once she is successful, the next heavier cone is used. The goal of the weight-graduated cones is to strengthen the pelvic muscle floor. This goal is achieved when the woman can maintain a 100-gm cone through pelvic muscle contraction in an upright position. This method is useful only for stress incontinence.

### 6. How do intraurethral plugs work?

Intraurethral plugs have been introduced as a measure to occlude the urethra in an attempt to prevent leakage. This technique requires a motivated patient who can insert the plug into the urethra. There are restrictions on the length of time that plugs can be left in place, and they are not intended for overnight use. Made of silicone, they easily conform to the urethra to create a seal at the bladder neck. At each voiding, the plug is removed, discarded, and replaced with a new intraurethral plug. Plugs are available commercially as Fem Soft (Rochester Medical Corporation; www.rocm.com). They are designed for women with stress incontinence.

### 7. Are penile clamps used often?

Also known as penile compression devices, padded clamps are applied externally on the penis to control male stress incontinence. They are recommended for temporary use and are not a permanent solution. Little scientific literature supports their use.

**8. What does a pessary accomplish?**

Pessaries, latex-free devices that are fitted by the clinician into the vagina, serve several purposes. By treating pelvic organ prolapse, stress incontinence is reduced or eliminated. Pessaries fit inside the vagina, using the pelvic bones to maintain position, much like a diaphragm. Once the prolapse is reduced, the pessary serves much like a dam to prevent the prolapse from recurring. The patient must make routine visits to her provider to have the pessary changed.

**9. Is periurethral collagen a surgical procedure?**

Yes and no. The procedure is usually done in an ambulatory surgical setting or outpatient basis with a local anesthetic and light sedation. Using liquid collagen, the clinician injects the material around the urethra until the lumen is occluded. This bulk reduces stress incontinence. In some instances, the procedure can be performed in the office by using a local anesthetic and bladder installation.

**10. What are the disadvantages of periurethral collagen injections?**

The collagen is reabsorbed through the body, thus requiring reinjection when bulk has diminished. Many patients seem to need additional injections annually. There are no long-term studies of the effects of exogenous collagen used in this matter, but most clinicians rate the safety profile high.

**11. Can medication improve stress incontinence?**

Depending on patient characteristics and exam findings, women with postmenopausal stress incontinence can be treated with local estrogen. Topical estrogen "bulks up" the urethra and bladder neck. Little systemic absorption occurs, making it safe for most women.

**12. How can topical estrogen be given?**

Estrogen cream can be delivered via applicator. Because of its propensity to cause transient burning when a full applicator is used, many clinicians recommend a fingertip length of cream in the applicator daily for 2 weeks, then 3 times/week thereafter.

**13. Are estrogen creams messy?**

For patients who find creams aesthetically unpleasant, an intravaginal estrogen tablet is available (Vagifem, Pharmacia). After 2 weeks, it is suggested that the pill be inserted vaginally twice a week. An estrogen-impregnated ring made of silicone can be placed in the vagina. Held in place by the pubic bones, it slowly releases estrogen over a period of 3 months. Commercially available as Estring (Pharmacia), it is well tolerated with few side effects.

**14. In women who take oral hormone replacement therapy, can topical estrogen be helpful?**

Yes. Local application appears beneficial with no additional side effects.

**15. List the contraindications to topical estrogen.**

- Breast or endometrial cancer
- Pregnancy
- Porphyria
- History of deep vein thrombosis or thrombophlebitis
- Hypersensitivity to cream or tablet components

**16. What other medications are available for stress incontinence?**

Alpha-adrenergic agonists increase urethral resistance to reduce stress incontinence. The usual agent is pseudoephedrine hydrochloride. Because preparations containing this agent can increase blood pressure significantly, they must be used with caution. Other side effects include tachycardia, nervousness, delirium, seizures, and hallucinations.

**17. What are the contraindications to any preparation containing this agent?**

- Hypertension
- Cardiac disease or arrhythmias
- [a] Concomitant administration with digoxin or beta blockers

**18. How does a tricyclic antidepressant help reduce stress incontinence?**
Imipramine (Tofranil), 10–50 mg/day titrating up to 3 times/day, causes urethral constriction.

**19. What are the side effects of this regimen?**
Postural hypotension and cardiac arrhythmias can occur with tricyclic antidepressant medications. Death can occur if given concurrently with a monoamine oxidase inhibitor. Patients with diabetes are instructed to monitor blood sugar more closely because glucose levels can be affected.

**20. What surgical procedures are available to treat stress incontinence?**
Although over 150 types of bladder suspension procedures have been described in the literature, the pubovaginal sling or transvaginal sling procedure is most commonly recommended. Of late, the transvaginal tape procedure has become more popular.

**21. What nonbehavioral treatments are available for urge incontinence?**
  • Implanted electrical stimulation
  • Pharmacologic therapy

**22. How does an implanted electrical stimulation unit work?**
The sacral nerves are stimulated by means of a small electrical current initiated by a neurostimulator. Looking much like a pacemaker, the lead wire is implanted at the sacral nerves. The operating unit is placed in the abdominal subcutaneous tissue. After the unit is implanted, the unit is turned on and adjustments in the strength and length of discharged currents are made to optimize continence. This device is marketed as InterStim Therapy (Medtronic). Studies have shown that about half of the patients with urge incontinence became entirely continent.

**23. Can implanted electrical stimulation help other types of incontinence?**
Patients with urinary retention can also benefit from InterStim Therapy. In one clinical study, over half of the patients responded well enough that indwelling catheterization was no longer necessary.

**24. Describe the pharmacologic therapy available for patients with urge incontinence.**
Drugs used to treat detrusor overactivity can be classified as anticholinergic agents:
  • Propantheline, 7.5–30 mg 3–4 times/day
  • Hyoscyamine (Levsin), 0.125 mg twice daily
  • Oxybutynin (Ditropan), 2.5–5 mg 3–4 times/day
  • Dicyclomine (Bentyl), 10–20 mg 3 times/day
  • Tolterodine (Detrol), 1–2 mg twice daily
  • Detrol LA, 4 mg/day
  • Ditropan XL, 5–15 mg/day

**25. How do anticholingergic drugs work?**
Relaxation of smooth muscle inhibits detrusor contractions via anticholinergic action.

**26. What are the most common side effects of anticholinergic medication?**
Dry mouth, constipation, restlessness, tachycardia, and gastroesophageal reflux.

**27. Are the side effects troublesome?**
Twenty percent of patients stop treatment because of side effects. Fortunately, the newer agents oxybutynin extended-release (Ditropan XL) and tolterodine long-acting (Detrol LA) significantly reduce side effects. Tolterodine has been shown to have significantly lower side effect incidence.

**28. What are the contraindications to anticholinergic medication use?**
  • Urinary retention               • Concomitant administration with other medications
  • Gastric retention               • Myasthenia gravis
  • Uncorrected glaucoma

**29. What other medications are helpful in treating urge incontinence?**
Imipramine at the same dose used in stress incontinence is helpful. Although it is considered a tricyclic antidepressant medication, it has high anticholinergic effects.

**30. Is surgery helpful?**
Surgery is a last resort for refractory urge incontinence unresponsive to other treatment methods. In this case an augmentation cystoplasty is performed.

**31. How is mixed incontinence treated?**
• Pharmacologic therapy
• Extracorporeal magnetic innervation

**32. What is the pharmacologic regimen for mixed incontinence?**
A combined approach with an anticholinergic plus one or more drug classes commonly used to treat stress incontinence. Many clinicians prefer to combine an anticholinergic with a topical estrogen when treating a postmenopausal woman with mixed incontinence.

**33. What is extracorporeal magnetic innervation (ExMI)?**
ExMI uses pulsing magnetic fields to stimulate pelvic nerves. The ensuing exercise improves strength and increases circulation. Studies report that one-half of all patients undergoing this therapy are continent after 6 weeks of therapy. An additional one-third of patients reported fewer incontinent episodes.

**34. What are the advantages of ExMI?**
Patients like this therapy because they can remain fully clothed during the 20-minute painless procedure. ExMI is manufactured by Neotonus as the NeoControl Pelvic Floor Therapy System.

**35. How is overflow incontinence treated?**
Treatment is aimed at the specific cause of overflow incontinence.

*Treatment Options in Overflow Incontinence*

| CAUSE | TREATMENT |
|---|---|
| Outflow obstruction caused by an enlarged prostate | Surgical intervention<br>Pharmacologic therapy |
| Outflow obstruction caused by urethral stricture | Surgical intervention followed by intermittent self-catheterization |
| Hypoactive bladder | Intermittent self-catheterization<br>Pharmacologic therapy |
| Detrusor sphincter dyssynergia | Intermittent self-catheterization combined with anticholinergic medication<br>Indwelling catheterization only as a last resort |

**36. What surgical procedures can be performed for an enlarged prostate?**
• Transurethral resection (TURP)
• Laser ablation of the prostate
• Open surgical removal
• Insertion of urethral stent
• Ablation by microwave hyperthermia
• Ablation by cryosurgery

**37. What surgical procedures are available to alleviate urethral strictures?**
Urethrectomy and laser incision. In both procedures, urethral patency is maintained by long-term intermittent self-catheterization.

**38. Describe pharmacologic therapy for an enlarged prostate.**

5-Alpha reductase inhibitors shrink prostate tissue. It is several months before any improvement in the voiding system is seen.

**39. What side effects are associated with 5-alpha reductase inhibitors?**

Impotence, decreased libido, and decreased ejaculate volume are the most common side effects. Because of its potential for causing birth defects, women of child-bearing potential should not handle crushed or broken tablets because absorption can occur through the skin.

**40. What other medication may be helpful in a patient with an enlarged prostate?**

Alpha-1 sympathetic blockers act by relaxing the smooth muscle in the bladder neck to relieve the obstruction. The most common medications used are:
• Doxazosin (Cardura), 1–8 mg/day
• Tamsulosin (Flomax), 0.4–0.8 mg/day
• Terazosin (Hytrin), 1–10 mg/day

**41. What side effects are common with alpha-1 sympathetic blockers?**

Orthostatic hypotension, syncope, dizziness, and somnolence.

**42. Do any natural remedies improve outlet obstruction?**

Saw palmetto, like the 5-alpha reductase inhibitors, slowly shrinks prostate tissue. The side-effect profile is low.

**43. Describe pharmacologic therapy for a patient with a hypotonic bladder.**

• Metoclopramide (Reglan) enhances detrusor contractility.
• Bethanechol chloride (Urecholine) stimulates the muscarinic acetylcholine receptors that initiate micturation.

**44. Does intermittent self-catheterization need to be done using sterile technique?**

Clean technique is acceptable. Patients are taught to wash their hands with soap and water prior to catheter insertion. The catheter is cleaned in warm soapy water and rinsed with running tap water after each procedure.

**45. How often is intermittent self-catheterization performed?**

Every 4 hours during the day and every 6 hours at night. It can be done more often if the patient feels bladder fullness.

**46. How is transient or functional incontinence best treated?**

Treating the underlying causes of the incontinence is the best approach.

**47. What treatment options are available for men experiencing postprostatectomy incontinence (PPI)?**

PPI is usually caused by detrusor instability, sphincter incompetence, or a combination of both. PPI is rare after TURP and most likely related to detrusor instability. PPI after radical prostatectomy is very common.

**48. How is PPI treated if behavioral methods are unsuccessful?**

When patients are unresponsive to behavioral treatment methods, periurethral bulking procedures with collagen injections are often helpful. Artificial urinary sphincter placement, an inpatient surgical procedure, can also be considered for intractable PPI.

**49. How is the artificial urinary sphincter placed?**

A cuff device is placed around the urethra. It is attached to a pump inserted in the scrotal sac. The patient presses the pump that then inflates the cuff to close off the bladder neck to maintain continence. By pressing on the pump a second time, the cuff deflates for urination.

**50. What treatments are available for childhood enuresis?**
Enuresis alarms coupled with nonpunitive measures are helpful. In intractable cases, intranasal antidiuretic hormone (DDAVP) can be helpful.

**51. Why is DDAVP not used in elderly patients with enuresis?**
Severe hyponatremia can occur.

**52. When should indwelling catheters be used to treat incontinence?**
- When incontinence is caused by obstruction and no other interventions are possible
- Patients with pressure ulcers as a short-term treatment when other options to reduce external contamination of the ulcer have failed
- In a severely incontinent person who lives alone without available alternative interventions and no available caregiver.

## BIBLIOGRAPHY

1. Agency for Health Care Policy and Research: Urinary Incontinence in Adults: Acute and Chronic Management. Rockville, MD, U.S. Department of Health and Social Services, AHCPR Publication No. 96-0682, 1996.
2. Harrison GL, Memel DS: Urinary incontinence in women: Its prevalence and its management in a health promotion clinic. Br J Gen Pract 44:149–152, 1994.
3. Roberts RG: Current management strategies for overactive bladder. Patient Care Nurse Pract Suppl Spring:22–30, 2001.
4. Newman D: The Urinary Sourcebook, 2nd ed. Los Angeles, Lowell House, 1999.
5. Springhouse Corporation: Clinical advances in incontinence management. Adv Skin Wound Care 13:290–292, 2000.
6. Payne CK: Advances in nonsurgical treatment of urinary incontinence and overactive bladder. Campbell's Urol 1(1):1–20, 1999.

# 81. TREATMENT OPTIONS IN FECAL INCONTINENCE

*Catherine T. Milne, APRN, MSN, CWOCN, CS, ANP,*
*and Lisa Q. Corbett, APRN, MSN, CWOCN, CS*

**1. What treatment options are available for patients suffering from fecal incontinence (FI)?**

As for urinary incontinence, behavioral and nonbehavioral treatments can be used to achieve favorable outcomes.

**2. What treatments should be tried first?**

Treatment is aimed at the factors contributing to FI. For example, an internal sphincter injury received during childbirth responds best to surgical repair. Lifestyles changes are reviewed with all patients, and compliance is encouraged.

*Treatment Options in Fecal Incontinence*

| CAUSE | TREATMENT OPTIONS |
| --- | --- |
| Pelvic muscle floor weakness | Pelvic floor muscle exercises, biofeedback |
| Pelvic floor muscle dyssynergia | Biofeedback |
| Anal sphincter injury | Surgical repair, artificial bowel sphincter implantation |
| Insensate rectum | Biofeedback with balloon distention training |
| Urge FI | Bowel habit training, biofeedback with balloon distention training, pharmacotherapy |
| Poor but intact sphincter function | Pelvic floor muscles exercises with biofeedback, sacral nerve stimulator |
| Severe neurogenic dysfunction with intact sphincter | Encirclement sphincter surgical procedure |
| Passive incontinence, loose or frequent stools | Pharmacotherapy |
| Inadequate sphincter muscle mass | Encirclement sphincter surgical procedure |
| Pelvic floor neuropathy | Post-anal surgical repair |

**3. Describe lifestyle changes that can be taught to a patient with FI.**

Little research has determined specific relationships between food and fecal incontinence. Obtaining a good history from the patient often reveals a food or drink pattern that the patient correlates with abnormal bowel function. Patient teaching should focus on the impact of the following:

- **Fiber intake.** Very soft stool is much more difficult to retain during times of fecal urgency. Many elderly patients ingest fiber supplements because they believe they have "constipation." Often, however, the stools are normal in consistency but decreased in frequency due to inadequate exercise or the effect of other medications. Fiber reduction is helpful in such cases. Conversely, increasing fiber intake is helpful in patients with mild, true constipation (hard stools) or those with loose stools.
- **Spicy foods** may increase bowel stimulation. In certain patients, they may be used to enhance bowel frequency; in others, the avoidance of spicy foods may promote continence.
- **Hot foods.** Encouraging the gastrocolic reflex, the consumption of hot foods promotes bowel function and evacuation.
- **Dairy products.** Known to have a negative effect on patients with irritable bowel syndrome, dairy products can lessen stool consistency. Lactose intolerance may be a contributing factor.

Yogurt or lactobacillus intake, especially during concurrent oral antibiotic dosing, can maintain the normal bowel flora and reduce the incidence of diarrhea.

- **Chocolate.** Many chocolate products are made with milk proteins, which may decrease stool consistency.
- **Artificial sweeteners.** Loose stools have been reported in patients with artificial sweetener intake. A well-known component of diet drinks, they are also an ingredient of other diet foods and sugarless gums and candies.
- **Bananas and arrowroot.** Both of these foods have demonstrated ability to firm stools. Bananas should be very ripe to gain maximal effects.
- **Caffeine.** A known bowel stimulant, it acts synergistically when combined in a hot liquid form, such as coffee or tea, to produce a movement.
- **Nicotine.** Although known to slow upper gastrointestinal motility and transit time, nicotine conversely increases rectosigmoid motility. Thus, nicotine in any form (patches, pills, or cigarette smoke) facilitates defecation. Elimination of nicotine can decrease rectal urgency.
- **Alcohol.** Some patients report increased fecal urgency with alcohol intake. Anecdotal reports suggest that beer is better tolerated than wine and that red wine causes more distress than white wine.
- **Routine exercise.** The benefits of exercise are numerous and include improved muscle tone and improve colonic transit.

### 4. What other lifestyle changes can be encouraged?

Skin care in the fecally incontinent patient is an important skill to teach (see Chapter 82). Patients also need to be taught how to manage an incontinent episode, if it should occur in public, while the process of restoring continence is under way. An extra change of clothes, disposable moist towelettes, and several plastic bags that are easy accessible at all times help reduce the possibility of prematurely ending an outing. If possible, any excursion should be timed before meals so that peristaltic waves are kept to a minimum to lessen FI.

Additionally, when patients feel the sudden urge to have a bowel movement in public, holding the breath and tensing muscles naturally occur. This natural response is actually counterproductive, because abdominal muscle wall tightening increases intra-abdominal pressures and rectal propulsive movements. Standing still, distraction techniques, and consciously contracting the external sphincter and pelvic muscle floor overcome the urge. This learned technique improves over time with repeated practice.

### 5. What is a bowel diary?

Similar to a bladder diary, a bowel diary notes the time, related activity, stool consistency, and presence or absence of an incontinent episode for each bowel movement. Clinicians can observe for incontinent patterns, use the diary as a diagnostic tool, and monitor response to treatment. Patients should complete a 7-day bowel diary when first evaluated and periodically thereafter.

### 6. How is bowel habit training performed?

Bowel habit training is designed to reduce urge. Using a behavior modification approach, the patient is first encouraged to sit on the toilet and contract the sphincter muscles and pelvic floor being careful not to hold their breath or tighten abdominal muscles. This position is held for 1 minute before defecation. Once the patient is successful at 1 minute, timing is gradually increased to 10 minutes over a period of several days.

The second stage begins when continence is achieved over the toilet for 10 minutes. The patient is expected to remain continent while in the bathroom but not over the toilet. Starting with 5 minutes, the "hold time" is slowly increased to 10 minutes.

The third and final stage is initiated after successful completion of the previous levels. The patient is instructed to slowly increase the distance away from the bathroom while maintaining continence for 10 minutes. Coupled with pelvic floor and sphincter strengthening exercises, bowel habit training may take up to several months. To avoid disappointment or nonadherence to the regimen, the patient should be informed before starting that results can take weeks or months.

**7. What medications can be used to treat fecal incontinence?**

Pharmacotherapy is limited to patients with loose or frequent stools. The most frequently used agent is loperamide hydrochloride (Imodium). This agent slows colonic transit, increases internal sphincter tone in the presence of stool, and may increase resting rectal pressures. By slowing peristaltic waves, increased water absorption occurs, thus increasing stool consistency. Although individual patients have various responses to the timing and dose of the medication, it is suggested that 1 mg 3 times/day before meals, be the initial starting point with upward or downward titration as appropriate. It is available as an over-the-counter preparation in either pill or syrup form.

Low-dose codeine phosphate can also be used to achieve continence. Although it is effective in some patients, its distinct disadvantages include increased expense, propensity toward addiction, and increased value when sold illegally on the black market.

**8. How does one perform pelvic muscle floor exercises (PFME) to reduce fecal incontinence?**

PFME is performed exactly as described under urinary incontinence (see Chapter 79).

**9. When are anal sphincter exercises appropriate?**

Anal sphincter exercises should be taught and performed with all PFME. Most patients cannot specifically identify the anal sphincter muscle and benefit greatly in learning these exercises using biofeedback. Anal sphincter exercises are actually a specific component of PFME but involve identifying and exercising a select muscle rather than the entire pelvic floor. All patients except those with known partial or full loss of anal sphincter muscle integrity can benefit.

**10. How does one perform anal sphincter exercises?**

The patient is instructed to sit comfortably, with legs uncrossed and knees slightly apart. The anal sphincter muscle can be described to the patient as the muscle that contracts to prevent passing flatus. The patient should feel as if the rectum is slightly lifting up and off the chair. Breath-holding and abdominal muscles are not involved. Once the muscle is identified, the patient is taught both "quick flicks" (strength) and endurance exercises. In performing "quick flicks," the anal muscle is contracted 5 times and held for a period of 5 seconds each, allowing a 10-second relaxation period between contractions. To increase endurance, the sphincter is squeezed in increments until full contraction is achieved. This position should be held as long as possible. Five repetitions with a 10-second rest period between each are suggested. For maximum benefit, the entire exercise process should be repeated 10 times daily.

**11. When can a patient expect to see improvement in incontinence when pelvic floor and anal sphincter exercises are used?**

Some improvement will be noticeable within 3–4 weeks of consistent exercise. This effect is thought to be related to enhanced neuromuscular coordination. Muscle strength through hypertrophy, the goal of pelvic floor and anal sphincter muscle exercises, is first apparent around 12 weeks of therapy.

**12. Discuss the role of biofeedback in the treatment of fecal incontinence.**

Many patients are unable to locate and control the pelvic muscle floor voluntarily. By giving the patient positive feedback through a technologic instrument that displays graphs, lights, or sounds with successful identification and contraction of the pelvic muscles floor (specifically, the anal sphincter muscle), repetitive exercises can be done in earnest.

**13. How is biofeedback performed in the fecally incontinent patient?**

Using externally placed sensors in addition to air-filled manometric balloons placed into the rectum that are connected to a visual response unit, the patient is taught to identify and squeeze specific pelvic floor or anal sphincter muscles. In patients with hypersensitive rectal vaults, the balloons are filled with air until the defecation sensation is felt. Sphincter exercises are performed to overcome the urge. At each successful session, the balloon is inflated more and the process is repeated until normal distention pressures are reached. Conversely, in patients with decreased rectal sensations the balloon is inflated until sensation is felt. Subsequent sessions have progressive declines in inflation until the patient can identify rectal distention at normal, rather than large, pressures.

**14. How long does it takes before results of biofeedback are seen?**

Most supervised sessions are completed weekly, although they can be scheduled as little as monthly, depending on patient response to therapy. Home biofeedback units are available for purchase, and the patient can perform the session at a convenient time. If the goal of therapy is to identify muscle groups and learn specific exercise, biofeedback results are seen after a few sessions at most. If the goal is to provide a feedback mechanism during exercise with the end result of continence, outcomes will not be seen for at least 12 weeks. Giving the patient a short-term goal in the meantime, in terms of number of days without an incontinent episode, is often helpful.

**15. What surgical procedures are available to treat fecal incontinence?**
- Sphincter repair
- Plication sphincteroplasty
- Post-anal repair
- Bilateral gluteus flap
- Encirclement sphincter procedure with gracilis muscle transfer
- Encirclement sphincter procedure with gracilis muscle transfer and permanent nerve stimulator implantation
- Artificial bowel sphincter
- Sacral nerve stimulator implant

**16. Why is the permanent nerve stimulator used in some cases but not others when an encirclement procedure with the gracilis muscle transfer is performed?**

The gracilis, a long thin muscle in the thigh, is brought around (encircles) the anus to "replace" muscle tone. In patients with no neurologic disorders, this transfer is adequate. However, in some underlying neurologic disorders, the gracilis muscle works for a time but then loses tone. The implantation of a nerve stimulator keeps the muscle in a contracted state. To perform defecation, the patient places a magnet over the stimulator, blocking input to the muscle. The muscle subsequently relaxes and defecation occurs. To resume continence, the magnet is removed.

**17. How does the artificial bowel sphincter work?**

This new device is an inflatable cuff surgically placed around the rectum. It is connected to a pump placed in the scrotal sac or, in women, the labia. A fluid reservoir is placed in the groin or fat pad above the symphysis pubis. The patient inflates the cuff to maintain continence by pumping fluid from the fluid reservoir to the cuff. To defecate, the pump is again squeezed to move the fluid from the cuff to the reservoir. Although this procedure is not 100% effective, most patients achieve continence.

**18. How does the sacral nerve stimulator help achieve continence?**

This treatment involves three separate surgical procedures. In the first, the sacral nerves are identified, and through electrical stimulation the nerve that exerts the greatest effect on anorectal functions is singled out. During the second procedure, a temporary electrode and stimulator are implanted, and the effect on continence is evaluated. The electrodes deliver continuous stimulation to cause sphincter contraction. If successful, the third procedure involves removal of the temporary stimulator and implantation of permanent electrodes and stimulator. This device is not yet approved in the United States but is currently undergoing multicenter clinical trials.

## BIBLIOGRAPHY

1. Jensen L: Fecal incontinence: Evaluation and treatment. J Wound Ostomy Contin Nurs 24(5):277–282.
2. Jensen L: Assessing and treating patients with complex fecal incontinence. Ostomy Wound Manage 46(12): 56–60, 2000.
3. Jensen L: Assessment and management: Patients with bowel dysfunction and fecal incontinence. In Doughty DB (ed): Urinary and Fecal Incontinence: Nursing Management, 2nd ed. St. Louis, Mosby, 2000.
4. Norton C, Chelvanayagam S: A nursing assessment tool for adults with fecal incontinence. J Wound Ostomy Contin Nurs 27(5): 279–291, 2000.
5. Perry JD, Perry LM: Advances in the diagnosis and treatment of fecal incontinence. Adv Nurs Pract 7(10):55–57, 1999.

# 82. PREVENTION AND TREATMENT OF PERINEAL SKIN BREAKDOWN

*Denise Henry Nix*, RN, BAN, MS, CWOCN

### 1. How common is perineal skin injury in incontinent patients?

Perineal skin injury has been found in as many as 33% of hospitalized adults. Products such as underpads and diapers commonly used with incontinent patients can contribute to perineal skin injury by trapping moisture against the skin.

### 2. What factors put a person at risk for developing perineal skin breakdown?

Characteristics of healthy skin and factors affecting skin barrier function such as pH and normal flora are covered in detail in Chapter 3. Incontinent substances on the skin cause an altered pH and microbial invasion. In addition, the skin is exposed to excessive moisture, enzymes, and friction. Exposure time, intensity of irritant, duration of irritant, and factors that cause diarrhea are significant risks for the development of perineal skin breakdown.

### 3. What is meant by duration of irritant?

Skin wetness has been defined as fluid in contact with the skin for 2 or more hours. The Braden Scale for predicting pressure ulcers has a subscale for moisture. The subscale definition for moisture is "degree to which skin is exposed to moisture." The Braden Scale further characterizes the degree to which skin is exposed by frequency of garment and linen change.

- Constantly moist: dampness is detected every time patient is moved or turned.
- Moist: skin is often but not always moist. Linen changes at least once a shift.
- Occasionally moist: linen is changed once a day.
- Rarely moist: skin is usually dry.

### 4. What is meant by intensity of irritant?

Intensity of irritant refers to the effluent's strength and ability to cause epidermal barrier disruption in human skin. Factors that correlate with barrier disruption include moisture, increased pH, and invasion of microorganisms. Wet skin has a higher pH than dry skin and is more permeable to irritants and bacteria than dry skin. Bacterial count of the irritant naturally influences intensity. Fewer bacteria are found in urine than in feces.

The consistency and characteristics of output from various locations in the GI tract have been described previously. The intestine is a natural reservoir of microorganisms exposed to the skin through feces. Stool from the large bowel is usually formed with less moisture. In contrast, small bowel discharge is liquid and reported to be a strong irritant to the skin. The skin irritation potential of digestive enzymes has also been reported. Studies show that prolonged occlusive exposure to digestive enzymes in feces causes erythema and epidermal barrier disruption in human skin. Increased pH is associated with more severe skin alterations.

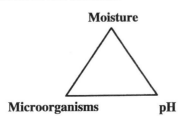

Irritant intensity factors.

### 5. What factors can result in diarrhea?

Low serum albumin, antibiotics and other medication, and tube feeding initiation have been associated with diarrhea. Sorbitol, a frequent additive in liquid medication, increases osmolality, thus increasing the risk of loose, frequent stools. Medications used to induce diarrhea purposefully place a patient at high risk. Such an example is Lactulose; the benefit of decreasing serum ammonia levels outweighs the risk for skin breakdown—at least from the physician's point of view! As nurses, we know that this condition is debilitating and painful. Other medical conditions, such as *Clostridium difficile* infection and ischemic bowel, can cause diarrhea. Factors contributing to diarrhea development put people at risk for developing perineal skin breakdown by increasing the intensity and frequency of the irritant.

### 6. Does intact erythema put a patient at higher risk for perineal skin breakdown?

Yes. Erythema and denudement are classic signs of tissue destruction. Once tissue damage is visible, barrier function is impaired. Visible changes indicate a decrease in tissue tolerance and susceptibility to microbial attack. Damaged skin can be indicative of the loss of collagen, blood flow, or elastic fibrous connective tissues. These important elements supply the skin with nutrients, elasticity, and strength. Algorithms for perineal skin condition have been defined in three stages: clear and intact, erythema, and denudement.

### 7. What tool is used for perineal risk assessment?

The Perineal Assessment Tool (PAT) is a four-item instrument. The framework for the PAT is based on four factors that are considered to be determinants in perineal skin breakdown: duration of irritant, intensity and type of irritant, perineal skin condition, and contributing factors causing diarrhea. Each subscale reflects degrees of risk factors. All subscales are rated from 1 (least risk) to 3 (most risk). Each rating has a descriptor and a description of each level of the scale. Total scores can range from 4 (least risk) to 12 (most risk). A designation of 7–8 distinguishes between high risk and low risk.

*Perineal Assessment Tool (PAT)*

| | 3 | 2 | 1 |
|---|---|---|---|
| **Intensity of irritant** | | | |
| Type and consistency of irritant | Liquid stool with or without urine | Soft stool with or without urine | Formed stool and/or urine |
| **Duration of irritant** | 3 | 2 | 1 |
| Amount of time that skin is exposed to irritant | Linen/pad changes at least every 2 hr | Linen/pad changes at least every 4 hr | Linen/pad changes every 8 hr or less |
| **Perineal skin condition** | 3 | 2 | 1 |
| Skin integrity | Denuded/eroded with or without dermatitis | Erythema/dermatitis with or without candidiasis | Clear and intact |
| **Contributing factors** | 3 | 2 | 1 |
| Low albumin, antibiotics, tube feeding, or *C. difficile* infection, other | 3 or more contributing factors | 2 contributing factors | 0–1 contributing factors |

Copyright © 2000 Denise Nix. Used with permission.

### 8. Has the PAT been validated?

Validity was established through a survey conducted with 102 wound, ostomy, continence (WOC) nurses averaging over 9 years of experience in skin and wound care in a diverse range of health care settings. Results revealed strong levels of agreement. The average level of agreement for PAT subscales ranged from 7.66 to 8.4 (range: 1 = strongly disagree to 10 = strongly agree). The median for all scales was 9. Interrater reliability of the PAT was examined by determining percentage agreement between a WOC nurse and 5 staff RNs or LPNs. PATs were completed on 20 patients at a long-term acute care hospital. Pearson product-moment correlation $r$ was used to measure interrater reliability. The calculated value of the Pearson product-moment correlation: $r = 0.970$, 95% confidence interval = 0.923–0.988, $p < 0.0001$.

**9. Is a perineal risk assessment tool useful in clinical practice?**

Time will tell. Currently the tool is used in research for assistance with inclusion-exclusion criteria. A valid and reliable risk assessment tool can assist nurses in identifying risk factors as well as the probability of skin breakdown. The assessment can enable caregivers to implement interventions that minimize or eliminate these factors to prevent skin breakdown. Researchers have identified the need for valid and reliable risk assessment methods for perineal skin breakdown. During validation of the PAT, overall reaction was positive. No large-scale changes were suggested to the tool. All WOCN respondents agreed that the four subscales were valid risk factors for perineal skin injury and that a perineal assessment tool would be useful in clinical practice. The market is saturated with various products for the prevention and treatment of perineal skin breakdown. Perhaps a tool such as the PAT could assist in product selection.

*How to use a risk assessment tool in product selection*
1. Cleanse with perineal cleanser containing proper pH.
2. Protect—choose product based on PAT score and presence/absence of candidiasis.

| LOW RISK: PAT 4–6* | HIGH RISK: PAT 7–12* |
|---|---|
| 3 in 1 product (can omit cleansing product if 3 in 1 is used)<br>*or* | Skin barrier paste (apply ostomy first if needed to help the barrier adhere to denuded skin)<br>*or* |
| Alcohol free liquid barrier film<br>*or* | Containment device with attached skin barrier |
| Barrier ointment or cream | |

\* If candidiasis is present, apply antifungal cream before the skin barrier.

**10. What additional tools are used to assess perineal skin?**

The literature includes two perineal skin assessment tools: the Perineal Dermatitis Grading Scale and the Perirectal Skin Assessment Tool (PSAT). The PSAT measures degree of skin breakdown. Multiple experts were consulted during its design, and interrater reliability was established at 87% agreement using 40 trials with 4 raters. The Perineal Dermatits Grading Scale resembles a wound and skin assessment. It specifies anatomic location, skin color, skin integrity, size in cm of skin damage, patient discomfort, and a description column. These tools are not commonly used in clinical practice.

*Perineal Dermatitis Grading Scale*

| DATE:_____<br>TIME:_____ | SKIN COLOR | SKIN INTEGRITY | SIZE IN CM<br>R & L | PATIENT<br>SYMPTOMS | DESCRIPTION |
|---|---|---|---|---|---|
| Buttocks | | | | | |
| Coccyx | | | | | |
| Rectal area | | | | | |
| Scrotum/<br>perineum | | | | | |
| Thighs | | | | | |

| **Skin Color** | **Patient Symptoms** | **Skin Integrity** |
|---|---|---|
| 0 = no erythema | 0 = none | 0 = intact |
| 1 = mild erythema | 1 = tingling | 1 = slight swelling, raised areas |
| 2 = moderate erythema | 2 = itching | 2 = swollen raised areas |
| 3 = severe erythema | 3 = burning | 3 = bullae or vesicles |
| | 4 = pain | 4 = open macerated areas |
| | | 5 = crusting or scaling |

From Storer-Brown D: Perineal dermatitis: Can we measure it? Ostomy Wound Manage 39(7):8–30, 32, 1993, with permission.

**11. What are some common types of perineal skin breakdown due to incontinence?**

Irritant and contact dermatitis, intertrigo, pruritus ani, candidiasis, tinea cruris.

**12. What less common dermatologic problems are associated with perineal skin breakdown?**

Herpes simplex virus, erythrasma, and herpes zoster.

**13. What are the primary goals for the prevention and treatment of perineal skin breakdown related to incontinence?**

Few clinical trials have addressed this issue in adults. In general, you want to cleanse, moisturize, and protect. Countless skin care products on the market are designed to accomplish one or more of these goals. Chapter 3 may be helpful in reviewing ingredients and their functions in the general skin care products discussed below.

**14. What factors and ingredients should be considered in the selection of a perineal skin cleanser?**

Comfort, pH, effectiveness, ease of application, removal time, and caregiver time are important considerations. Irritants such as effluent and bacteria should be removed from the perineal region as soon and as gently as possible. A good cleanser should loosen soil without the need for aggressive scrubbing. Sometime odor and bacterial control is a desirable characteristic if the ingredient used for odor and bacterial control is not itself an irritant. The pH of the product should range from 4 to 7 for best compatibility with the skin. Bar soap is more likely to have an alkaline pH. Therefore liquids and foams are thought to be more desirable than bars. Choice between rinse and no-rinse cleansers depends on preference. The ingredient responsible for the actual cleansing is the surfactant.

**15. What factors should be considered in the selection of a perineal skin barrier?**

Comfort, pH, effectiveness, ease of application, removal time, and caregiver time for use (similar to the characteristics examined for the perineal cleanser). Ingredients most commonly found in perineal barrier are petrolatum, dimethicone, and zinc oxide. These products range from creams to thick ointments and barrier pastes. Creams, which are the most esthetically pleasing, can be either water-in-oil or oil-in-water emulsions. Ointments are less preferred by patients because of the consistency. Barrier pastes are ointments mixed with a fine powder. The powder is placed in the ointment to help absorb weepy moisture from denuded skin. Fiers and Theyer suggest the use of a skin barrier paste for significant perineal erosion or ulceration to absorb drainage and provide an effective barrier against irritants.

**16. What are skin sealants? Can they be used for perineal skin care?**

Skin sealants are liquid barrier films made of polymers and solvents. The solvent evaporates after the product is applied to the skin leaving behind a protective film. The product can be used effectively in the perineal region *only* if it is alcohol-free to prevent pain and irritation. Think about your clinical practice and what it felt like when the alcohol swab touched a break in your skin. The clinician should check with the manufacturer for a list of the ingredients before using a liquid barrier film in combination with ointments or creams.

**17. Which skin care products cleanse, moisturize, and protect all in one step?**

Often referred to as "3-in-1" products, they are packaged in one container and designed to cleanse, moisturize, and leave a barrier. One of the few published clinical trials related to these products showed a reduction in cost and caregiver time when the 3-in-1 product was used on 20 patients in two clinical settings. The study also showed that 100% of the subjects experienced reduction of pain and erythema.

**18. Do wound dressings, topical antimicrobials, steroids, and burrows solution have a place in incontinent perineal skin care?**

Not routinely. Wound dressings are generally not useful for perineal skin breakdown related to incontinence because of problems with excessive moisture, stabilization, and frequent soiling.

Antimicrobials are present in skin care products to prevent spoilage but do not kill bacteria on the skin. Topical steroids may help to decrease inflammation but over time can actually thin the epidermis and are to be used only for the short term. Burrows' solution or aluminum acetate compresses 3 times/day may temporarily soothe and dry large weepy areas of epidermal loss related to incontinence. A skin barrier must be applied after each compress to provide a barrier against urine and feces. The ease of use is an important consideration if you are teaching a patient or caregiver how to perform perineal skin care. Making the regimen too complex often results in no care at all.

**19. What devices are available for containment of urine and feces?**

External urinary catheters and fecal incontinent collectors can be selected to contain urine and feces. If the products are chosen carefully and applied properly, they can prevent and treat perineal skin breakdown. Factors to consider when selecting these devices include comfort, cost, anatomy, cognitive and sensory status, mobility, dexterity, as well as patient or caregiver ability and motivation to use the product successfully.

## CONTROVERSY

**20. What is the role of antimicrobials?**

The use of antimicrobial agents for skin care products is controversial. Some researchers suggest that the use of antimicrobial-based skin products may be beneficial in the management of patients colonized with methicillin-resistant *Staphylococcus aureus* (MRSA). Others contend that little convincing evidence supports routine use of an antimicrobial product as effective or necessary. Researchers raise concerns that regular use of an antimicrobial may increase the risk of selecting for resistant organisms. The area of greatest agreement is in the use of antimicrobial agents for hand-washing by health care personnel. Several studies have compared the benefits of antimicrobial cleansers in hand washing among health care personnel (see Chapter 3).

## BIBLIOGRAPHY

1. Agency for Health Care Policy and Research: Clinical Practice Guideline: Urinary Incontinence in Adults. Rockville, MD, U.S. Department of Health and Human Services, AHCPR, 1992.
2. Bergstrom N, Braden B: A conceptual schema for the study of the etiology of pressure sores. Rehabil Nurs 12(1):8–12, 1987.
3. Storer-Brown D, Sears M: Perineal dermatitis: A conceptual framework. Ostomy Wound Manage 39(7):20–26, 1993.
4. Faria DT, Shwayder T, Krull EA: Perineal skin injury: Extrinsic environmental risk factors. Ostomy Wound Manage 42(7):28–30, 32–34, 36–37, 1992.
5. Fiers S, Thayer D: Management of intractable incontinence. In Doughty DB: Urinary and Fecal Incontinence: Nursing Management, 2nd ed. St. Louis, Mosby, 2000, pp 183–207.
6. Haugen V: Perineal skin care for patients with frequent diarrhea or fecal incontinence. Gastroenterol Nurs 20(3):87–90, 1997.
7. Lyder CH: Perineal dermatitis in the elderly. A critical review of the literature. J Gerontol Nurs 23(12):5–10, 1997.
8. Nix, DP: Factors to consider when selecting skin cleansing products. J Wound Ostomy Contin Nurs 27:260-268, 2000.
9. Nix DP: Validity and reliability of the Perineal Assessment Tool (PAT). Ostomy Wound Manage [accepted for publication].
10. Storer-Brown D: Perineal dermatitis: Can we measure it? Ostomy Wound Manage 39(7):8–30, 32. 1993.
11. Warshaw E, Kula J, Nix DP, Markon C: A multicentered product evaluation of a cleanser protectant lotion containing 2% dimethicone in the treatment of perineal skin breakdown in low risk incontinent patients from long term acute care and skilled long term care [submitted].

# IV. Essential Resources

## 83. LEGAL ISSUES IN WOUND, OSTOMY, AND CONTINENCE CARE

*Sharon A. Aronovitch, PhD, RN, CETN*

### 1. How do nurses avoid legal problems in wound, ostomy, and continence practice?

By understanding basic legal principles, such as negligence, standards of care, and malpractice, nurses can structure their practice to lessen the chance of being named in a civil or criminal suit.

### 2. When a patient has a wound, ostomy or incontinence problem, what documentation should be kept in the record?

Documentation, no matter what the diagnosis or care the patient is receiving, should be complete and follow publicized, nationally recognized standards of care. Short cuts in documentation should be avoided. Hand written notes should be legible with minimal abbreviation. Use only the recognized abbreviations within your facility of employment and within the practice of nursing.

### 3. What are the statistics related to medical malpractice?

The Harvard Medical Malpractice Study reported that over 180,000 deaths occur each year as a result of a medical mistake. Eighteen to 36% of hospitalized patients suffer from a medical mistake that leads to either injury or death.

Beckmann analyzed a database of 747 cases between the years of 1988 and 1993 to develop a comprehensive picture of nursing malpractice in hospitals. The primary situations cited for malpractice were communication with the physician about a change in the patient's condition and medication administration. Others areas of nursing practice that were found to be problematic include:
- Failure to perform a nursing intervention or procedure correctly
- Failure to assess the patient systematically
- Failure to provide a safe environment
- Failure to obtain help for a patient receiving inadequate physician care
- Failure to use equipment and products properly
- Failure to prevent infection

The areas of practice most at risk for nursing negligence are the emergency department, operating room, medical and surgical units, pediatrics, labor and delivery unit, and the newborn nursery. Unfortunately, data for long-term, subacute, and home health care are sparse. However, there is a definite trend toward an increase in malpractice claims in long-term care. In wound, ostomy, and continence (WOC) practice, wounds carry the greatest risk of legal liability.

### 4. What are the most common errors of malpractice in wound care?

In wound care cases reviewed by the author as an expert witness for both plaintiffs and defendants, the most common areas of negligence involved documentation in meeting standards of care. If you have been consulted to provide a patient with expertise in wound care, it is not enough simply to advise which wound care products should be used. According to the standards of care established by the WOC Nurses Society, one should also address the patient holistically with a thorough review of nutritional status, assess the patient's skin risk potential using a valid and reliable tool, determine the need for specialty devices (e.g., support surfaces), and suggest appropriate referrals to another medical specialty practice such as a dietician, plastic surgeon, or infectious disease specialist. It is your responsibility to determine how the care that the patient is receiving contributes to complications related to surgery and wound healing. Should a patient with diabetes and uncontrolled blood sugar receive $D_5W$ for hydration after a cardiac catheterization? How would the continued uncontrolled glucose levels during $D_5W$ administration affect the healing of a surgical incision after coronary bypass graft? Even though you are not the diabetic nurse specialist caring for the patient, it is within your scope of practice as a wound care nurse to advocate for appropriate care.

### 5. Do all malpractice cases go to a civil trial?

No. Many times malpractice cases are decided during mediation, arbitration, or conciliation. Mediation is an informal process that permits both parties (plaintiff and defense) to resolve their differences using a third party, the mediator. Arbitration is a more formal process in which the third party reviews the material and renders a decision. Conciliation is used to improve communication and decrease tension between the two parties by interpreting issues and providing suggestions to potential solutions. Conciliation is often a part of both mediation and arbitration.

### 6. Why should professional registered nurses carry their own malpractice insurance, even though they are covered through their employer?

The reasoning is simple. The malpractice insurance provided by your employer covers you only for the position and job description for which you were hired. The hospital's malpractice insurance does not provide coverage off the premises of your employment. There is the possibility (although rare) that if both you and the employer are involved in the same lawsuit, your employer may chose not to support your legal fees and initiate an lawsuit against you in a separate negligence case related to the original malpractice case. If this scenario were to happen, you would no longer be protected under your employer's malpractice insurance.

You can decide whether to carry personal professional malpractice insurance based on your assets. For example, if your personal assets make you "worth suing," you are strongly advised to have your own malpractice policy separate from your employers.

### 7. What does negligence mean in regard to professional practice as a nurse?

Negligence is defined as "conduct which falls below the professional standard of due care." It is further defined as a "standard minimum of special knowledge and ability." For negligence to be proved, there must be evidence that the nurse's conduct deviated from the conduct of a reasonably well-qualified professional in the same field. Any purported negligent activity must also meet all of the following criteria to be considered negligence by law:

- There must be a bond of duty between the injured party and the person alleged to cause the injury.
- A breach of duty must have occurred.
- The breach of duty must be the cause of the injury.
- The damages, injuries or both are recognized and compensable by law and must be experienced by the injured party.

Negligent behavior by a professional nurse can occur either by commission (an act that an ordinary, reasonable, and prudent person would not do) or omission (failure to perform a duty, such as an assessment or referral to another professional for management of a specific patient need).

### 8. How can a nurse prevent professional negligence?

The professional nurse always provides patient care that meets established standards. In addition, prudent nurses continually evaluate and improve their skills to maintain current knowledge of their practice area through continuing education and reading journal articles.

### 9. What role does certification play?

Certification within a specialty practice demonstrates basic competency above the level of general practice. Certification is another means by which the professional nurse can demonstrate competency within a specialty practice, such as certification through the WOC Nurses Society.

**10. What is a preventative behavior?**

Documentation of competency and working within the assigned job description are important preventive behaviors, not always followed in this age of nursing shortage. Another example is adherence to established patient care policies and procedures, which includes accurate documentation.

**11. Why can I be found negligent when a patient is deemed "at risk" for developing a wound if I signed the appropriate medical records for documentation of care?**

Documentation can prove or disprove the care provided to a patient based on the patient's outcome. For example, the nurse signs a document indicating that she has provided care related to preventing potential alteration in skin integrity. However, during hospitalization the patient develops a stage IV pressure ulcer. A review of the medical record may determine that the nurse did not complete all areas of care compared with the standard of care for preventing a potential alteration in skin integrity. This issue can be determined by assessing whether any or all of the individual activities of care outlined within this standard, such as monitoring serum albumin level or risk assessment by means of the Braden Scales, were not performed. It may be determined that the patient's serum albumin levels were drawn but not reviewed by the nurse, who thereby missed the opportunity to "fulfill a duty to the patient" to contact a registered dietician to assist in nutritional management. Another possibility is that the nurse completed the skin risk assessment tool but failed to contact a WOC nurse for further evaluation of the patient's needs related to preventing the occurrence of a pressure ulcer, if the institutional policy indicates that such an action should occur.

**12. If I am served with legal papers for a lawsuit, what should I do?**

Immediately contact your professional liability insurance carrier. In many instances, the malpractice insurance firm will assist you in obtaining legal counsel. Never try to handle your own legal case because you do not have the skills or expertise to obtain important papers such as medical records or depositions and negotiate a decrease in monetary settlement or a reduction in charges or penalties.

**13. What should I do if I am called to give a deposition or testify in court?**

Whether you are contacted to provide a deposition as a defendant or an expert witness, you will be accompanied to the hearing by your attorney. An expert witness represents the attorney's client. In either case, you should answer only questions posed to you and provide no additional information. Answer all questions clearly. Only after you have answered the question should you provide an explanation. Keep your "cool" during questioning by the opposing attorney. It is a part of the opposing attorney's job to make you mad. Never nod your head in affirmation to a question, because a court typist must document all that is said during the deposition and trial. The court typist cannot transcribe a physical response as either yes or no. You will be provided with a copy of your typed deposition before it becomes a final document to correct any misspelling and clarify any statements given during the deposition.

**14. What is an expert witness? For whom does the expert witness work?**

An expert witness is someone within your profession who has special knowledge of the subject and is formally involved in a medical malpractice case. This status enables the expert witness to express opinions and draw conclusions in testimony and trial. For example, an expert witness in a malpractice case related to complications of a revascularized lower extremity postoperative wound is most likely to be a WOC nurse, not a nurse with experience in perioperative or vascular practice. The expert witness reviews all pertinent medical records, including depositions or other material provided by the attorney of hire. The expert witness's job, based on the review of the facts, is to present an opinion as to the merit of the case to the judge, jury, or other arbitrator. The expert witness is most commonly asked, "Were the damages alleged by the plaintiff the direct result of negligence of the defendant?"

The expert witness is hired by either the injured party's (plaintiff's) attorney or the defense attorney. The selection of an expert witness by the hiring attorney is based on the individual's knowledge of the area of nursing practice involved in the malpractice case. Therefore, the attorney of hire will review the proposed expert witness's curriculum vitae for education, experience, certification, relevant publications, and teaching as well as for any hints of impropriety. References will also be reviewed to determine whether the proposed expert witness is the best fit for the malpractice case in question. Expert witnesses must be currently involved in the practice area for which they have been hired to provide medical review and testimony.

## CASE EXAMPLES

**Case 1. The patient is a morbidly obese man with a history of diabetes, hypertension, sleep apnea, and coronary artery disease. He is followed by a home care agency for management of his diabetes and hypertension. The patient experiences chest pain during a stress test and is admitted to the hospital for cardiac catheterization. During the procedure he experiences several episodes of hypotension and respiratory distress, which are appropriately managed; however, the usual time for an uneventful cardiac catheterization is exceeded. The patient develops a sacral pressure ulcer and ultimately requires flap surgery to close the ulcer. Nursing staff followed appropriate standards of care for treating an alteration in skin. The patient and family sue the hospital, physician, and nursing staff providing care. Is there evidence of negligence on the part of the hospital or nursing staff?**

According to the opinion submitted by the expert witness, based on the medical records and other documents, the hospital was not at fault because appropriate management of the patient's presenting problem in the cardiac catheterization unit was followed by all staff. In addition, the patient himself created negligence by continued noncompliance with his medical care regimen before the cardiac catheterization. He had not maintained a diet to meet the physiologic changes in his body due to diabetes and hypertension and was morbidly obese. Simply put, the patient was his own worst enemy.

**Case 2. You are the newest member of a wound care team as well as the only member certified in wound care. As you become familiar with the patient population, you discover that most patients with leg and foot ulcers are treated with a topical growth factor. Most of these patients also have diabetes. The average length of time for this modality of care is 7 months. You review the patients' medical records and note minimal to no progression in wound healing. What should you do?**

The first step is to look at what other modalities were tried before use of the growth factor. Were these products used appropriately? Your next step is to review the literature to see what other options are available and appropriate for each patient's particular wound. A good presentation to advocate a change in care to the members of the interdisciplinary team includes product information and a cost comparison. For example, if the patient had been using a tube of Regranex each month for 6 months, the cost to the patient is approximately $2,400, excluding dressings. Your presentation to the team would reflect this cost compared with the replacement that you are suggesting, such as an alginate, foam, or a polysaccharide gel/powder (Multidex). Always present a change in practice as a mini-educational program, because your colleagues will find this approach less threatening than telling them that they were wrong.

## BIBLIOGRAPHY

1. Beckmann JP: Nursing Negligence: Analyzing Malpractice in the Hospital Setting. Thousands Oaks, CA, Sage Publications, 1996.
2. Bogart JB: Legal Nurse Consulting Principles and Practice. New York, CRC Press, 1998.
3. Brent NJ: Nurses and the Law: A Guide to Principles and Application, 2nd ed. Philadelphia, W.B. Saunders, 2001.
4. Dempski K: Serving as an expert witness. RN 63(2):65–68, 2000.
5. Grensing-Pophal L: Here comes the judge. Nursing 30(6):80–81, 2000.
6. Laduke S: Tips for coping with legal trouble. Nursing 31(9):54–57, 2001.
7. Murphy E: Individual malpractice insurance decisions revisited. AORN J 67(6):1234–1236, 1998.
8. Wilkinson AP: Nursing malpractice. Nursing 26(8):80–81, 1998.

# 84. CERTIFICATION IN WOUND, OSTOMY, OR CONTINENCE SPECIALTIES

*Catherine T. Milne, APRN, MSN, CWOCN, CS, ANP, and Lisa Q. Corbett, APRN, MSN, CWOCN, CS*

**1. How do I become certified?**

A decision must first be made in *which* specialty you want to be certified. You may choose any one or all three: wound, ostomy, or continence nursing certification.

**2. What organizations offer wound certification?**

Wound certification is available from two organizations: the Wound, Ostomy, Continence Nurses Society Certification Board (WOCNCB) and the American Academy of Wound Management (AAWM).

**3. What is the difference between the two?**

Both organizations have information about specific criteria necessary to become certified in wound management. The AAWM offers a program for the certified wound specialist (CWS). Many different health care professionals can take the CWS exam. Most are physicians, nurses, dietitians, and physical therapists. The WOCNCB is focused on nursing practice of wound management. Thus only registered nurses are allowed to take the examination. The WOCNCB awards successful candidates with the title of certified wound care nurse (CWCN). The Wound, Ostomy, and Continence Nurses Society also gives the title of CWOCN to a nurse who has met the criteria for all three specialties: wound, ostomy, and continence.

**4. What about ostomy certification?**

Ostomy certification is available only through the WOCNCB. The certification title for this section only is certified ostomy care nurse (COCN). The United Ostomy Association, an organization for health care professionals and laypersons with and without ostomies, does not provide certification.

**5. What about continence certification?**

Certification can be obtained through the WOCNCB as a certified continence care nurse (CCCN). Many nurses with an interest in urology become certified as a CURN (certified urological registered nurse) through the Certification Board of Urologic Nurses and Associates (CBSUNA). Both the WOC Nurses Society and the Society of Urological Nurses and Associates (SUNA) are professional organizations with separate entities to deal strictly with certification.

**6. What is the difference between SUNA and the WOCN?**

SUNA expertise involves a variety of urologic nursing issues. WOCN focuses specifically on continence in addition to wound and ostomy management as a nursing specialty.

**7. What other organizations include continence in the forefront of their agenda?**

The National Association for Continence, National Bladder Foundation, and the Simon Foundation. In addition, the Association for Women's Health, Obstetric and Neonatal Nurses, is spearheading efforts to educate clinicians about women's incontinence. These organizations currently do not offer certification in continence practice.

**8. What formal training is involved in WOC nursing?**

Several schools offer education that qualifies a student to sit for the WOCN exams in all three areas. These sites are listed in the monthly WOCN journal and at the WOCN website (www.wocn. org). A few schools offer education and training only in wound management.

*Schools Offering Programs in Wound, Ostomy, and Continence Specialties*

| NAME | CONTACT | CONTENT OFFERED |
|---|---|---|
| Emory University School of Medicine Wound Ostomy Continence Nursing Education Center | 404-778-4067 | Wound, ostomy, continence |
| Harrisburg Area WOC Nursing Education Program by Wicks Educational Associates | 717-737-2770<br>800-807-WICKS<br>www.igateway.com/clients/weai | Wound, ostomy, continence |
| La Salle University School of Nursing | 212-951-1413<br>www.lasalle.edu | Wound, ostomy, continence |
| Rupert B. Turnbull, Jr. School of ET Nursing | 216-444-5966<br>www.clevelandclinic.org/cors/etschool.htm | Wound, ostomy, continence |
| University of Southern California ET Nursing Education Program | 323-442-2028<br>www.usc.edu | Wound, ostomy, continence |
| New Mexico School of ET Nursing | 800-472-3060<br>www.nmia.com/~paumer | Wound, ostomy, continence |
| University of Texas M.D. Anderson Cancer Center– Wound, Ostomy, Continence Nurse Education Program | 713-745-0219<br>swoolems@mdanderson.org | Wound, ostomy, continence |
| Medical University of South Carolina | 843-792-2651 | Wound |
| Web WOCN Nursing Education Program | 612-331-4601<br>www.webwocnurse.com | Wound, ostomy, continence |

### 9. What should I look for in these schools?

If you plan to take the WOCN certification exam, you should choose a school that is accredited by the WOCN.

### 10. Are opportunities for formal training available on the Internet?

New methods of distance learning are now available through the Internet. Although these types of programs are in their infancy, they are fast becoming popular. At the time of publication, there is only one WOCN-accredited web based program (see table above). Check current journal listings and websites frequently for updated information. See Appendix B for greater detail.

### 11. How do I know whether I qualify to sit for a certification exam?

It is best to contact the certification board directly to inquire about current prerequisites for a certification exam. Certification organizations are listed below.

| ORGANIZATION | CONTACT | CERTIFICATION |
|---|---|---|
| Wound, Ostomy, Continence Certification Board | www.wocncb.org or www.goamp.com for eligibility and requirements for certification | Wound, ostomy, continence |
| Certification Board of Urologic Nurses and Associates | www.suna.org | Continence |
| American Academy of Wound Management | www.aawm.org | Wound |

## 12. What are the benefits of certification?

The most important benefit of certification is to the patient. Certification is designed to protect the patient. The organization providing the credential can assure patients and the general public that successful candidates have the theoretical knowledge basic for a specific area of practice. In reality, the "basic" concepts tested during the certification process in a specialty nursing practice can be considered "expert" knowledge compared with a clinician who is not practicing in this area.

Many institutions and agencies pay certified staff at a higher base rate. Some start certified staff at higher pay levels and offer opportunities for larger raises and bonuses. Clinical promotions via career ladders or other mechanisms reward staff who earn and maintain certification. Many employers would rather offer a job to a certified person than a noncertified person if all other characteristics are equal between the two candidates.

Finally, certification can give a sense of accomplishment. Meeting the demands of certification is not always easy. However, once completed, it is a feather in one's cap. Certification is one hallmark of professional practice.

## BIBLIOGRAPHY

1. American Academy of Wound Management: www.aawm.org
2. Society of Urological Nurses and Associates: www.suna.org
3. Wound, Ostomy, Continence Nurses Certification Board: www.wocnb.org
4. Wound, Ostomy, Continence Nurses Society: www.wocn.org

# APPENDIX A: Resources for Ostomates

*Compiled by Debra L. Dubuc*, APRN, CS, CWCN, COCN

## MAJOR OSTOMY EQUIPMENT MANUFACTURERS

Bard Medical Division
8195 Industrial Blvd.
Covington, GA 30013

Coloplast Corporation
5610 W. Sligh Ave, Suite 100
Tampa, FL 33634-4468
1-800-533-0464
1-800-237-4555

ConvaTec
A Bristol-Myers Squibb Company
P.O. Box 5254
Princeton, NJ 08543-5254
1-800-422-8211

Cymed Inc.
Micro Skin Ostomy Pouching Systems
1336-A Channing Way
Berkeley, CA 947402

Hollister, Inc.
200 Hollister Dr.
Libertyville, IL 60048-3746
1-800-323-4060

Marlen Manufacturing & Development Co.
5150 Richmond Road
Bedford, OH 44146

Nu-Hope Laboratories, Inc.
P.O. Box 331150
Pacoima, CA 91333-1150
1-800-899-5017

Perma-Type Company, Inc.
83 Northwest Drive
Plainville, CT 06602
1-800-242-4234

VPI Non-Adhesive Systems
A Cook Group Company
127 South Main Street
P.O. Box 266
Spencer, IN 47460
1-800-843-4851

## OSTOMY ASSOCIATIONS AND RESOURCE GROUPS

American Cancer Society
1599 Clifton Road, NE
Atlanta, GA 30329
1-800-ACS-2345
www.cancer.org

Crohn's and Colitis Foundation of America
386 Park Avenue South, 17th Floor
New York, NY 10016
www.ccfa.org

Digestive Diseases National Coalition
507 Capital Court, NE, Suite 200
Washington, DC 21006-7374
1-202-544-7497

United Ostomy Association
19772 MacArthur Blvd., Suite 200
Irvine, CA 92612-2405
1-800-826-0826
www.uoa.org

World Council of Enterostomal Therapists
6 Ferrands Close
Hardin Bingley
W. Yorkshire BD16 1JA, UK

Wound, Ostomy, Continence Nurses Society
2755 Bristol Street, Suite 110
Costa Mesa, CA 92626
1-714-476-0268
www.wocn.org

National Digestive Diseases Information
  Clearinghouse
2 Information Way
Bethesda, MD 20892-3570
1-301-654-3810

National Institute of Diabetes, Digestive
  and Kidney Diseases
2 Information Way
Bethesda, MD 20892

Young Ostomy United, Inc. (YOU)
P.O. Box 1433
Narre Warren N.D.C.
VIC 3805
Australia
www.youinc@bigpond.com

## PLACES TO OBTAIN OSTOMY SUPPLIES

AARP Pharmacy Service
Ostomy Care Center
P.O. Box 40011
Roanoke, VA 24022-0011

American Ostomy Supply (AOS)
W223 N777 Saratoga Drive, Suite 2001
Waukesha, WI 53186
1-800-858-5858

Bruce Medical Supplier
411 Waverly Oaks Road
P.O. Box 9166
Waltham, MA 02454
1-800-225-8466

Edgepark Surgical, Inc.
1810 Summit Commerce Park
Twinsburg, OH 44087
1-800-321-0591

Express Medical Supply, Inc.
P.O. Box 1164
Fenton, MO 63026
1-800-633-2139

Fittleworth Medical Ostomy Supplies
1 Racetrack Road
East Brunswick, NJ 08816
1-800-686-1377

Parthenon Ostomy Supplies
3311 W. 2400S
Salt Lake City, UT 84119
1-800-453-8898

Perma-Type Company, Inc.
83 Northwest Drive
Plainville, CT 06602
1-800-243-4234

Sterling Medical Services
2 Twosome Drive
Moorsetown, NJ 08057
1-800-216-5500

## RECOMMENDED READING WRITTEN BY AN OSTOMATE

Barbara Barrie: Second Act: Life After Colostomy. New York, Scribner, 1997.

Barbara Barrie: Don't Die of Embarrassment: Life After Colostomy and Other Adventures. New York, Fireside, 1999.

# APPENDIX B: Resources in Wound, Ostomy, and Continence Specialties

*Compiled by Catherine T. Milne, APRN, MSN, CWOCN, CS, ANP, and Lisa Q. Corbett, APRN, MSN, CWOCN, CS*

## PROFESSIONAL ORGANIZATIONS

Wound, Ostomy, and Continence
  Nurses Society
4700 W. Lake Ave.
Glenview, IL 60025-1485
www.wocn.org
Membership: nurses

National Lymphedema Network
1611 Telegraph Ave.
Suite 1111
Oakland, CA 94612-2138
www.lymphnet.org
Memberships: occupational therapists,
  physical therapists, nurses, physicians,
  industry representatives, laypersons

Tissue Viability Society
Glanville Centre
Salisbury District Hospital
Salisbury, UK SP2 8BJ
www.tvs.org.uk
Membership: occupational therapists,
  physical therapists, nurses, physicians,
  industry representatives, laypersons

Wound Healing Society
13355 Tenth Avenue North
Suite 108
Minneapolis, MN 55441
www.woundheal.org
Membership: occupational therapists,
  physical therapists, nurses, physicians,
  industry representatives, podiatrists,
  laypersons

Association for the Advancement of Wound Care
83 General Warren Blvd.
Malvern, PA 19355
aawc.org
Membership: occupational therapists,
  physical therapists, nurse,physicians,
  industry representatives, podiatrists,
  laypersons

Biofeedback Foundation of Europe
P.O. Box 75416
1020 AK Amsterdam
The Netherlands
www.bfe.org
Membership: occupational therapists,
  physical therapists, nurses, physicians,
  industry representatives

National Association for Continence (NFAC)
P.O. Box 8310
Spartenburg, NC 29305
Membership: occupational therapists,
  physical therapists, nurses, physicians,
  industry representatives, laypersons

National Pressure Ulcer Advisory Panel (NPUAP)
11250 Roger Bacon Dr.
Suite 8
Reston, VA 20190-5202
www.npuap.org
Membership: occupational therpists,
  physical therapists, nurses, physicians,
  industry representatives, podiatrists,
  laypersons

United Ostomy Association (UOA)
19772 MacArthur Blvd.
Suite 220
Irvine, CA 92612-2405
www.uoa.org
Membership: ostomates, nurses, other health
  care professionals

Simon Foundation for Continence
P.O. Box 815
Wilmette, IL 60091
www.simonfoundation.org
Membership: occupational therapists,
  physical therapists, nurses, physicians,
  industry representatives, laypersons

# CLASSIC BOOKS

## Wounds

AHRQ: Prevention of Pressure Ulcers (1992) and Treatment of Pressure Ulcers (1994). Available online at AHRQ.gov. These clinical practice guidelines are frequently referenced by experts in the field. Note: Also used by members of the legal profession to enhance their cases—no matter what side they are on!

Bryant R (ed): Acute and Chronic Wounds: Nursing Management. St. Louis, Mosby, 2000.

Frykberg R, Gibbons G, Veves A, Harkless L: The High Risk Foot in Diabetes, 2nd ed. New York, Elsevier Science, 2002.

Hess CT (ed): Clinical guide to Wound Care, 4th ed. Springhouse, PA, Springhouse Corporation, 2002.

Krasner D, Rodeheaver G (eds): Chronic Wound Care: A Clinical Source Book for Healthcare Professionals, 3rd ed. Wayne, PA, HMP Communications, 2001.

Kloth L, McCulloch J (eds): Wound Healing Alternatives in Management, 3rd ed. Philadelphia, F.A. Davis, 2001.

Maklebust J, Sieggreen M: Pressure Ulcers: Guidelines for Prevention and Nursing Manangement, 3rd ed. Springhouse, PA, Springhouse Corporation, 2002.

Mulder G, Haberer P (eds): Clinician's Pocket Guide to Wound Care, 4th ed. Springhouse, PA, Springhouse Corporation, 1998.

Sussman C, Bates-Jensen B (eds): Wound Care: A Collaborative Practice Manual for Physical Therapists and Nurses, 2nd ed. Gaithersburg, MD, Aspen Publications, 2002.

## Ostomy

MacKeighan J, Cataldo P (eds): Intestinal Stomas: Principles and Managment. St. Louis, Quality Medical Publishing, 1993.

Hampton B, Bryant R (eds): Ostomies and Continent Diversions: Nursing Management. St. Louis, Mosby, 1992.

## Continence

AHRQ: Urinary Incontinence: Acute and Chronic Managment–1996. Available online at AHRQ. gov. These clinical practice guidelines are frequently referenced by experts in the field.

Doughty D (ed): Urinary and Fecal Incontinence: Nursing Management. St. Louis, Mosby, 2000.

Kaschak Newman D, Dzurinko MK, Diokno AC: The Urinary Sourcebook, 2nd ed. New York, McGraw-Hill, 1999.

Newman D: Continence for Women: Research-Based Practice. Washington, DC, Association of Women's Health, Obstetric and Neonatal Nurses, 2000.

## JOURNALS

Advances in Wounds and Skin Care: Springhouse Corporation.
Journal of Wound, Ostomy, Continence Nursing: the official publication of the WOCN.
Ostomy Wound Managment: an official publication of the AAWC.
Urologic Nursing: the official publication of SUNA.
Wounds: A Compendium of Research: an official publication of the AAWC.

## RESOURCE BOOKS BY PRODUCT NAME, FUNCTION, AND MANUFACTURER

Kestrel Wound Product Sourcebook. www.woundsource.com
Kestrel Health Information, P.O. Box 961, Williston, VT. 05495

Kestrel Incontinence Product Sourcebook. www.incontinencesource.com
Kestrel Health Information, P.O. Box 961, Williston, VT. 05495

NAFC Resource Guide. www.nafc.org

National Association for Continence, P.O. Box 8310, Spartenburg, NC 29305

Ostomy Wound Management Buyers Guide. www.o-wm.com
HMP Communications, 83 General Warren Blvd., Malvern, PA 19355

## INTERNET SITES

There are so many reliable, informative sites. Caution, however, is the word. The wild, wild west-like atmosphere has spawned many sites and chat rooms that spout unresearched methods for improving wound, ostomy, or incontinence conditions. Some make no sense physiologically. Other sites are vendor-sponsored with the goal of selling products. Although many vendors are reliable and have good material, the buyer must beware. Of course, all of the usual Internet cautions must be heeded in dealing with any site. Information posted by nonprofit organizations and educational institutions rather than vendors tends to have links to credible sites. The following sites are a good place to start.

Association of Advancement in Wound Care: awcone.org

National Bladder Foundation: bladder.org

Food and Drug Administration: clinical trials.gov lists FDA-approved clinical trials in wound care along with other drug studies. This site does not include trials for non-drug research studies, which do not have to go through as rigorous a process. An examples of this type of clinical trial is one associated with a new wound dressing or urinary catheter design.

Natinoal Lymphedema Network: lymphnet.org

National Association for Continence: nafc.org

National Pressure Ulcer Advisory Panel: npuap.org

Society of Urological Nurses and Associates: suna.com

United Ostomy Association: uoa.org

Access to Continence Care and Treatment: wellweb.com/INCONT/acct/contents.htm

Wound, Ostomy, Continence Nurses Society: wocn.org

Wound Healing Society: woundheal.org

## CONSULTANTS

Many organizations that accept membership also provide a list of consultants. The WOCN lists consultants on its web site, wherease others (SUNA, AAWC) have printed rosters available. Consulting activities are varied, depending on the interests and abilities of the consultant. Some listings are clinically oriented for providing patient care, whereas others offer education, research activities, and general consultation to recommend improvements in care.

## BIBLIOGRAPHY

1. Ambre J, Guard R, Perveller F, Renner J, Rippen, H: Criteria for assessing the quality of health information on the internet. Mitretek Systems Health Information Technology Institute. www.mitretek.org/hiti/showcase/documents/criteria.html. 1999.
2. Diering C, Palmer MH: Professional information about urinary incontinence on the world wide web: Is it timely? Is it accurate? J Wound Ostomy Contin Nurs 28(1):55–62, 2001.
3. Fikar CR, Corral OL: Wound-care resources on the internet. J Am Podiatr Med Assoc 90(2):93–97, 2000

# INDEX

Page numbers in **boldface type** indicate complete chapters.